UROLOGICAL EMERGENCIES

CURRENT CLINICAL UROLOGY

Eric A. Klein, MD, SERIES EDITOR

Urological Emergencies: A Practical Guide, edited by **Hunter Wessells and Jack W. McAninch**, 2005

Advanced Endourology: The Complete Clinical Guide, edited by **Stephen Y. Nakada and Margaret S. Pearle**, 2005

Oral Drug Therapy of Male Sexual Dysfunction: A Guide to Clinical Management, edited by **Gregory A. Broderick**, 2005

Management of Prostate Cancer, Second Edition, edited by **Eric A. Klein**, 2004

Essential Urology: A Guide to Clinical Practice, edited by **Jeannette M. Potts**, 2004

Management of Benign Prostatic Hypertrophy, edited by **Kevin T. McVary**, 2004

Essential Urologic Laparoscopy: The Complete Clinical Guide, edited by **Stephen Y. Nakada**, 2003

Laparoscopic Urologic Oncology, edited by **Jeffrey A. Cadeddu**, 2004

Pediatric Urology, edited by **John P. Gearhart**, 2003

Urologic Prostheses: The Complete Practical Guide to Devices, Their Implantation, and Patient Follow-Up, edited by **Culley C. Carson, III**, 2002

Male Sexual Function: A Guide to Clinical Management, edited by **John J. Mulcahy**, 2001

Prostate Cancer Screening, edited by **Ian M. Thompson, Martin I. Resnick, and Eric A. Klein**, 2001

Bladder Cancer: Current Diagnosis and Treatment, edited by **Michael J. Droller**, 2001

Office Urology: The Clinician's Guide, edited by **Elroy D. Kursh and James C. Ulchaker**, 2001

Voiding Dysfunction: Diagnosis and Treatment, edited by **Rodney A. Appell**, 2000

Management of Prostate Cancer, edited by **Eric A. Klein**, 2000

UROLOGICAL EMERGENCIES

A PRACTICAL GUIDE

Edited by

HUNTER WESSELLS, MD, FACS

*University of Washington School of Medicine
and Harborview Medical Center, Seattle, WA*

JACK W. MCANINCH, MD, FACS

*University of California School of Medicine
and San Francisco General Hospital, San Francisco, CA*

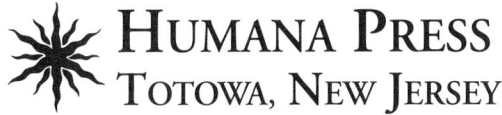

HUMANA PRESS
TOTOWA, NEW JERSEY

© 2005 Humana Press Inc.
999 Riverview Drive, Suite 208
Totowa, New Jersey 07512

humanapress.com

For additional copies, pricing for bulk purchases, and/or information about other Humana titles, contact Humana at the above address or at any of the following numbers: Tel.: 973-256-1699; Fax: 973-256-8341; E-mail: orders@humanapr.com; or visit our Website: www.humanapress.com

All rights reserved.

No part of this book may be reproduced, stored in a retrieval system, or transmitted in any form or by any means, electronic, mechanical, photocopying, microfilming, recording, or otherwise without written permission from the Publisher.

All articles, comments, opinions, conclusions, or recommendations are those of the author(s), and do not necessarily reflect the views of the publisher.

Due diligence has been taken by the publishers, editors, and authors of this book to assure the accuracy of the information published and to describe generally accepted practices. The contributors herein have carefully checked to ensure that the drug selections and dosages set forth in this text are accurate and in accord with the standards accepted at the time of publication. Notwithstanding, as new research, changes in government regulations, and knowledge from clinical experience relating to drug therapy and drug reactions constantly occurs, the reader is advised to check the product information provided by the manufacturer of each drug for any change in dosages or for additional warnings and contraindications. This is of utmost importance when the recommended drug herein is a new or infrequently used drug. It is the responsibility of the treating physician to determine dosages and treatment strategies for individual patients. Further it is the responsibility of the health care provider to ascertain the Food and Drug Administration status of each drug or device used in their clinical practice. The publisher, editors, and authors are not responsible for errors or omissions or for any consequences from the application of the information presented in this book and make no warranty, express or implied, with respect to the contents in this publication.

Production Editor: Robin B. Weisberg
Cover Illustration: From Figure 4, Chapter 14, "Priapism," by Ricardo Munarriz, Noel N. Kim, Abdul Traish, and Irwin Goldstein.
Cover design by Patricia F. Cleary

This publication is printed on acid-free paper. ∞
ANSI Z39.48-1984 (American National Standards Institute) Permanence of Paper for Printed Library Materials.

Photocopy Authorization Policy:
Authorization to photocopy items for internal or personal use, or the internal or personal use of specific clients, is granted by Humana Press Inc., provided that the base fee of US $30.00 per copy is paid directly to the Copyright Clearance Center at 222 Rosewood Drive, Danvers, MA 01923. For those organizations that have been granted a photocopy license from the CCC, a separate system of payment has been arranged and is acceptable to Humana Press Inc. The fee code for users of the Transactional Reporting Service is: [1-58829-256-8/05 $30.00].

Printed in the United States of America. 10 9 8 7 6 5 4 3 2

eISBN 1-59259-886-2

Library of Congress Cataloging-in-Publication Data

Urological emergencies : a practical guide / edited by Hunter Wessells, Jack W. McAninch.
   p. ; cm. -- (Current clinical urology)
  Includes bibliographical references and index.
  ISBN 1-58829-256-8 (hardcover : alk. paper) -- ISBN 1-59259-886-2 (eISBN)
  1. Urological emergencies.   I. Wessells, Hunter. II. McAninch, Jack W. III. Series.
  [DNLM: 1. Urologic Diseases--diagnosis. 2. Emergencies.
3. Urogenital System--injuries. 4. Urologic Diseases--therapy.
WJ 141 U777 2005]
RC874.8.U76 2005
616.6'025--dc22

2004013202

Dedication

To B.C. and C.L.W.

Preface

The changing paradigms of health care delivery require that the management of more and more complex problems takes place in the emergency department and the offices of primary care providers. A cadre of emergency physicians with limited urological training is being called upon to diagnose and treat many acute conditions of the genitourinary tract. Furthermore, the anticipated shortage of urologists, in conjunction with increased use of physician extenders within the urological community, will further limit the availability of urgent urological consultation. *Urological Emergencies: A Practical Guide* is intended to summarize the optimal management of urgent and emergent urological conditions so that the incredible improvements in the acute management of urological problems gained over the last decades can be easily accessible in one volume.

Injury is the leading cause of death in people younger than 44 years of age. The worldwide burden of disease resulting from trauma will increase immensely in the 21st century as a result of wartime injuries and motor vehicle accidents in all parts of the globe. Few nations have trauma systems in place that can rival our own, and thus mortality and disability resulting from trauma in nations with sudden expansion in vehicular traffic will be far higher than in North America. Severe renal injuries are immediately life threatening, and proper recognition of these requires appropriate criteria for staging and the availability of accurate imaging modalities. Lower urinary tract trauma, if unrecognized or mismanaged, can lead to early complications as well as permanent disability and dysfunction from disruption of essential neural, anatomical, and vascular structures of the pelvis.

Mortality from acute injury and infection is so rare in the developed world that the main causes of death in adults are cardiovascular disease and cancer. As a result of the aging of the adult population and the epidemic of obesity and type 2 diabetes mellitus, a dramatic increase in infectious, vascular, and obstructive urological emergencies in the United States is expected. In the developing world, obstructive uropathy, infected stones, and urosepsis remain major sources of morbidity and mortality. Differentiating between acute pyelonephritis and infection caused by an obstructed ureter is essential for proper triage and successful treatment. Identifying Fournier's gangrene in a timely fashion is of paramount importance.

Surgical error remains an irreducible feature of urological practice. Although simulators and systems-based approaches may one day reduce complication rates, iatrogenic injuries are an important problem in ureteral, bladder, and urethral diseases. Lessons from trauma management as well as innovations in endoscopic techniques have allowed urologists to avoid surgical solutions in many cases. The appropriate supportive and medical care must be understood by those in direct contact with the patient.

Congenital anomalies of the genitourinary tract carry a disproportionate risk of coexisting organ system abnormalities that require a highly multidisciplinary team approach to avoid death, permanent disfigurement, or irreversible cosmetic consequences. Despite prenatal sonography, many lower urinary tract anomalies are discovered only at birth. New concepts in the assignment of gender and the basis of gender have dramatically changed the landscape for cases of ambiguous genitalia.

The chapters in *Urological Emergencies: A Practical Guide* are organized by pathophysiology rather than organ system, which allows the reader to develop approaches to the care of patients with acute urological conditions based on mechanism of disease. Nationally and internationally recognized experts have provided up-to-date, evidence-based descriptions of the appropriate diagnostic and therapeutic considerations on topics of traumatic, infectious, obstructive, hemorrhagic, iatrogenic, vascular, and congenital urological emergencies. The relevant pathophysiological background and epidemiology are reviewed, necessary diagnostic tests are recommended, and detailed medical, surgical, and endourological management approaches are provided. These include advances in diagnostic testing and radiographic imaging, nonoperative treatment of acute injuries, endoscopic, angiographic, and percutaneous interventions for obstruction, bleeding, and abscess.

It is hoped that *Urological Emergencies: A Practical Guide* will serve as an authoritative bedside resource for urology residents, practicing urologists, emergency medicine trainees and practitioners, and primary care providers without immediate access to urological consultation.

ACKNOWLEDGMENTS

I would like to acknowledge Richard Drews for his diligence and persistence.

Hunter Wessells, MD, FACS
Jack McAninch, MD, FACS

Contents

Preface vii
Contributors xi

PART I: UROGENITAL TRAUMA

1 Diagnosis and Treatment of Renal Trauma 3
   Dan Rosenstein and Jack W. McAninch

2 Ureteral Trauma 25
   Noel A. Armenakas

3 Bladder Trauma 39
   Steven B. Brandes and Jay S. Belani

4 Urethral Trauma 57
   Eric R. Richter and Allen F. Morey

5 Trauma to the External Genitalia 71
   George W. Jabren and Wayne J. G. Hellstrom

6 Blunt and Penetrating Trauma to the Penis 95
   Jack H. Mydlo

PART II: INFECTION

7 Infection of the Upper Urinary Tract 115
   Maxwell V. Meng and Jack W. McAninch

8 Genital and Infectious Emergencies: *Prostatitis, Urethritis, and Epididymo-Orchitis* 135
   Khoa B. Tran and Hunter Wessells

9 Penile Prosthesis Infection 147
   Dominick J. Carbone, Jr.

10 Fournier's Gangrene 157
   Peter C. Black and Hunter Wessells

PART III: VASCULAR AND HEMORRHAGIC EMERGENCIES

11 Renal Artery Embolism and Renal Vein Thrombosis 171
   Edward J. Yun and Christopher J. Kane

12 Retroperitoneal and Upper Tract Hemorrhage 181
   Atul D. Rajpurkar and Richard A. Santucci

13 Hemorrhagic Cystitis 201
   Kian Tai Chong and John M. Corman

14 Priapism 213
    Ricardo Munarriz, Noel N. Kim, Abdul Traish, and Irwin Goldstein

15 The Acute Scrotum 225
    Gerald C. Mingin and Hiep T. Nguyen

PART IV: ACUTE URINARY TRACT OBSTRUCTION

16 Renal Colic Resulting From Renal Calculus Disease:
    Diagnosis and Management 241
    Rajveer S. Purohit and Marshall L. Stoller

17 Nonurolithic Causes of Upper Urinary Tract Obstruction 263
    Roger K. Low

18 Urgent and Emergent Management of Acute Urinary Retention ... 281
    Ugur Yilmaz and Claire C. Yang

PART V: IATROGENIC COMPLICATIONS

19 Vesicovaginal Fistula and Ureteral Injury During Pelvic Surgery ... 295
    Craig V. Comiter and Christina Escobar

20 Endoscopic Perforation and Complications of BCG Therapy 315
    Nathan F. E. Ullrich, Sanjay Ramakumar, and Bruce L. Dalkin

PART VI: NEWBORN UROLOGICAL EMERGENCIES

21 The Exstrophy–Epispadias Complex 329
    Richard W. Grady

22 Intersex Conditions 339
    Richard W. Grady

23 Posterior Urethral Valves 349
    Hiep T. Nguyen

24 Spina Bifida 363
    Hiep T. Nguyen

    Index 375

Contributors

NOEL A. ARMENAKAS, MD, FACS • *Section of Urology, Lenox Hill Hospital, New York, NY*
JAY S. BELANI, MD • *Division of Urologic Surgery, Washington University School of Medicine, St. Louis, MO*
PETER C. BLACK, MD • *Department of Urology, University of Washington School of Medicine, Seattle, WA*
STEVEN B. BRANDES, MD • *Division of Urologic Surgery, Washington University School of Medicine, St. Louis, MO*
DOMINICK J. CARBONE, JR., MD • *Department of Urology, Wake Forest University School of Medicine, Winston-Salem, NC*
KIAN TAI CHONG, MBBS, MRCS(Ed) • *Section of Urology and Renal Transplantation, Virginia Mason Medical Center, Seattle, WA*
CRAIG V. COMITER, MD • *Section of Urology, University of Arizona Health Sciences Center, Tucson, AZ*
JOHN M. CORMAN, MD • *Section of Urology and Renal Transplantation, Virginia Mason Medical Center, Seattle, WA*
BRUCE L. DALKIN, MD • *Section of Urology, University of Arizona, Tucson, AZ*
CHRISTINA ESCOBAR, MD • *Section of Urology, University of Arizona Health Sciences Center, Tucson, AZ*
RICHARD W. GRADY, MD • *Department of Urology, University of Washington School of Medicine and Children's Hospital and Regional Medical Center, Seattle, WA*
IRWIN GOLDSTEIN, MD • *Department of Urology, Boston University School of Medicine, Boston, MA*
WAYNE J. G. HELLSTROM, MD, FACS • *Department of Urology, Tulane University School of Medicine, New Orleans, LA*
GEORGE W. JABREN, MD • *Department of Urology, Tulane University School of Medicine, New Orleans, LA*
CHRISTOPHER J. KANE, MD • *Department of Urology, University of California, San Francisco, San Francisco, CA*
NOEL N. KIM, MD • *Department of Urology, Boston University School of Medicine, Boston, MA*
ROGER K. LOW, MD • *Department of Urology, University of California, Davis, Sacramento, CA*
JACK W. MCANINCH, MD • *Department of Urology, University of California San Francisco, San Francisco, CA and San Francisco General Hospital, San Francisco, CA*
MAXWELL V. MENG, MD • *Department of Urology, University of California San Francisco, San Francisco, CA*
GERALD C. MINGIN, MD • *Department of Urology, University of California, San Francisco Children's Hospital, San Francisco, CA*
ALLEN F. MOREY, MD • *Urology Service, Brooke Army Medical Center, Fort Sam Houston, TX*

RICARDO MUNARRIZ, MD • *Department of Urology, Boston University School of Medicine, Boston, MA*
JACK H. MYDLO, MD • *Department of Urology, Temple University Hospital, Philadelphia, PA*
HIEP T. NGUYEN, MD, FAAP • *Department of Urology, Harvard Medical School and Children's Hospital, Boston, MA*
RAJVEER S. PUROHIT, MD, MPH • *Department of Urology, University of California, San Francisco, CA*
ATUL D. RAJPURKAR, MD • *Department of Urology, Wayne State University School of Medicine, Detroit, MI*
SANJAY RAMAKUMAR, MD • *Section of Urology, University of Arizona, Tucson, Arizona*
ERIC R. RICHTER, MD • *Urology Service, Brooke Army Medical Center, Fort Sam Houston, TX*
DAN ROSENSTEIN, MD, FRC(SC) • *Division of Urology, Santa Clara Valley Medical Center, Santa Clara and Department of Urology, Stanford University, Palo Alto, CA*
RICHARD A. SANTUCCI, MD • *Department of Urology, Wayne State University School of Medicine, Detroit, MI*
MARSHALL L. STOLLER, MD • *Department of Urology, University of California, San Francisco, San Francisco, CA*
ABDUL TRAISH, MD • *Department of Urology and Biochemistry, Boston University School of Medicine, Boston, MA*
KHOA B. TRAN, MD • *Department of Urology, University of Washington School of Medicine, Seattle, WA*
NATHAN F. E. ULLRICH, MD • *Section of Urology, University of Arizona, Tucson, AZ*
HUNTER WESSELLS, MD, FACS • *Department of Urology, University of Washington School of Medicine and Harborview Medical Center, Seattle, WA*
CLAIRE C. YANG, MD • *Department of Urology, University of Washington School of Medicine, Seattle, WA*
UGUR YILMAZ, MD • *Department of Urology, University of Washington School of Medicine, Seattle, WA*
EDWARD J. YUN, MD • *Department of Urology, University of California, San Francisco, San Francisco, CA*

I Urogenital Trauma

1 Diagnosis and Treatment of Renal Trauma

Dan Rosenstein, MD, FRCSC
and Jack W. McAninch, MD

CONTENTS

INTRODUCTION
CLASSIFICATION AND INITIAL EVALUATION
RADIOGRAPHIC STAGING
INDICATIONS FOR SURGICAL EXPLORATION
RENAL VASCULAR INJURIES
PEDIATRIC RENAL TRAUMA
RENAL EXPLORATION AND RECONSTRUCTION
VASCULAR INJURY AND REPAIR
POSTOPERATIVE CARE AND COMPLICATIONS
SUMMARY
REFERENCES

INTRODUCTION

The kidney is the most frequently injured genitourinary organ because of external trauma and is involved in as many as 5% of abdominal trauma cases. Although the majority of injuries are minor contusions, renal trauma may occasionally represent a true life-threatening emergency. Advances in staging techniques (resulting from increased use of computed tomographic [CT] scanning) as well as increased awareness of the kidney's capacity for healing have permitted the majority of these injuries to be successfully managed nonoperatively.

Nonetheless, certain severely injured kidneys are best managed by exploration and reconstruction, with nephrectomy reserved for life-threatening hemorrhage or kidneys injured beyond repair. The urologist as well as the emergency medicine physician may thus be required to participate in the care of a patient with a suspected renal injury and should be up to date on staging and imaging of suspected renal injuries, indications for operative intervention, and reconstructive techniques for the management of renal trauma. Ultimately, the objective of managing these patients is to prevent significant hemorrhage and retain enough functioning nephron mass to avoid end-stage kidney

From: *Urological Emergencies: A Practical Guide*
Edited by: H. Wessells and J. W. McAninch © Humana Press Inc., Totowa, NJ

failure. A secondary goal is to avoid complications specifically attributable to the traumatized kidney.

This chapter reviews current recommendations for evaluating the patient with suspected renal trauma, highlighting the indications for exploration and the role of nonoperative management. Renovascular injuries as well as pediatric renal trauma are also highlighted. Finally, complications associated with operative and nonoperative management are discussed.

CLASSIFICATION AND INITIAL EVALUATION

Approximately 90% of renal injuries result from blunt trauma, usually falls from great heights, motor vehicle crashes, and violent assaults. Most of these injuries are minor and rarely require exploration. At San Francisco General Hospital, only 2% of all bluntly injured kidneys have required exploration or repair *(1)*. Pediatric kidneys as well as congenitally abnormal kidneys (cystic kidneys, hydronephrotic kidneys) are more susceptible to major injury secondary to blunt mechanisms *(2)*. Although only 10% of renal injuries result from penetrating trauma, up to 55% of these injuries will require exploration or repair. This is usually consequent to more severe renal injury, associated intraabdominal injuries, incomplete preoperative radiographic staging, or a combination of these factors *(3)*.

The American Association for the Surgery of Trauma (AAST) has created an organ injury scale for renal injuries; the scale correlates with patient outcomes and permits appropriate and selective management to be undertaken *(4)* (Fig. 1). This is one of the few classification trees prospectively validated and found to correlate directly with need for surgical intervention *(5)*. Grade I injuries include subcapsular hematomas and renal contusions. Grade II injuries involve small parenchymal lacerations into the renal cortex. Grade III parenchymal lacerations extend through the corticomedullary junction. Grade IV injuries involve violation of the collecting system and include vascular injuries such as main renal artery or vein injury with contained hemorrhage. Grade V injuries include kidneys with pedicle avulsion off the great vessels as well as completely shattered kidneys. This final category of injury is life threatening by definition.

Clinical staging begins with careful history and physical examination, including the determination of the presence of hematuria. Based on these criteria, a subset of patients likely to have significant renal injury may be identified. This subset may then undergo radiographic staging to stage the injury completely and determine whether operative management is indicated.

History should focus on the mechanism of trauma (blunt or penetrating), as well as presence of significant deceleration, which should raise suspicion for significant renal injury. In penetrating trauma, knowledge of type of bullet (high vs low velocity) or knife used in the assault may assist in prediction of degree of renal injury. On physical examination, the presence of shock (defined as systolic blood pressure [SBP] below 90 mmHg) should be recorded. The lowest recorded SBP is critical in determining the need for radiographic imaging in adult blunt renal trauma *(6)*.

A patient in shock who cannot be resuscitated may require urgent laparotomy, thus bypassing radiographic staging of suspected renal injury. This patient will require intraoperative staging (*see* "Indications for Surgical Exploration"). The abdomen, flank, and

FIGURE 2
AAST renal injury classification scheme

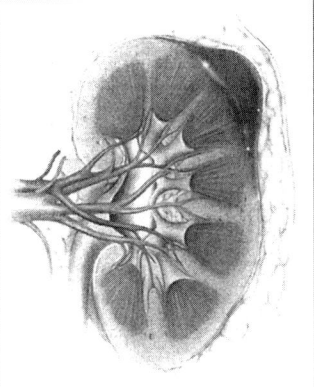

Grade I
Renal contusion: Microscopic or gross hematuria, urologic studies normal
Subcapsular hematoma: Nonexpanding without parenchymal laceration

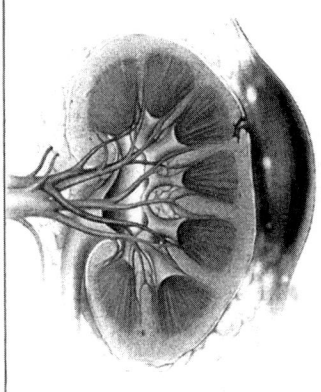

Grade II
Cortical laceration: <1 cm parenchymal depth of renal cortex without urinary extravasation
Perirenal hematoma: Nonexpanding, confined to renal retroperitoneum

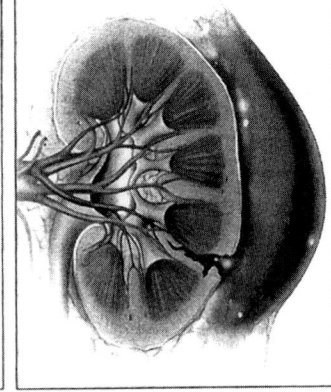

Grade III
Parenchymal laceration: Deep, >1 cm parenchymal depth of renal cortex without collecting system rupture or urinary extravasation

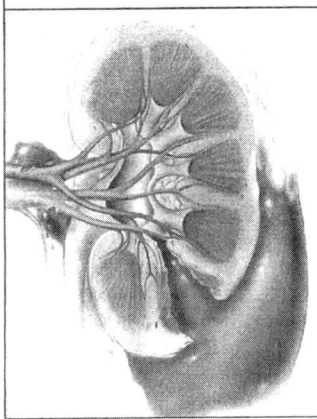

Grade IV
Parenchymal laceration: Involving the collecting system, with or without a devascularized segment
Vascular: Main renal artery or vein injury with contained hemorrhage

Grade V
Laceration: Completely shattered kidney
Vascular: Renal artery thrombosis, avulsion of the renal pedicle

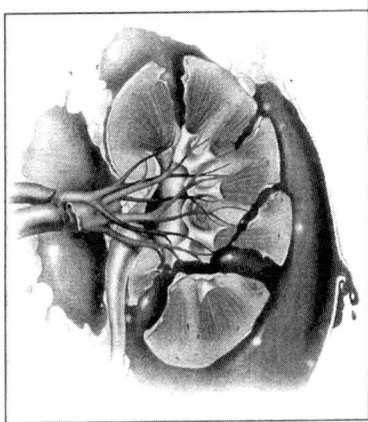

Fig. 1. American Association for the Surgery of Trauma classification of renal injuries. (From ref. *61*, p. 47.)

back should be carefully examined. Flank tenderness or ecchymosis as well as lower rib fractures may indicate underlying renal injury. In penetrating trauma, entry and exit wounds may point to a transrenal course.

Hematuria is the most common sign of penetrating and blunt renal trauma. However, the presence of hematuria does not correlate consistently with degree of renal injury *(7)*. This is particularly true in penetrating injuries, for which a high percentage of patients with significant renal injuries may have no hematuria. The first voided or catheterized specimen should be analyzed because hematuria may clear rapidly. Either dipstick or microscopic analysis may be performed.

RADIOGRAPHIC STAGING

Using the clinical information outlined above, the indications for radiographic imaging may be tailored to detect patients with a significant chance of having a major renal laceration (considered grades III–V). Based on our experience at San Francisco General Hospital, we recommend imaging patients *(8)* with the following categories of injuries:

1. Penetrating trauma: abdomen, flank or back injury with *any* degree of hematuria, particularly when the course of the missile appears to involve the kidney or ureter.
2. Blunt trauma with either gross hematuria or microhematuria associated with *shock* (defined as any recorded SBP below 90 mmHg.). Patients who sustain blunt trauma and have microhematuria without associated shock can safely avoid renal imaging *(9)*.
3. Blunt trauma in the setting of significant deceleration injury, such as falls from heights *(10)* or high-speed motor vehicle crashes. This mechanism of injury has been associated with a higher incidence of ureteropelvic junction disruption as well as renovascular trauma.
4. Pediatric penetrating injury or blunt trauma with microhematuria greater than 50 red blood cells per high-power field (RBC/HPF) *(11)*. There is mounting evidence that the adult imaging criteria outlined above will identify the majority of significant renal lacerations in children *(12)*, but this remains a controversial topic (*see* later). The clinician should continue to maintain a low threshold for renal imaging in the pediatric population.

Contrast-enhanced CT scanning has replaced intravenous pyelography (IVP) as the imaging modality of choice in renal trauma patients. CT is noninvasive and offers rapid and accurate detection of renal injuries as well as associated injuries to other organs *(13)*. CT defines depth and extent of lacerations, a functioning contralateral kidney, the presence of associated hematoma and contrast extravasation (suggesting collecting system violation), as well as any devitalized renal parenchyma (Fig. 2). Consideration must be given to each of these factors when deciding on a treatment plan.

Helical (spiral) CT scanning has been used because of its speed in the trauma setting. The patient may pass through the scanner in a few minutes. It has limited use in fully staging renal injuries because contrast may not have reached the renal calyces or renal pelvis before the images are procured. Significant collecting system injuries may thus be missed *(14)*. We routinely obtain a set of delayed images at 10 to 20 min to visualize the entire collecting system to the bladder. A plain radiograph (kidneys, ureter, bladder [KUB]) at this time may add complementary information to the CT scan. CT is also accurate in demonstrating renovascular injuries, when present. Renal artery occlusion as well as active bleeding may be accurately detected *(15)*.

CT findings consistent with main renal artery injury include lack of renal enhancement or abrupt cutoff of an enhancing artery (Fig. 3). Segmental arterial injuries typically appear as wedge-shaped infarcts with the apex facing the renal hilum *(1)*. Isolated main or segmental renal arterial thrombosis typically arises secondary to deceleration trauma, causing the disruption of the inelastic intimal layer with subsequent irreversible parenchymal ischemia and infarction. A renal vein laceration may be suspected by the finding of hematoma medial to the renal hilum, but similar findings may occur with lumbar vein injuries.

Adjunctive radiographic imaging techniques include renal ultrasound, nuclear scintigraphy, and magnetic resonance imaging, and retrograde pyelography. Ultrasound is readily available and noninvasive. Although it is an operator-dependent study, it will usually identify significant parenchymal lacerations *(16)*. It

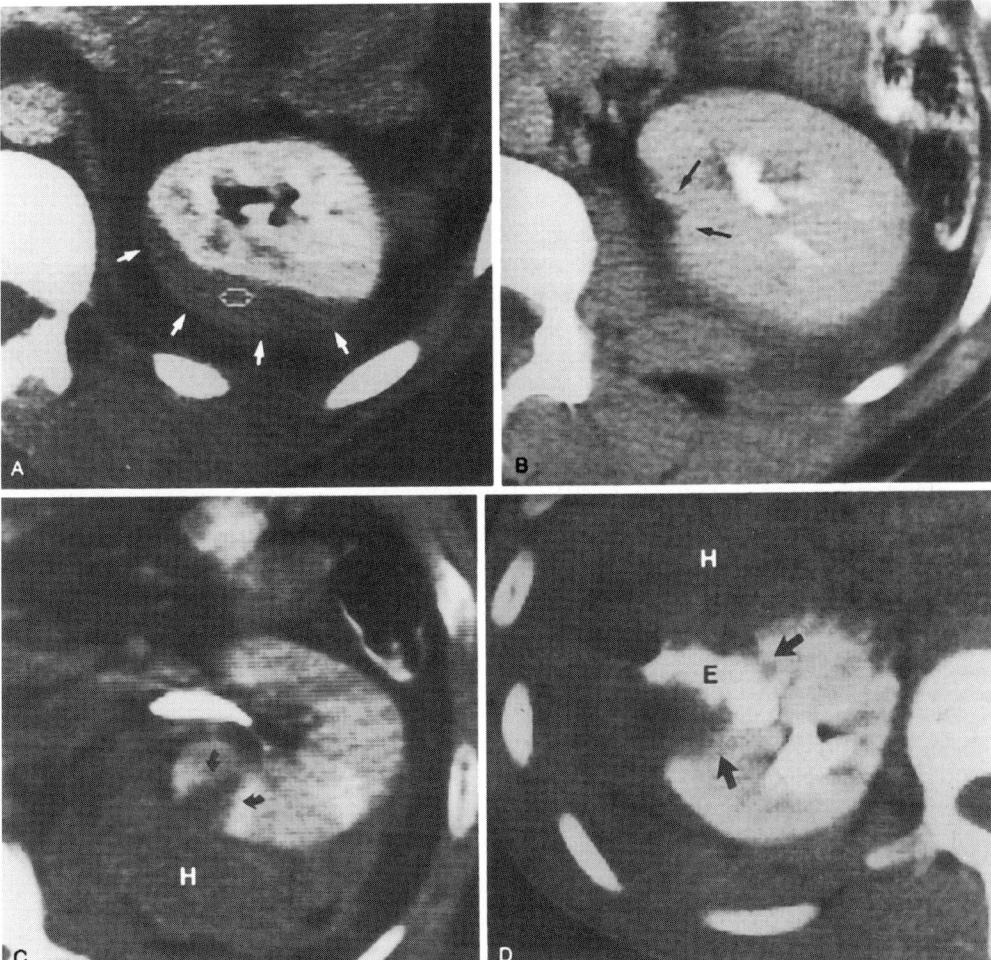

Fig. 2. The spatial resolution of computed tomography (CT) allows it to identify clearly the subcapsular hematoma (**A**) (arrows outline renal capsule) and differentiate superficial (**B**) from deep (**C**) lacerations, without (**C**) and with (**D**) extravasation of opacified urine (arrows identify laceration margins, and the letters H and E indicate perirenal hematoma and urinary extravasation, respectively. (From ref. *25*, p. 99.)

may be used to assess injuries to other associated organs. Ultrasound has limited ability to assess the renal vasculature, however. Doppler ultrasound may increase the sensitivity of this modality in detecting renal vascular injuries, but it appears to have no significant benefit over CT scan.

Renal nuclear scintigraphy has a limited role in the acute trauma setting. Although it provides accurate functional information with less radiation exposure (compared to CT or IVP), nuclear scans provide limited anatomic detail and are inferior to CT regarding regional anatomy. Nuclear scans are of value when following the function of a traumatized kidney following nonoperative or operative management *(17)*. None of these are recommended as first-line studies in the acute setting.

Arteriography is diagnostic of renovascular injury and may occasionally be used therapeutically (*see* later), specifically in cases requiring renal arterial embolization or

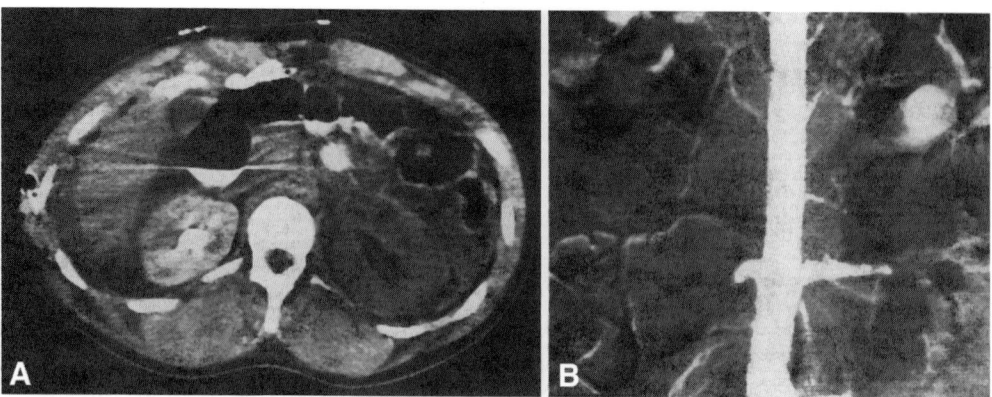

Fig. 3. Left renal arterial thrombosis secondary to blunt renal trauma. Note the intact renal contour with no parenchymal enhancement. (From ref. *62*, p. 122.)

stenting of a thrombosed renal artery. Patients with renovascular injuries have usually sustained other significant visceral injury requiring laparotomy and will only rarely be stable enough to undergo selective renal angiography.

INDICATIONS FOR SURGICAL EXPLORATION

The vast majority of renal injuries are contusions or minor lacerations and may thus be managed nonoperatively if adequately staged. Based on mechanism of injury, presence of hematuria, and radiographic staging, we have created and successfully employed an algorithmic approach to adult renal injuries (Fig. 4). Appropriate radiographic staging has also permitted selective nonoperative management of major lacerations in both blunt and penetrating trauma. In a recent series of grade IV lacerations at San Francisco General Hospital, 22% were successfully managed nonoperatively *(18)*.

Penetrating injuries more commonly require laparotomy because of associated injuries or hemodynamic instability. In our experience, however, 55% of stab wounds and 24% of gunshot wounds were successfully managed expectantly using careful selection and complete clinical and radiographic staging *(19)*. If expectant management is selected for a major renal laceration, close monitoring with serial hematocrit measurements and liberal use of repeat imaging are indicated. The expectant approach thus does *not* imply nonsurgical management, and the urologist must be prepared to intervene surgically when necessary.

The only absolute indication for surgical exploration in renal trauma is massive and potentially life-threatening hemorrhage from a severely injured kidney (grade V injuries) *(20)*. These patients often present in deep shock, and it is thus rare for them to have undergone radiographic staging prior to emergency celiotomy. The typical intraoperative finding of a pulsatile or expanding retroperitoneal hematoma usually signifies a major renal vascular or parenchymal injury, and exploration and reconstruction should be performed expeditiously. In the setting of renal pedicle avulsion or severely shattered kidney, reconstruction may be impossible, and nephrectomy may be lifesaving *(21)*. Some studies have attempted to manage grade V renal injuries in a nonoperative/expectant fashion *(22)*. On careful review, many of the kidneys so managed involved multiple deep lacerations without pedicle avulsion or a truly shattered kidney with massive bleeding. We believe that the grade V classification should be reserved for kidneys that require urgent operative intervention *(23)*.

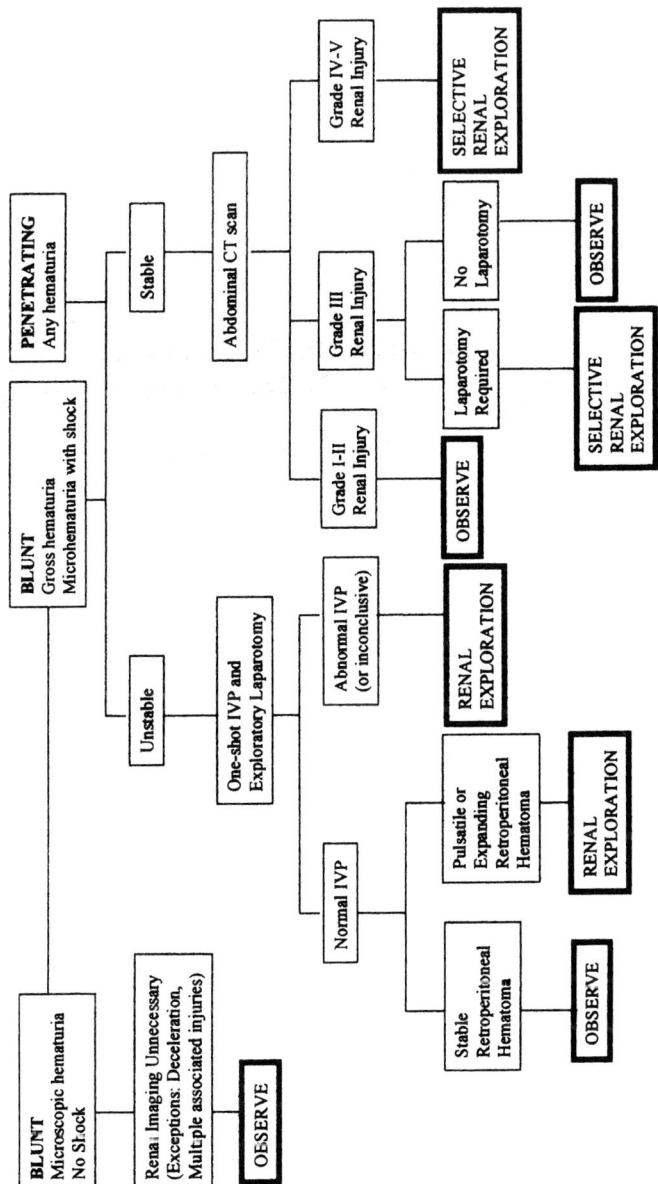

Fig. 4. Algorithm for patients with adult renal trauma. IVP, intravenous pyelogram. (From ref. 8, p. 445.)

Relative indications for renal exploration include incomplete staging, devitalized renal parenchyma, vascular injury, and urinary extravasation *(24)*. In cases of the critically injured patient, complete preoperative radiographic staging is usually not possible prior to laparotomy. The urologist may also be called for an unexpected retroperitoneal hematoma found at the time of laparotomy in the trauma patient. An intraoperative "one-shot" high-dose IVP is an invaluable study in this setting *(25)*. A single abdominal plain film is obtained 10 min following the push injection of a 2-cc/kg bolus of intravenous contrast material. This film confirms the presence of a normally functioning contralateral kidney and helps stage the injury of the affected renal unit. Any abnormality on the intraoperative IVP should prompt renal exploration and repair.

In addition, all patients with penetrating trauma and incomplete preoperative staging and a retroperitoneal hematoma require exploration. Although the one-shot IVP may be indeterminate, a study found that it successfully obviated renal exploration in 32% of patients in whom it was required *(26)*. Furthermore, this approach has not been found to increase the rate of unnecessary nephrectomy *(1)*. The initial celiotomy is the optimal time for any required renal reconstruction. Delayed exploration has resulted in nephrectomy rates as high as 50% *(16)*.

Significant amounts of devitalized renal parenchyma are often best managed by early surgical debridement. Expectant management of patients with devitalized fragments and associated intraabdominal injury may lead to a higher rate of abscess and infected urinoma formation as well as delayed bleeding, all of which may require open surgical management *(27)*. Immediate exploration in this setting reduced the post-trauma complication rate from 82 to 23% *(28)*. This finding suggests that major renal lacerations with devitalized fragments and associated intraabdominal injuries should be immediately repaired, particularly if a laparotomy is already planned by the trauma surgeon. We also feel that patients with a major devitalized fragment associated with urinary extravasation and a significant hematoma are ultimately best treated by early exploration and reconstruction, even without concomitant intraperitoneal injury. However, the nonoperative approach in this situation may be more prudent for the urologist who rarely undertakes renal exploration in the trauma setting.

Urinary extravasation signifies collecting system violation secondary to a major renal laceration, but does not specifically mandate surgical repair. The collecting system may be violated at a fornix, a minor or major calyx, or most significantly, through the renal pelvis and ureteropelvic junction (UPJ). Although the majority of lacerations into fornices and minor calyces will seal spontaneously, larger degrees of extravasation may leak for a prolonged period and are less likely to resolve spontaneously *(29)*. Serial CT scans are mandatory in the management of these patients. The first scan should be obtained at approx 36–48 h postinjury to rule out the development of significant new complications *(30)*.

Intervention is indicated for sepsis, ongoing leakage, or significant urinoma formation. In these cases, placement of an indwelling ureteral (double J) stent may speed resolution of extravasation *(31)*. Lacerations of the renal pelvis usually do not resolve spontaneously and should be surgically repaired. Similarly, UPJ avulsion mandates surgical repair. These unusual injuries are more commonly found in deceleration injury of children. CT findings that suggest UPJ avulsion include nonvisualization of the ipsilateral ureter and medial extravasation of contrast material *(32)* (Fig. 5). The urologist should also maintain a low threshold for repair of an extravasating kidney associated with a gunshot wound. These are often associated with significant

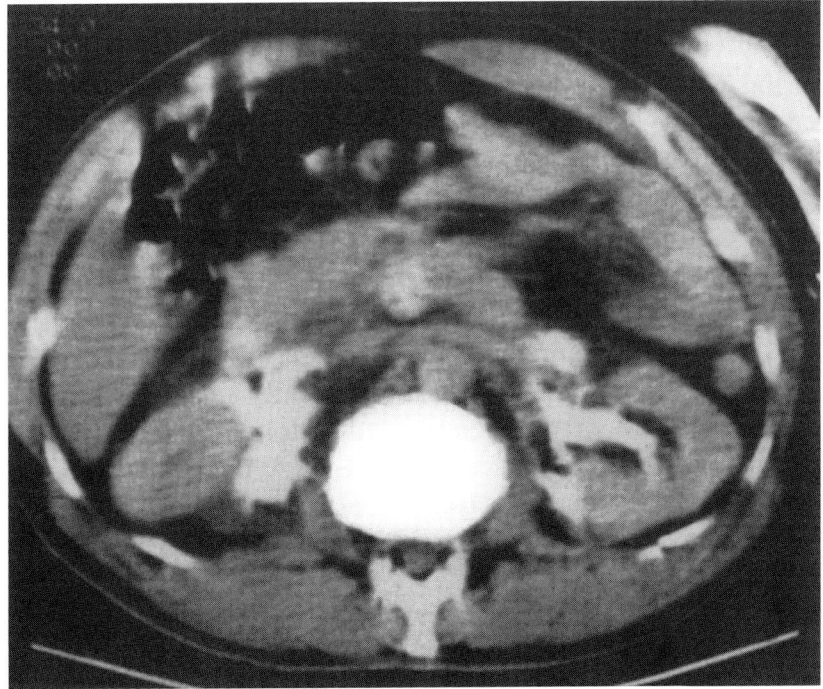

Fig. 5. Abdominal computed tomographic (CT) scan of a patient who sustained bilateral ureteropelvic junction injuries. (From ref. *63*, p. 173.)

devitalized parenchyma secondary to blast effect, particularly when a high-velocity missile has been used.

RENAL VASCULAR INJURIES

The estimated incidence of renal vascular injuries is variable, but typically involves approx 25% of all major renal injuries. Major injury to the main renal artery or vein usually requires operative management. Of reported cases of renal vascular injuries, 60% involve renal arterial injury, 30% involve renal venous injury, and 10% involve both *(33)*. The left renal artery is more prone to deceleration injury/thrombosis than the right. Physical examination is not usually specific for renal vascular injury, and gross hematuria may be absent in as many as 40% of cases *(34)*. These patients have higher rates of complications, renal loss, and mortality compared to those with nonvascular renal injuries *(35)*.

Despite the ongoing advances in trauma care, successful renal salvage after major renovascular injury only occurs in 25 to 35% of cases *(36)*. A recent multicenter review of outcomes following major renovascular trauma found that grade V injuries, blunt trauma, and attempted arterial repair all correlated with a poor result (renovascular hypertension, renal dysfunction) *(37)*. Time to reperfusion is the major factor in determining the ultimate outcome. Renal function is significantly impaired following 3 h of total and 6 h of partial ischemia. Despite a technically successful repair, late hypertension occurs frequently in these cases. It appears to complicate 50% of renal arterial injuries managed nonoperatively *(38)*, compared with 57% that were revascularized *(39)*. We thus reserve renal arterial repair for solitary kidneys, bilaterally injured kidneys, and in the rare situation of detection within 6 h of injury.

There have been encouraging early results in the use of endovascular techniques to place wall stents in select cases of renal artery thrombosis *(40)*, but long-term results have yet to be reported. In the uncommon young trauma patient without atherosclerotic disease, hemodynamic instability, or associated organ injury, this may be an attractive option for addressing isolated arterial thrombosis. Similarly, selective renal embolization may play an important role in obtaining hemostasis in major renal vascular injury, particularly if no other injuries are present. Subselective catheterization and embolization of the lacerated vessel may minimally compromise the remaining normal parenchyma *(41)*.

If detection of renal artery thrombosis is delayed and celiotomy is otherwise indicated, nephrectomy should be performed at that time. Otherwise, the kidney may be allowed to atrophy, with delayed nephrectomy performed if hypertension develops.

PEDIATRIC RENAL TRAUMA

The pediatric kidney is more susceptible to injury than the adult kidney. The pediatric kidney has less protective perinephric fat and occupies a larger portion of the retroperitoneum than does the adult kidney. There is also less protection from blunt trauma secondary to less-developed back and chest wall musculature. A child's kidney is also more mobile, and deceleration forces put significant shearing stress on the renal pedicle. Renal congenital anomalies (including UPJ obstruction, malrotation, and duplex collecting systems) appear to predispose the kidney to greater risk of injury *(42)*. Motor vehicle crashes and falls are the most common causes of renal trauma in the preadolescent age group, with penetrating trauma increasing in prevalence in the adolescent years.

The imaging criteria for children with suspected renal injuries are less well established. Because children may dramatically increase systemic vascular resistance, hypotension may not occur with a significant renal laceration *(43)*. Although some have argued that significant renal injuries may present without any hematuria *(44)*, it has been our experience that major renal injuries are unlikely in children with blunt injury without gross or microhematuria (>50 RBC/HPF) *(45)*. The history, clinical status, and mechanism of injury all play key roles in the decision to image a child with suspected renal trauma. CT scan with intravenous contrast and delayed images has become the study of choice in imaging pediatric renal trauma. As in the adult population, most lacerations are minor and will be successfully treated nonoperatively, with exploration reserved for major renal injuries or incomplete staging.

RENAL EXPLORATION AND RECONSTRUCTION

Proximal Vascular Control

Historically, renal exploration in the trauma setting usually resulted in total nephrectomy. Using a refined approach to proximal vascular control and a meticulous approach to reconstruction, we have successfully repaired 87% of kidneys requiring surgical exploration *(1)*. Our primary goals for reconstruction include control of renal hemorrhage, preservation of maximal parenchyma, and reduction of potential complications attributable to the injured kidney *(46)*.

The main indication for unplanned nephrectomy in the trauma setting is uncontrolled hemorrhage. We therefore routinely obtain proximal vascular control prior to opening

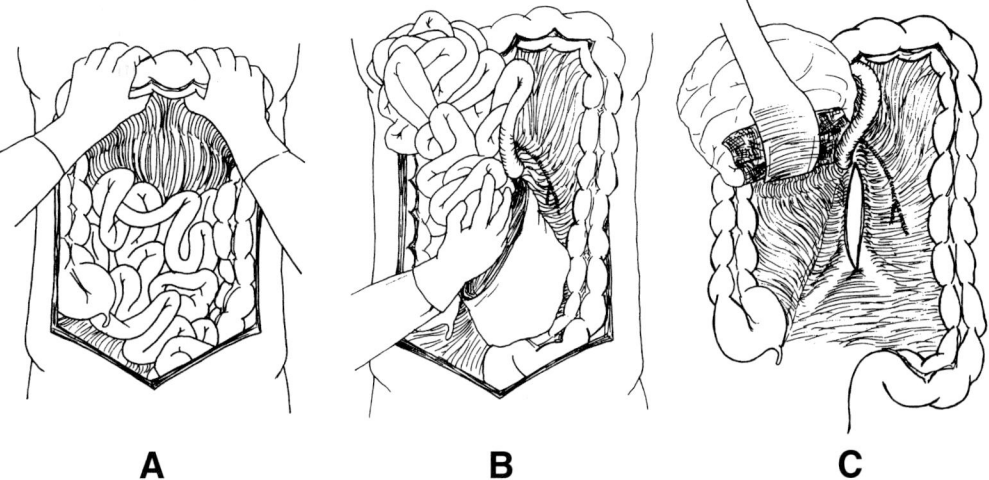

Fig. 6. Exposure for proximal vascular control in renal trauma. (From ref. *46*, pp. 32–33.)

the retroperitoneal hematoma *(47)*. Although temporary vascular occlusion is rarely necessary (approx 13% of our renal explorations), there is no accurate method of determining which kidneys will require this maneuver during the subsequent reconstruction. Those who have presented series suggesting pedicle control can be safely obtained if necessary following release of the perinephric hematoma have reported nephrectomy rates approximately three times higher than those recorded at San Francisco General Hospital *(48,49)*.

The traumatized kidney should be explored through a midline transperitoneal incision extending from the xiphoid process to the pubic symphysis. Except in cases of renal pedicle avulsion, all associated intraabdominal injuries (spleen, liver, pancreas, small and large intestines) should be addressed before renal exploration, thus allowing Gerota's fascia to maintain its natural tamponade effect on the hematoma.

The approach to the injured kidney begins with proximal vascular control. The transverse colon is wrapped in moist laparotomy sponges and placed on the chest (Fig. 6). The small intestine is placed in a bowel bag and retracted superiorly and to the right. This exposes the root of the mesentery, the ligament of Treitz, and the underlying great vessels. The retroperitoneal incision is made over the aorta superior to the inferior mesenteric artery and extending up to the ligament of Treitz. If a large retroperitoneal hematoma obviates easy palpation of the aorta at the level of the ligament of Treitz, the incision may be made medial to the inferior mesenteric vein. This vein is an important guide, located a few centimeters left of the aorta. It is easily identifiable, even in the presence of a large hematoma *(50)*.

Dissection should be carried superiorly along the anterior wall of the aorta until the left renal vein is identified crossing anterior to it (Fig. 7). This vessel is encircled (but *not* occluded) with a vessel loop, allowing it to be retracted cephalad. It serves as a guide to the remaining renal vessels, each of which is then encircled in vessel loops. These vessels are all left unoccluded unless heavy bleeding is encountered during the renal dissection. In our experience, most bleeding is successfully controlled with manual compression alone. Temporary renal vascular occlusion should be less than 30 min to minimize warm ischemic damage *(51)*.

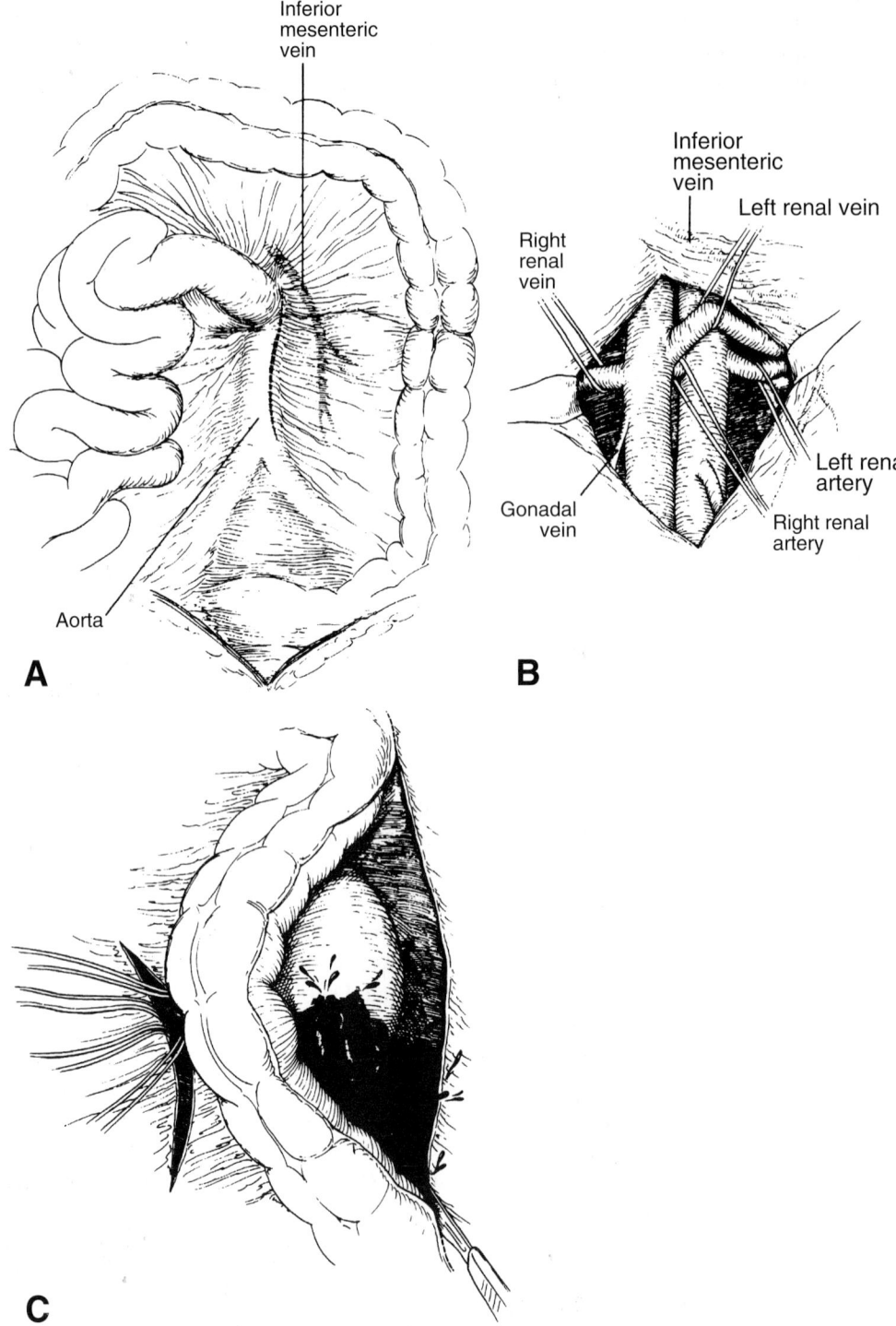

Fig. 7. The renal vasculature is approached medially after incising over the aorta. Note the anatomic relationships of the renal vessels. (From ref. *53*, p. 107.)

After vascular control has been successfully achieved, the injured kidney may be exposed by mobilizing the ipsilateral colon along the white line of Toldt and reflecting it medially. Gerota's fascia is then incised along the lateral aspect of the kidney to expose the kidney completely. Care should be taken to maintain the integrity of the renal capsule as the kidney is mobilized to decrease hemorrhage and preserve the capsule for later closure.

Principles of Reconstruction

The general principles applicable to all renal reconstructions include the following: (1) broad exposure of the entire kidney; (2) temporary vascular occlusion for bleeding not arrested by manual compression of the parenchyma; (3) sharp debridement of nonviable parenchyma; (4) meticulous hemostasis; (5) watertight collecting system closure; (6) primary reapproximation of the parenchymal edges (renorrhaphy) or coverage of the parenchymal defect; (7) omental interposition flap placement to separate reconstructed kidney from surrounding pancreatic, colonic, or vascular injuries; and (8) retroperitoneal drain placement *(52)*.

The kidney should be debrided sharply back to viable, bleeding parenchyma (Fig. 8). To avoid dialysis, 30% of one normally functioning kidney is required; this should serve as a guideline in determining whether renal salvage should be undertaken *(53)*. Major polar injuries are best managed with partial nephrectomy; lacerations to the midkidney should undergo renorrhaphy (*see* later). Hemostasis is then performed by individually suture-ligating arterial vessels with 4-0 chromic sutures. We then place hemostatic agents such as thrombin-soaked Gelfoam bolsters or Flo-Seal® between the cut parenchymal edges.

The collecting system is then inspected for obvious tears. Injection of 2–3 cc methylene blue into the renal pelvis (using a 27-gage needle) may demonstrate these openings more clearly. They are then oversewn with running 4-0 chromic suture. We place a double-J stent only in significant renal pelvis or ureteral injuries, but not in simple calyceal injuries *(54)*. In a deep, slitlike parenchymal laceration from a knife or sword, the thin parenchymal defect will not permit easy access to the collecting system, and we rely on closure of the overlying parenchyma to seal the collecting system *(9)*.

If the renal capsule is intact and viable, it should be used to close the parenchymal defect primarily without tension. If the capsule has been destroyed or the defect is too large to close primarily without causing ischemia, we routinely harvest an omental pedicle flap. The omentum is ideal for coverage because it imports its own vascular supply and lymphatic drainage, which will promote healing. Knowledge of omental anatomy and vasculature are critical to the dissection (Fig. 9).

Harvest begins by dissecting the greater omentum from its attachments to the transverse colon. If additional length is needed, the omentum may then be detached from the stomach and basing the flap on the right gastroepiploic artery. The omentum is guided through the paracolic gutter to reach the kidney and sutured to the defect with 3-0 absorbable sutures. If omentum is not available, the defect may be covered with perinephric fat or a peritoneal free graft; however, these are less-desirable options. For a shattered kidney or multiple deep lacerations, the kidney may be placed in an envelope of Vicrylmesh to stabilize the repair *(55)* (Fig. 10).

Following reconstruction involving the collecting system, a 1-in. Penrose drain is placed adjacent to the kidney and connected to a urostomy bag to drain any leak if necessary. Alternatively, a Jackson-Pratt (JP) drain may be used as long as it is *not* connected to suction, which would promote prolonged urinary drainage. These drains

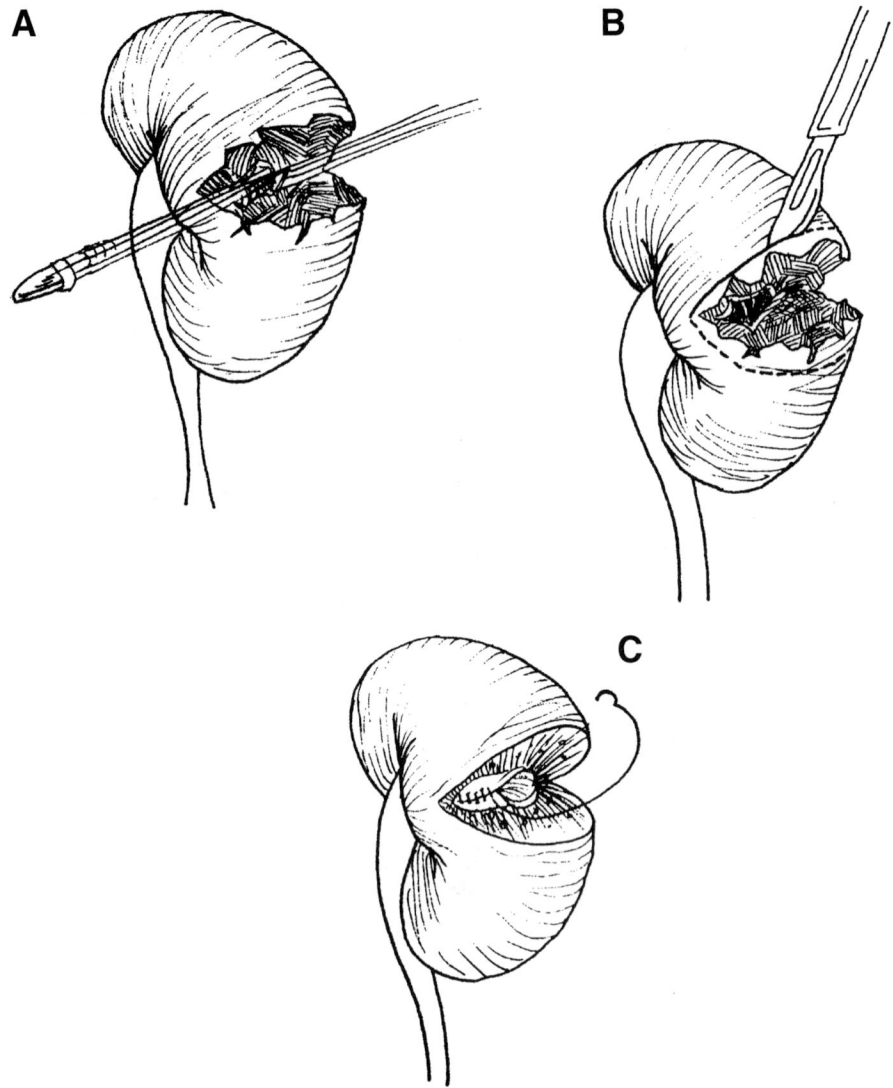

Fig. 8. Principles of renal reconstruction following a gunshot wound through the midpolar region. (From ref. *46*, p. 43.)

are typically removed after 48 to 72 h unless output is high, in which case the drainage creatinine should be measured. If the creatinine value suggests a urine leak, the drain is left in place for a more prolonged period. Placement of an indwelling ureteral stent may help expedite sealing of a persistent urine leak.

Specific Techniques

Renorrhaphy is appropriate for lacerations involving the interpolar aspect of the kidney (Fig. 11), or polar lacerations with a limited amount of devitalized tissue. This technique employs all the principles outlined in the preceding section. Following debridement and hemostasis, the collecting system is closed. The residual wedge-shaped defect is then closed over an absorbable thrombin-soaked Gelfoam bolster. Omental

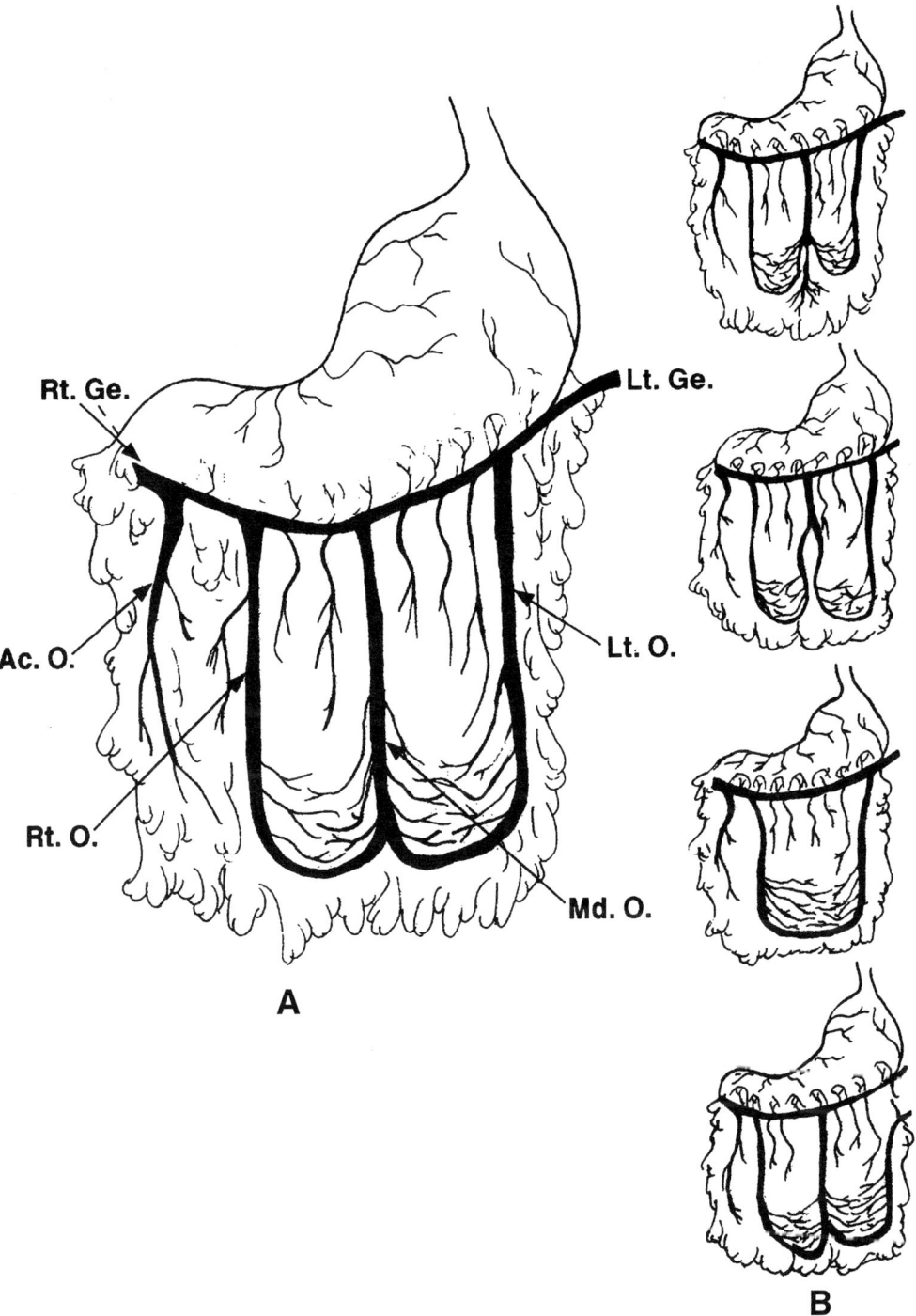

Fig. 9. Arterial blood supply of the greater omentum, key in mobilization of omental pedicle flaps. Rt. Ge., right gastroepiploic artery; Lt. Ge., left gastroepiploic artery; Rt. O., right omental artery; Lt. O., left omental artery; Md. O., middle omental artery; Ac. O., accessary omental artery. (From ref. *46*, p. 41.)

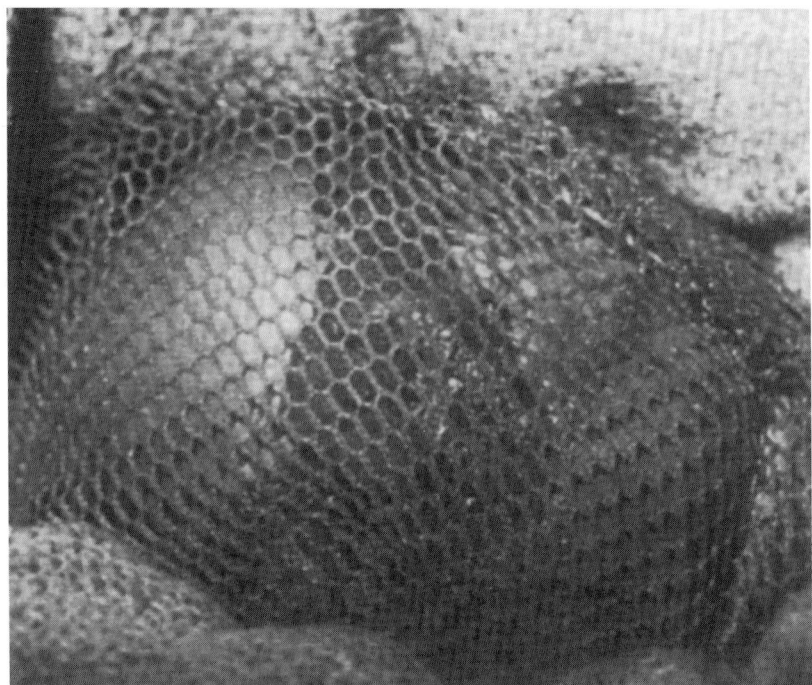

Fig. 10. Absorbable mesh placed around kidney serves as support for renorrhaphy. (From ref.*53*, p. 111.)

flaps are used for large parenchymal defects. To identify the site of the repair on subsequent imaging studies, we place small titanium surgical clips on the sutures that approximate the capsular edges.

Extensive damage to the upper or lower renal poles usually requires partial nephrectomy (Fig. 12). The capsule should be dissected off the fractured parenchyma for use in defect coverage. Following hemostasis and collecting system closure as outlined in the preceding section, the defect may be covered by capsule (if available) or by an omental pedicle flap.

VASCULAR INJURY AND REPAIR

Unlike parenchymal lacerations, renovascular injuries are frequently irreparable and may result in nephrectomy. Proximal vascular control is particularly critical in these cases. Injury to the main renal vein typically results in significant hemorrhage and may require ligation. If reconstruction is feasible, the partially lacerated vein may be repaired with 5-0 prolene suture following appropriate vascular clamping. Injuries to segmental veins may be safely ligated because of the extensive renal venous collateral circulation.

As mentioned, the ultimate outcome of attempted renal arterial reconstruction is time dependent. Segmental arterial injuries may be safely ligated, with few complications arising from the subsequently devascularized renal parenchyma *(56,57)*. Alternatively, a partially lacerated segmental artery may be repaired with 5-0 or 6-0 prolene suture.

In cases of main renal artery injury, the type of repair indicated relates to the extent and mechanism of injury *(58)*. Penetrating injuries with incomplete transection may be

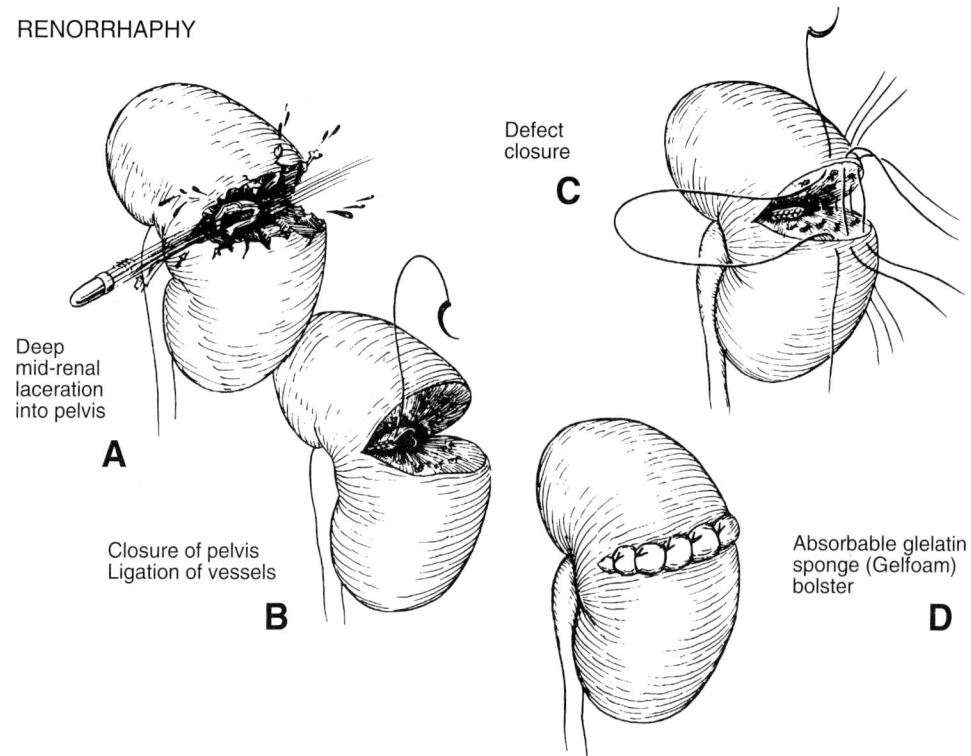

Fig. 11. Technique of renorrhaphy after midpolar penetrating injury into collecting system. (From ref. *4*, p. 447.)

primarily repaired using 5-0 prolene sutures. Blunt injuries typically require thrombectomy and debridement of the damaged arterial segment. Ideally, a primary tension-free reanastomosis of the injured artery should be undertaken. If this is not feasible, we recommend a hypogastric artery interposition vascular graft. Less-attractive graft alternatives include reversed saphenous vein, Dacron®, or other vascular prosthetic materials. Although technically feasible, ex vivo renal reconstruction and autotransplantation into the iliac fossa are rarely indicated in the critically injured patient with multiple associated injuries *(59)*.

POSTOPERATIVE CARE AND COMPLICATIONS

A urethral catheter should be maintained until the patient is hemodynamically stable and mobile enough to void. The patient should be kept on bed rest until gross hematuria clears. We recommend obtaining an abdominal CT scan and radionuclide renal scan at approx 3 mo to quantify the function of the injured/reconstructed kidney. In our series of traumatically injured and subsequently reconstructed kidneys, the average differential renal function was 39%, corresponding to two-thirds of one kidney.

The reported complication rate following renal injury ranges between 3 and 20% *(37)*. Complication rates increase proportionately with increasing grade of injury and appear to be higher in kidneys managed nonoperatively *(22)*. Our complication rate is approx 10%. Interestingly, our complication rate (attributable specifically to the kidney) for grade IV injuries was similar for nonoperative and operative management, 5 and 4%,

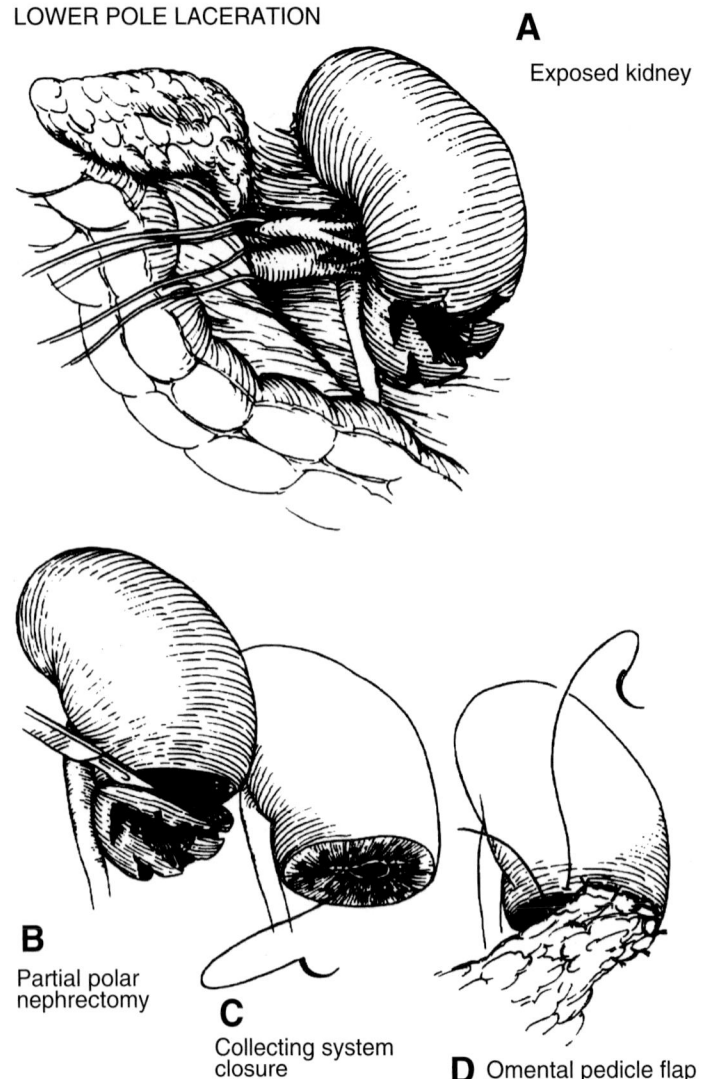

Fig. 12. Technique of partial nephrectomy following blunt trauma to the lower pole. Note complete debridement of devitalized parenchyma down to viable tissue, followed by hemostasis and collecting system closure. The defect may then be covered with capsule, Vicryl mesh, or an omental pedicle flap. (From ref. 53, p. 108.)

respectively (1). This is likely because of our higher rate of renal exploration (78% of grade IV injuries) than other series, as well as our patient selection for nonoperative management.

Complications may be divided into early (within 1 mo) and late complications. Early complications include urinomas, delayed bleeding, urinary fistulas, abscesses, and hypertension. Urinomas are the most common complication and are usually successfully managed by endoscopic stenting or percutaneous drainage. Delayed bleeding typically occurs within 1–2 wk of injury and is more commonly associated with stab wounds.

Angiography and selective embolization are both diagnostic and therapeutic in this case *(60)*.

Long-term complications include hydronephrosis, renal failure, delayed hypertension, and arteriovenous fistulas. The first two complications are uncommon, but hypertension may be seen in untreated arterial thrombosis and devitalized parenchyma. This has been documented in approx 0.2% of cases in our experience *(2)*. Post-traumatic hypertension is mediated by the renin–angiotensin system, and delayed nephrectomy is indicated in this setting if medical management fails. An arteriovenous fistula may present with hemorrhage, hypertension, or high-output cardiac failure following a stab wound. Arteriography and fistula embolization usually characterize and treat the fistula successfully. Long-term follow-up is critical to check for development of hypertension, which may develop slowly.

SUMMARY

The recommendations presented in this review are based on our experience in managing more than 3000 renal trauma patients during the past 25 yr at San Francisco General Hospital. The development and ongoing refinement of the treatment algorithms presented here provide validated guidelines for the general urologist who manages trauma infrequently. Although the majority of renal injuries may be successfully managed nonoperatively, certain well-defined relative and absolute indications demand operative intervention. Early vascular control has significantly increased the renal salvage rate at our center, and we strongly recommend it for all renal explorations. Adherence to the reconstructive techniques outlined will serve the urologist well in successfully repairing the traumatically injured kidney.

REFERENCES

1. Brown SL, Elder JS, Spirnak JP. Are pediatric patients more susceptible to major renal injury from blunt trauma? A comparative study. J Urol 1998; 160: 138–140.
2. Wessells H, McAninch JW, Meyer A. Criteria for management of significant penetrating renal lacerations. J Urol 1997; 157: 24–27.
3. Moore EE, Shackford SR, Pachter HL. Organ injury scaling; spleen, liver, kidney. J Trauma 1989; 29: 1664.
4. Santucci RA, McAninch JW, Safir MH, Mario LA, Service S, Segal MR. Validating the American Association for the Surgery of Trauma Organ injury severity scale for the kidney. J Trauma 2001; 50: 195–200.
5. Mee SL, McAninch JW, Robinson AL. Radiographic assessment of renal trauma: a 10 year p Segal MR, Segal MR,rospective study of patient selection. J Urol 1989; 141: 1095–1098.
6. Bright TC, White K, Peters PC. Significance of hematuria after trauma. J Urol 1978; 120: 455.
7. Miller KS, McAninch JW. Radiographic assessment of renal trauma: our 15-year experience. J Urol. 1995; 154: 352–355.
8. Santucci RA, McAninch JW. Diagnosis and management of renal trauma: past, present and future. J Am Coll Surg 2000; 191: 443–451.
9. Brandes SB, McAninch JW: Urban free falls and patterns of renal injury: a 20 year experience with 396 cases. J Trauma Injury Infect Crit Care 1999; 47: 643–649.
10. Morey AF, Bruce JE, McAninch JW. Efficacy of radiographic imaging in pediatric blunt renal trauma. J Urol 1996; 156: 2014–2018.
11. Santucci RA, Wessells H, Bartsch G, et al. Evaluation and management of renal injuries: consensus statement of the renal trauma subcommittee. BJU Int 2004; 93: 937–954.

12. Bretan PN, McAninch JW, Federle MP, Jeffrey RB. Computerized tomographic scanning of renal trauma: 85 consecutive cases. J Urol 1986; 136: 561–565.
13. Brown SL, Hoffman DM, Spirnak JP. Limitations of routine spiral computerized tomography in the evaluation of blunt renal trauma. J Urol 1998; 160: 1979–1981.
14. Kawashima A, Sandler CM, Ernst RD, et al. CT evaluation of renovascular disease. Radiographics 2000; 20: 1321–1340.
15. Steinberg DL, Jeffret RB, Federle MP, et al. The computerized tomographic appearance of renal pedicle injury. J Urol 1984; 132: 1163.
16. Jaske G, Furtschegger A, Egender G. Ultrasound in patients with blunt renal trauma managed by surgery. J Urol 1987; 138: 21.
17. Wessells H, Deirmenjian J, McAninch JW.. Preservation of renal function after reconstruction for trauma: quantitative assessment with radionuclide scintigraphy. J Urol 1997; 157: 1583–1586.
18. Santucci RA, McAninch JW. Grade 4 renal injuries: evaluation, treatment and outcome. World J Surg 2001; 25: 1565–1572.
19. McAninch JW, Carroll PR, Klosterman PW. Renal reconstruction after injury. J Urol. 1991; 145: 932–937.
20. Holcroft JW, Trunkey DD, Minagi H. Renal trauma and retroperitoneal hematomas: indications for exploration. J Trauma 1975; 15: 1045.
21. Nash PA, Bruce JE, McAninch JW. Nephrectomy for traumatic renal injuries. J. Urol 1995; 153: 609–611.
22. Altman AL, Haas C, Dinchman KH, Spirnak JP. Selective nonoperative management of blunt grade 5 renal injury. J Urol 2000; 164: 27–31.
23. McAninch JW. Editorial comment to selective nonoperative management of blunt grade 5 renal injury. J Urol 2000; 164: 31.
24. Meng MV, Brandes SB, McAninch JW. Renal trauma: indications and techniques for surgical exploration. World J Urol 1999; 17: 71–77.
25. Nash PA, Carroll PR. Staging of renal trauma. In Traumatic and Reconstructive Urology. (McAninch JW, Carroll PR, Jordan GH, eds.) Saunders, Philadelphia, PA, 1996, pp. 95–104.
26. Morey AF, McAninch JW, Tiller BK, Duckett CP, Carroll PR. Single shot intraoperative excretory urography for the immediate management of renal trauma. J Urol 1999; 161: 1088–1092.
27. Hussmann DA, Morris JS. Attempted non-operative management of blunt renal lacerations extending through the corticomedullary junction: the short-term and long-term sequelae. J Urol 1990; 143: 682–684.
28. Hussmann DA, Gilling PJ, Perry MO, Morris JS, Boone TB. Major renal lacerations with a devitalized fragment following blunt abdominal trauma: a comparison between non-operative (expectant) vs surgical management. J. Urol 1993; 150: 1774–1777.
29. Mathews LA, Smith EM, Spirnak JP. Non-operative treatment of major blunt renal lacerations with urinary extravasation. J Urol 1997; 157: 2056–2058.
30. Wessells H. Evaluation and management of renal trauma in the 21st century. AUA Update Ser 2002; 21: 233–240.
31. Glenski WJ, Hussmann DA. Non-surgical management of major renal lacerations associated with urinary extravasation. J Urol 1995; 153: 315A.
32. Townsend M, DeFalco AJ. Absence of ureteral opacification below ureteral disruption: a sentinel CT finding. AJR Am J Roentgenol 1995; 164: 253–254.
33. Clark DE, Georgitis JW, Ray FS: Renal arterial injuries caused by blunt trauma. Surgery 1981; 90: 87–96.
34. Dinchman KH, Spirnak JP. Traumatic renal artery thrombosis: evaluation and treatment. Semin Urol 1995; 13: 90–93.
35. Carroll PR, McAninch JW, Klosterman P, Greenblatt M. Renovascular trauma: risk assessment, surgical management and outcome. J Trauma 1990; 30: 547.
36. Tillou A, Romero J, Asensio JA, Best CD, Petrone P, Roldon G. Renal vascular injuries. Surg Clin North Am 2001; 81(6): 1417–1430.
37. Knudson MM, Harrison PB, Hoyt DB, devilliers van Nickerk JP, Cremin BJ, Holt SA, Peterson NE. Outcome after major renovascular injuries: a Western Trauma Association Multicenter report. J Trauma 2000; 49(6): 1116–1122.

38. Stables DP, Fouche RF, deVillers van Niekerk JP, Cremin BJ, Holt SA, Peterson NE. Traumatic renal artery occlusion: 21 cases. J Urol 1976; 115: 229–233.
39. Maggio AJ, Brosman S. Renal artery trauma. Urology 1978; 11: 125–130.
40. Villas PA, Cohen G, Putnam SG III, et al. Wallstent placement in a renal artery after blunt abdominal trauma. J Trauma 1999; 46: 1137–1139.
41. Hoffer EK, Sclafani SJA. Interventional radiology in urologic trauma. In: Traumatic and Reconstructive Urology (McAninch JW, Carroll PR, Jordan GH, eds.), Saunders, Philadelphia, PA, 1996, pp. 157–170.
42. McAleer IM, Kaplan GW. Pediatric genitourinary trauma. Urol Clin North Am 1995; 22(1): 177–188.
43. Medica J, Caldamone A. Pediatric renal trauma: special considerations. Semin Urol 1995; 13: 73.
44. Nguyen MM, Das S. Pediatric renal trauma. Urology 2002; 59(5): 762–767.
45. Morey AF, Bruce JE, McAninch JW. Efficacy of radiographic imaging in pediatric blunt renal trauma. J Urol 1996; 156: 2014–2018.
46. Brandes SB, McAninch JW. Surgical exposure and repair of the traumatized kidney. Atlas Urol Clin North Am 1998; 6(2): 31–45.
47. McAninch JW, Carroll PR. Renal trauma: kidney preservation through improved vascular control—a refined approach. J Trauma 1982; 22: 285–290.
48. Atala A, Miller FB, Richardson JD, et al. Preliminary vascular control for renal trauma. Surg Gynecol Obstet 1991; 172: 386.
49. Corriere JN, McAndrew JD, Benson GS. Intraoperative decision making in renal trauma surgery. J Trauma 1991; 31: 1390.
50. Brandes SB, McAninch JW. Reconstructive surgery for trauma of the upper urinary tract. Urol Clin North Am 1999; 26(1): 183–199.
51. Carroll PR, McAninch JW, Wong A, Wolf JS, Newton C. Outcome after temporary vascular occlusion for the management of renal trauma. J Urol 1994; 151: 1171–1173.
52. Brandes SB, McAninch JW. Renal trauma: a practical guide to evaluation and management. Digital Urology Journal on-line. Available at: http://www.duj.com/Article/McAninch/McAninch.html.
53. Carroll PR, McAninch JW. Renal exploration after trauma: indications and reconstructive techniques. In: Traumatic and Reconstructive Urology (McAninch JW, Carroll PR, Jordan GH, eds.), Saunders, Philadelphia, PA, 1996, pp. 105–112.
54. Presti JC, Carroll PR, McAninch JW. Ureteral and renal pelvic injuries from external trauma: diagnosis and management. J Trauma 1989; 29: 370.
55. Mounzer AM, McAninch JW, Schmidt RA. Polyglycolic acid mesh in repair of renal injury. Urology 1986; 28: 127.
56. Bertini JE, Flechner SM, Miller P, et al. The natural history of traumatic branch renal artery injury. J Urol 1986; 135: 228.
57. Cass AS. Renovascular injuries from external trauma. Urol Clin North Am 1989; 16: 213.
58. Alexander JJ. Renal pedicle injury: vascular reconstruction. Atlas Urol Clin North Am 1998; 6(2): 47–58.
59. Brown M, Graham JM, Mattox KL. Renovascular trauma. Am J Surg 1980; 140: 802.
60. Sclafani SJA, Becker JA, Shaftan GW. Strategies for the management of genitourinary trauma. Urol Radiol 1985; 7: 231.
61. Rosenstein D, McAninch JW. Update on the management of renal trauma. Contemp Urol 2003; 15(7): 47.
62. Carroll PR. Injuries to major abdominal arteries, veins and renal vasculature. In: Traumatic and Reconstructive Urology. (McAninch JW, ed.), Saunders, Philadelphia, PA, 1996, p. 122.
63. Presti JC, Carroll PR. Ureteral and renal pelvic trauma: diagnosis and management. In: Traumatic and Reconstructive Urology (McAninch JW, ed.), Saunders, Philadelphia, PA, 1996, p. 173.

2 Ureteral Trauma

Noel A. Armenakas, MD, FACS

CONTENTS
    INTRODUCTION
    DIAGNOSIS
    INJURY CLASSIFICATION
    ANATOMIC CONSIDERATIONS
    MANAGEMENT CONSIDERATIONS
    SURGICAL TECHNIQUES
    DRAINAGE ISSUES
    POSTOPERATIVE EVALUATION
    COMPLICATIONS
    SUMMARY
    REFERENCES

INTRODUCTION

The ureter serves as the sole source of urinary transport from the kidney. Any injury to this delicate tubular structure poses a potential risk to the ipsilateral renal unit. Ureteral injuries may be classified etiologically as *surgical* or *external*. Surgical injuries are the most common. During abdominal surgery, the ureter is vulnerable to inadvertent injury because of its inconspicuous retroperitoneal location, adjacent to the iliac vessels, colon, and uterus. In addition, various abdominal disease processes can affect the normal ureteral course, causing it to deviate and making it more difficult to identify.

Factors that predispose to surgical ureteral trauma are listed in Table 1. In the past, the majority of surgical ureteral injuries occurred during gynecological procedures, most frequently during abdominal hysterectomies (1–6). The most common site was at the pelvic brim where the ovarian vessels cross the ureter in the infundibular pelvic ligament. With the advent of ureteroscopic surgery, however, urological procedures now cause most ureteral injuries; fortunately, the majority of these are minor injuries and can be safely treated nonsurgically (7,8). Other surgical procedures that may injure the ureter include aortoiliac and aortofemoral arterial bypass surgery, low anterior bowel resection, and, rarely, lumbar laminectomy (Table 2). Mechanisms of injury include kinking, crushing, electrocoagulation, devascularization, ligation, perforation, transection, and excision.

From: *Urological Emergencies: A Practical Guide*
Edited by: H. Wessells and J. W. McAninch © Humana Press Inc., Totowa, NJ

Table 1
Factors That Predispose to Surgical Ureteral Trauma

- Prior surgery
- Infection or Inflammation (e.g., diverticulitis, pelvic inflammatory disease, endometriosis)
- Radiation therapy
- Malignancy
- Uterine size >12-wk gestation
- Ovarian mass >4 cm
- Obesity
- Massive bleeding

Table 2
Causes of Surgical Ureteral Trauma, by Procedure

Reference	Gynecologic	Urological	Colon	Vascular	Spinal	Total
Higgins (1967) (1)	60	5	12	7	2	86
Ihse (1975) (2)	23	13	6	0	0	42
Dowling (1986) (4)	14	8	3	1	1	27
Gangai (1986) (3)	9	10	3	0	2	24
Assimos (1984) (7)	11	12	4	0	0	27
Seltzman (1996) (8)	56	70	28	10	1	165
Total	173	118	56	18	6	371
	(46.6%)	(31.8%)	(15.1%)	(4.9%)	(1.6%)	

Ureteral injuries constitute up to 3% of all genitourinary injuries from external trauma (9). The ureter's mobility and anatomic characteristics protect it from trauma; its narrow diameter and retroperitoneal location between major muscle groups and the spine make it an unlikely target. Most external ureteral injuries occur from gunshot wounds; stab wounds are infrequent (Table 3) (10–15). The bullet does not need to transect the ureter; if its path is simply near the ureter, the temporary cavitation created by the missile can cause significant tissue destruction and delayed necrosis. These injuries can be very difficult to identify and often present with delayed sequelae. Penetrating ureteral injuries are almost always associated with multiple organ injuries. The most common sites, in order of decreasing frequency, include the small bowel, colon, liver, and iliac vessels (14–22). The location of ureteral injuries is fairly evenly distributed, with the upper ureter slightly more prone to trauma (Table 4) (11,15–18,22–25).

Ureteral injuries from blunt trauma are rare. They usually occur in children or young adults during rapid deceleration, which causes excessive hyperextension of the vertebral column and disruption at the ureteropelvic junction (UPJ). They also are associated with multiple organ injuries, most commonly to the liver, spleen, and skeletal system (26–31). In general, UPJ disruptions occur almost exclusively in polytraumatized patients, with most presenting in shock.

Table 3
Mechanism of Ureteral Injury From External Trauma[a]

Injury mechanism	No. patients (%)
Gunshot wounds	227 (81.9)
Stab wounds	14 (5.1)
Blunt	36 (13.0)
Total	277

[a]Results of combined series from refs. *10, 11, 15, 17–19, 23–25, 28–30,* and *32*.

Table 4
Sites of Penetrating Ureteral Trauma[a]

Ureteral sites	Injuries (%)
Upper	126 (38.9)
Middle	107 (33.1)
Lower	91 (28.0)
Total	324

[a]Results of combined series from refs. *11, 15–18,* and *22–25*.

DIAGNOSIS

Clinical

Prompt diagnosis is the first step toward a successful outcome. With external ureteral trauma, this is complicated by the presence of multiple organ injuries and the absence of early clinical and laboratory findings specific for ureteral trauma. Indeed, hematuria, which is a reliable indicator of renal trauma, is absent in approx 30% of ureteral injuries *(10–15,19,21,22,25,28,29,31)*. Early clinical indicators of ureteral trauma are vague or nonexistent.

To avoid the additional morbidity associated with a delay in diagnosis, it is imperative that the evaluating physician maintains a high index of suspicion based on injury mechanism and location. Whether from an external or surgical cause, delayed signs or symptoms of a ureteral injury include prolonged ileus, urinary obstruction, urinary leakage, azootemia, fever, persistent flank pain, fistula formation, and eventually sepsis. After abdominal or pelvic surgery, any patient presenting with these signs or symptoms that suggest the possibility of a ureteral injury should be thoroughly evaluated. In addition, all patients with penetrating abdominal or flank trauma should be suspected of having a ureteral injury and appropriately assessed. Similarly, children and young adults with significant blunt abdominal trauma and multiple associated injuries, especially from a mechanism of rapid deceleration, should undergo radiographic ureteral assessment regardless of the findings on urinalysis.

Table 5
Injury Recognition in Penetrating Ureteral Trauma

Reference	Delayed	Immediate	Intraoperative (%)[a]
Liroff (1977) *(21)*	0	20	9 (45)
Pitts (1981) *(19)*	3	15	7 (38.9)
Franco (1988) *(24)*	2	19	11 (52.4)
Presti (1989) *(12)*	2	14	12 (75)
Rober (1990) *(20)*	0	16	8 (50)
Brandes (1994) *(14)*	1	11	11 (91.7)
Azimuddin (1998) *(15)*	1	20	20 (95.2)
DiGiacomo (2001) *(32)*	0	23	23 (100)
Total	9 (6.1%)	138 (93.9%)	101 (68%)

[a]Represents percentage of the total injuries.

Table 6
Injury Recognition in Surgical Ureteral Trauma

Reference	Delayed	Immediate
Ihse (1975) *(2)*	31	11
Dowling (1986) *(4)*	23	4
Daly (1988) *(5)*	8	8
Selzman (1996) *(8)*	80	85[a]
Total	142 (56.8%)	108 (43.2%)

[a]Composed primarily of urological injuries.

Overall, more than 90% of ureteral injuries from external trauma are identified immediately (defined as during the first 24-h period) *(11,15,16,18,24,25,32)*, whereas less than half of surgical ureteral injuries are identified immediately (Tables 5 and 6) *(4,5,8)*. Laparoscopic injuries result in the highest incidence of delay *(33,34)*. This can be ascribed to the mechanism of these injuries, usually by electrocoagulation or ligation, which can lead to delayed tissue necrosis and consequent delayed recognition.

Radiographic

Initial urinary tract imaging can be obtained in the resuscitation suite with computed tomography (CT) of the abdomen and pelvis or a complete high-dose (2-mL contrast/kg body weight) intravenous urogram (IVU). Contrast extravasation is the *sine qua non* of any ureteral injury. On IVU, the findings are often subtle, including delayed function or mild ureteral dilation or deviation. The most consistent CT finding in an upper ureteral transection or UPJ avulsion is extravasation of contrast confined predominantly to the medial perirenal space; urinary ascites is a less-frequent presentation *(35,36)*.

Table 7
Organ Injury Scale for Ureteral Injuries

AAST grade	Ureteral injury
I	Contusion or hematoma without devascularization
II	<50% transection
III	≥50% transection
IV	Complete transection with >2 cm devascularization
V	Avulsion with >2 cm devascularization

AAST, American Association for the Surgery of Trauma. (From ref. *38*.)

In addition, on *delayed* CT images, with a complete ureteral injury there is absence of distal ureteral opacification. When rapid-sequence spiral CT is used, this lack of distal ureteral filling cannot be accurately evaluated unless delayed films are explicitly requested *(37,38)*. Typically, a repeat CT scan should be performed 15 to 20 min after the initial study to assess ureteral filling. If the results of the CT and IVU are inconclusive, a retrograde ureterogram may be performed. Although it is the most accurate ureteral imaging study, it is often impractical in the acute trauma setting.

A one-shot IVU is unreliable and nondiagnostic for ureteral injuries. The role of ultrasonography is limited in the acute setting, with insufficient data available.

Intraoperative

Direct visual inspection is the most reliable method of assessing ureteral integrity. The bowel should be reflected sufficiently to expose the ureter(s) and an attempt made at tracing the missile's path. Urinary extravasation, ureteral discoloration or bruising, and lack of bleeding are indicative of ureteral trauma; decreased peristalsis is a more subtle finding. Intraoperative recognition can be facilitated by the intravenous or intraureteral injection of indigo carmine or methylene blue. This should be used as a last step in the intraoperative evaluation of the ureter as the bluish dye somewhat obscures the surgical field.

INJURY CLASSIFICATION

Ureteral injuries are classified according to the organ injury scaling system of the committee of the American Association for the Surgery of Trauma (Table 7) *(39)*.

ANATOMIC CONSIDERATIONS

The ureter is a thick-walled, narrow tube measuring approx 25 to 30 cm long and varying in diameter from 1 to 10 mm. It has three distinct layers: an outer adventitial sheath, through which the vessels course; a medial layer made of longitudinal and circular smooth muscle fibers; and an inner mucosal lining consisting of transitional epithelium. The ureter derives its blood supply from an anastomotic network, within the adventitia, arising from multiple vessels. The upper ureter receives its blood supply mainly from the renal arteries, its midportion receives it from the aorta and iliac arteries, and the lower segment receives it from the superior and inferior vesical, middle hemorrhoidal, and uterine arteries.

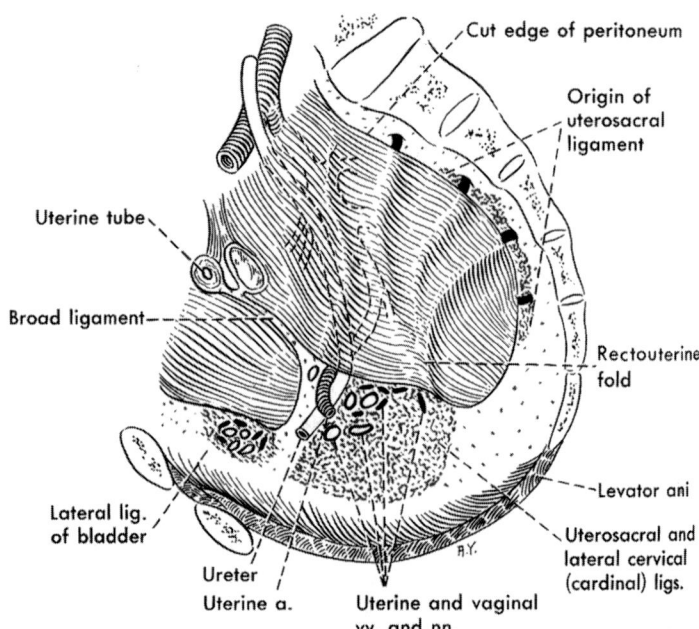

Fig. 1. Female pelvic ureteral anatomy.

The vessels to the upper two-thirds and lower third of the ureter emanate medially and laterally, respectively. Because these vascular sources can be variable, ureteral dissection always should be performed cautiously to avoid inadvertent devascularization. Additional obstacles that need to be recognized include ureteral anomalies, which may alter its course (retrocaval, ectopic), size (megaureter, diverticulum), or number (duplication).

In the female, the pelvic portion of the ureter courses posterior to the infundibular pelvic ligament and then passes anteromedially at the base of broad ligament, lateral to the uterosacral ligament. At this level, it is crossed anterosuperiorly by the uterine artery; this occurs 1.5 cm lateral to the uterus, but can vary markedly when pathological conditions have distorted the anatomic relationships. The uterine artery then runs medially to ascend alongside the uterus. The ureter continues distally, coursing medially and then passing anterior to the vagina prior to traversing the bladder wall obliquely (Fig. 1) *(40)*.

MANAGEMENT CONSIDERATIONS

Selection

Selection of the appropriate management depends on the patient's condition (including the associated organ injuries), promptness in injury recognition, and location and grade of the ureteral injury. Most patients with external ureteral injuries require prompt operative exploration for management of their associated abdominal injuries. If suspected intraoperatively, the injured ureter should be carefully inspected for evidence of ischemia. Concomitant intraabdominal organ or vascular injuries should not preclude ureteral reconstruction in an otherwise stable patient *(15,41,42)*. In these cases, the appropriate reconstructive procedure can be safely performed and an omental flap interposed to protect the repair.

Temporary Urinary Diversion

Ureteral injuries with a significant delay in diagnosis or in an unstable patient are best managed initially by percutaneous nephrostomy drainage or endoscopic ureteral stenting. Percutaneous nephrostomy placement is safer and more universally applicable, whereas retrograde ureteral stenting should be attempted only for certain low-grade injuries. For select grade I–III surgical injuries, these minimally invasive techniques alone may be therapeutic *(7,8,43)*. Similarly, grade I external ureteral injuries can be successfully managed in this way.

In an intraoperative situation in which a high-grade ureteral injury is identified but the patient's precarious condition does not permit immediate ureteral reconstruction, ureteral ligation with placement of a percutaneous nephrostomy tube serves as an expedient "bail-out" procedure. Open nephrostomy should not be used because this is more invasive and consumes precious operating time, further jeopardizing patient outcome. The goal in this setting is to ensure hemodynamic and metabolic homeostasis prior to addressing the ureteral injury.

Most high-grade injuries will eventually require reconstruction. This should be deferred until the patient has healed from any associated injuries and the acute periureteral inflammatory response has resolved. The appropriate procedure should be planned only after compiling the necessary functional and anatomic radiographic information. Besides antegrade or retrograde ureteral imaging, a cystogram should always be obtained when the bladder is under consideration for the reconstructive procedure.

Incisions

With external trauma, the ureter is explored through a midline transperitoneal incision as part of the laparotomy. Surgical injuries identified intraoperatively can be repaired through the original incision, which may be extended as needed to optimize exposure. With planned ureteral reconstruction, the incision can be tailored to the specific procedure. In general, a midline abdominal incision allows complete exposure of the ureter and bladder. Alternatively, select proximal or distal ureteral injuries can be exposed through a subcostal or a Gibson incision, respectively.

SURGICAL TECHNIQUES

General principles of ureteral reconstruction *(44)* include careful debridement, creation of a watertight, tension-free, spatulated anastomosis; isolation of the anastomosis from associated injuries; and adequate ureteral and retroperitoneal drainage. Minimal handling of the adventitia and careful periureteral dissection are paramount in preserving ureteral vasculature. The appropriate reconstructive procedure should be performed based on the location and grade of the ureteral injury (Fig. 2). A description of the various techniques follows.

Disligation

Select surgical injuries that are identified intraoperatively and felt to be simply caused by inadvertent ureteral ligation can be managed by disligation. Once this is done, the ureter must be observed carefully for any signs of devascularization and, at least, stented. If there is any suggestion of irreversible ischemia, the appropriate reconstructive procedure should be performed.

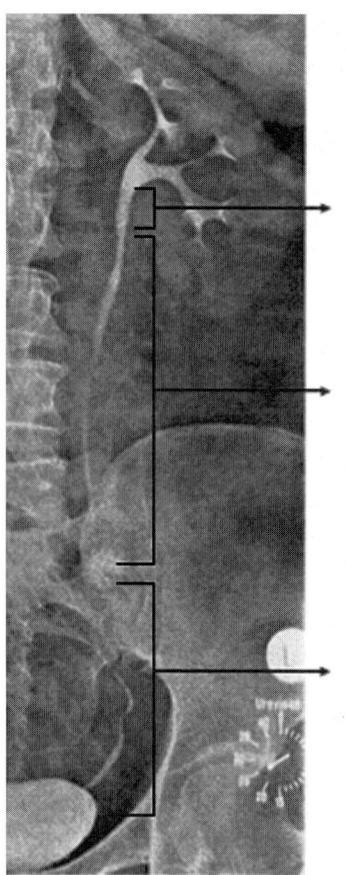

Ureteropelvic Junction (UPJ)
Reanastamosis

Proximal and Mid Ureter
Short defects: end-end anastamosis
Long defects: vesico-psoas hitch, Boari flap or Transureteroureterostomy (TUU)

Distal Ureter
Short defects: reimplantation
Long defects: vesico-psoas hitch or Boari flap reimplantation

Fig. 2. Reconstructive techniques by injury location.

Primary Closure

This technique has limited use for external ureteral injuries. Occasionally, it can be considered in the management of grade II stab wounds. It should never be used for gunshot wounds as these injuries require careful debridement to avoid delayed tissue breakdown as a consequence of the underestimated thermal damage created by the missile's cavitation. Select grade II or III clean surgical ureteral lacerations, when identified promptly, can be managed by primary closure.

Interrupted fine absorbable sutures are used to reapproximate the ureter carefully, and a ureteral stent is placed to protect the repair. Care is taken to avoid inadvertent narrowing of the suture line.

Reimplantation

Injuries to the distal lower third of the ureter are best managed by submucosal bladder reimplantation. This is done using a combined intra- and extravesical approach, bringing the ureter through the posterior bladder wall just medial to the original hiatus. A submucosal tunnel is created based on the standard 3:1 ratio (tunnel length:ureteral diameter). The distal ureter is then spatulated and secured to the bladder wall with interrupted fine absorbable sutures. The repair is stented, and the bladder closed in two layers. Attention to adequate ureteral mobilization without excessive adventitial dissection or ureteral kinking will limit potential postoperative problems, including reflux, obstruction, and extravasation.

Psoas Hitch

Injuries involving the entire lower third of the ureter are best managed by a psoas hitch in conjunction with ureteral reimplantation. Preoperative cystography is helpful in ensuring normal bladder capacity.

The proximal ureteral end is debrided, and a traction suture is placed distally to facilitate handling. The bladder fundus is mobilized by dissecting it away from the peritoneal reflection. The contralateral superior vesical pedicle is ligated; when needed, bilateral superior pedicle ligation affords improved bladder mobilization. An oblique anterior cystotomy is then made perpendicular to the involved ureter. Using the index and middle fingers, the bladder dome is guided over the ipsilateral iliac vessels toward the psoas tendon and anchored to this with three interrupted sutures. Care is taken to avoid entrapping the genitofemoral nerve. The ureter is then reimplanted, as previously described in the section on reimplantation, and the bladder wall is closed perpendicular to the cystotomy, in two layers, leaving a suprapubic tube for drainage. Occasionally, *de novo* detrusor instability can occur.

Anterior Bladder Wall Flap

Injuries encompassing the entire lower two-thirds of the ureter are best managed with an anterior bladder wall flap in conjunction with a psoas hitch. This procedure should not be used in patients with prior pelvic irradiation or neurogenic bladder disease.

The bladder is mobilized as described in the section on psoas hitch, and a full-thickness U incision is made in its anterior wall; for longer defects, additional length can be obtained using an L configuration. The width of the flap should be approximately three to four times the ureteral diameter, maintaining a wider base to ensure an adequate blood supply. The flap is raised toward the involved ureter, and the bladder wall is hitched to the psoas tendon. The ureter is reimplanted submucosally into the flap, which is then closed in a tubular configuration. Bladder closure is completed as described in the section on psoas hitch. Accurate flap dissection with maintenance of a wide base can minimize flap complications and avoid significantly decreasing bladder capacity.

Using this technique, ureteral defects of up to 15 cm can be easily bridged. The ureteral defect can be further decreased by up to 3 to 4 cm by performing a reverse nephropexy. Dissecting the kidney away from Gerota's fascia and fixing the renal capsule caudally to the underlying retroperitoneal muscles accomplishes this. Extensive dissection or tension can result in renal hemorrhage or vascular injury, respectively.

Ureteroureterostomy

Most grade II–IV lacerations involving the middle or upper third of the ureter can be best managed by primary ureteroureterostomy. The ureteral ends are carefully dissected and debrided to viable tissue. Each end is spatulated on opposite sides, and a watertight, tension-free anastomosis is fashioned over a ureteral stent using fine absorbable sutures. Optical loop magnification is helpful in achieving optimal suture placement. Maintaining ureteral vascularity minimizes postoperative stricture and fistula formation.

With concomitant intraabdominal organ injury, the greater omentum can be used to exclude the ureter and protect the repair. This is dissected from the greater curvature of the stomach and sustained on either the right or the left gastroepiploic vessels. The short gastric vessels are then divided, and the flap is transferred retroperitoneally and wrapped around the ureteral anastomosis, isolating it from the abdominal contents.

Transureteroureterostomy/Transureteropyelostomy

Alternatively, injuries involving the distal two-thirds of the ureter with insufficient bladder capacity or severe pelvic scarring can be managed by transureteroureterostomy. The posterior peritoneum is incised, exposing both ureters. The diseased ureter is brought through a retroperitoneal window carefully, avoiding any angulation. A 1.5-cm longitudinal ureterotomy is made on the medial surface of the recipient ureter, and an end-to-side anastomosis is created with interrupted fine absorbable sutures. The donor ureter should course above the inferior mesenteric artery to avoid inadvertent ureteral impingement. For more extensive injuries, a transureteropyelostomy can be performed by anastomosing the involved ureter to the medial aspect of the contralateral renal pelvis.

These procedures can potentially jeopardize the integrity of the normal ureter or pelvis and should be used selectively. In addition, they are contraindicated in patients with upper tract transitional cell carcinoma or recurrent urolithiasis.

Ureterocalycostomy

An ureterocalycostomy can be used for extensive injuries to the ureteropelvic junction and proximal ureter. The lower pole of the involved kidney is amputated, exposing the infundibulum of the inferior calyx. The ureter is generously spatulated, allowing a direct end-to-end ureterocalyceal anastomosis over an internal stent.

This procedure should be used as a last resort because it involves excessive renal dissection and is fraught with a high incidence of anastomotic stricture.

Ileal Interposition

For complete ureteral avulsion, a segment of ileum may be interposed as a ureteral substitute. This cannot be done acutely because it requires a standard mechanical and antibiotic bowel preparation. Moreover, it should be used exclusively in patients with relatively normal renal function (serum creatinine <2.5 mg/dL).

A 20- to 25-cm segment of ileum is chosen 15 cm proximal to the ileocecal junction. The bowel mesentery is divided, maintaining vascular integrity, and the appropriate segment of ileum is resected using a linear anastomotic stapler. Bowel continuity is resumed by creating a stapled functional end-to-end enteric anastomosis; the mesenteric window is closed to prevent internal visceral herniation. The ileal neoureter is then positioned posteriorly in an isoperistaltic fashion. An end-to-end pyeloileal anastomosis is completed using a nephrostomy to maintain a low-pressure system during healing. Distally, the ileal segment is anastomosed to the bladder dome without tunneling. This can be accomplished by opening the bladder anteriorly in the midline and completing the end-to-side ileovesical anastomosis using a combined intra- and extravesical approach. Although bacteriuria and vesicoileal reflux are common, they have not been shown to have a deleterious effect on renal function *(45–47)*. In addition, the ileum can be tapered to decrease its absorptive surface area, potentially limiting the incidence of metabolic derangements arising from urinary absorption. Because it is an infrequent occurrence, this maneuver may be superfluous.

For extensive bilateral ureteral injuries, a segment of ileum can be tailored as a conduit for both kidneys. This can be used alone or in conjunction with a psoas hitch or anterior bladder wall flap to minimize the segment of ileum used. Alternatively, in select grade V ureteral injuries for which the urinary tract cannot be used for reconstruction, partial ureteral replacement can be achieved using a shorter segment of ileum.

Potential long-term complications of ileal interposition include hyperabsorption of electrolytes, which is manifested by hyperchloremic metabolic acidosis. Patients who are symptomatic should be treated with oral alkalizing agents. Other postoperative problems include anastomotic leaks, obstruction, prolonged mucus formation, recurrent infection, and ischemic ileal necrosis.

Renal Autotransplantation

In patients with a solitary kidney or compromised renal function, complete ureteral avulsions can be managed by renal autotransplantation. The affected kidney is transplanted into the iliac fossa with vascular anastomoses of the renal and iliac vessels; urinary continuity is restored with a pyelovesicostomy. Although this is a more formidable surgical procedure that requires comfort with vascular techniques, it can achieve excellent long-term preservation of renal function *(48)*.

DRAINAGE ISSUES

All ureteral injuries should be stented to maximize urinary diversion. An internal double-J or exteriorized pediatric feeding or single-J tube can be used for this purpose. A retroperitoneal drain should be placed at the site of reconstruction to limit urinoma formation. A passive drain (e.g., penrose) is preferable because suction drains can prolong leakage by exerting negative pressure on the suture line. The bladder should be decompressed using a transurethral Foley catheter or a suprapubic Malecot tube, alone or in combination. Both tubes are usually used when the bladder has been opened, although in female patients, the suprapubic tube may be foregone. The retroperitoneal drain is maintained for at least 48 h or until urinary extravasation subsides. The bladder catheter is removed in 2 to 7 d, depending on the type of ureteral repair and the extent of bladder dissection. The ureteral stent usually is maintained for 4 to 6 wk.

POSTOPERATIVE EVALUATION

Once the patient is tube free, ureteral patency and renal function are evaluated using CT, IVU, or radionuclide scanning. This should be repeated at 3 and 6 mo to ensure proper healing. In addition, after ileal interposition periodic assessment of blood chemistries is essential to identify any potential metabolic complications.

COMPLICATIONS

Complications of ureteral injuries include prolonged urinary extravasation, infection, urinoma, fistula, and stricture. Progressive renal failure with acidosis and upper urinary tract decompensation can complicate a failed repair. Complications specific to each reconstructive procedure are discussed in the Surgical Techniques section.

SUMMARY

With surgical ureteral injuries, prevention is the goal. An understanding of ureteral anatomy and location at all times during abdominal or pelvic surgery is paramount to avoid inadvertent injury to the ureter. When a ureteral injury is suspected, vigilant intraoperative inspection and immediate implementation of corrective measures will minimize complications. With all ureteral injuries, the clinical and radiographic evaluations are often indeterminate; consequently, maintaining a high index of suspicion is paramount in making the diagnosis promptly. A delay in diagnosis is the most important contributory factor in morbidity related to ureteral injury. The decision when to repair the ureteral injury is based on the patient's overall condition and associated organ injuries, promptness of injury recognition, and type of ureteral injury. In an unstable patient, restoring hemodynamic and metabolic stability takes precedence over definitive ureteral repair. Successful surgical management, whether performed immediately or in a delayed fashion, requires familiarity with the broad reconstructive armamentarium, as well as meticulous attention to the specific details of each procedure. Adhering to these diagnostic and therapeutic principles will serve to minimize complications and maximize renal preservation in patients who sustain ureteral injuries.

REFERENCES

1. Higgins CC. Ureteral injuries during surgery. JAMA 1967; 199: 82.
2. Ihse I, Arnesjö B, Jönsson G. Surgical injuries of the ureter. Scand J Urol Nephrol 1975; 9: 39.
3. Gangai MP, Agee RE, Spence CR. Surgical injury to the ureter. Urology 1976; 8: 22.
4. Dowling RA, Corriere JN, Sandler CM. Iatrogenic ureteral injury. J Urol 1986; 135: 912.
5. Daly JW, Higgins KA. Injury to the ureter during gynecologic surgical procedures. Gynecol Obstet 1988; 167: 19.
6. St. Lezin MA, Stoller ML. Surgical ureteral injuries. Urology 1991; 38: 497.
7. Assimos DG, Patterson LC, Taylor CL. Changing incidence and etiology of iatrogenic ureteral injuries. J Urol 1994; 152: 2240.
8. Selzman AA, Spirnak JP. Iatrogenic ureteral injuries: a 20-year experience in treating 165 injuries. J Urol 1996; 155: 878.
9. Fried FA, Rutledge R. A statewide, population-based analysis of the frequency and outcome of genitourinary injury in a series of 215,220 trauma patients. J Urol 1995; 153: 314A.
10. Carlton CE Jr, Scott R Jr, Guthrie AG. The initial management of ureteral injuries: a report of 78 cases. J Urol 1971; 105: 335.
11. Bright TC, Peters PC. Ureteral injuries due to external violence: 10 years' experience with 59 cases. J Trauma 1977; 17: 616.
12. Presti JC Jr, Carroll PR, McAninch JW. Ureteral and renal pelvic injuries from external trauma: diagnosis and management. J Trauma 1989; 29:370.
13. Campbell EW Jr, Filderman PS, Jacobs SC. Ureteral injury due to blunt penetrating trauma. Urology 1992; 40: 216.
14. Brandes SB, Chelsky MJ, Buckman RF, Hanno PM. Ureteral injuries from penetrating trauma. J Trauma 1994; 36: 766.
15. Azimuddin K, Milanesa D, Ivatury R, Porter J, Ehrenpreis M, Allman DB. Penetrating ureteric injuries. Injury 1998; 29: 363.
16. Albert DJ, Banks DE, Persky L. Civilian ureteral gunshot injuries. Ohio State Med J 1970; 66: 479.
17. Eickenberg H, Amin M. Gunshot wounds to the ureter. J Trauma 1976; 16: 562.
18. Holden S, Hicks CC, O'Brien DP, Stone HH, Walker JA, Walton KN. Gunshot wounds of the ureter: a 15 year review of 63 consecutive cases. J Urol 1976; 116: 562.
19. Pitts JC, Peterson NE. Penetrating injuries of the ureter. J Trauma 1981; 21: 978.
20. Rober PE, Smith JB, Pierce JM Jr. Gunshot injuries of the ureter. J Trauma 1990; 30: 83.
21. Liroff SA, Pontes JES, Pierce JM Jr. Gunshot wounds of the ureter: 5 years of experience. J Urol 1977; 118: 551.
22. Perez-Brayfield MR, Keane TE, Krishnan A, Lafontaine P, Feliciano DV, Clarke HS. Gunshot wounds to the ureter: a 40-year experience at Grady Memorial Hospital. J Urol 2001; 166: 119.

23. Evans RA, Smith MJV. Violent injuries of the upper ureter. J Trauma 1976; 16: 558.
24. Franco I, Eshghi M, Schutte H, et al. Value of proximal diversion and ureteral stenting in management of penetrating ureteral trauma. Urology 1988; 32: 99.
25. Ghali AMA, El Malik EMA, Ibrahim AIA, Ismail G, Rashid M. Ureteric injuries: diagnosis, management and outcome. J Trauma 1999; 46: 150.
26. Laberge I, Homsy YL, Dadour G, Beland G. Avulsion of ureter by blunt trauma. Urology 1979; 13: 172.
27. Giyanani VL, Gerlock AM, Grozinger KT, Venable DD, Mirfakhraee M. Trauma of occult hydronephrotic kidney. Urol 1985; 15: 8.
28. Beaumud-Gomez A, Martinez-Verduch M, Estornell-Moragues F, Olague-Ros R, Garcia-Obarra F. Rupture of the ureteropelvic junction by nonpenetrating trauma. J Pediatr Surg 1986; 21:702, 1986.
29. Boone TB, Gilling PJ, Husmann DA. Ureteropelvic junction disruption following blunt abdominal trauma. J Urol 1993; 150: 33.
30. Kawashima A, Sandler CM, Corriere JN, Rogers BM, Goldman SM. Ureteropelvic junction injuries secondary to blunt abdominal trauma. Radiology 1997; 205: 487.
31. Kattan S. Traumatic pelvic-ureteric junction disruption. How can we avoid delayed diagnosis? Injury Int J Care Injured 2001; 32: 797.
32. DiGiacomo JC, Frankel H, Rotondo MF, Schwab CW, Shaftan GW. Preoperative radiographic staging for ureteral injuries is not warranted in patients undergoing celiotomy for trauma. Am Surg 2001; 67: 969.
33. Grainger DA, Soderstrom RM, Schiff SF, Glickman MG, DeCherney AH, Diamond MP. Ureteral injuries at laparoscopy: Insights into diagnosis, management, and prevention. Obstet Gynecol 1990; 75: 839.
34. Oh BR, Kwon DD, Park KW, Ryu SB, Park YI, Presti JC. Late presentation of ureteral injury after laparoscopic surgery. Obstet Gynecol 2000; 95: 337.
35. Kenney PJ, Panicek DM, Witanowski LS. Computed tomography of ureteral disruption. J Comput Assist Tomogr 1987; 11: 480.
36. Gayer G, Zissin R, Apter S, et al. Urinomas caused by ureteral injuries: CT appearance. Abd Imag 2002; 27: 88.
37. Mulligan JM, Cagiannos I, Collins JP, Millward SF. Ureteropelvic junction disruption secondary to blunt trauma: excretory phase imaging (delayed films) should help prevent a missed diagnosis. J Urol 1998; 159: 67.
38. Brown SL, Hoffman DM, Spirnak JP. Limitations of routine spiral computerized tomography in the evaluation of blunt renal trauma. J Urol 1998; 160: 1979.
39. Moore EE, Cogvill TH, Jurkovich GJ, et al. Organ injury scaling III: chest wall, abdominal vascular, ureter, bladder and urethra. J Trauma 1992; 33: 337.
40. The pelvis and perineum. In Hollinshead's Textbook of Anatomy, 5th ed. (Rosse C, Gaddum-Rosse P, eds.), Lippincott Raven, Philadelphia, 1997, 1985, pp. 639–701.
41. Spirnak JP, Hampel N, Resnick MI. Ureteral injuries complicating vascular surgery: is repair indicated? J Urol 1989; 141: 13.
42. Blasco FJ, Saladie JM. Ureteral obstruction and ureteral fistulas after aortofemoral or aortoiliac bypass surgery. J Urol 1991; 145: 237.
43. Lask D, Abarbanel J, Luttwak Z, Manes A, Mukamel E. Changing trends in the management of iatrogenic ureteral injuries. J Urol 1995; 154: 1693.
44. Armenakas NA. Ureteral trauma: surgical repair. Atlas Urol Clin North Am 1998; 6: 71.
45. Boxer RJ, Fritzsche P, Skinner DG, et al. Replacement of the ureter by small intestine: clinical application and results of the ileal ureter in 89 patients. J Urol 1979; 121: 728.
46. Bejany DE, Lockhart JL, Politano VA. Ileal segment for ureteral substitution or for improvement of ureteral function. J Urol 1991; 146: 302.
47. Verduyckt FJH, Heesakkers JPFA, Debruyne FMJ. Long-term results of ileum interposition for ureteral obstruction. Eur Urol 2002; 42: 181.
48. Bodie B, Novick AC, Rose M, Straffon RA. Long-term results with renal autotransplantation for ureteral replacement. J Urol 1986; 136: 1187.

3 Bladder Trauma

Steven B. Brandes, MD and Jay S. Belani, MD

CONTENTS
- INCIDENCE
- ANATOMY
- MECHANISM OF INJURY
- SIGNS AND SYMPTOMS
- ASSOCIATED INJURIES
- EVALUATION
- CLASSIFICATION
- MANAGEMENT
- IATROGENIC INJURIES
- AUGMENTATION CYSTOPLASTY RUPTURE
- NEOBLADDER RUPTURE
- COMPLICATIONS OF BLADDER TRAUMA
- SUMMARY
- REFERENCES

INCIDENCE

Of trauma visits to the emergency room (ER), injury to the urinary bladder is not a common occurrence. Major bladder trauma accounts for fewer than 2% of injuries requiring surgical exploration. Mortality can be as high as 22% because of associated multiple organ injuries rather than the extent of bladder injury *(1)*. Overall, roughly 60% of injuries are extraperitoneal, 30% are intraperitoneal, and 10% occur concomitantly *(2)*.

Blunt external trauma accounts, either from a direct blow to the abdomen or because of shearing forces, for the majority of bladder injuries presenting through the ER. The most common cause of penetrating bladder injury is iatrogenic. Most of these injuries occur as a result of surgery, with the greatest incidence from pelvic surgery. Injury can also occur (although rare) as a result of migration and erosion of foreign bodies, such as surgical drains, intrauterine devices, or long-term Foley catheters *(3)*. Of ER visits, in the civilian population, penetrating trauma accounts for about 14 to 33% of bladder rupture, usually as a result of gunshot wounds (GSWs) or stab wounds from sharp objects *(1)*.

From: *Urological Emergencies: A Practical Guide*
Edited by: H. Wessells and J. W. McAninch © Humana Press Inc., Totowa, NJ

ANATOMY

In adults, the bladder is an extraperitoneal organ well protected deep within the retropubic space and surrounded by the pelvis. Its anatomic position changes with its extent of distention. An empty bladder is bounded superiorly by the peritoneum, which passes into the median umbilical ligament. Inferolaterally, it is bounded by the pelvic floor fascia, levator ani musculature, and pelvic wall. Posteriorly, in males, it is bounded by Denonvillier's fascia and the rectum. In females, it is closely related to the anterior wall of the vagina. Last, at the neck of the bladder (where it opens to the prostate in males), it is bounded anteriorly by the pubic symphysis and held in place by the puboprostatic ligaments *(3)*.

As the bladder fills, the dome exits the protective confines of the retropubic space and rises to become an intraperitoneal organ. On overfilling, it can even reach the level of the umbilicus. If the bladder is full at the time of rupture, it is more likely to result in an intraperitoneal injury; an extraperitoneal injury is more likely when the bladder is empty. In children, however, the bladder is largely an intraperitoneal organ and is more vulnerable to trauma. As the child grows, the pelvis enlarges, protecting the bladder from injury *(3)*.

MECHANISM OF INJURY

Blunt injury to the bladder can result from sudden deceleration in a high-speed motor vehicle crash or from an external blow to the lower abdomen. Seat belts can cause injury to a full bladder during a motor vehicle crash *(4)*. Penetrating trauma can occur as a result of GSW or stab wound to the bladder. Intraperitoneal bladder rupture occurs in a fully distended bladder because the sudden increase in intravesical pressure from blunt lower abdominal trauma results in injury to its weakest portion, the dome. The dome of the bladder is protected only by the peritoneal reflection; the rest of the bladder is secured by ligamentous attachments. These injuries are usually several centimeters long, and an empty bladder is usually not injured in this way *(2)* (Fig. 1). There may be multiple sites of injury, and the extent of extravasation on cystography does not usually correlate with the extent of bladder injury.

In contrast, extraperitoneal bladder injuries are nearly always associated with pelvic fracture. Injuries are commonly anterolateral and near the bladder base and primarily felt because of shearing or bursting forces and to a lesser degree because of perforation by bony spicules. There are varying older studies that concluded that the main mechanism of extraperitoneal bladder injury from blunt trauma is laceration from a bony fragment because the site of most (up to 76%) of the bladder injuries were proxal to the fracture site *(5,6)*.

In contrast, contemporary series have demonstrated rather that most bladder ruptures occur away from the pelvic fracture as a result of a bursting-type injury or shearing force from the disruption of the ligamentous attachments of the bladder to the pelvis *(1,7)*. Carrol and McAninch reported that 63% of blunt injuries occurred in the dome or sidewall, 20% at the anterior or posterior bladder, and only 14% proximal to the pelvic fracture (near the bladder neck) *(1)*. Moreover, other contemporary series also reported that most areas of extravasation on cystogram were away from the site of pelvic fracture, and on exploration, bony spicules were never found at the site of bladder injury *(7)*.

Extravasated urine is confined to the pelvis when the urogenital diaphragm is intact. When the superior fascia of the urogenital diaphragm (which is contiguous with Dartos,

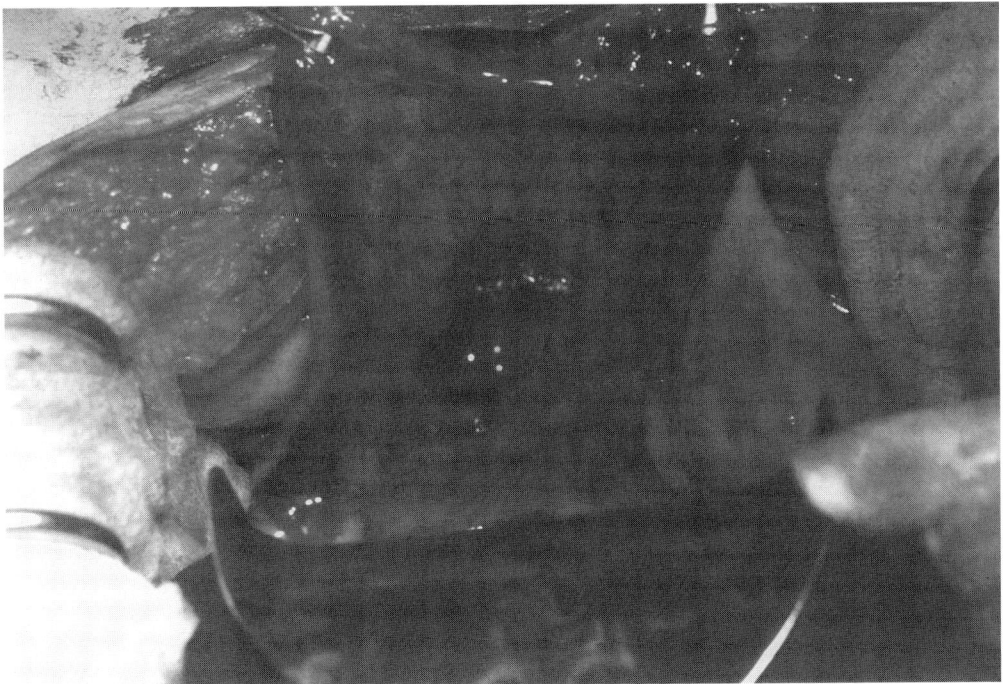

Fig. 1. Intaperitoneal bladder rupture at the dome caused by external trauma to a full bladder. Note the laceration is long, nearly 10 cm.

Colles', and Scarpa's fasciae) is ruptured, urine can infiltrate the scrotum, perineum, and abdominal wall. When the inferior fascia is disrupted, urine can also infiltrate the penis or thigh *(8)*.

SIGNS AND SYMPTOMS

All patients who present with lower abdomen trauma, whether blunt or penetrating, are at risk for bladder injury. Symptoms are typically nonspecific. Patients commonly complain of pelvic or lower abdominal pain and inability to void. On physical examination, the patients may have lower abdominal bruising or tenderness over the suprapubic (SP) region or pubic symphysis. Other signs of potential bladder injury are a distended abdomen, absent bowel sounds (secondary to an intraperitoneal bladder rupture and urinary ascites), or low urine output. Women with bladder rupture should undergo careful vaginal (pelvic) examination to assess for concomitant vaginal or urethral lacerations or palpable bony spicules. Gross blood in the vaginal vault suggests such injury and warrants a thorough examination. A rectal examination is essential to assess for rectal tone (loss of tone suggests spinal cord injury), blood in the rectal vault (suggesting rectal laceration), palpable bony spicule, or a "high-riding" or nonpalpable prostate (suggesting urethral injury). The associated large pelvic hematoma, however, often makes rectal landmarks indistinct and the prostate difficult to palpate.

The hallmark of bladder injury is hematuria. Gross hematuria is found in more than 95% of blunt bladder ruptures, and the remaining 5% have microscopic hematuria *(1,9)*. In contrast, one-half of penetrating bladder injuries present with microscopic hematuria, and the other half present with gross hematuria. A concomitant pelvic fracture injury may be the sole manifestation of a bladder injury. Pelvic disruption is associated with about 90% of bladder ruptures, but only 9 to 16% of pelvic fractures have a concomitant bladder rupture *(2,8)*. There is usually no association between the type of pelvic fracture and type of bladder injury *(7)*.

Bladder ruptures that are initially missed and diagnosed late often present with the signs of elevated levels of serum blood urea nitrogen or creatinine, hyperchloremic metabolic acidosis, hypernatremia, or hyperkalemia or on physical exam as abdominal distention, hypoactive bowel sounds, or prolonged ileus *(10)*.

ASSOCIATED INJURIES

Bladder injuries from external blunt trauma are rarely isolated, with 94 to 97% with associated injuries, mainly pelvic and long-bone fractures and head/spinal and visceral injuries. Mortality rates are high (16–53%), primarily caused by severe pelvic fracture and hemorrhage and late multisystem organ failure. In 10% and less than 2% of bladder ruptures, male urethral and renal injuries occur, respectively. Most urethral injuries are type III posterior injuries. In women with a bladder injury or pelvic fracture, a thorough pelvic exam is important to determine any concomitant vaginal or urethral laceration. When GSWs cause bladder rupture, more than 80% of the individuals have associated visceral injuries *(4)*.

EVALUATION

Imaging

Suspected bladder injury warrants conventional cystography or computed tomographic (CT) cystography. The usual indications for imaging are gross hematuria or combined pelvic fracture and microscopic hematuria. When performed properly, either imaging technique is highly sensitive and specific in identifying bladder injury *(11–13)*. In general, for reliable results, formal retrograde bladder filling with contrast is warranted. Antegrade bladder filling by Foley catheter clamping is unreliable because of inadequate bladder distention.

Conventional Cystography

A proper conventional cystogram is performed by filling the bladder with dilute contrast via a Foley catheter under gravity to at least 300 cc or until contrast extravasation (in adults) or to urgency or leakage around the catheter (in children). Films are taken before filling, when the bladder is full, and after the contrast is drained and the bladder empty. Films in at least two projections are preferred, but are often not possible because of concomitant pelvic fracture. Inadequate bladder filling is demonstrated by folds in the bladder lining. Postdrainage films are essential to avoid missing roughly 13% of injuries, especially for small extraperitoneal bladder lacerations and for penetrating bladder injuries *(11,12)*. The degree of contrast extravasation does not commonly correspond to the extent of bladder injury.

Findings on cystography that distinguish each bladder injury are as follows:
1. Bladder contusion is a bladder mucosa or muscle wall injury without loss of wall continuity. The bladder outline is commonly distorted, but there is no contrast extravasation. The diagnosis is mainly one of exclusion, with no noted associated upper tract injury

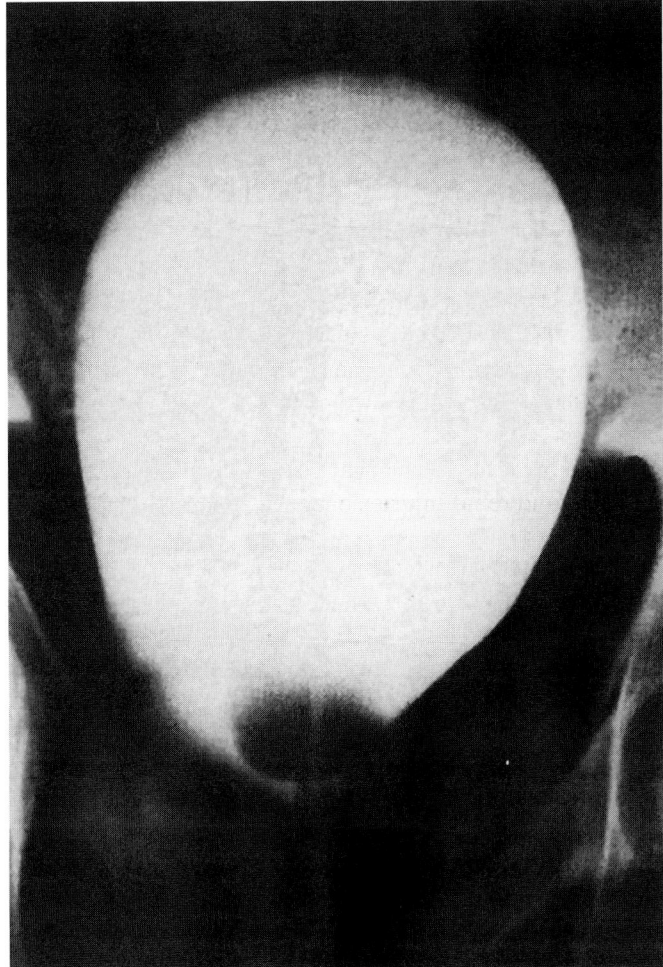

Fig. 2. Cytography demonstrating an interstitial bladder rupture. Note the distorted bladder outline at the right base, near the bladder neck, without extravasation of contrast.

   (normal abdominal CT or intravenous pyelogram) and urethral injury (normal retrograde urogram) to explain the presenting hematuria.
2. Interstitial bladder rupture is a tear of the bladder wall that is not full thickness. The bladder outline is commonly distorted, but there is no extravasation of contrast (Fig. 2).
3. Intraperitoneal bladder ruptures are distinguished by contrast extravasation, which outlines loops of bowel or fills the cul-de-sac or paracolic gutters. Such contrast is usually all above the superior margin of the acetabulum (Fig. 3).
4. Extraperitoneal bladder ruptures are characterized by flamelike or starburst contrast extravasation. Typically, such contrast extravasation is all below the superior margin of the acetabular line (Fig. 4).
5. Large pelvic hematoma typically results in "teardrop"-shaped bladder because the pelvic hematoma compresses the bladder from both sides. Aside from elongation, the bladder is lifted out of the pelvis. The degree of bladder distortion often corresponds to the severity of the pelvic hemorrhage (Fig. 5).

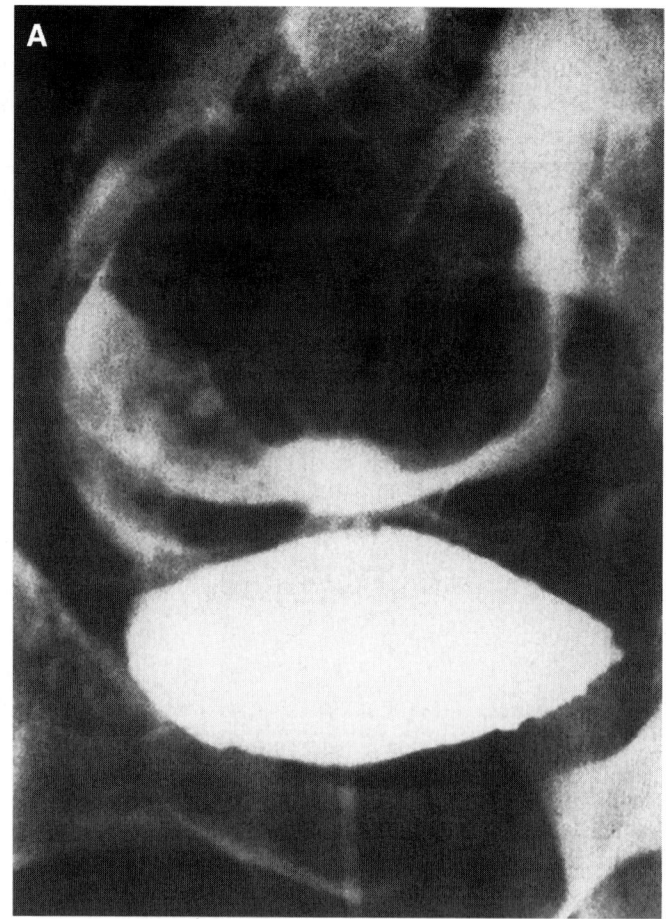

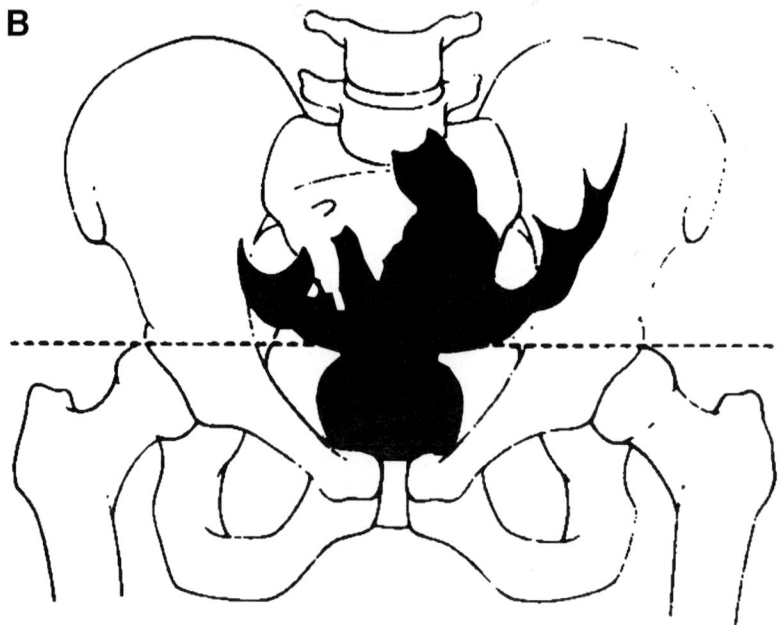

Fig. 3. (**A**) Cystography demonstrating an intraperitoneal bladder rupture by contrast extravasation outlining loops of bowel. (**B**) Illustration that intraperitoneal bladder rupture contrast extravasation is usually all above the superior margin of the acetabulum. (Reproduced with permission from ref. *37*, p. 119.)

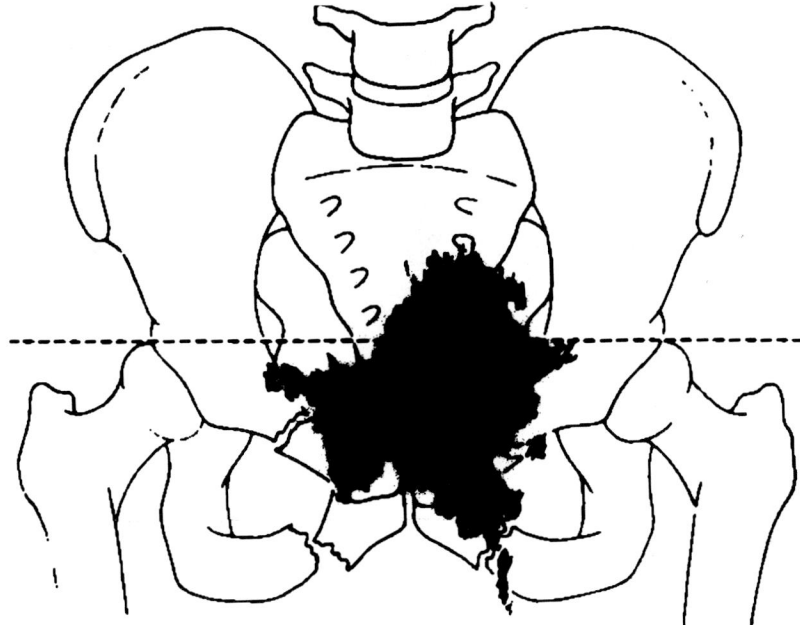

Fig. 4. Illustration of the starburst contrast extravasation pattern of extraperitoneal bladder ruptures. Note that contrast extravasation is typically below the superior margin of the acetabular line. (Reproduced with permission from ref. *37*, p. 119.)

CT CYSTOGRAPHY

Pelvic CT without contrast bladder filling is not accurate in diagnosing bladder injury *(14)*. Delayed films after intravenous contrast and Foley clamping are not adequate because the bladder may not be completely distended, thus injuries can be missed *(14)*. However, when CT cystography is performed by retrograde instillation of contrast material into the bladder via a Foley catheter, it is equally as accurate and reliable as conventional cytography. At least 300 cc of a dilute contrast material must be instilled (i.e., 50 mL of Hypaque in 450 cc of normal saline) and the catheter clamped *(15)*. Spiral pelvic CT is then performed. Postdrainage films are not needed because the CT scan can accurately image the posterior bladder when the bladder is full of contrast.

Further advantages of CT cystography over plain film cystography are that it can be combined with other CT imaging for assessing associated injuries to the head, chest, abdomen, or pelvis; has equivalent sensitivity and specificity; and can be easily be performed in 10 min, at the same time as other CT studies, which saves time and saves the patient (with a potentially unstable pelvic or spine fracture) from transfer to the fluoroscopy suite. Interpreting CT cystography is also less affected by overlying bone fragments caused by pelvic fracture, spine boards, or military antishock trousers. CT also provides more information about the surrounding pelvic structures and can more accurately assess the associated pelvic hematoma volume and extent *(13)*. Images illustrating intraperitoneal bladder injuries diagnosed by CT cystography are shown in Fig. 6.

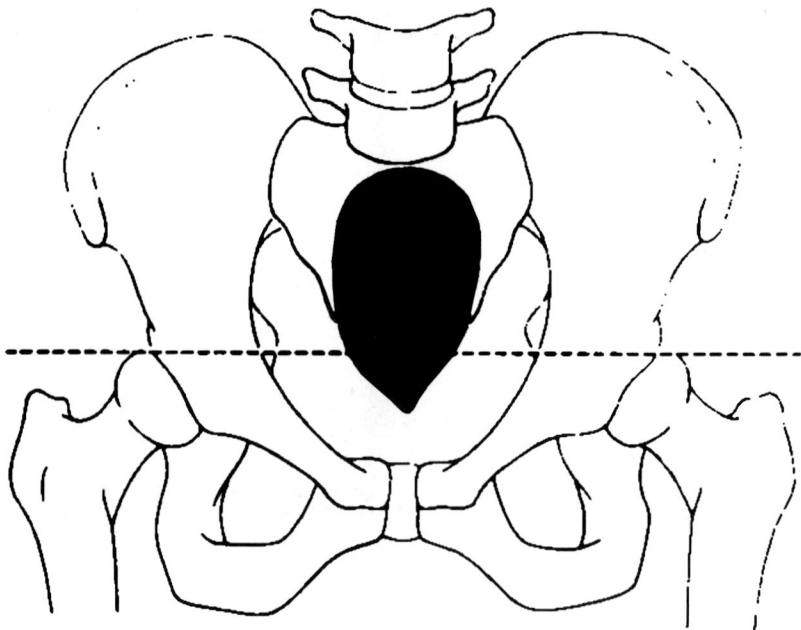

Fig. 5. Illustration of the cystographic appearance of the classic "teardrop"-shaped bladder caused by pelvic hematoma compression of the bladder from both sides. Aside from elongation, the bladder is lifted out of the pelvis.

Indications for Imaging

After a penetrating trauma to the lower abdomen, all patients should have imaging of the urinary bladder, either by CT cystogram or plain film cystogram. In cases of blunt trauma, most recommend that all patients who have gross hematuria, microscopic hematuria and pelvic fracture, or suspected bladder injury undergo cystography *(5)*. Others *(9)* have demonstrated that gross hematuria and pelvic fracture are the only absolute indication for radiographic imaging of the bladder. In general, more than 95% of blunt bladder ruptures present with gross hematuria, and about 88% present with a concomitant pelvic fracture *(10)*. Relative indications for cystography include gross hematuria without pelvic fracture, microhematuria with pelvic fracture, or isolated microhematuria. In addition, Fuhrman et al. *(16)* argued that performing cystography only in patients who have gross hematuria is safe and provides a significant cost savings. Although there are prospective reports correlating pelvic fracture type to urethral injury, no specific pelvic fracture pattern or type is associated with bladder rupture.

CLASSIFICATION

Bladder injuries can be divided into five types based on the extent of injury seen radiographically (traditionally by plain film cystography) and have been extrapolated to similar findings on CT cystogram *(17)*.

Type 1 injuries are defined as a bladder contusion. Radiographic imaging either is normal or the bladder is medially deviated because of an extravesical pelvic hematoma *(17,18)*.

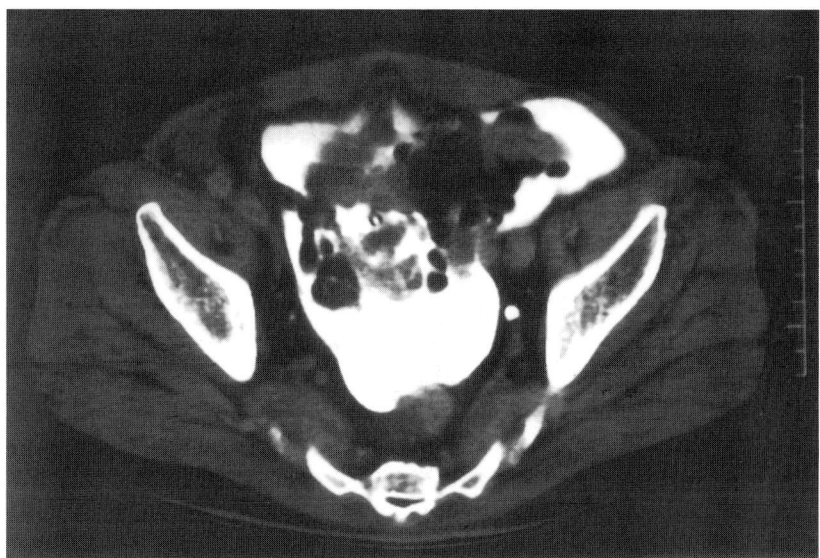
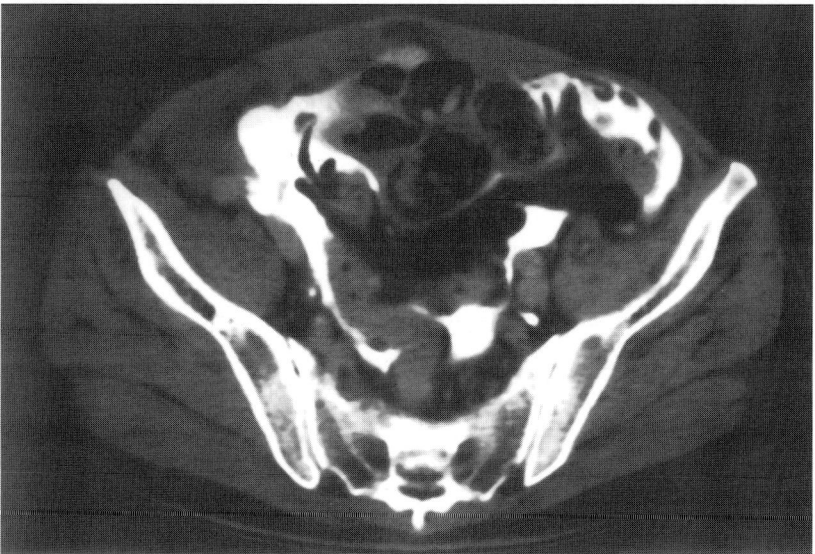

Fig. 6. Computed tomographic cystography illustrating intraperitoneal bladder laceration after a blow to the abdomen with a full bladder. Note the contrast extravasation outlining the bowel and free in the abdomen.

Type 2 injuries represent an intraperitoneal rupture. Radiographically, contrast may be seen outlining bowel loops. On CT, contrast can be seen between mesenteric folds or in the paracolic gutters *(15)*.

Type 3 injuries are defined as interstitial bladder injuries, with contrast dissecting into the bladder wall.

Type 4 injuries show an extraperitoneal bladder rupture in which contrast is seen in the perivesical space. On plain cystogram, evidence of an extraperitoneal rupture may be seen on the postdrainage films only, especially if the rupture is posterior to the bladder.

Table 1
Organ Injury Scale for Bladder Injuries

AAST Grade	Bladder injury
I	Contusion, intramural hematoma; or partial-thickness laceration
II	Extraperitoneal bladder wall laceration <2 cm
III	Extraperitoneal bladder wall laceration >2 cm or intraperitoneal bladder wall laceration <2 cm
IV	Intraperitoneal bladder wall laceration >2 cm
V	Intraperitoneal or extraperitoneal bladder wall laceration extending into bladder neck or ureteral orifice (trigone)

AAST, American Association for the Surgery of Trauma. (From ref. *19.*)

Type 5 injuries are concomitant intraperitoneal and extraperitoneal injuries. Contrast will be seen both retropubically in the prevesical space and intraperitoneally outlining loops of bowel.

The other commonly employed bladder injury grading system is the Organ Injury Scale of the American Association for the Surgery of Trauma *(19)*. The advantages of this grading system include (1) a correlation between grade and injury severity and (2) predictive value in patient outcomes (the Organ Injury Scale is used to calculate the Abbreviated Injury Scale and Injury Severity Score; *see* Table 1).

MANAGEMENT

The evaluation and treatment methods we employ for lower urinary tract trauma are summarized in Fig. 7. The size and number of intraperitoneal ruptures can only be reliably assessed by surgical exploration, not by cystography. For penetrating injuries, each missile tract should be explored, all foreign bodies and debris removed, all devitalized tissue debrided, and the cystotomy closed. In iatrogenic penetrating injuries, the entire bladder should be thoroughly inspected for more than one injury.

After formal bladder repair, the urine is diverted by Foley or SP tube. Large-bore catheters are used to facilitate bloody drainage. Reports showed that, with adequate bladder repair, complication rates are the same for either method (Foley or SP tube) of bladder drainage *(20)*. It is thus a matter of preference to place either or both. However, many orthopedic surgeons feel that SP tubes should be avoided when possible because they compromise anterior exposure for internal fixation of an associated bladder injury and may increase the rate of pelvic and hardware infection *(21)*. If both are placed, then the Foley is usually removed once the urine clears. After 10 to 14 d, the SP tube or Foley is commonly removed, after cystography.

Blunt extraperitoneal bladder injuries or interstitial ruptures that are isolated injuries can be successfully managed by Foley catheter drainage. As long as the patient has uninfected urine and appropriate catheter care, all patients with an extraperitoneal bladder injury can be managed with simple catheter drainage despite the amount of extravasation seen on cystography *(7)*. All patients managed nonoperatively should have a large-bore SP tube or Foley catheter placed and should be maintained on prophylactic antibiotics to cover both Gram-positive and Gram-negative bacteria.

The greatest risks to proper and expeditious healing are a urinary tract infection and bladder distention from inadequate bladder drainage *(22)*. Most patients have concomi-

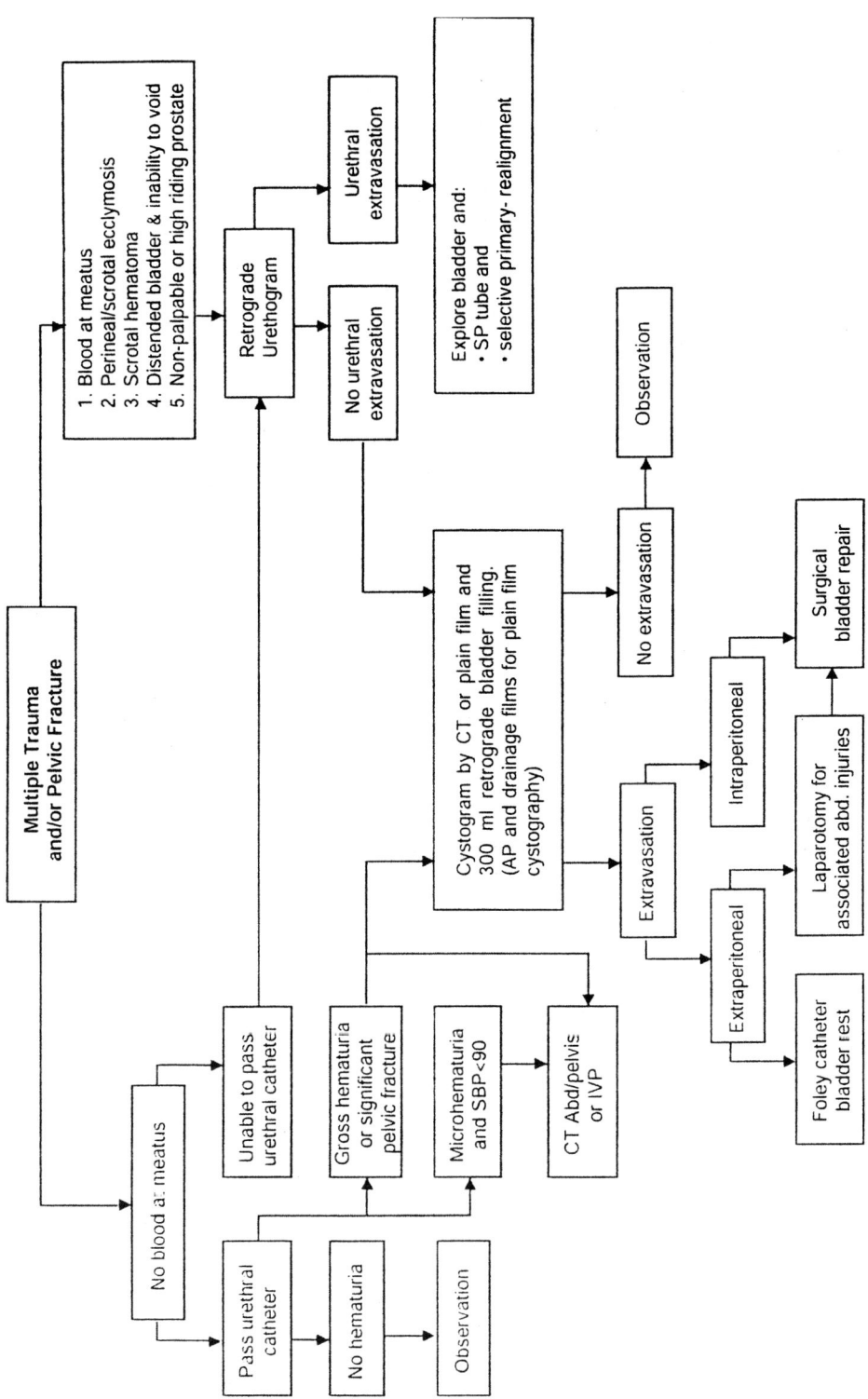

Fig. 7. Evaluation and treatment methods for blunt lower urinary tract trauma.

tant pelvic hematomas, and improper drainage can lead to bacterial colonization of the hematoma, abscess formation, and poor bladder wall healing. After 10 to 14 d of drainage, retrograde cystography should be performed to evaluate for persistent urinary extravasation. Spontaneous healing occurs in 74 to 87% of patients after 2 wk of bladder rest *(7,22)*. Another 11 to 13% will heal with prolonged drainage for 2 to 13 wk.

Patients at greatest risk for impaired healing include those with more severe concomitant injuries, worse pelvic fractures, and a higher transfusion requirement *(22)*. However, when the abdomen is explored for associated injuries, most recommend that extraperitoneal bladder ruptures also be repaired at the same time. Also, if the patient was too unstable for cystography, but intraoperatively there are suggestions of a bladder injury, the bladder should be explored. The bladder should be exposed through a midline abdominal incision, with the bladder opened at the dome to avoid the lateral pelvic hematomas. Opening the pelvic hematoma may cause bacterial contamination and release the tamponade effect. Bladder lacerations are then oversewn from within the bladder. The bladder neck and ureteral orifices need inspection for possible injury. To assess for ureteral integrity, the ureteral orifices can be either gently cannulated with a pediatric feeding tube or observed for blue urine after the administration of intravenous indigo carmine. To avoid potential contamination of the pelvic hematoma, some surgeons do not place drains. However, use of a closed suction drain is well tolerated, even in the presence of orthopedic hardware.

All bladder lacerations that extend into the bladder neck demand formal and prompt repair because if unrepaired the majority of individuals will have fixed incontinence. Other indications for immediate repair include urethral disruption that precludes urethral catheterization and concomitant rectal injury.

All intraperitoneal bladder ruptures should be explored through either a lower midline incision or a formal laparotomy incision if other intraabdominal injury is suspected. The dome of the bladder should be opened via a midline cystotomy, and the bladder mucosa should be inspected. Each ureteral orifice should be inspected for signs of injury. Any areas of devitalized tissue should be excised, and all lacerations identified should be closed in two or three layers of absorbable suture *(1)*. The bladder should be drained with a SP tube or Foley catheter. If a SP tube is placed, it should be through a separate cystotomy and brought out obliquely through a separate skin incision.

On abdominal exploration, if persistent and uncontained pelvic bleeding is found, a "damage control" management should be employed. Damage control entails a staged, planned reexploration with the pelvis packed, abdomen closed, and the bleeding pelvic vessels embolized in the angiography suite. Ligating the hypogastric arteries or attempting to find any venous bleeding is often of little benefit in controlling bleeding and often releases the tamponade effect. After 24 to 48 h of stabilization in the intensive care unit, the patient should be reexplored, and the laparotomy packs should be removed.

IATROGENIC INJURIES

The bladder is organ most frequently injured during pelvic surgery. The greatest risk factors for iatrogenic injury to the urinary bladder are poor visibility and anatomic distortion. Such risk factors are typically present with large pelvic masses, pregnant uterus, obesity, pelvic hemorrhage, malignant disease, or inadequate surgical exposure, small incision size, or poor wound illumination. The risk factor of anatomic distortion may occur as a result of adhesions/previous pelvic surgery, pelvic organ prolapse, congenital anomalies, radiation therapy, chronic inflammatory pelvic disease, en-

Table 2
Incidence of Bladder Injury by Surgical Procedure

Surgery	Per 1000 procedures
Vaginal delivery	0.1
Cesarean section	1.8
Gynecologic surgery (open)	1.5
Vaginal hysterectomy	9
Radical cancer hysterectomy	14
Obstetric hysterectomy	61
Gynecologic surgery (laparoscopic)	3
Lap assist vaginal hysterectomy	28
Transurethral resection of a bladder tumor	25
Bladder neck suspension	9
Inguinal herniorrhaphy	1.5

Modified with permission from ref. *18.*

dometriosis, malignant infiltration, or a distended, thin-walled bladder. Table 2 provides a detailed list of bladder injury by surgical procedure *(18).*

Bladder injury during a surgical procedure may be evident by clear fluid draining into the operative field or a visible laceration of the bladder. When bladder injury is suspected, the entire bladder walls should be thoroughly inspected. Another method to assess for bladder injury is to retrograde fill the bladder with methylene blue-tinged saline. Blue dye in the pelvis indicates a bladder laceration. Cystoscopy can be performed, particularly to assess the location of the bladder injury and proximity to the trigone or ureteral orifices. To facilitate locating the bladder injury, if the abdomen is already open, the bladder can be opened at the dome, and the bladder can be explored. Bladder injuries in proximity to the ureteral orifices may require ureteral reimplantation.

When a bladder injury is discovered during pelvic surgery, it is wise also to investigate for a concomitant ureteral injury. Direct inspection of the surgically exposed ureter or after indigo carmine administration is often sufficient and prudent. If the patient had received prior pelvic irradiation such as for cervical cancer, all bladder injuries should be covered with omentum or peritoneum (if available) to prevent possible fistulization.

Principles for bladder management and repair are the same as for injuries from external trauma. Bladder rest by Foley catheter is typically for 7 to 14 d. An SP tube is generally unnecessary unless there is considerable gross hematuria that could obstruct the catheter. A suction drain should also be placed in the prevesical space for a few days until drainage is minimal. If drainage output remains high, the drainage fluid should be sent for creatinine concentration. Creatinine levels greater than that of serum indicate a urine leak; levels equal to that of serum indicate peritoneal or lymphatic fluid. Persistent leakage typically resolves with prolonged bladder drainage *(23).*

Undiagnosed intraoperative injuries to the bladder typically present days to weeks after surgery. In patients with prior pelvic irradiation, fistulas can present months to even years after hysterectomy. Typical signs of missed injury are hematuria, oliguria, an elevated serum urea nitrogen/creatinine ratio, lower abdominal pain and distension, peritonitis or sepsis, or a urinary fistula. When signs and symptoms suggest a missed bladder injury, CT or plain film cystography with drainage films should be performed. Proper retrograde bladder filling to 300–350 cc of contrast is essential for reliable results.

Laparoscopic procedures have a 2- to 10-fold greater risk of bladder injury than the open surgical counterpart. When injured, the bladder is usually penetrated by and on initial placement of the Veress needle or trocar (typically by trocar placement in the midline and lower abdomen). Trocar injuries are typically to the bladder dome and have entry and exit wounds. Laproscopically, bladder injuries occur most often with a full bladder or a bladder with distorted anatomy from previous pelvic surgery, endometriosis, or adhesions *(24)*.

Intraoperatively, the diagnosis of bladder injury is suggested by the presence of gas insufflation of the Foley bag or gross hematuria. Other signs of injury are urinary/fluid drainage from an accessory trocar site incision or fluid (urinary ascites) pooling in the abdomen/pelvis. Because of the pneumoperitoneum, the borders of the bladder tear are often easy to visualize because the bladder is also distended from the insufflating gas *(25)*. If the bladder injury site is not obvious, the bladder should be filled retrograde with methylene blue-colored saline. Extravasation of dye notes an intraperitoneal bladder injury *(24,25)*.

Veress needle injuries and other small injuries to the bladder can be successfully managed conservatively by prolonged catheter drainage followed by cystography. Large bladder injuries, such as by trocar or surgical dissection, require suturing the injuries closed (either laparoscopically or by open repair). Laparoscopic repair of such bladder injuries should be performed only if the laceration is small, there is adequate exposure and visualization of the cystotomy, the ureters and bladder neck are not compromised, and the surgeon has adequate expertise in intracorporeal suturing *(24,25)*.

AUGMENTATION CYSTOPLASTY RUPTURE

Augmentation enterocystoplasty has been an effective method to achieve urinary incontinence for patients with poorly compliant, low-volume neurogenic bladders. Typically, such patients are children with myelomeningocele or adults with neurological disorders such as multiple sclerosis or spinal cord injury. However, because they are typically insensate, if the augmented bladder is not drained frequently enough it can potentially be overdistended and rupture.

Usually, signs of rupture include abdominal pain with rebound tenderness, decreased or absent bowel sounds, or microscopic or gross hematuria *(26)*. Many symptoms are nonspecific and may vary from shoulder pain (caused by diaphragmatic irritation from extravasated urine) to septic shock. Radiographic studies often do *not* show any urinary extravasation. In only one-half of cases will a cystogram show urinary extravasation *(27,28)*. Others have reported that ultrasound and CT are more likely to show extravasated urine than conventional cystography *(29)*. However, it is difficult to differentiate between extravasated urine and cerebrospinal fluid, which is seen with most patients with meningomyelocele patients (i.e., because of a ventriculoperitoneal shunt) *(28)*. Therefore, radiographic imaging is unreliable, and a high index of suspicion is required to diagnose an augmented bladder rupture. The decision to explore the abdomen is often based on the clinical history and physical exam and not radiological imaging.

Enterocystoplasty rupture may occur as a result of catheter trauma, chronic infection, or chronic overdistention. There are only two reports of rupture as a result of blunt trauma *(27,28)*. Bladder rupture may occur as a result of ischemia in parts of the bowel after detubularization. As the bladder is chronically distended, areas of vascular insufficiency can occur, weaken the wall, and lead to delayed rupture of the bladder wall *(26)*.

The gold standard treatment for augmentation cystoplasty rupture is surgical exploration *(26–28)*. Management includes broad-spectrum antibiotics, identification and repair of the laceration, and catheter drainage and prevesical drain *(27)*. In highly select cases, catheter drainage alone (without surgical intervention) can be attempted. There are case reports of successful conservative management with serial abdominal exams, broad-spectrum intravenous antibiotics, and catheter drainage for stable patients without peritoneal signs. However, for patients who do not improve within 48 hs or who have peritoneal signs, abdominal exploration is warranted *(28)*.

NEOBLADDER RUPTURE

In the last decade or so, continent, orthotopic bladder replacement has become a common surgical operation for patients undergoing radical cystectomy for bladder cancer. Up to 20% of patients with a neobladder are unable to void by Valsalva and require clean intermittent catheterization. Rupture occurs as a result of overdistention of the neobladder from either mucus plug or infrequent catheterization. The neobladder wall may be weakened from ischemic changes to the detubularized bowel segment, transmural infection, or intraperitoneal adhesions that result in impaired flexibility *(30)*.

According to Laplace's law, wall tension is proportional to the radius. As the bladder distends, the radius and wall tension increase, and blood flow decreases. In turn, a decrease in blood flow can lead to ischemia and bladder wall weakness *(26,30)*. Usual sites of perforation include the dome or upper side wall, which have a compromised blood supply and lack mesenteric support *(30,31)*.

Presenting signs and symptoms and efficacy of cystographic imaging for diagnosing rupture are the same for both augmented bladders and neobladders. Management of neobladder rupture involves exploratory laparotomy and repair of the injury. All areas of devitalized bowel should be excised and primarily repaired, and there should be prolonged bladder drainage *(31)*. Anecdotal reports of conservative management with catheter drainage alone have been described in stable patients, along with broad-spectrum antibiotics, bowel rest, and prolonged Foley catheter use *(32)*. Conservative management, however, is clearly not the standard of care because Fournier's gangrene and death have also been reported with nonoperative management *(33)*.

COMPLICATIONS OF BLADDER TRAUMA

After bladder injury repair, long-term voiding dysfunction is usually not significant *(12,22)*. The most common complications after repair include urinary tract infections and bladder spasms. However, more severe complications can occur, including incontinence, abscess formation, or fistula.

Incontinence

Lacerations away from the bladder neck may lead to transient urge incontinence once the Foley catheter is removed. Urgency is often caused by bladder mucosal irritation from the wound itself or the indwelling catheter and balloon, and it usually only lasts for several days. Transient stress incontinence may also occur in women and usually lasts a few days or weeks *(1)*.

Injuries involving the bladder neck, especially if it extends into the membranous urethra, can result in total urinary incontinence, especially in women. Bladder neck injuries are diagnosed by cystography or by direct exploration by palpation or visualization. All bladder neck injuries, therefore, should be repaired carefully with interrupted sutures around a Foley catheter. Persistent incontinence after bladder trauma should be evaluated with a careful voiding history, physical examination, cystoscopy, and urodynamic testing. Improvement in urinary control can occur for up to 1-yr postinjury. Thus, surgical intervention should be postponed until after that time. In patients who fail conservative management or medical therapy (with α–adrenergic agonists), continence may be achieved with an artificial urinary sphincter or urethral sling. Bulking agents to the bladder neck typically have poor durable results (particularly because the incompetent bladder neck is scarred) *(12)*.

Pelvic Infection/Abscess

Overall, up to 6% of patients develop an abscess after bladder trauma *(1)*. Abscess usually occurs as a result of infection of the pelvic hematoma in association with pelvic fracture. To avoid infection of the hematoma, prevesical drains should be avoided because drains act more as a path for bacterial colonization than hematoma drainage *(12)*.

In patients with extraperitoneal rupture who are managed with Foley catheter alone, abscess may occur as a result of retrograde colonization of the hematoma from the catheter and urinary leakage *(22)*. This risk is minimized by keeping the patient on broad-spectrum antibiotics and using a large-bore catheter (greater than 22 French) to maximally drain the bladder. If a pelvic infection is suspected after catheter removal, the patient should be placed on broad-spectrum antibiotics and the size and location of the abscess determined by CT or ultrasound *(12)*. In male patients, epididymoorchitis may occur as a result of prolonged transurethral catheterization. We minimize this complication by placing a SP tube and a Foley catheter. The Foley catheter is removed as soon as the urine clears.

Fistula

Urinary fistulas often develop as a delayed complication after bladder injury. The bladder injury is initially not recognized, the repair is improper, or urinary infection resulted in suture breakdown. Additional risk factors for fistula formation include bladder outlet obstruction, urethral stricture disease, neurogenic bladder, diabetes mellitus, long-term steroid use, malignancy, prior pelvic irradiation, or foreign body presence *(12,34)*.

Vesicovaginal fistulas (VVFs) may form as a result of concomitant vaginal laceration at the time of bladder injury. Each woman who presents with a pelvic fracture, bladder injury, or blood in the vaginal vault should undergo a thorough pelvic examination, speculum examination, or vaginoscopy to rule out a vaginal wall injury. If a vaginal injury is found, it should be closed in two layers, usually in the lithotomy position. Concomitant bladder injury should be closed in two layers from within the bladder because exposure is better, and the ureteral orifices can be visualized *(12,35)*.

Bladder fistulas are typically recognized in a delayed fashion with painless, constant incontinence. Severity of the leakage is proportional to the size and location of the fistula. Diagnosis can be made by simultaneous retrograde bladder filling, cystoscopy, and vaginal speculum examination. In addition, a standard "pad" test can be performed with methylene-blue instilled in the bladder, oral Pyridium, and pads or tampons placed in the vagina to evaluate for staining of the pads. An intravenous urogram should also be performed to rule out a ureteral injury. If there is a high index of suspicion of a ureterovaginal fistula or the intravenous urogram is equivocal, a retrograde urogram should be performed *(12)*. VVFs, when small and oblique, can sometimes be successfully managed with catheter drainage alone. Most posttraumatic VVFs, however, require surgical repair after 3 to 6 mo of tract maturing. If the fistula is diagnosed early (within 48 h after injury), immediate repair can be performed. In addition, if possible, omentum, peritoneum, or labial fat pad (Martius flap) should be interposed between the lacerations for maximal prevention of fistula formation *(12,36)*.

Vesicocutaneous fistulas can also occur, usually along the tract of a prior SP site. Other commonly occurring nonhealing bladder fistulas are caused by a foreign body, a penetrating bony spicule, or bladder entrapment from pelvic fracture. Bladder fistulas usually close with prolonged Foley catheter bladder rest, unless they are very large, contain a foreign body, or there is significant obstructive voiding dysfunction. Persistent fistulas require formal excision of the fistula tract, bladder repair, and removal of the foreign body (i.e., bony spicule); correction of any outlet obstruction is warranted.

SUMMARY

Bladder injuries typically occur as the result of external force and are often associated with pelvic fracture, and/or gross hematuria. Iatrogenic injuries may result from gynecological or other extensive pelvic procedures. Reliable imaging for bladder rupture is conventional cystography with adequate filling and postdrainage films, or antegrade bladder filling and CT cystography. Most extraperitoneal bladder injuries can be managed effectively by prolonged catheter bladder drainage. Intraperitoneal bladder or bladder neck injuries typically demand prompt exploration and repair. On repairing bladder injuries, the midline pelvic hematoma should be avoided, and the bladder lacerations typically closed from within.

REFERENCES

1. Carroll PR, McAninch JW. Major bladder trauma: mechanisms of injury and a unified method of diagnosis and repair. J Urol 1984; 132: 254.
2. Brandes S, Borrelli J Jr. Pelvic fracture and associated urologic injuries. World J Surg 2001; 25: 1578.
3. Corriere JN Jr. Trauma to the lower urinary tract. In: Adult and Pediatric Urology, 3rd ed. (Gillenwater JY, ed.), Mosby, St. Louis, MO, 1996, Vol. 1, pp. 563–585.
4. Sivit CJ, Taylor GA, Newman KD, et al. Safety-belt injuries in children with lap-belt ecchymosis: CT findings in 61 patients. AJR Am J Roentgenol 1991; 157: 111.
5. Cass AS, Luxenberg M. Features of 164 bladder ruptures. J Urol 1987, 138: 743.
6. Clark SS, Prudencio RF. Lower urinary tract injuries associated with pelvic fractures. Diagnosis and management. Surg Clin North Am 1972; 52: 183.
7. Corriere JN Jr, Sandler CM. Mechanisms of injury, patterns of extravasation and management of extraperitoneal bladder rupture due to blunt trauma. J Urol 1988; 139: 43.
8. Thomas CL, McAninch JW. Bladder trauma. AUA Update Ser 1989; 8: 242.
9. Iverson AJ, Morey AF. Radiographic evaluation of suspected bladder rupture following blunt trauma: critical review. World J Surg, 2001; 25: 1588.
10. Morey AF, Iverson AJ, Swan A, et al. Bladder rupture after blunt trauma: guidelines for diagnostic imaging. J Trauma 2001; 51: 683.
11. Carroll PR, McAninch JW. Major bladder trauma: the accuracy of cystography. J Urol 1983; 130: 887.
12. Brandes S, McAninch JW. Complications of genitourinary trauma. In: Complications of Urologic Surgery. (Taneja SS, Smith RB, Erlich RM, eds.), Saunders, Philadelphia, PA, 2001, pp. 205–225.

13. Deck AJ, Shaves S, Talner L, et al. Computerized tomography cystography for the diagnosis of traumatic bladder rupture. J Urol 2000; 164: 43.
14. Mee SL, McAninch JW, Federle MP. Computerized tomography in bladder rupture: diagnostic limitations. J Urol 1987; 137: 207.
15. Vaccaro JP, Brody JM. CT cystography in the evaluation of major bladder trauma. Radiographics 2000; 20: 1373.
16. Fuhrman GM, Simmons GT, Davidson BS, Buerk CA. The single indication for cystography in blunt trauma. Am Surg 1993; 59(6): 335–337.
17. Sandler CM, Hall JT, Rodriguez MB, et al. Bladder injury in blunt pelvic trauma. Radiology 1986; 158: 633.
18. Gomez RG, Ceballos L, Coburn M, et al. Bladder Trauma 2002 SIU Genitourinary Trauma Consensus Conference, Stockholm, Sweden.
19. Moore EE, Cogbill TH, Malgoni, MA, et al. Organ injury scaling. Surg Clin North Am 1995; 75: 293.
20. Parry NG, Rozycki GS, Feliciano DV, et al. Traumatic rupture of the urinary bladder: is the suprapubic tube necessary? J Trauma 2002; 54(3): 431–436.
21. Patterson BM: Pelvic ring injury and associated urologic trauma; an orthopedic perspective. Semin Urol 1995; 13: 25.
22. Kotkin L, Koch MO. Morbidity associated with nonoperative management of extraperitoneal bladder injuries. J Trauma 1995; 38: 895.
23. Williams RD. Urologic complications of pelvic surgery. In: Urologic Complications of Pelvic Surgery and Radiotherapy. (Jewett MAS, ed.), Isis Medical Media, Oxford, UK, 1995, pp. 1–39.
24. Saidi MH, Sadler RK, Vancaillie TG, Akright BD, Farhart SA, White AJ. Diagnosis and management of serious urinary complications after major operative laparoscopy. Obstet Gynecol 1996; 87: 272–276.
25. Appeltans BM, Schapmans S, Willemsen PJ, et al. Urinary bladder rupture: laparoscopic repair. Br J Urol 1998; 81: 764.
26. Crane JM, Scherz HS, Billman GF, et al. Ischemic necrosis: a hypothesis to explain the pathogenesis of spontaneously ruptured enterocystoplasty. J Urol 1991; 146: 141.
27. Elder JS, Snyder HM, Hulbert WC, et al. Perforation of the augmented bladder in patients undergoing clean intermittent catheterization. J Urol 1988; 140: 1159.
28. Slaton JW, Kropp KA. Conservative management of suspected bladder rupture after augmentation enterocystoplasty. J Urol 1994; 152: 713.
29. Glass RB, Rushton HG. Delayed spontaneous rupture of augmented bladder in children: diagnosis with sonography and CT. AJR Am J Roentgenol 1992; 158: 833.
30. Desgrandchamps F, Cariou G, Barthelemy Y, et al. Spontaneous rupture of orthotopic detubularized ileal bladder replacement: report of five cases. J Urol 1997; 158: 798.
31. Nippgen JB, Hakenberg OW, Manseck A, et al. Spontaneous late rupture of orthotopic detubularized ileal neobladders: report of five cases. Urology 2001; 58: 43.
32. Parsons JK, Schoenberg MP. Successful conservative management of perforated ileal neobladder. J Urol 2001; 165: 1214.
33. Kyriakidis A. Fournier's gangrene following delayed rupture of an ileal neobladder (Hautmann). Br J Urol 1995; 76: 668.
34. Bockrath JM, Nanninga JB, Lewis VL Jr, et al. Extensive suprapubic vesicocutaneous fistula following trauma. J Urol 1981; 125: 246.
35. Labasky RF, Leach GE. Prevention and management of urovaginal fistulas. Clin Obstet Gynecol 1990; 33: 382.
36. Kursh ED, Morse RM, Resnick MI, et al. Prevention of the development of a vesicovaginal fistula. Surg Gynecol Obstet 1988; 166: 409.
37. Wyker AW, Gillenwater JY. Method of Urology. Williams and Wilkins, Baltimore, MD, 1975.

4 Urethral Trauma

Eric R. Richter, MD and Allen F. Morey, MD

CONTENTS

    INTRODUCTION
    ANTERIOR URETHRA
    POSTERIOR URETHRA
    SUMMARY
    REFERENCES

INTRODUCTION

Urethral injuries are uncommon yet potentially devastating, leading often to sequelae such as strictures, impotence, infertility, and incontinence. Anterior urethral trauma usually occurs in conjunction with straddle-type injuries to the perineum; the fixed bulbar urethra is crushed. The pendulous urethra is less susceptible to traumatic injury because of its mobility, although penile rupture during intercourse may extend into the urethra. Posterior urethral injuries are those located near the external sphincter mechanism, occurring exclusively as a result of pelvic fracture. Urological management differs depending on the location of injury.

ANTERIOR URETHRA

The anterior urethra is divided into two segments, the bulbar and the pendulous. The pendulous urethra extends from the external meatus to the penoscrotal junction. The bulbar urethra is located just proximal, between the inferior margin of the urogenital diaphragm and the penoscrotal junction.

The incidence of anterior urethral injuries is low, comprising only 10% of lower urinary tract injuries *(1)*. Of these, bulbar urethral injuries comprise 85% *(2)*. Blunt trauma typically affects the bulbar urethra as a result of a straddle injury from a fall, crush, or motor vehicle accident *(3)*. The bulbar area is susceptible to injury because of its fixed position beneath the inferior pubis *(4)*.

Penetrating urethral injuries may occur because of gunshot wounds or stab injuries to the penis, buttock, abdomen, or scrotum. Iatrogenic anterior urethral injury is associated with traumatic endoscopic procedures or catheter placement. Delayed injury may arise from a chronic indwelling urethral catheter, secondary to pressure necrosis, infection, or chemical irritation *(5)*.

From: *Urological Emergencies: A Practical Guide*
Edited by: H. Wessells and J. W. McAninch © Humana Press Inc., Totowa, NJ

Pendulous urethral injury occurs in 15 to 37% of penile fractures *(6,7)*. Most cases occur during intercourse, with the erect penis striking the pubic ramus of the female pubis. The patient reports a history of a popping sound, followed by severe pain and immediate detumescence. Penile swelling and ecchymosis are usually striking. A corporal defect may be palpable, but is usually obscured by hematoma.

Diagnosis

Any blunt or penetrating injury to the perineum, genitalia, or pelvis should suggest the possibility of urethral injury, and severity can be suggested by information about the type of weapon used or the object or force that struck the perineum. A complete voiding history should be obtained, including ability to void spontaneously, time of last void, hematuria, dysuria, and caliber of stream.

The extent of injury is best determined radiographically prior to transurethral catheterization. Any patient with blood at the urethral meatus warrants an immediate retrograde urethrogram.

Genital swelling and hematoma not only suggest urethral trauma, but also its distribution aids in determination of which anatomic boundaries have been violated *(8)*. If Buck's fascia is ruptured, blood and urine can extravasate around Colles' fascia, giving a characteristic "butterfly" sign in the perineum *(9)*. A sleeve distribution limited to the penile shaft indicates that the injury is confined within Buck's fascia. When extravasation of blood or urine surrounds the prostate, typically from blunt urethral trauma, a palpable soft rectal mass may also be appreciated on the anterior rectal surface. Unlike posterior urethral injuries, the prostate will be in its normal position *(4)*.

Dynamic retrograde urethrography (contrast injected during film exposure) is preferable to static urethrography because it produces urethral distention, which facilitates visualization *(5)*. Urethrography should be performed with the penis on stretch and the patient in the oblique position. Contrast may be injected using a Brodney clamp, a catheter-tip syringe, or a Foley catheter inserted far enough (2–3 cm) for the balloon to be lodged within the fossa navicularis. Extravasation of contrast material is diagnostic of urethral injury, although the quantity and location of extravasated contrast material is a function of the volume and rate of contrast infusion.

Armenakas and McAninch *(4)* proposed the following simple, practical classification scheme based on radiographic findings for anterior urethral injuries:

1. Contusion. Retrograde urethrogram normal with clinical features suggestive of anterior urethral injury.
2. Incomplete disruption. Retrograde urethrography demonstrates urethral extravasation, with contrast material entering the bladder, thus indicating partial urethral continuity.
3. Complete disruption. Retrograde urethrography demonstrates extravasation without filling of the proximal urethra or bladder.

Initial Management

The goal of initial management is to provide urinary drainage and minimize potential complications, such as stricture, fistula, and infection. Typically, if the patient is unstable, it is not as a result of urethral injury, so resuscitation is primarily directed at associated injuries to other organs.

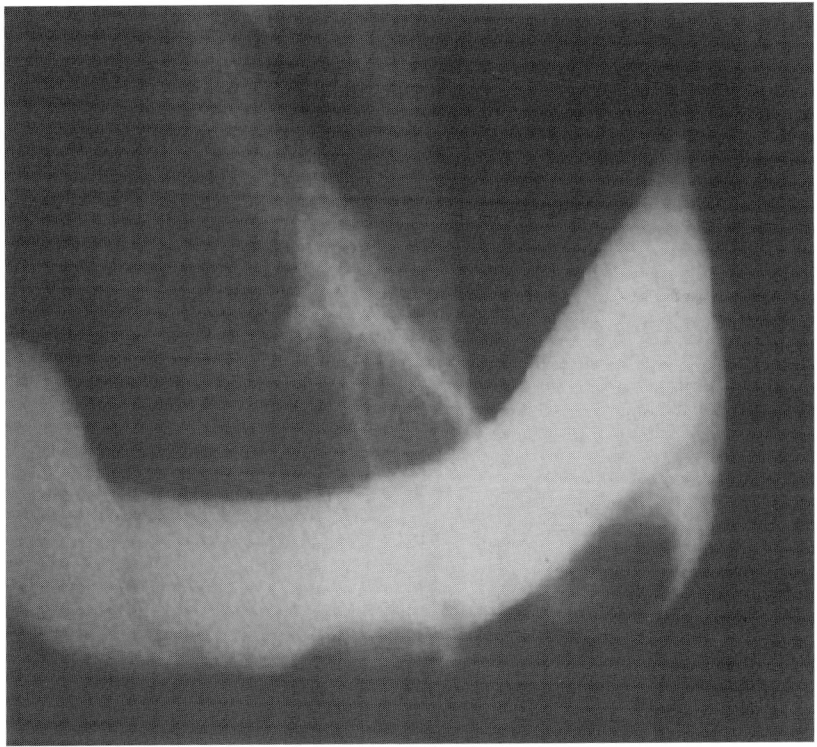

Fig. 1. Retrograde urethrography after perineal trauma caused by bicycle injury demonstrates extravasation from ventral aspect of deep bulbar urethra. Note that the dorsal urethra is intact. This patient was successfully managed by Coude catheter placement alone.

Management of contusions is straightforward, consisting of urethral catheterization alone. The catheter is removed 10 to 14 d after injury and is followed by voiding cystourethrography at the time of removal. Partial disruptions contained within Buck's fascia can also be managed with transurethral catheterization alone *(10)*. A Coude catheter or flexible cystoscope is often useful to bypass the attenuated area safely. Successful outcome with realignment is dependent on the preservation of a partially intact mucosa, which allows for urethral regeneration (Fig. 1).

Suprapubic cystostomy is a practical, simple solution for acute management of major injuries. It is familiar to all urologists and avoids urethral manipulation. Although percutaneous placement may be more efficient in most cases, open cystostomy may be preferable if the bladder is not palpable suprapubically. Transabdominal sonography can be used to guide the catheter's placement. When suprapubic cystostomy is used as the primary treatment option, the cystotomy tube is maintained for approx 4 wk to allow urethral healing. It is then clamped, and voiding cystourethrography is performed. Once normal micturition is confirmed, the tube can be safely removed *(4)*.

Massive blunt urethral injuries may be associated with extensive soft tissue destruction, making evaluation of the extent of injury difficult. Extensive debridement of the urethra and corpus spongiosum is not advised because bruised, otherwise viable erectile tissue can appear ischemic acutely. Overzealous debridement may result in large wounds that require major delayed reconstruction *(11)*. Significant urethral injury associated

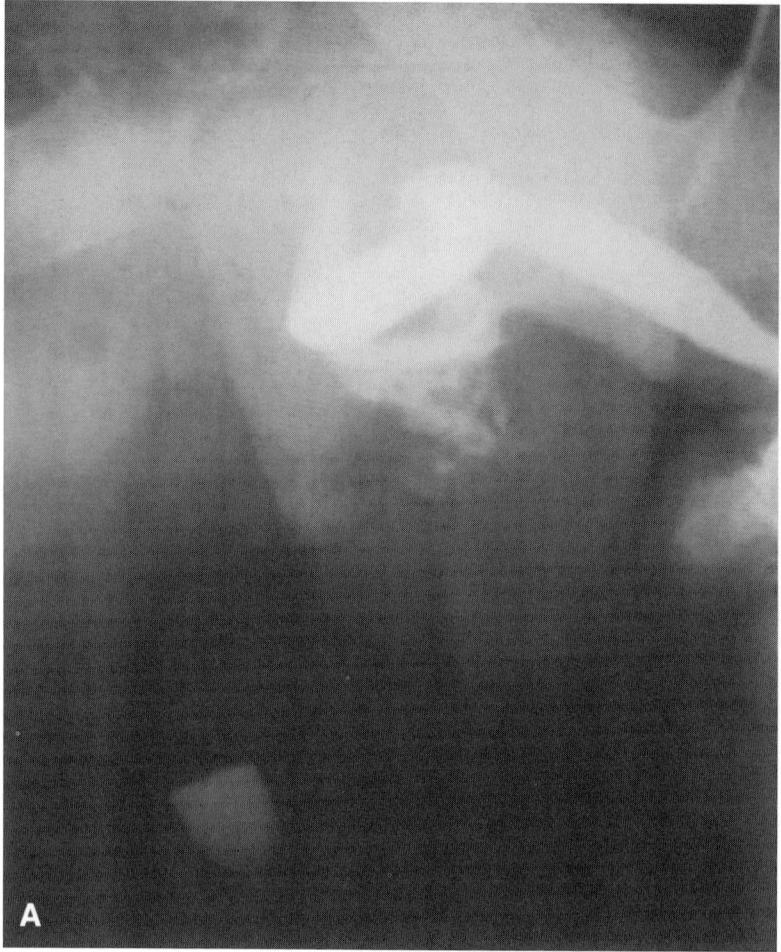

Fig. 2. (**A**) Retrograde urethrography obtained after gunshot wound to buttock demonstrates extravasation from bulbar urethra and bullet retained within scrotum. Primary repair was performed acutely. (**B**) Voiding cystourethrogram 2 wk after repair reveals completely normal urethra.

with loss of corpus spongiosum usually results in significant stricture that requires formal urethral reconstruction (*12*). Broad-spectrum antibiotics should be started in all patients with extensive extravasation of blood or urine.

Urethral injuries occurring in the context of penile fracture or penetrating trauma are best managed with primary repair (Fig. 2). Complications such as penile deformity, abscess, dyspareunia, and erectile dysfunction are less likely when immediate surgical repair with fine absorbable suture is instituted (*7,9*). Stricture rates after suprapubic diversion are 66 to 78% compared to 12 to 20% for primary repair (*13,14*).

Primary repair is probably not justified for transections of the urethra following high-velocity penetrating trauma given the likely extensive amount of surrounding tissue damage. Treatment should be suprapubic diversion, local wound care, and consideration for a proximal urethostomy with delayed urethral reconstruction (*15*).

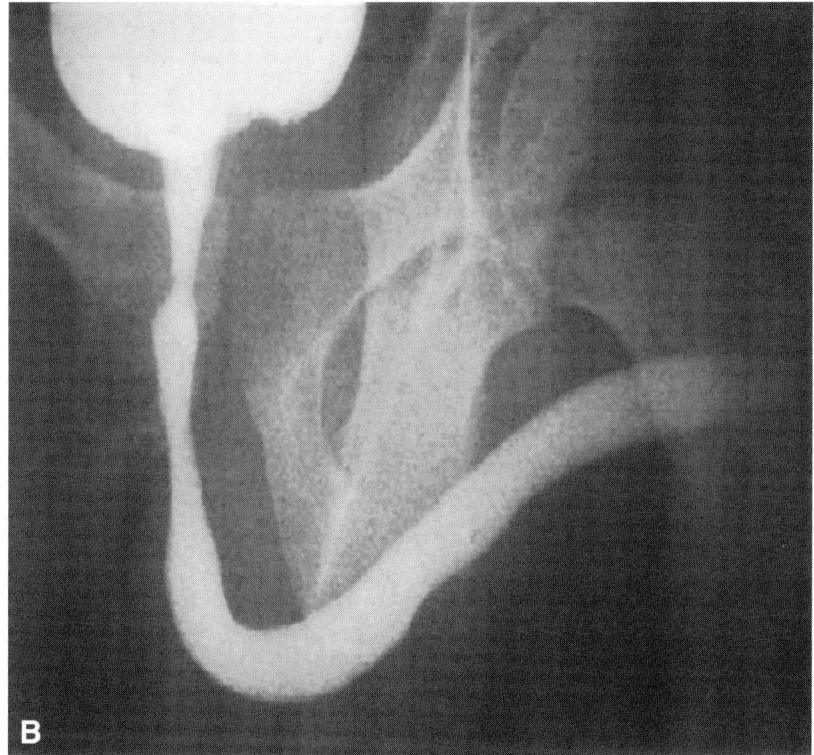

Fig. 2. *Continued*

Delayed Reconstruction

Stricture management depends on location, severity, and extent of the stricture. Options include dilation, internal urethrotomy, excision with primary end-to-end anastomosis, single-stage flap or graft urethroplasty, and two-stage urethroplasty.

Repair of a traumatic stricture should be delayed at least 2 mo after the initial injury *(16)*. Bulbar urethral strictures smaller than 2.5 cm are usually amenable to resection and primary end-to-end anastomosis. Strictures of the pendulous urethra and those in the bulbar urethra that are longer than 2.5 cm will likely require substitution urethroplasty with a flap or graft. Most posttraumatic strictures that require grafting have failed previous dilations or endoscopic treatments.

Preoperative imaging of anterior urethral strictures via retrograde urethrography combined with voiding cystourethrography delineates the location and severity of the stricture in most cases. Repeat imaging may be required to guide selection of an appropriate reconstructive procedure. Sonourethrography is an ancillary staging technique that may complement traditional imaging techniques. Stricture length and diameter may be more precisely measured using ultrasound, resulting occasionally in selection of a different reconstructive procedure than that originally suggested by conventional urethrography *(17)*. Specifically, for intermediate-length strictures (11–25 mm) of the bulbar urethra, preoperative sonourethrography can prospectively identify strictures too long for resection and end-to-end anastomosis *(18)*.

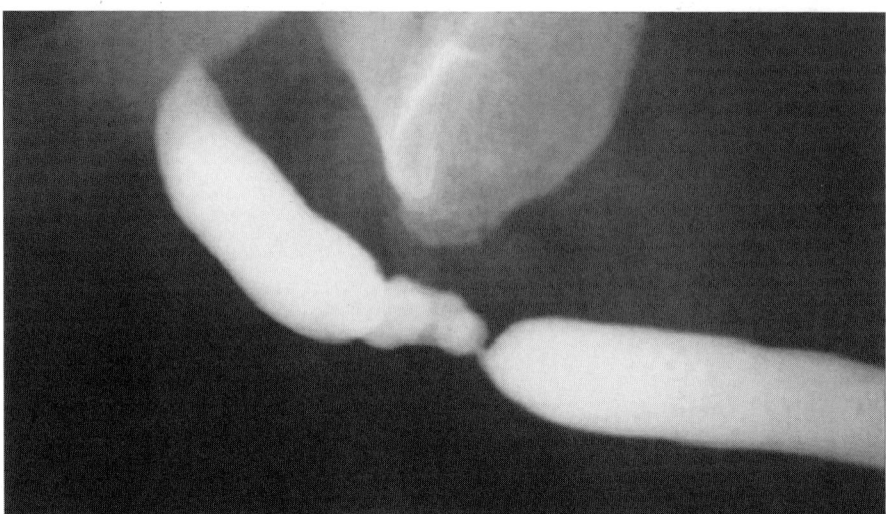

Fig. 3. Retrograde urethrography shows 4.5-cm bulbar stricture. Patient had failed several prior endoscopic treatments. Augmented anastomotic urethroplasty with buccal mucosa graft was successful.

Most traumatic strictures are dense and recur after dilation or endoscopic urethrotomy. Because of its high failure rate, urethrotomy is best reserved for patients who cannot tolerate urethroplasty or for thin diaphragmatic strictures that arise occasionally after formal repair *(19)*.

Primary end-to-end urethroplasty offers patients the best opportunity for a stricture-free outcome. Long-term cure rates approach 100% when properly selected patients are treated with excision and primary anastomosis *(20)*. Patients best suited for primary end-to-end anastomosis are those who have strictures of the bulbar urethra that are less than 2.5 cm *(18)*. For longer bulbar strictures, the augmented anastomotic urethroplasty (graft combined with partial dorsal wall excision) has been shown to have a stricture-free rate of 93% *(21)*. In the augmented anastomotic urethroplasty, the most severe area of stricture is excised and combined with a graft only (Fig. 3). Excessive urethral excision can result in chordee, penile shortening, or a repair that is under tension.

Strictures of the pendulous urethra are rarely amenable to excision and primary anastomosis. Pendulous strictures tend to be more diffuse than bulbar strictures, and their excision is more likely to produce chordee. As a result, onlay procedures involving a graft or flap will be required in most cases *(20)*. Full-circumference replacement is less successful than an onlay procedure, and aggressive efforts should be employed to preserve or salvage the urethral plate *(22)*.

Graft survival requires a well-vascularized bed. Because the intrinsic blood supply of the distal urethra is less robust than that in the bulb, penile skin flap reconstruction is preferable to graft procedures in the pendulous area. Wessels and McAninch demonstrated that grafts placed in the bulbar urethra have a greater success rate than those placed in the penile urethra *(23)*.

Buccal mucosa has become the most commonly used urethral graft because it is reliable, resilient, hairless, easy to handle, and highly vascular. These practical and theoretical advantages over other graft materials allow excellent results in appropriately selected patients, even in those with refractory strictures *(24)*. Alternative graft choices

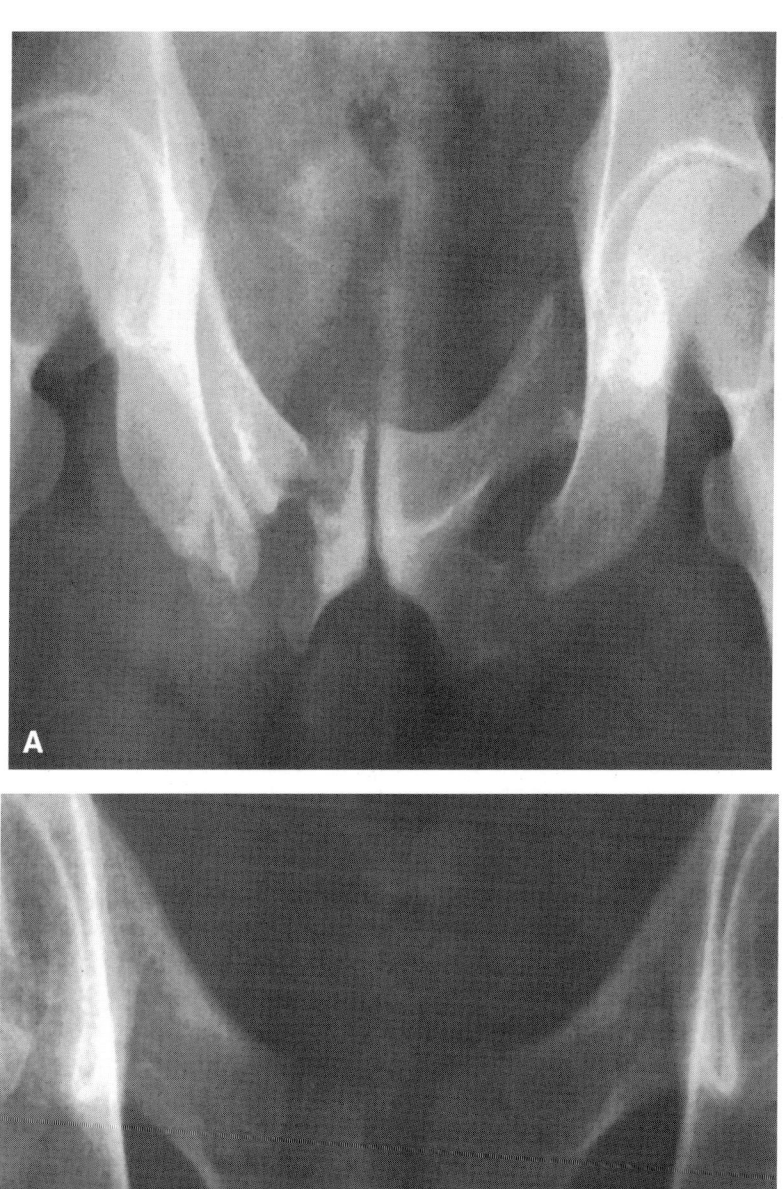

Fig. 4. Posterior urethral distraction injury occurred in conjunction with a crush injury to the pubic area in these two cases. (**A**) "Straddle" fracture involving bilateral superior and inferior pubic rami and (**B**) barely perceptible pubic diastasis are two examples of the spectrum of pubic injuries that may be implicated.

include penile skin and bladder epithelium. Graft procedures are more efficient for complex bulbar strictures, especially in sexually active men, because they involve a less-extensive genital dissection than penile skin flaps.

POSTERIOR URETHRA

The posterior urethra consists of the prostatic and membranous urethra; injuries occur in conjunction with pelvic fracture and commonly lead to stricture, impotence, and incontinence. Traumatic disruption of the posterior urethra occurs in 10% of all cases of pelvic fractures (25). The type of fracture that most frequently causes urethral injury is a Malgaigne fracture (fracture of both ischiopubic rami with disruption of ipsilateral sacrum, sacroiliac joint, or ilium), although others may be implicated (Fig. 4) (26). Other causes of posterior urethral injury include perineal penetrating trauma, self-instrumentation, and pelvic diastasis without fracture (27). Concomitant bladder injury occurs in 18% of patients with urethral disruptions (28).

Diagnosis

The diagnosis of posterior urethral injury is suggested by a history of pelvic fracture, most commonly following a motor vehicle accident or pedestrian injury, but also after a fall or work-related crush injury. Like anterior urethral injuries, blood at the meatus and inability to void warrant complete urological evaluation. Other significant diagnostic findings are a palpably full bladder and an elevated prostate on rectal examination. Typically, the prostate will be indistinguishable from the pelvic hematoma. Retrograde urethrogram should always be performed prior to transurethral catheterization when urethral injury is suspected.

Initial Management

Initial management depends on the patient's hemodynamic stability and the status of associated orthopedic and nonorthopedic injuries. Two options now exist for the management of posterior urethral injury: primary realignment or suprapubic cystostomy with delayed repair. In the past, immediate open repair with pelvic hematoma evacuation was suggested (29). Immediate suture repair can no longer be recommended because delayed elective reconstruction is associated with superior outcomes.

Proponents of immediate suprapubic cystostomy alone note the benefits of avoiding the retroperitoneal hematoma and expediting treatment in the severely traumatized patient. As the hematoma resorbs and the prostate settles into its normal position, a 1- to 2-cm stricture typically results. Complete excision of the scar during elective perineal repair is performed when the patient has recovered from major associated injuries, usually after 3 mo (30).

Primary realignment implies stenting the disrupted area with a transurethral catheter. Realignment procedures may be performed either immediately or subacutely, several days after the initial injury, when the patient is more stable. A variety of techniques, including interlocking or magnetic sounds ("railroading"), retrograde passage of a catheter through cystotomy under direct vision, and endoscopically assisted catheter realignment, have been advocated (27,31). Cystostomy is usually performed via a suprapubic incision to enable combined antegrade and retrograde access to the urethra (Fig. 5).

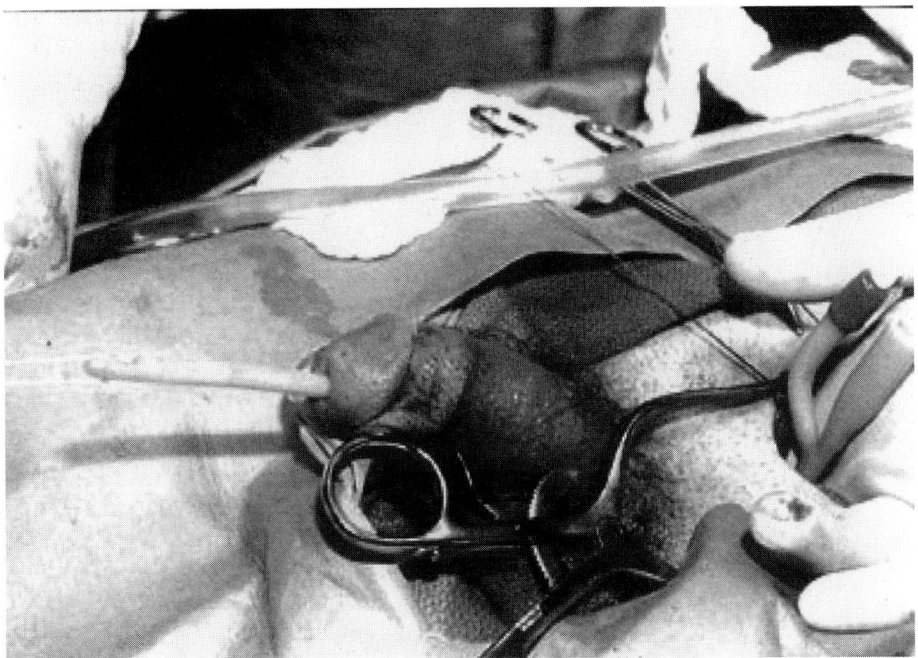

Fig. 5. Posterior urethral realignment is performed by passing a urethral catheter antegrade through a infraumbilical approach to the bladder. A urethral catheter was tied to the end of this catheter and drawn retrograde into the bladder. Suprapubic tube was also placed. This patient went into urinary retention almost immediately after the urethral catheter was removed 1 mo after injury. Subsequent posterior urethroplasty was successful.

The benefit of a minimally invasive approach (realignment) is the potential avoidance of a subsequent posterior urethroplasty, which is near uniform for suprapubic cystostomy. Although most patients require repeated instrumentation or self-catheterization to maintain patency long term, many can be treated with Van Buren sounds, internal urethrotomy, or laser ablation; some require multiple procedures and eventual urethroplasty *(32)*. Prolonged endoscopic realignment procedures may cause infectious complications and should therefore be avoided.

Potency and continence rates with primary realignment have been comparable to those achieved by delayed repair *(27,32–34)*. Most authorities now believe that impotence and incontinence result from the injury, not secondary to surgical management *(35)*. Delayed return of potency is not uncommon, occurring as late as 3 yr after injury *(36)*.

Primary realignment may be of specific benefit when there is wide separation of urethral ends, bladder neck or rectal injury, and pelvic fractures that will require open reduction and internal fixation. Suprapubic cystostomy affords an advantage when there is minimal or incomplete urethral rupture, the patient is critically unstable, or when realignment cannot easily be performed *(37)*.

Delayed Reconstruction

Retrograde urethrography with simultaneous cystography determines the length of the defect and competency of the bladder neck. Alternatively, flexible antegrade cystos

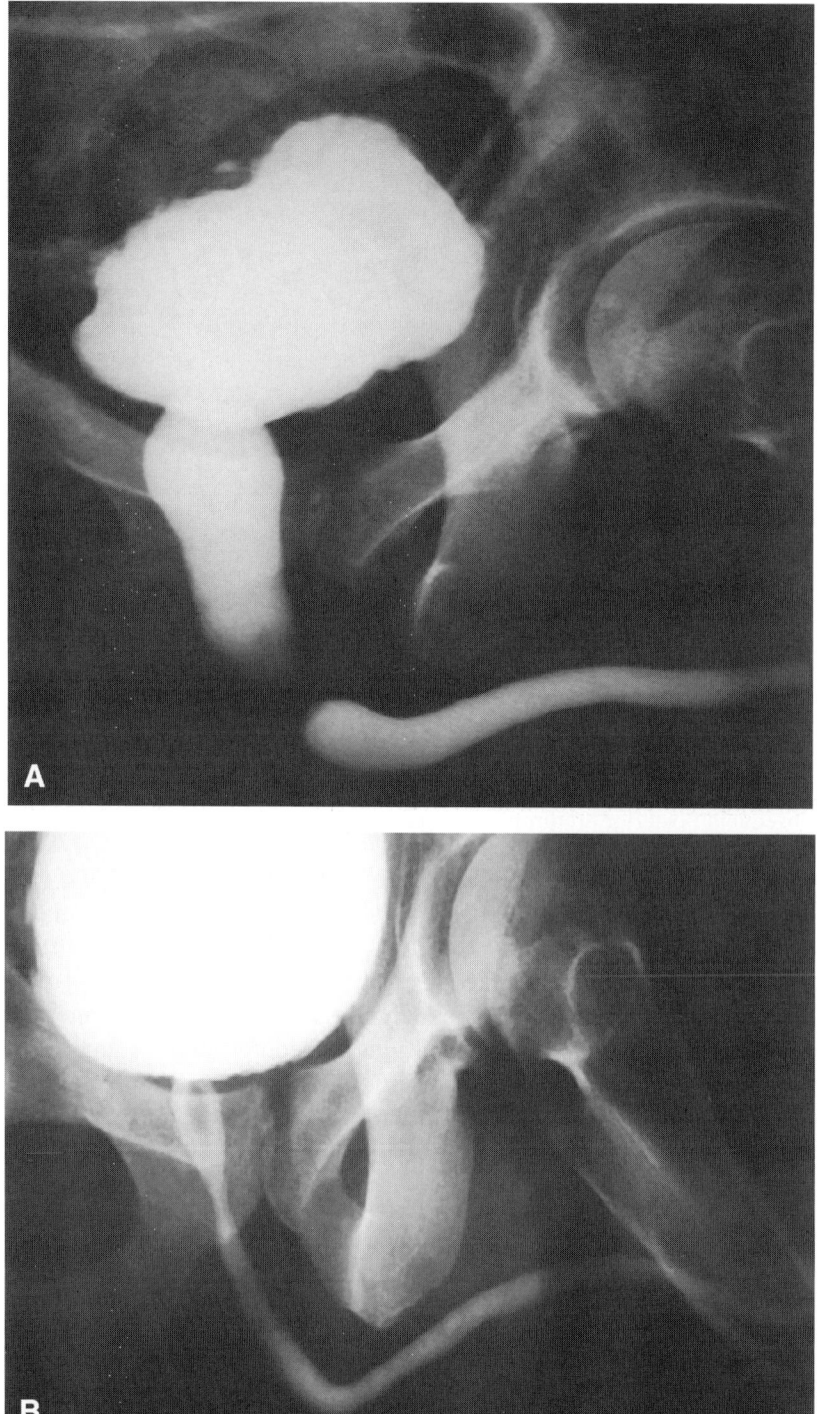

Fig. 6. (**A**) Combined retrograde urethrography/voiding cystourethrogram reveals dense urethral stenosis 3 mo after posterior urethral disruption. (**B**) Postoperative voiding cystourethrogram after successful posterior urethral reconstruction via excision/primary anastomosis technique reveals completely normal urethral lumen.

copy may be combined with retrograde urethrography to delineate the magnitude of fibrosis. Magnetic resonance imaging can provide additional information in selected complex or reoperative cases *(38)*.

Posterior urethroplasty success rates above 90% have been reported (Fig. 6) *(36)*. Reconstruction is delayed until it can be performed under ideal conditions, when associated injuries are stabilized. A perineal approach is adequate in most cases; transpubic procedures are reserved for complex or reoperative cases in which a tension-free bulboprostatic anastomosis is not otherwise possible *(39,40)*.

Complete resection of the fibrotic segment with end-to-end anastomosis is the most successful method for posterior urethral reconstruction *(41)*. Distal urethral mobilization is routinely accomplished to the level of the suspensory ligament of the penis. If necessary, corporal body separation, inferior pubectomy, or supracrural urethral rerouting may be utilized in sequential fashion to bridge the defect *(42)*. Continence after posterior urethral reconstruction relies on the bladder neck and prostate. An open bladder neck on a preoperative cystogram, however, does not prove functional incompetence *(43,44)*.

SUMMARY

Urethral injury may be of secondary importance at the time of presentation of the acute trauma victim. However, devastating urological complications such as sexual dysfunction, incontinence, and stricture disease may drastically impair quality of life in the long term. A high index of suspicion is necessary to ensure early, accurate diagnosis and prompt, effective treatment of urethral injuries.

Urethral injury should be considered in the setting of penile fracture, pelvic fracture, or penetrating trauma to the genitalia, pelvis, or perineum. Blood at the meatus always indicates the need for retrograde urethrogram in the trauma setting. Suprapubic cystostomy with delayed reconstruction is a safe, proven strategy, although primary realignment is reasonable when it is possible without heroic measures. Continence and potency rates seem to be associated more with the nature of the injury than with the method of urological management.

ACKNOWLEDGMENT

The views expressed in this chapter are those of the authors and do not reflect the official policy of the US Department of Defense or other departments of the US government.

REFERENCES

1. Mitchell JP. Injuries to the urethra. Br J Urol 1968; 40: 649–670.
2. Badenoch AW. Traumatic stricture of the urethra. Br J Urol 1968; 40: 671–676.
3. Pierce JM. Disruptions of the anterior urethra. Urol Clin North Am 1989; 16: 329–334.
4. Armenakas NA, McAninch JW. Acute anterior urethral injuries: diagnosis and initial management. In: Traumatic and Reconstructive Urology. (McAninch JW, ed.), Saunders, Philadelphia, PA, 1996, pp. 543–550.
5. Hernandez J, Morey AF. Anterior urethral injury. World J Urol 1999; 17: 96–100.
6. Mydlo JH. Surgeon experience with penile fracture. J Urol 2001; 166: 526–528.
7. Fergany AF, Angermeier KW, Montague DK. Review of Cleveland Clinic experience with penile fracture. Urology 1999; 54: 352–355.
8. Kiracofe HL, Pierce JM, Peterson NE. Management of non-penetrating distal urethral trauma. J Urol 1975; 114: 57–62.

9. Gottenger EE, Wagner JR. Penile fracture with complete urethral disruption. J Trauma 2000; 49: 339–341.
10. Pontes JE, Pierce JM. Anterior urethral injuries: four years of experience at the Detroit General Hospital. J Urol 1978; 120: 553–564.
11. Corriere JN. Editorial page 72 in Hussman DA, Boone TB, Wilson WT. Management of low velocity gunshot wounds in the anterior urethra: the role of primary repair vs urinary diversion alone. J Urol 1993; 150: 70–72.
12. Chapple CR, Png D. Contemporary management of urethral trauma and the post-traumatic stricture. Curr Opin Urol 1998; 9: 253–260.
13. Hussmann DA, Boone TB, Wilson WT. Management of low velocity gunshot wounds to the anterior urethra: the role of primary repair vs urinary diversion alone. J Urol 1993; 150: 70–72.
14. Miles BJ, Poffenberger RJ, Farah RN, Moore S. Management of penile gunshot wounds. Urology 1990; 36: 318–321.
15. Hussman DA, Wilson WT, Boone TB, Allen TD. Prostomembranous urethral disruptions: management by suprapubic cystostomy and delayed urethroplasty. J Urol 1990; 144: 76.
16. Devine PC, Devine CJ, Horton CE. Anterior urethral injuries: secondary reconstruction. Urol Clin North Am 1977; 4: 157–162.
17. Nash PA, McAninch JW, Bruce JE, Hanks DK. Sonourethrography in the evaluation of anterior urethral strictures. J Urol 1995; 154: 72–76.
18. Morey AF, McAninch JW. Role of preoperative sonourethrography in bulbar urethral reconstruction. J Urol 1997; 158: 1376–1379.
19. Albers P, Fitchner J, Bruhl P, Muller SC. Long-term results of internal urethrotomy. J Urol 1996; 156: 1611–1614.
20. Rosen MA, McAninch JW. Stricture excision and primary anastomosis for reconstruction of the anterior urethral stricture. In: Traumatic and Reconstructive Urology. (McAninch JW, ed.), Saunders, Philadelphia, PA, 1996, pp. 565–569.
21. Guralnick ML, Webster GD. The augmented anastomotic urethroplasty: indications and outcome in 29 patients. J Urol 2001; 165: 1496–1501.
22. Wessells H, Morey AF, McAninch JW. Single stage reconstruction of complex anterior urethral strictures: combined tissue transfer techniques. J Urol 1997; 157: 1271–1274.
23. Wessells H, McAninch JW. Use of free grafts in urethral stricture reconstruction. J Urol 1996; 155: 1912–1915.
24. Morey AF, McAninch JW. When and how to use buccal mucosal grafts in adult bulbar urethroplasty. Urology 1996; 48: 194–198.
25. Follis HW, Koch MO, McDougal WC. Immediate management of prostomembranous urethral disruptions. J Urol 1992; 147: 1259–1262.
26. Koraitim MM, Marzouk ME, Atta MA, Orabi SS. Risk factors and mechanism of urethral injury in pelvic fractures. Br J Urol 1996; 77: 876–880.
27. Elliott DS, Barrett DM. Long-term followup and evaluation of primary realignment of posterior urethral disruptions. J Urol 1997; 157: 814–816.
28. Webster GD. Perineal repair of membranous urethral stricture. Urol Clin North Am 1989; 16: 303–312.
29. Dixon CD. Diagnosis and acute management of posterior urethral disruptions. In: Traumatic and Reconstructive Urology. (McAninch JW, ed.), Saunders, Philadelphia, PA, 1996, pp. 347–355.
30. McAninch JW. Traumatic injuries to the urethra. J Trauma 1981; 21: 291.
31. Moudouni SM, Patard JJ, Manunta A, Guiraud P, Lobel B, Guille F. Early endoscopic realignment of post-traumatic posterior urethral disruption. Urology 2001; 57: 628–632.
32. Jepson BJ, Boullier JA, Moore RG, Parra RO. Traumatic posterior urethral injury and early primary endoscopic realignment: evaluation of long-term follow-up. Urology 1999; 53: 1205–1210.
33. Porter JR, Takayama TK, Defalco AJ. Traumatic posterior urethral injury and early realignment using magnetic urethral catheters. J Urol 1997; 158: 425–430.
34. Follis HW, Koch MO, McDougal WS. Immediate management of prostatomembranous urethral disruptions. J Urol 1992; 147: 1259–1262.

35. Kotkin L, Koch MO. Impotence and incontinence after immediate realignment of posterior urethral trauma: result of injury or management? J Urol 1996; 155: 1600–1603.
36. Morey AF, McAninch JW. Reconstruction of posterior urethral disruption injuries: outcome analysis in 82 patients. J Urol 1997; 157: 506–510.
37. Koraitim MM. Pelvic fracture urethral injuries: evaluation of various methods of management. J Urol 1996; 156: 1288–1291.
38. Dixon CM, Hricak H, McAninch JW. Magnetic resonance imaging of traumatic posterior urethral defects and pelvic crush injuries. J Urol 1992; 148: 1162–1165.
39. Morey AF, McAninch JW. Reconstruction of traumatic posterior urethral strictures. Tech Urol 1997; 3: 103–107.
40. Koraitim MM. The lessons of 145 posttraumatic posterior urethral strictures treated in 17 years. J Urol 1995; 153: 63–55.
41. Mundy AR. Urethroplasty for posterior urethral strictures. Br J Urol 1996; 78: 243–247.
42. Webster GD, Ramon J. Repair of pelvic fracture posterior urethral defects using an elaborated perineal approach: experience with 74 cases. J Urol 1991; 145: 744–748.
43. Mundy AR. Pelvic fracture injuries of the posterior urethra. World J Urol 1999; 17: 90–95.
44. Iselin CE, Webster GD. The significance of the open bladder neck associated with pelvic fracture urethral distraction defects. J Urol 1999; 162: 347–351.

5 Trauma to the External Genitalia

*George W. Jabren, MD
and Wayne J. G. Hellstrom, MD, FACS*

CONTENTS

INTRODUCTION
TESTIS
EPIDIDYMIS
SCROTUM
MANAGEMENT
OUTCOME
SUMMARY
REFERENCES

INTRODUCTION

Genitourinary injuries occur in approx 10 to 15% of patients who suffer abdominal and pelvic injuries. Trauma to the external genitalia is uncommon. Whenever trauma to the genitalia occurs, consideration of a urethral injury is prudent. Prompt diagnosis and treatment of external genital trauma aims to preserve organ structure and function and complications such as infection, hemorrhage, and urinary extravasation. In general, the ample blood supply serving the external genitalia encourages healing and prevents infection. In cases of significant genital injury and organ loss, the likelihood for severe emotional distress may warrant early psychiatric consultation.

Anatomy

The scrotum is composed of eight testis-protecting layers: skin, dartos, external spermatic fascia, cremasteric layer, internal spermatic fascia, parietal and visceral layers of the tunica vaginalis, and the tunica albuginea (Fig. 1). The dartos is a continuation of Camper's fascia. The external spermatic fascia extends from the external oblique aponeurosis, the cremasteric layer derives from the internal oblique aponeurosis, and the internal spermatic fascia continues from the transversus abdominis aponeurosis. The tunica vaginalis covers the anterior, lateral, and medial aspects of the testis. The superficial external pudendal artery divides and supplies the dartos; the scrotal artery, a branch of the internal pudendal artery, also sends collaterals to the dartos.

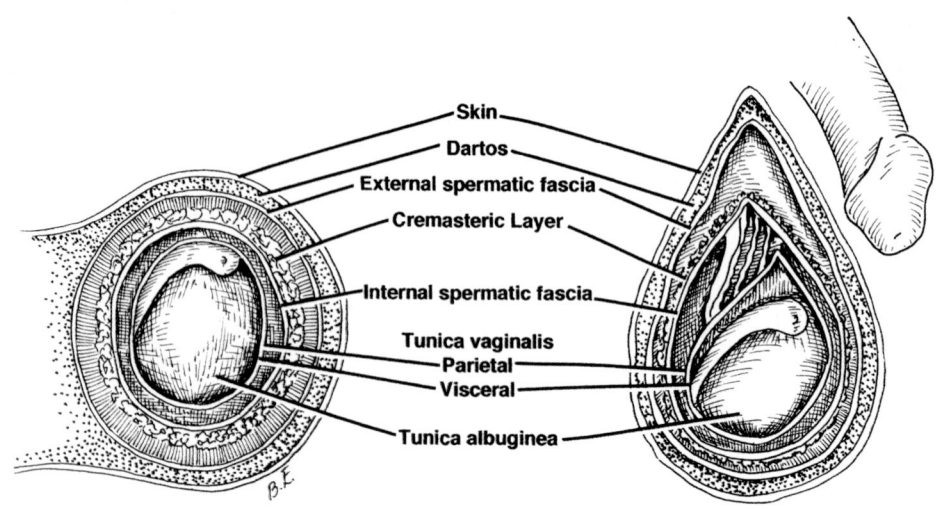

Fig. 1. Anatomical diagram of the scrotum's eight testis-protecting layers.

The main blood supply to the testis originates from the testicular artery, with additional contributions from the cremasteric and deferential arteries. The cremasteric artery is derived from the inferior epigastric artery; the deferential artery originates from the superior vesical artery. Both arteries anastomose with the testicular artery at the level of the spermatic cord near the epididymis. The paired testicular arteries originate from the aorta below the renal arteries, course down their respective spermatic cords, and enter the individual testes at the level of the mediastinum testis, where they branch to become the subcapsular tunica vascularis, which provides a capillary network to the seminiferous tubules. The testicular artery also sends a branch as the superior epididymal artery to the globus major of the epididymis. The cremasteric artery contributes perforating branches into the tunica albuginea. In addition to supplying the vas deferens, the deferential artery sends a branch as the inferior epididymal artery to the globus minor of the epididymis. The venous drainage system of the testicle generally parallels the arterial system.

History and Physical

A careful history and physical examination are mandatory after trauma to the external genitalia. A history of nausea, emesis, syncope, extreme pain, swelling, or bruising may suggest a more extensive injury than what is superficially observed. Any palpable testicular injury warrants surgical exploration. If the physical exam is equivocal, scrotal ultrasonography may provide exquisite anatomic detail of an injured genital site. However, imaging studies should not significantly delay treatment of a severe genital injury that intuitively requires surgical exploration and repair.

Physical exam may be limited by extreme swelling and pain. In rare circumstances, a spermatic cord nerve block with lidocaine injection may aid in evaluation *(1)*.

TESTIS

The natural position and structure of the testis provide protection against most episodes of trauma in life. The durability of the tunica albuginea, the mobility of the testis, and the contraction of the cremasteric muscle that results in testicular withdrawal help to circumvent injury *(2)*. Studies have shown the tunica albuginea is durable enough to withstand 50 kg of blunt trauma before rupture *(3)*.

Many cases of testicular trauma go unreported because the injured party considers the injury either minor or a source of embarrassment. Most testicular injuries are accidental blunt blows that occur during sports contests, such as from bicycle handlebars or other related straddle-type injuries. Blunt trauma is more common than penetrating trauma. The most common causes of documented trauma to the scrotum are motor vehicle accidents and gunshot wounds (GSWs)*(4)*. Cass and Luxenberg reviewed 86 patients with testicular trauma and noted 72 cases of blunt trauma and 14 GSWs *(5)*. Bilateral testicular injury represents 6% of testicular injuries *(6)*. It is 15 times more likely that bilateral testicular injuries are caused by penetrating rather than blunt trauma *(5)*.

Moore et al. *(7)* composed the Testis Injury Scale to grade the severity of testicular trauma (Table 1). Approximately 5% of cases of torsion are associated with trauma, and even minor traumatic events can initiate an episode of testicular torsion in susceptible patients. Viability remains for 96% of testicles if surgical detorsion is undertaken within 12 h of the onset of acute pain, but spermatogenesis may undergo irreversible damage if no intervention occurs within 6 h of torsion *(8–11)*. For this reason, any suspicion of torsion in these circumstances warrants prompt exploration.

Approximately 10 to 15% of testicular tumors present incidentally after scrotal trauma; however, testicular injury in itself has not been a causative agent for cancer *(12)*. Testicular neoplasms are susceptible to rupture even by minor scrotal trauma *(13)*.

Blunt Trauma

The testicular insult from blunt trauma can range from contusion to complete rupture. The most severe examples of blunt testicular trauma are crushes of the testis against the pubic bone, the thigh, or both *(14)*. Antibiotics are generally not necessary for cases of blunt trauma. Of unilateral injuries, 50% cause testicular atrophy, with resulting organ volumes measuring less than half the size of the nontraumatized testis *(15)*. Testicular atrophy occurs from a combination of resorption of necrotic tissues and ischemia induced by pressure from the edema and hematoma confined by the tunica albuginea. Atrophy can lead to a loss of spermatogenesis and reduced hormonal secretion. In addition, vas deferens obstruction occurs in up to 10% of such trauma cases *(16)*.

The most common etiology of blunt trauma to the testes is sports-related injuries and assaults *(14,17,18)*. An often-overlooked cause of blunt testicular trauma is breech vaginal delivery, especially when the birth weight is greater than 2500 g and the mother is primiparous*(19)*. Therefore, a birth history can provide important information in adult males who present with anorchia, hypogonadism, or unexplained male infertility. In addition, blunt genital self-mutilation has been documented in cases of autocastration by transsexuals and psychotic patients *(20,21)*.

Testicular Dislocation

Traumatic dislocation of the testis is the displacement of one or both testes to a position other than in the scrotum *(22)*. This phenomenon was first described by Claubry in 1818 *(23)*. This condition is distinct from retractile testis or the testis exposed from open trauma. Approximately 100 cases of testicular dislocation have been reported in the literature *(24,25)*. Sites of dislocation include pubic, superficial or deep inguinal canal, penile, preputial, perineal, superficial to the fascia lata, femoral

Table 1
American Association for the Surgery of Trauma (AAST) Organ Injury Scale
for Testicular Injury

AAST grade	Testicular injury
I	Contusion or hematoma
II	Subclinical laceration of tunica albuginea
III	Laceration of tunica albuginea with <50% parenchymal loss
IV	Major laceration of tunica albuginea with ≥50% parenchymal loss
V	Total testicular destruction or avulsion

From ref. 7.

canal, abdominal cavity, and the acetabulum *(26)*. The patient typically complains of severe pain, and examination reveals an empty hemiscrotum and abnormal testicular location. Dislocation can result in torsion of the testis, testicular rupture, and intratesticular hemorrhage.

Sports-Related Injury

Although sports activities are common causes of blunt trauma to the external genitalia, testis injuries are somewhat rare in team sports. McAleer et al. reviewed 14,763 trauma cases and noted 0.11% testicular injuries *(27)*. Of these testicular injuries, only 25% were caused by team sports. All testicular injuries in this study were explored and repaired if indicated, with a 100% salvage rate.

The American Academy of Pediatrics guidelines for sports participation incur no restrictions on the patient with a solitary testis for both contact and noncontact sports except for the use of a protective genital cup in certain high-risk sports *(28)*. Dorsen, on the contrary, in 1986 recommended that young patients with a solitary testis engage only in noncontact sports because of the higher risk of anorchia if severe trauma were to occur *(29)*. Medicolegal aspects are an issue that need to be discussed with each patient individually.

Besides team sports, aggressive bicycle riding has been associated with trauma to the external genitalia.

Using scrotal ultrasound, Frauscher et al. showed a higher prevalence of extratesticular and testicular disorders in extreme mountain cyclists (94%) compared with noncyclists (16%) *(30)*. Of noncyclists, 16% demonstrated benign epididymal cysts; the extreme mountain cyclists more often had scrotal calculi (81%), epididymal cysts (46%), epididymal calcifications (40%), testicular calcifications (32%), hydroceles (28%), varicoceles (11%), and testicular microlithiasis (1%). Calcifications within the scrotum may be a consequence of tunica vaginalis inflammation, appendix testis or appendix epididymis torsion, or hematomas resulting from microtrauma induced from bicycle seat vibration and shocks *(31)*.

Penetrating Trauma

Assault Related

The most common cause of penetrating injury to the external genitalia is GSWs *(4,32)*. Approximately 35% of GSWs result in genital injury *(33)*. Bilateral testicular injuries occur in as many as 31% of penetrating trauma cases to this region of the body *(34)*.

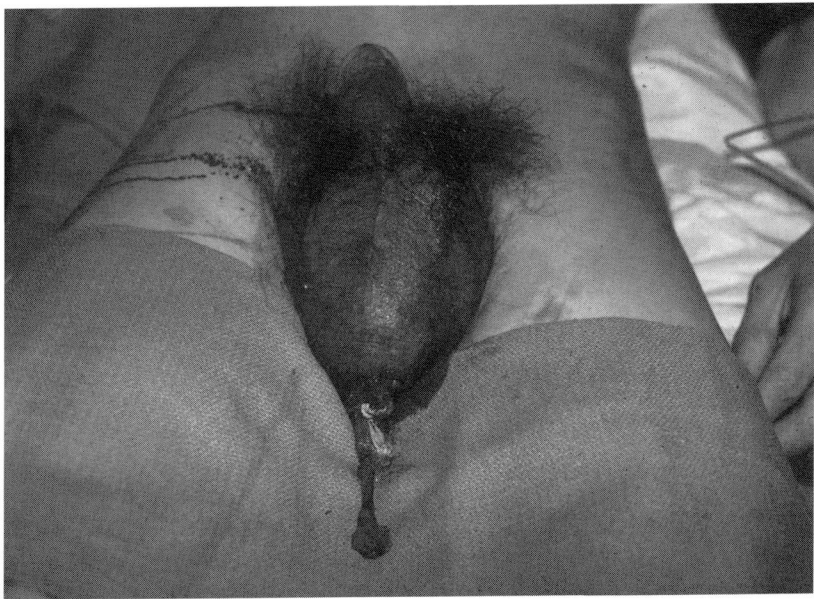

Fig. 2. A gunshot wound to the scrotum with a low-velocity projectile.

Most civilian GSWs involve handguns with low-velocity projectiles (>1000 ft/s), which possess only enough energy to damage tissue within their trajectory (Fig. 2). High-velocity weapons of war (>1000 ft/s) cause significant destruction to surrounding tissues because the projectile transmits radially emitted energy along its pathway. Shotguns are considered low-velocity weapons with projectiles that possess high mass. Thus, they can potentially damage more tissue than a single low-velocity missile.

Bickel et al. reported a 94% rate of associated injuries with penetrating scrotal trauma *(35)*; Monga et al. revealed that 50% of GSW victims suffered associated injuries *(33)*. The most commonly associated injuries involve the thigh (75%), penis (37%), perineum (25%), urethra (18%), abdomen, femoral vein, femur, and extraperitoneal bowel in the form of a direct inguinal hernia *(16,35)*. Hence, appropriate consultation with a general or vascular surgeon is prudent in these cases.

Although it is rare for mortality to occur among civilians who suffer from isolated GSWs to the external genitalia or genital injuries associated with soft tissue damage, the mortality rate has been reported as high as 24.7% when high-velocity weapons of war are involved, mainly because of associated major injuries to the thorax, abdomen, and limbs *(36–41)*. During the Vietnam War, of 214 patients documented at four hospitals with genitourinary injuries, the scrotal injury rate was 25.4%; the scrotal injury rate was 1.06% of all injuries reported at these hospitals *(36)*. Of 24,865 hospitalized patients from 1991 to 1993 in the war in Croatia, 2.4% of injuries were to the genitourinary system, with 22.7% of these scrotal and genital injuries *(42)*.

SELF-MUTILATION

Testicular injuries can be caused by genital self-mutilation *(43)*. In fact, 50% of individuals in these cases are successful in removing one or both testicles (Fig. 3) *(44)*. Lewis termed autocastration the "Eshmun complex" after the Phoenician god of spring, who castrated himself to avoid the advances of the mother goddess Astronae *(45,46)*.

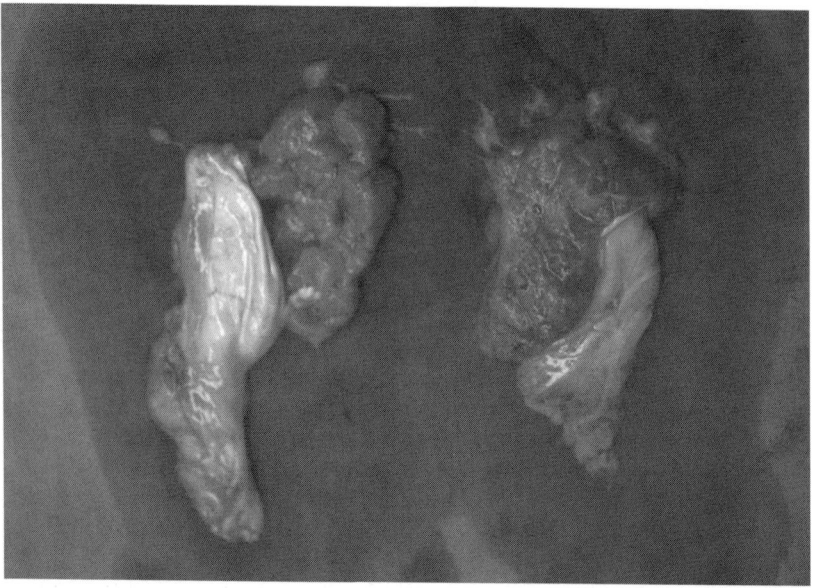

Fig. 3. Genital self-mutilation often involves unilateral or even bilateral autocastration.

Genital self-mutilation injuries are generally isolated, but on occasion have been associated with injury to other body parts *(47)*.

Greilsheimer and Groves reviewed 52 cases of genital self-mutilation and noted that 87% of patients suffered from psychosis, ranging from functional psychosis to brain damage. Of the cases, 13% were nonpsychotic individuals with fanatical cultural or religious beliefs, character disorders, or transvestitism *(48)*. Interestingly, 20% of these patients presented with a prior history of self-destruction involving their external genitalia.

Aboseif et al. reviewed 14 patients with 19 self-inflicted injuries, ranging from simple genital skin lacerations to penectomy and orchiectomy *(43)*. Of the patients in this study, 65% had psychosis, and 55% had a history of alcohol or drug abuse. Three patients had performed a unilateral orchiectomy, and 5 patients succeeded at bilateral orchiectomy. Management of these complex patients requires the combined efforts of both urologists and psychiatrists.

Testicular Rupture

The first report of traumatic testicular rupture was by Cotton in 1905 *(49)*. This occurs more commonly with penetrating (31%) than with blunt trauma (1.5%) *(6,50,51)*. One study by Cass and Luxenberg documented that the risk of rupture after blunt testicular trauma was as high as 50% *(5)*. In blunt trauma, the mechanism involves the testis pressing against the thigh or pubic arch, with subsequent tunica albuginea rupture and extrusion of seminiferous tubules *(14)*. Disruption of the tunica albuginea can result in solitary longitudinal or transverse tears, stellate tears, or complete destruction of the testis. Traumatic fractures of the testis most often occur in 10- to 30-yr-old males involved in sports-related activities *(2,16)*. All cases of suspected testicular fracture need expedient surgical exploration to preserve both anatomy and function *(14)*.

Chapter 5 / External Genital Trauma 77

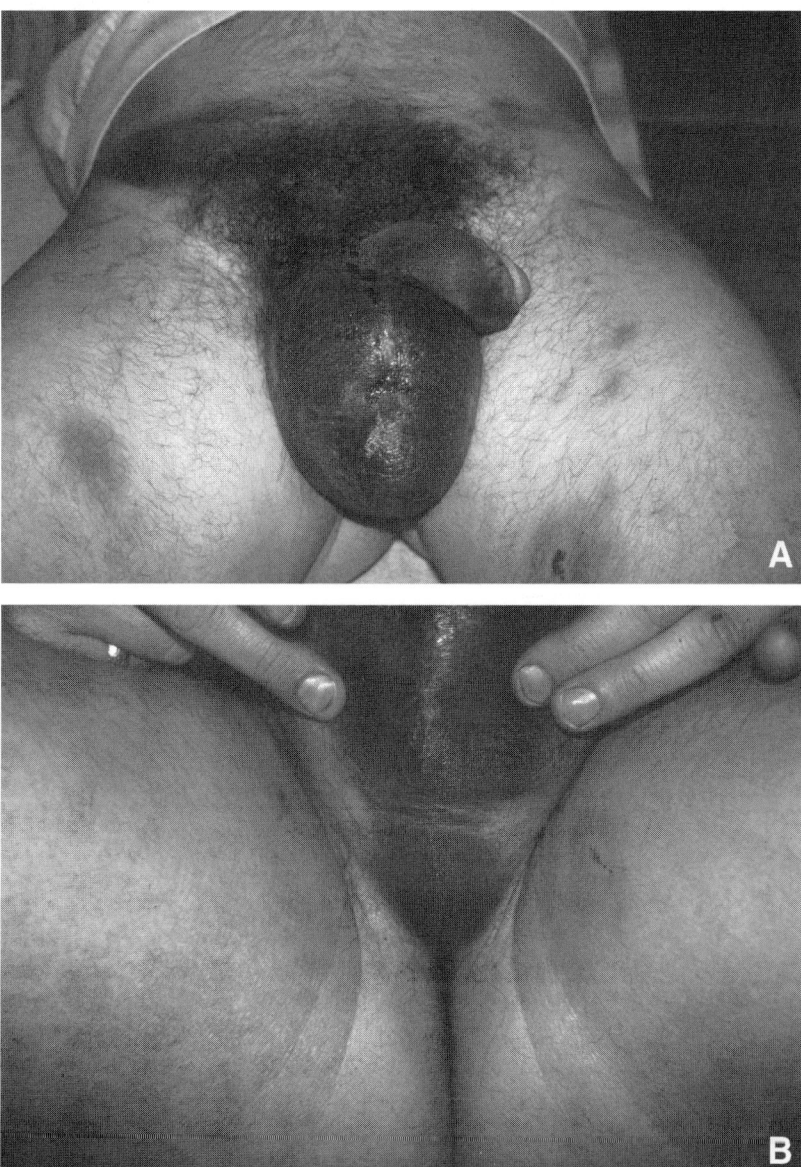

Fig. 4. A patient with blunt trauma to the external genitalia. Intrascrotal bleeding confined by Colles' fascia can be seen extending into (**A**) the lower abdomen and (**B**) perineum after Buck's fascia was perforated.

Hematocele

Approximately 80% of hematoceles are caused by testicular rupture *(16)*. With fracture of the tunica albuginea, delicate vessels located within the testicular parenchyma leak blood between the visceral and parietal layers of the tunica vaginalis to cause a hematocele. Large hematoceles usually complicate testicular palpation. After scrotal trauma, a tender, firm scrotal mass on physical exam that fails to transilluminate suggests a hematocele *(52)*. If the parietal layer ruptures as well, both blood and seminiferous tubules can extend into the groin and perineum (Fig. 4) *(53)*. If the blood dissects into the dartos and skin, scrotal ecchymosis will be present. In this circumstance, the examiner cannot assume that scrotal ecchymosis after trauma is caused by damage only to the superficial skin and dartos tissues. Further imaging studies are warranted in these situations to rule out rupture of the tunica albuginea.

Imaging

SCROTAL ULTRASOUND

Despite the use of analgesia or anesthesia in a stable patient, physical examination after trauma to the external genitalia may remain equivocal because of swelling. In these situations, use of scrotal ultrasonography with color Doppler can provide the urologist with invaluable information for deciding between conservative and surgical management *(54)*. This imaging modality is noninvasive and readily available and can be performed with minimal discomfort to the patient. First-hand review of the ultrasound studies by the clinician is imperative because ultrasonography is operator dependent.

Of the 17 testicular injuries caused by GSWs reported by Monga et al., two patients had a normal physical exam but had abnormal scrotal ultrasound studies *(33)*. A few authorities regard ultrasound as unreliable and inconsistent *(55,56)*. However, most consider scrotal ultrasound to have superior sensitivity *(57,58)*. In a number of studies, this imaging modality has correctly predicted normality and abnormality of the testis in up to 94% of patients with scrotal trauma *(59)*.

Although loss of tunica albuginea continuity may be assessed by ultrasound, a discrete testicular rupture through the tunica albuginea is demonstrated in only 20% of ruptures because of the thin nature of this layer *(60)*. A normal testicle has evidence of smooth parenchyma, but internal echoes and testicular heterogeneity is usually seen in cases of testicular rupture in addition to the irregular testicular margin because of intratesticular hemorrhage, ischemia, infarct, or tissue disruption (Fig. 5) *(61,62)*. Moreover, a hematocele can be easily identified with ultrasound. In the patient with a history of prior orchidopexy or hydrocelectomy, a testicular rupture may not present as easily with an associated hematocele *(12)*. Color Doppler can evaluate perfusion to the testis in these circumstances.

NUCLEAR MEDICINE

Technetium 99m pertechnetate radionuclide imaging has been used for evaluation of external genital trauma. However, this nuclear medicine scan is not routinely utilized for trauma evaluation because of time factors that may delay exploration and emergent management *(63)*. With this imaging modality, testicular rupture presents with increased uptake in the surrounding soft tissues, which represents inflammation and hyperemia; the central photodeficient area corresponds to a hematocele and necrosis of the parenchymal tissues *(64)*.

EPIDIDYMIS

After blunt or penetrating trauma, epididymitis or a hematoma of the epididymis may occur. Both epididymal ruptures *(18)* and epididymal avulsion injuries are rare *(65,66)*.

SCROTUM

Scrotal injury can range from contusion to complete avulsion of the overlying skin. The severity of scrotal injury can be gauged by Moore's Scrotal Injury Scale *(7)* and is based on the potential threat to the patient's life (Table 2).

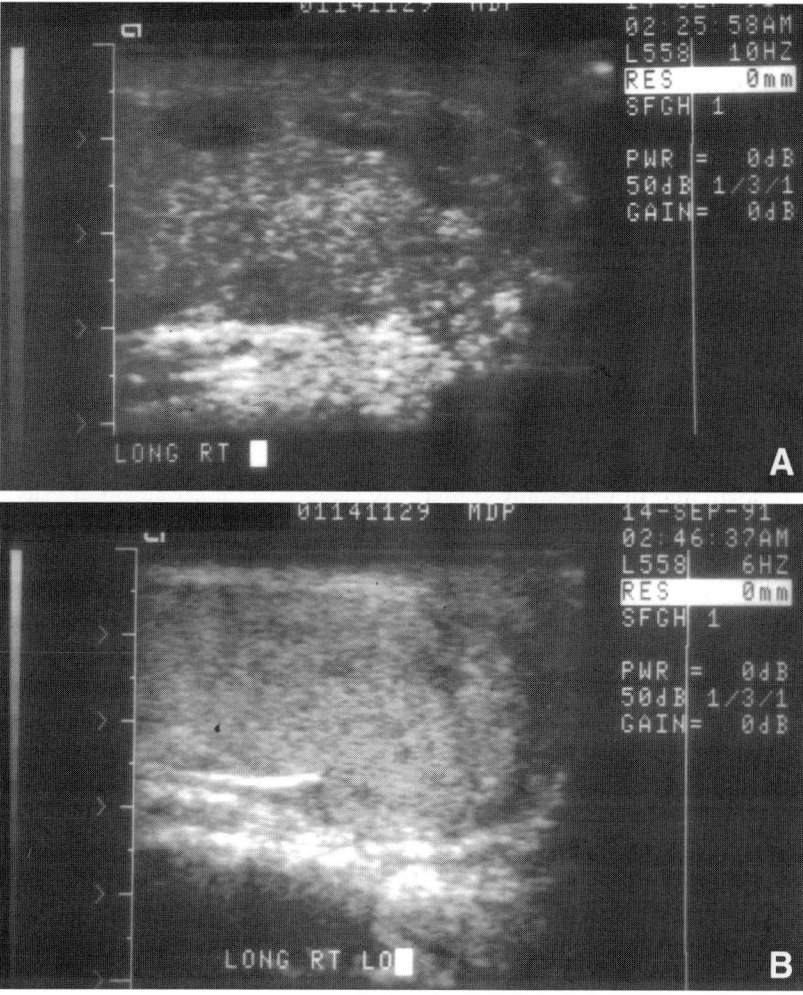

Fig. 5. (A) and (B) Ultrasound findings of testicular rupture include heterogeneous echogenicity of testicular parenchyma and a disruption in the tunica albuginea border.

Intrascrotal Hematoma

The scrotum is a unique anatomic structure because its inherent distensibility and viscoelasticity prevent intrascrotal bleeding to be adequately tamponaded. These same properties, in addition to its native location between the thighs, help to protect the scrotum and its contents from injury. Intrascrotal hematoma is a common postoperative complication that can occur after any scrotal procedure, including hydrocelectomy, orchiectomy, and epididymectomy. Even minor capillary bleeding, if left untreated, can evolve into a major intrascrotal hematoma with the potential for significant pain and infection.

Scrotal hematomas have even been reported after extracorporeal shock wave lithotripsy of distal ureteral calculi *(67)*. Hematomas in these cases resolve spontaneously with conservative management. Prevention against intrascrotal hematomas with this modality can be accomplished by maintaining the water level in the bath above the level of the scrotum or by altering the air–fluid interface at the scrotum with a wet towel *(67)*.

Table 2
American Association for the Surgery of Trauma (AAST) Organ Injury Scale
for Scrotal Injury

AAST grade	Scrotal injury
I	Contusion
II	Laceration <25% of scrotal diameter
III	Laceration ≥25% of scrotal diameter
IV	Avulsion <50%
V	Avulsion = 50%

From ref. 7.

Bites to Genitalia

Patients bitten in the genital region by animals or humans need prompt attention (Fig. 6). Approximately 85% of bites harbor pathogens *(68)*. Canine bites affect 129 of every 10,000 individuals in the United States *(69)*. Dog attacks lead to 10 to 20 deaths in the United States each year, and the victims are usually children *(68)*. Cummings and Boullier reported on seven patients with scrotal dog bites, but none of the patients had involvement of the testes or spermatic cords, and no major reconstruction was required *(70)*.

Infection occurs in 6 to 13% of all dog bites and 20 to 25% of puncture wounds *(71)*. *Pasteurella* organisms are the most common pathogens cultured from dog and cat bites, but anaerobic organisms may also be present *(72)*. Although *Staphylococcus aureus* and *Streptococcus pyogenes* are common pathogens in cutaneous infections, they are uncommon in bites *(72)*. Dog bites are known to transmit blastomycosis, brucellosis, cat scratch disease, erysipeloid, lymphocytic choriomeningitis, leptospirosis, melioidosis, pasteurellosis, rabies, tetanus, tularemia, and yersiniosis *(73)*. When fever occurs in an immunocompromised patient after a dog bite, *Capnocytophaga canimorsus* is the likely responsible pathogen *(68)*. Thus, consultation with an infectious disease specialist may be warranted in such circumstances.

Infections occur more often from human bites than from dog bite wounds. *Eikenella corrodens* is commonly cultured in human bite wounds *(72)*. Moreover, human bites have been reported to spread actinomycosis, hepatitis B and C, herpes simplex virus, human immunodeficiency virus (HIV), tetanus, toxic shock syndrome, and tuberculosis *(74)*.

Laceration/Avulsion

Scrotal trauma can vary in severity from abrasions, to lacerations, to complete avulsion. Forms of trauma involving the scrotum range from blunt trauma to penetrating trauma, sometimes involving off-label sexual devices. Avulsion of the scrotum has been reported both with power machinery, when clothing may become entrapped in moving parts, and with deceleration injuries involving bicycles, motorcycles, and other motorized vehicles, in which the scrotum becomes trapped by a stationary object. Because of the viscoelastic nature of the scrotum, most cases of scrotal avulsion involve only the skin and dartos, leaving the external spermatic fascia intact over the testes. Hence, avulsions rarely affect the testis or spermatic cord. During some aberrant sexual practices, scrotal skin injury occurs from constricting bands involving the scrotum or scrotal weighted harnesses.

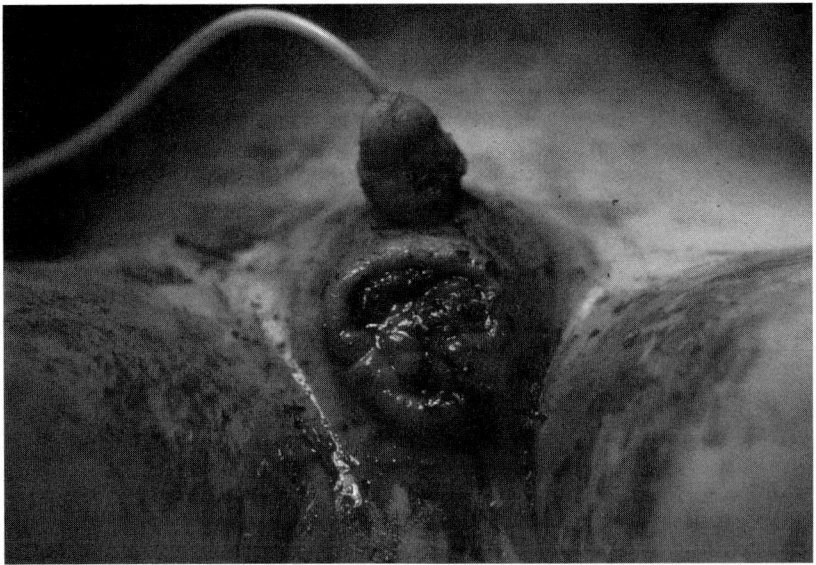

Fig. 6. A dog bite wound to the scrotum.

Burns

Between 2.8 and 5% of patients hospitalized for burns have genital and perineal involvement *(75,76)*. The percentage (13%) of perineal burns requiring hospitalization is higher in the military *(77)*. Fortunately, burn deaths are rarely related only to genital or perineal locations *(75)*.

The depth of the burn is important in management of these injuries and can be classified by three degrees of severity. First-degree burns manifest with erythema and involve only the epidermis, which allows for some maintenance of protection. Second-degree burns involve all of the epidermis and part of the dermis and often present with blisters. Both first- and second-degree burns possess viable tissue, which over time will reepithelialize. Third-degree burns are full-thickness injuries involving all of the epidermis and dermis. There is no evidence of capillary refill or sensation. These burns present as white, brown, black, or red and in essence are nonviable tissues in need of debridement and grafting.

Three main types of scrotal burns are encountered in clinical practices: thermal, chemical, and electrical. Thermal flame and scald burns account for the majority of these injuries *(75)*. Unfortunately, the urologist must be made aware that child abuse has been identified in 46% of boys and 48% of girls younger than 2 yr old who present with scald burns involving the perineum or external genitalia *(78)*. Although thermal and chemical burns can cause significant damage to the skin, it is the injury from electrical burns, which can affect deeper layers and organs of tissue, that can be most problematic. Electricity passes through the body from an initial contact focus to an area of exit. Although electrical burns may have the appearance of only a small superficial skin injury, the energy involved may destroy the organs and vessels deep within the scrotum by coagulative necrosis.

Radiation-Induced Injury

Penoscrotal edema is recognized to occur in up to 1% of cases of external beam radiotherapy. This prevalence can increase to between 5 and 20% if the patient has had prior pelvic lymphadenectomy *(79,80)*. The perilymphatic fibrosis obliterates lymphatic vessels and veins, causing a state of chronic lymphedema.

MANAGEMENT

Conservative Therapy

For uncomplicated scrotal contusion consisting of intrascrotal hematoma and ecchymosis without injury to the scrotal contents, treatment involves compression with a scrotal support, elevation, ice packs, and analgesics *(4)*. Attempts at evacuating posttraumatic scrotal hematomas are fraught with more bleeding and difficulties because of blood infiltration through the many scrotal layers rather than formation of a defined collection. An exception is the large scrotal hematoma that occurs after transcrotal surgery. In this postoperative situation, the hematoma can be evacuated by opening up the prior scrotal incision, and the active bleeding site can be identified and controlled.

Prevention of postoperative hematomas can be accomplished by using a tight scrotal support. Some choose to use an X-shaped scrotal dressing. Oesterling described a method to decrease postoperative scrotal hematomas and edema substantially by suturing the scrotal skin to the lower abdominal wall over a 4-in. gauze roll with polypropylene sutures for a period of 24 h with subsequent use of a scrotal support *(81)*. A number of authors have described circumferential and turban dressings to accomplish this same goal *(82–84)*. Others routinely use open or closed drainage systems after transcrotal surgery to obliterate the dead space and drain any accumulated blood. For the most part, drains do not necessarily prevent the occurrence of scrotal hematomas postoperatively.

Scrotal Laceration/Avulsion

Superficial scrotal lacerations involving only the skin and dartos are easily debrided and closed primarily (Fig. 7). Perioperative antibiotics are commonly used. Penetration deep to the dartos layer necessitates surgical exploration. Broad-spectrum antibiotics are given to all penetrating injury cases. Gross contamination of the wound involves debridement, copious irrigation, routine dressing changes, and delayed closure of the scrotum.

Scrotal avulsions with less than 60% superficial skin loss are treated like lacerations with primary or delayed closure (Fig. 8). Avulsed tissue can be salvaged if a vascularized pedicle remains after debridement. In severe scrotal avulsions, saline packs are placed on the affected area emergently, and an attempt is made to determine the demarcation between viable and nonviable tissue, which will require excision. If the area of demarcation is not apparent, reevaluation after 48 h may be necessary. Once demarcation is identified, debridement and primary skin closure are accomplished. Urinary and fecal diversion are sometimes needed in complex scrotal avulsion cases to prevent wound contamination.

If an avulsed scrotum cannot be closed primarily, the testicles can be placed in the superiomedial thigh by creating subcutaneous pouches *(85)*. The testes must be placed as posterior as possible in these thigh pouches to prevent pulling on the spermatic cords. Bertini and Corriere, on the contrary, recommended saline-moistened gauze only to cover exposed testes in cases of scrotal avulsion to provide a cool, protected environment *(4)*.

Chapter 5 / External Genital Trauma

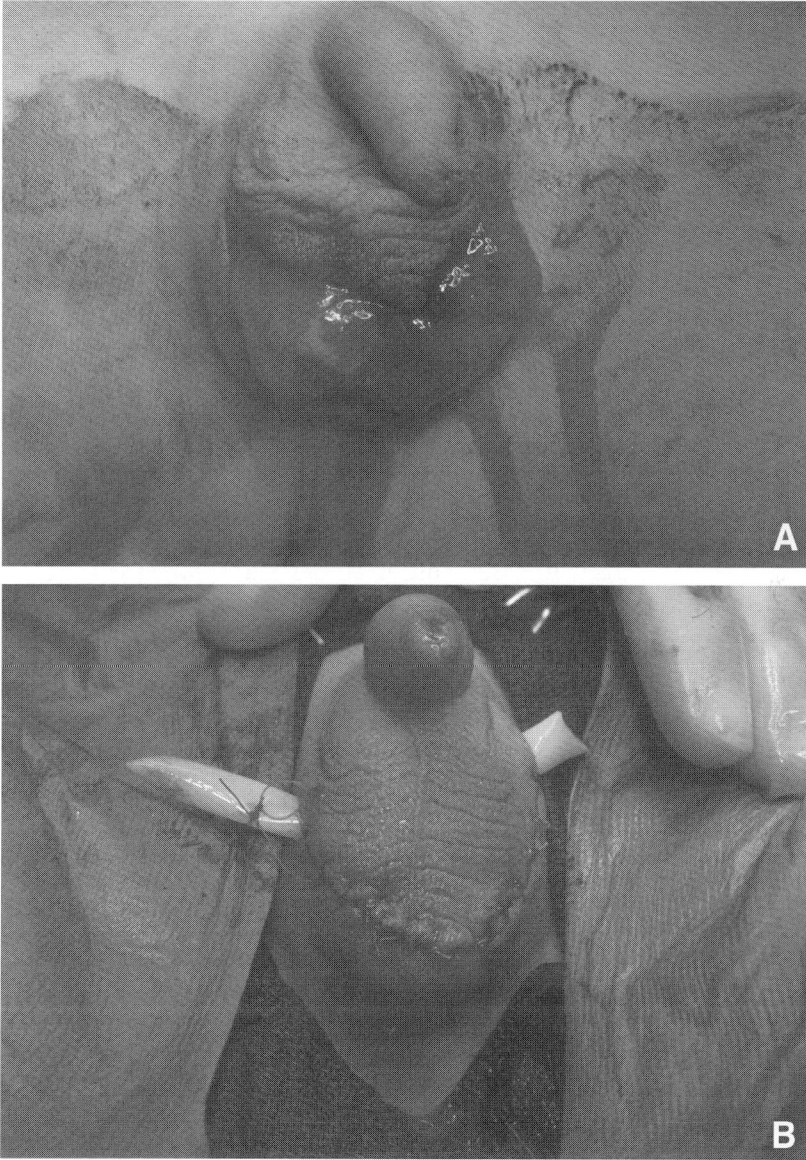

Fig. 7. (**A**) A child's scrotal laceration caused by blunt trauma from a fall. (**B**) The wound is closed primarily, and a penrose drain is left in place.

In cases of avulsions involving more than 60% of the scrotum, scrotal reconstruction is performed using either a meshed split-thickness skin graft (STSG) or a flap. If these severe cases were allowed to heal by only secondary intention, the testes would become immobile in scar tissue. Covering such a large defect can be executed primarily or delayed for 2 wk, depending on the patient's condition and the viability of the remaining scrotal tissue.

SPLIT-THICKNESS SKIN GRAFT

Balakrishnan first reported the use of the STSG to cover scrotal defects in 1956 *(86)*. The STSG contains epidermis and part of the dermis. The take or viability of an STSG depends

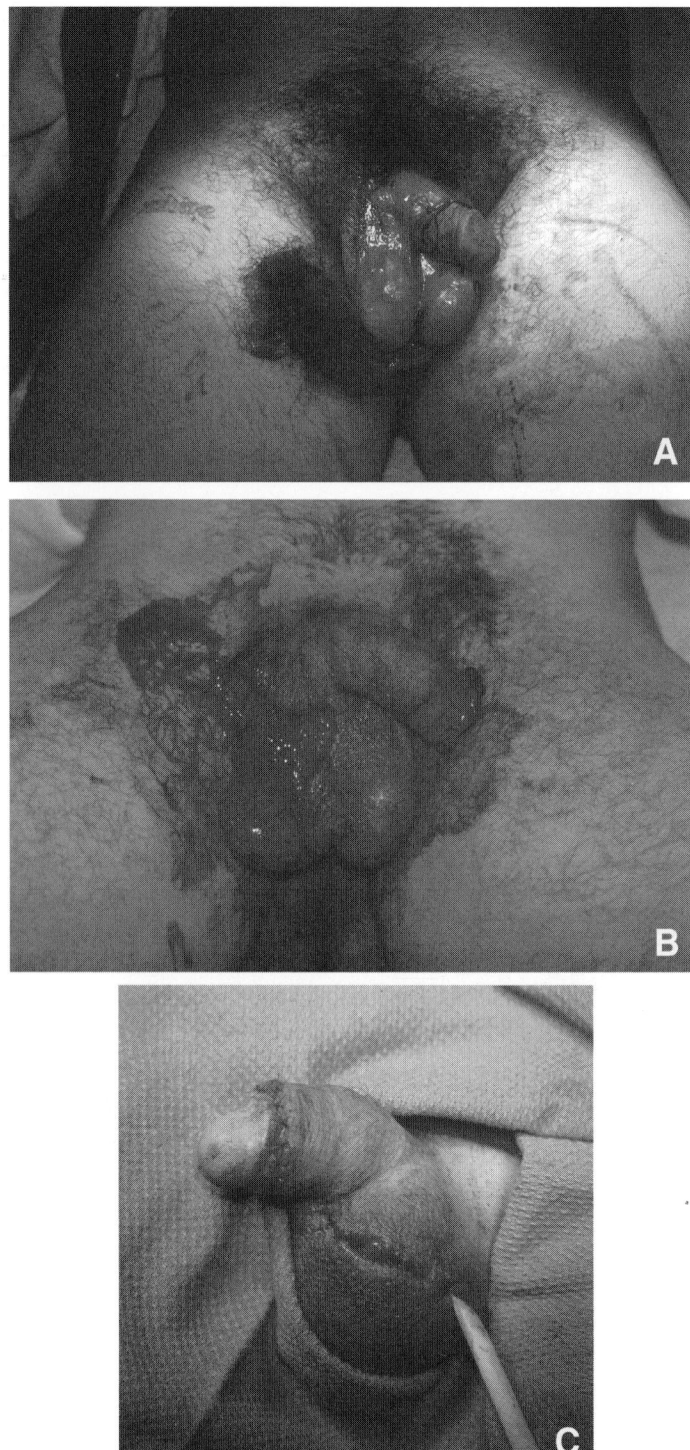

Fig. 8. (**A**) Avulsion of the external genitalia caused by farm power machinery. (**B**) Injury to the scrotum and penis from a circular saw with the defect reapproximated primarily and (**C**) with a penrose drain left in place.

on plasmatic inhibition and inosculation. During plasmatic inhibition, which lasts approx 48 h, the graft absorbs nutrients and water from its host plasma bed and remains relatively dry and hypothermic. During inosculation, the host bed and graft vessels make contact, allowing angiogenesis to begin, hydrating the graft, and ensuring isothermia.

Using a pneumatic dermatome, anterior thigh STSGs are harvested at 0.014 to 0.018 in. thickness, and the tissue is meshed 2:1 *(87)*. Meshing the STSG has a number of benefits:

1. It mimics the scrotal rugae on healing.
2. It increases the graft surface area without compromising donor site pain and cosmesis.
3. It allows exudates to drain from the host bed.

Any granulation tissue is excised from the testes, and the testes are sutured together in the midline to prevent migration from the graft. The testes are placed dependently to encourage expansion of the graft into the form of a scrotum. The STSG covers the anterior and posterior aspects of the testicles and is pexed to both the perineum and the ventral penis. After application of the meshed STSG, antibiotic petroleum gauze is applied to the wound and covered by dry fluff gauze for 5 d to ensure its take. On the fifth day, the dressing is removed.

Bed rest generally is required for 5 d postoperatively to provide for graft immobilization. Urinary diversion via urethral catheter or suprapubic cystostomy is employed for 2 wk after grafting to prevent graft contamination. The patient is not allowed to engage in any strenuous activity for at least 6 wk, and he should refrain from sexual intercourse for 3 mo.

FLAPS

In special cases, a superomedial thigh flap or a gracilis myocutaneous flap can be used to reconstruct the scrotum. The testes are ideal to expand the neoscrotum. Some surgeons have used tissue expanders to form a two-compartment scrotum, but these are time-consuming maneuvers *(88)*.

Bilateral superomedial thigh flaps are advantageous because of the excellent blood supply and similar innervation and hair-bearing appearance to the native scrotum *(87)*. These pedicles are based on the external pudendal, obturator, and medial circumflex arteries, as well as the genitofemoral and the ilioinguinal nerves. These flaps require loose thigh skin and only a small amount of subcutaneous tissue, and the testes are sutured in the midline as in the placement of STSGs *(87)*.

The gracilis myocutaneous flap has also been used to reconstruct the scrotum *(89,90)*. However, this particular procedure is more difficult to perform and gives a poorer cosmetic result for the neoscrotum.

Burns

Assessment of both burn depth and type is important in determining management. Initial treatment begins with fluid resuscitation and infection control. Urethral catheterization is used to measure urine output, but is discontinued as soon as the initial resuscitation is completed. Few complications occur when catheters are used in patients with genital and perineal burns *(91)*. Fecal diversion is not generally needed. Tetanus immunization status should not be omitted. For first- and second-degree thermal burns, conservative therapy is recommended. Treatment requires gentle irrigation of the affected area with cool water. All hair in affected areas is shaved, and bullae greater than 2 cm are excised to prevent infection. Antibiotic creams (1% silver sulfadiazine, 0.5% silver nitrate, or mafenide acetate) are needed for both deep second- and third-degree burns. If there is uncertainty whether the burn is second or third degree, the wound can be conservatively managed for up to 3 wk and then reevaluated.

Third-degree burns will not heal spontaneously and will require eschar excision and STSG. Third-degree burns to the external genitalia are managed in a similar manner to third-degree burns in other areas of the body. In a study by Michielsen et al., only 9.9% of patients with perineal and genital burns required STSG (75).

Chemical burns are copiously irrigated with saline to remove any substances not yet fixed to the tissues. Sodium bicarbonate is used if the burn is caused by an acid, and dilute acetic acid is used if it is caused by an alkaline agent. Subsequent treatment of chemical burns is similar to that for thermal burns.

Conservative management should be employed with electrical burns for the first 24 h to identify viable tissue and nonviable eschar. Further treatment of these wounds is similar to that for thermal burns.

Radiation-Induced Injury

For chronic lymphedema caused by radiation therapy, conservative management is recommended in the majority of cases. Initial treatment consists of scrotal elevation and a firm scrotal support. If the scrotal edema becomes unmanageable or there is evidence of necrosis, the affected tissue may be excised and STSG employed.

Bites

The initial treatment of bites includes local debridement of devitalized tissue, irrigation with normal saline or povidone-iodine, antibiotic prophylaxis, tetanus immunization, and in certain cases, rabies immunization (92). High-pressure irrigation with copious volumes of irrigant decreases the concentration of bacteria. Wound cultures after bites are of little value because they rarely correlate with an infection if it does develop (68). Amoxicillin-clavulanic acid or a first-generation cephalosporin is commonly used for antibiotic prophylaxis (70,93).

Patients who have had two or fewer primary tetanus immunizations receive both tetanus immunoglobulin and tetanus toxoid (68). For those patients who completed a primary immunization series but had not had a booster within 5 yr, tetanus toxoid alone is needed (68). When rabies prophylaxis is indicated because an animal was either rabid or not captured, the rabies immunoglobulin and five doses of human rabies vaccine are given (68). In human bites, HIV, hepatitis, and syphilis screens need to be tested and prophylaxis initiated if there is a high risk of transmission.

Bite wounds are closed primarily if there is minimal skin loss, but are left open if they occurred more than 6 to 12 h prior to presentation (68). If there is significant tissue loss and no infection presents after a few days of observation, a meshed STSG can be used (73).

Scrotal Exploration

The goals of scrotal exploration are hemostasis, prevention of infection, and preservation of hormonal function, fertility, micturition, and psychological well-being of the patient. Hematoceles, intratesticular hematomas, and testicular ruptures are explored and repaired (14,94–98). Early operative intervention in such cases is recommended because of higher rates of testicular salvage, lower incidences of infection and necrosis, decreased pain, shorter hospital stays, and more rapid recovery (2,5,15,17,34,95,97–101).

In theory, early exploration may diminish the risk of immune reactions to testicular tissue with subsequent formation of antisperm antibodies.

Cass documented an orchiectomy rate of only 9% for early exploration and repair vs 45% in delayed procedures (2). In another series, testicular salvage was 80% if exploration occurred within 3 d of the injury, but less than 33% when more than 9 d had passed (95). Schuster showed that a delay in diagnosis and surgery increased the orchiectomy rate eightfold (18).

As a rule, penetrating scrotal traumas that enter deep to the dartos fascia or are associated with scrotal swelling need to be explored. In the study by Monga et al., only 8% of a series of 36 scrotal GSWs had injury that would have been ruled out by physical exam alone, and all patients underwent exploration (33). Testicular salvage is between 35 and 65% when the GSW involves the spermatic cord (16,35,102). When injury to the vas deferens and epididymis is encountered, most experts suggest delayed microsurgical repair to allow for inflammation to subside (16,99).

A transverse scrotal skin incision is commonly used for unilateral exploration, but a longitudinal median raphe approach is used for a bilateral scrotal exploration. During exploration, the testes, epididymes, and spermatic cords are completely exposed and examined (Fig. 9). For all penetrating injuries, irrigation with normal saline and sometimes bacitracin, as well as a search for any foreign bodies, must be performed because penetrating wounds can bring dirt, clothing, and other materials into the scrotum. Draining sinuses are consequences of residual foreign materials (4).

If the tunica vaginalis is injured without damage to the tunica albuginea, a penrose drain is placed, and the skin is closed primarily. Hematoceles are drained to prevent compression injury to the testicular parenchyma, which can lead to subsequent atrophy and necrosis. In 1937, Campbell first described debridement of necrotic tubules with reapproximation of the tunica albuginea for testicular rupture (103). For testicular disruptions, the extruded seminiferous tubules are debrided, any intratesticular hematoma is drained, and the tunica albuginea is closed with a running 4-0 absorbable suture. Even small tunical tears without appearance of testicular extrusion need to be repaired because intratesticular swelling after trauma can cause further extrusion of seminiferous tubules (14). If the tunica albuginea cannot be reapproximated after debridement, intratesticular tissue may be shaved off or a small patch of the tunica vaginalis can be used to cover the defect (104). If there is complete testicular destruction, testicular abscess, or ischemic necrosis of the testis, orchiectomy is the only option.

Some surgeons leave a drain in all explorations; others use drains only when hemostasis is an issue (105). Closure with 3-0 or 4-0 absorbable vertical mattress sutures is optimal for skin closure, with overlying scrotal fluff gauze and a scrotal support. If a penrose drain is placed, it can usually be removed 24 h postoperatively. Postoperative antibiotics are continued as long as the drain is left in.

The Dislocated Testis

Immediate surgical relocation is recommended for the dislocated testis because delayed treatment may be associated with testicular atrophy and infertility (106–108). Manual reduction is often difficult because of associated local edema unless the testis is palpable in the upper scrotum; in this instance, an attempt may be made for manual reduction after sedating the patient (109). If this maneuver fails or the testis is nonpalpable, exploration, relocation, and orchidopexy are recommended (110).

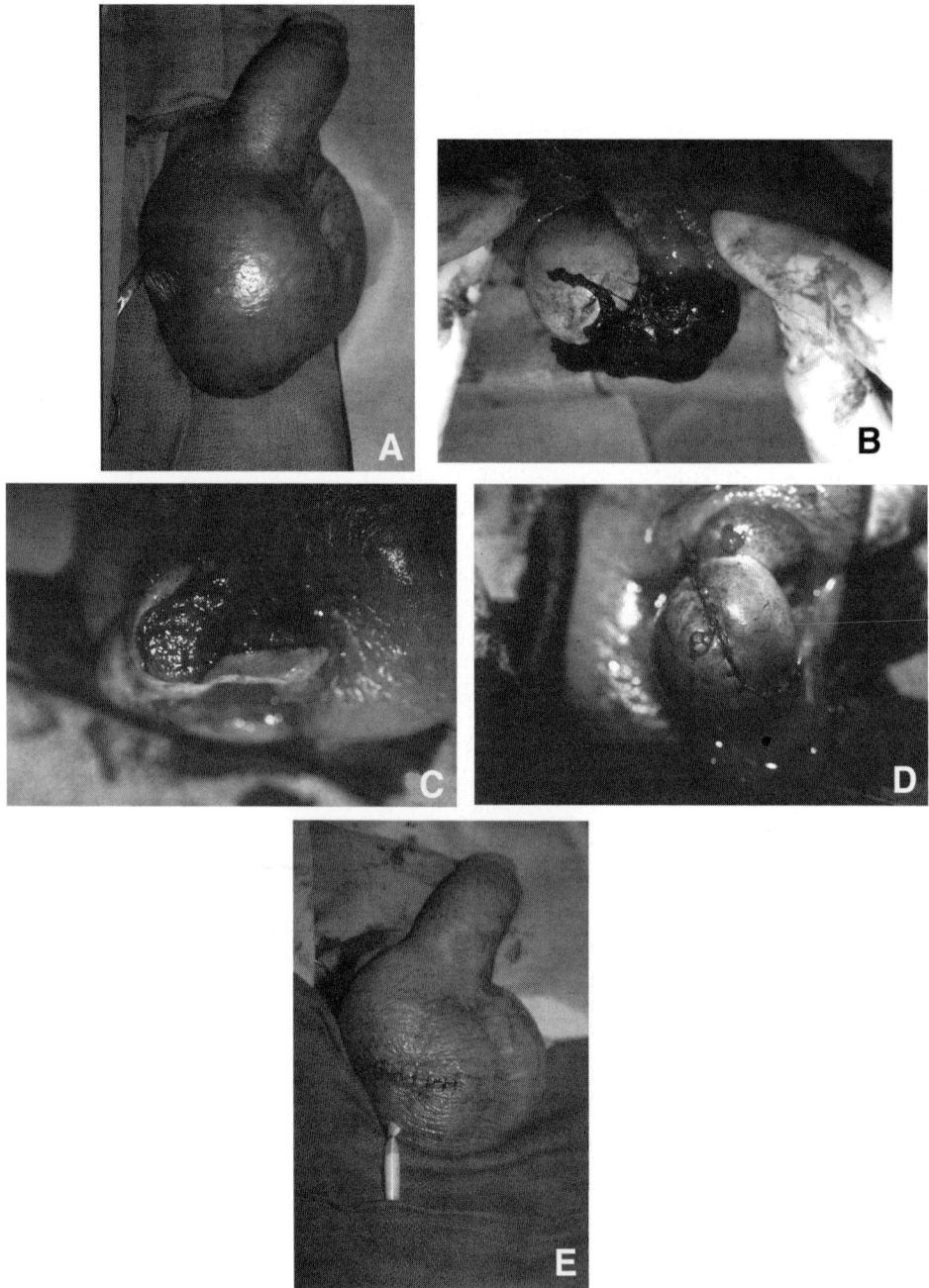

Fig. 9. (A) Blunt scrotal trauma, resulting in testicular rupture **(B)** with extrusion of necrotic seminiferous tubules. **(C)** Necrotic tubules have been debrided. **(D)** The tunica albuginea is closed primarily with running 4-0 absorbable suture. **(E)** The scrotal skin is then reapproximated, and a 0.25-in. penrose drain is left in place.

Testicular Reimplantation

In the case of traumatic orchiectomy with a sharply cut spermatic cord, an attempt can be made for reimplantation with the use of an operating microscope *(111)*. Success is more likely if there is little devitalized tissue and if the amputation occurred within 6 h.

If the testis is not available or the injury was longer than 6 h prior, the vessels of the spermatic cord are simply ligated. If the injury occurred during an episode of scrotal avulsion, the testis can rarely be reimplanted because of severe stretching and snapping apart of the spermatic cord and its vessels.

If recovered, an amputated testis should be preserved using the "bag-within-a-bag" technique. The organ is placed in saline-soaked gauze inside a clean bag, and this bag is then sealed and placed in a bag of ice. At the time of surgery, the spermatic cord stumps are debrided, and the testicular vessels are reanastomosed using 10-0 and 11-0 nylon sutures. The vas deferens can then be reanastomosed in a modified one- or two-layer closure using 10-0 and 9-0 nylon sutures. If the scrotum also needs reconstruction, the reimplanted testes are placed in thigh pouches until a later time *(85)*.

OUTCOME

Abnormal semen parameters that cause infertility (which is not immune related) and testicular atrophy can follow genital trauma *(112)*. In theory, unilateral testis trauma can have bilateral testicular effects. Even minor trauma can impair testicular blood flow and affect reproductive function *(113)*. Early attention to scrotal trauma with an emphasis on testicular salvage may preserve spermatogenesis and testosterone production. Adequate spermatogenesis often can be maintained even after salvage in cases of bilateral testicular rupture *(50)*.

If testicular parenchyma is preserved after trauma, there is usually a rapid return to normal endocrine function *(16)*. Surprisingly, long-term endocrine studies in male testicular trauma and torture cases exhibited no significant changes in prolactin, follicle-stimulating hormone, luteinizing hormone, or testosterone levels *(112,114)*. Although serum testosterone levels are usually initially depressed after trauma, they eventually normalize after placement of testes in thigh pouches and with reconstruction of a neoscrotum *(87,99)*.

SUMMARY

Management of trauma to the external genitalia needs to be a systematic process with an emphasis on early intervention if indicated. A thorough knowledge of anatomy, clinical signs and symptoms, and imaging findings of organ damage are essential. The optimal goal of organ salvage allows the maintenance of fertility, endocrine function, sexual health, micturition, and cosmesis. Although conservative management is appropriate in many situations, a high suspicion of a serious injury mandates immediate surgical intervention. When trauma involves multiple organ systems, the urologist needs to work closely with experts from other medical and surgical teams for the patient's ultimate rehabilitation benefit.

ACKNOWLEDGMENT

Special thanks to Hunter Wessells for providing some of the figures used in this chapter.

REFERENCES

1. Bertini JE, Corriere JN. Male genital trauma: evaluate promptly, treat with restraint. Contemp Urol 1992; 4:13.
2. Cass AS. Testicular trauma. J Urol 1983; 129:299–300.

3. Wesson MB. Traumatism of the testicle: report of a case of a rupture of a solitary testicle. Urol Cutaneous Rev 1946; 50: 16.
4. Bertini JE, Corriere JN. The etiology and management of genital injuries. J Trauma 1988; 28: 1278–1281.
5. Cass AS, Luxenberg M. Testicular injuries. Urology 1991; 37: 528–530.
6. Cass AS, Ferrara L, Wolpert J, Lee J. Bilateral testicular injury from external trauma. J Urol 1988; 140: 1435–1436.
7. Moore EE, Malangoni MA, Cogbill TH, et al. Organ injury scaling VII: cervical vascular, peripheral vascular, adrenal, penis, testis, and scrotum. J Trauma 1996; 41: 523–524.
8. Lrhorfi H, Manunta A, Rodriguez H, Lobel B. Trauma-induced testicular torsion. J Urol 2002; 168: 2548.
9. Elsaharty S, Pranikoff K, Magoss IV, Sufrin G. Traumatic torsion of the testis. J Urol 1984; 132: 1155–1156.
10. Sanders LM, Premkumar A, Amis ES Jr, Cohen M, Newhouse JH. Trauma-induced testicular torsion: ultrasonographic features and pathologic correlation. J Clin Ultrasound 1989; 17: 538–541.
11. Manson AL. Traumatic testicular torsion: case report. J Trauma 1989; 29: 407–408.
12. Tumeh SS, Bensen CV, Richie JP. Acute diseases of the scrotum. In: Semin Ultrasound, CT, MR. Saunders, Philadelphia, PA, 1991, Vol. 2, pp. 115–130.
13. Cassie GF. Rupture of the testis: seminoma. Br J Urol 1956, 28: 283.
14. MacDermott JP, Gray BK, Hamilton Stewart PA. Traumatic rupture of the testis. Br J Urol 1988; 62: 179–181.
15. McCormack JL, Kretz AW, Tocantins R. Traumatic rupture of the testicle. J Urol 1966; 96: 80–82.
16. Gomez RG, Castanheira AC, McAninch JW. Gunshot wounds to the male external genitalia. J Urol 1993; 150: 1147–1149.
17. Vaccaro JA, Davis R, Belville WD, Kieshing VJ. Traumatic hematocele: association with rupture of the testicle. J Urol 1986; 136: 1217–1218.
18. Schuster G. Traumatic rupture of the testicle and a review of the literature. J Urol 1982; 127: 1194–1196.
19. Tiwary, C. M. Testicular injury in breech delivery: possible implications. Urology 1989; 34: 210–212.
20. Master VA, McAninch JW, Santucci RA. Genital self-mutilation and the Internet. J Urol 2000; 164: 1656.
21. Money J, DePriest M. Three cases of genital self-surgery and their relationship to transexualism. J Sex Res 1976; 12: 283–294.
22. Ockuly EA. Traumatic luxation of the testis. Am J Surg 1946; 71: 93.
23. Claubry EG. Observations sur une retrocession subite des deux testicules dans l'abdomen, á la suite d'une violente compression de la partie inferieure de la paroi abdominale par une roué de charrette. J Gen Med Chir Pharm 1818; 64: 325.
24. Mikami O, Fujita I, Doi T, Kawamura H, Matsuda T, Komatz Y. Traumatic dislocation of the testis. Acta Urol Jpn 1992; 38: 1075–1078.
25. Madden JF. Closed reduction of a traumatically-dislocated testicle. Acad Emerg Med 1994; 1: 272–275.
26. Alyea EP. Dislocation of the testis. Surg Gynecol Obstet 1929; 49: 600–615.
27. McAleer IM, Kaplan GW, LoSasso BE. Renal and testis injuries in team sports. J Urol 2002; 168: 1805–1807.
28. American Academy of Pediatrics, Committee on Sports Medicine and Fitness. Medical conditions affecting sports participation. Pediatrics 1994; 84: 757–760.
29. Dorsen PJ. Should athletes with one eye, kidney, or testicle play contact sports? Phys Sportsmed 1986; 14: 130–138.
30. Frauscher F, Klauser A, Stenzl A, Helweg G, Amort B, zur Nedden D. Ultrasound findings in the scrotum of extreme mountain bikers. Radiology 2001; 219: 427–431.
31. Linkowski GD, Avellone A, Gooding GAW. Scrotal calculi: sonographic detection. Radiology 1985; 156: 484.
32. Cass AS, Gleich P, Smith C. Male genital injuries from external trauma. Br J Urol 1985; 57: 467–470.

33. Monga M, Moreno T, Hellstrom WJG. Gunshot wounds to the male genitalia. J Trauma 1995; 38: 855–858.
34. Cass AS, Luxenberg M. Value of early operation in blunt testicular contusion with hematocele. J Urol 1988; 139: 746–747.
35. Bickel A, Mata J, Hochstein L M, Ladreneau MD, Aultman DF, Culkin DJ. Bowel injury as a result of penetrating scrotal trauma: review of associated injuries. J Urol 1990; 143: 1017–1018.
36. Salvatierra O, Rigdon WO, Norris DM, Brady TW. Vietnam experience with 252 urologic war injuries. J Urol 1969; 101: 615–620.
37. Busch FM, Chenault OW, Zinner NR, Clarke BG. Urologic aspects of Vietnam War injuries. J Urol 1967; 97: 763–765.
38. Miles BJ, Poffenberger RJ, Farah RN, Moore S. Management of penile gunshot wounds. Urology 1990; 36: 318–321.
39. Selikowitz SM. Penetrating high velocity genitourinary injuries. Urology 1977; 9: 371–376.
40. Tucak A, Lukacevic T, Kuvezdic H, Petek Z, Novak R. Urogenital wounds during the war in Croatia in 1991/1992. J Urol 1995; 153: 121–122.
41. Umhey CE. Experience with genital wounds in Vietnam: a report of 25 cases. J Urol 1968; 99: 660–661.
42. Vuckovic I, Tucak A, Gotovac J, et al. Croatian experience in the treatment of 629 urogenital war injuries. J Trauma 1995; 39: 733–736.
43. Aboseif S, Gomez R, McAninch JW. Genital self-mutilation. J Urol 1993; 150: 1143–1146.
44. Romilly CS, Isaac MT. Male genital self-mutilation. Br J Hosp Med 1996; 55: 427–431.
45. Lewis NDC. The psychobiology of the castration reaction. Psychoanal Rev 1928; 15: 53–84.
46. Lewis NDC. Additional observations on castration reaction in males. Psychoanal Rev 1931; 18: 146–165.
47. Tenzer JA, Orozco H. Traumatic glossectomy. Report of a case. Oral Surg 1970; 30: 182–184.
48. Greilsheimer H, Groves JE. Male genital self-mutilation. Arch Gen Psychiatry 1979; 36: 441–446.
49. Cotton FJ. Explosive rupture of the testis from trauma. J Urol 1905; 2: 587.
50. Pohl DR, Johnson DE, Robison JR. Bilateral testicular rupture: report of a case. J Urol 1968; 99: 772–773.
51. Bernardi R, Agugliaro JP. Rupture traumatica de ambos testiculos. Rev Argent Urol 1959; 28: 81–84.
52. Senger FL, Bottone JJ, Ittner WF. Traumatic rupture of the testicle. J Urol 1947; 55: 451–452.
53. Holder LE, Melloul M, Chen D. Current status of radionuclide scrotal imaging. Semin Nucl Med 1981; 11: 232–249.
54. Watson LR, Older RA. Scrotal ultrasonography: technique and interpretation. Contemp Urol 1994; 23–35.
55. Corrales JG, Corbel L, Cipolla B, et al. Accuracy of ultrasound diagnosis after blunt testicular trauma. Urology 1993; 150: 1834–1836.
56. Ugarte R, Spaedy M, Cass AS. Accuracy of ultrasound in diagnosis after blunt testicular rupture. Urology 1990; 36: 253–254.
57. Friedman SG, Rose JG, Winston MA. Ultrasound and nuclear medicine evaluation in acute testicular trauma. J Urol 1981; 125: 748–749.
58. Anderson KA, McAninch JW, Jeffrey RB, Laing FC. Ultrasonography for the diagnosis and staging of blunt scrotal trauma. J Urol 1983; 130: 933–935.
59. Fournier GR Jr, Laing FC, Jeffrey RB, McAninch JW. High resolution scrotal ultrasonography: a highly sensitive but nonspecific diagnostic technique. J Urol 1985; 134: 490–493.
60. Jeffrey RB, Laing FC, Hricak H, McAninch JW. Sonography of testicular trauma. Am J Roentgenol 1983; 141: 993–995.
61. Micallef M, Ahmad I, Ramesh N, Hurley M, McInerney D. Ultrasound features of blunt testicular injury. Injury Int J Care Injured 2001; 32: 23–26.
62. Hamm B. Differential diagnosis of scrotal masses by ultrasound. Eur Radiol 1997; 7: 668–679.
63. Barloon TJ, Weissman AM, Kahn D. Diagnostic imaging of patients with acute scrotal pain. Am Fam Phys 1996; 53: 1734–1750.
64. McConnell JD, Peters PC, Lewis SE. Testicular rupture in blunt scrotal trauma: review of 15 cases with recent application of testicular scanning. Urology 1982; 128: 309–311.

65. Redman JF, Rountree GA, Bissada NK. Injuries to scrotal contents by blunt trauma. Urology 1976; 7: 190–191.
66. Ashkar LN, Schreck WR. Traumatic rupture of the testis and epididymis. J Urol 1968; 99: 774–775.
67. Kaye MC, Streem SB, Yost A. Scrotal hematoma resulting from extracorporeal shock wave lithotripsy for a distal ureteral calculus. J Urol 1993; 150: 481–482.
68. Fleisher GR. The management of bite wounds. N Engl J Med 1999; 340: 138–140.
69. Weiss HB, Friedman DI, Coben JH. Incidence of bite injuries treated in emergency departments. JAMA 1998; 279: 51–53.
70. Cummings JM, Boullier JA. Scrotal dog bites. J Urol 2000; 164: 57–58.
71. Callaham ML. Domestic and feral mammalian bites. In: Management of Wilderness and Environmental Emergencies. (Auerbach PS, Geehr EC, eds.), Macmillan, New York, 1983; pp. 31–351.
72. Talan DA, Citron DM, Abrahamian FM, Moran GJ, Goldstein EJC. Bacteriologic analysis of infected dog and cat bites. N Engl J Med 1999; 340: 85–92.
73. Wolf JS Jr, Turzan C, Cattolica EV, McAninch JW. Dog bites to the male genitalia: characteristics, management and comparison with human bites. J Urol 1993; 149: 286–289.
74. Wolf JS Jr, Gomez R, McAninch JW. Human bites to the penis. J Urol 1992; 147: 1265–1267.
75. Michielsen D, Van Hee R, Neetens C, Lafaire C, Peeters R. Burns to the genitalia and perineum. J Urol 1998; 159: 418–419.
76. Peck MD, Boileau MA, Grube BJ, Heimbach DM. The management of burns to the perineum and genitals. J Burn Care Rehab 1990; 11: 54–56.
77. McDougal WS, Peterson HD, Pruitt BA, Persky L. The terminally injured perineum. J Urol 1979; 121: 320–323.
78. Angel C, Shu T, French D, Orihuela E, Lukefar J, Herndon DN. Genital and perineal burns in children: 10 years of experience at a major burn center. J Ped Surg 2002; 37, 99–103.
79. Lawton CA, Won M, Pilepich MV, et al. Long term treatment sequelae following external beam irradiation for adenocarcinoma of the prostate: analysis of RTOG studies 7506 and 7706. Int J Radiat Oncol Biol Phys 1991; 21: 935–939.
80. Solsona E, Ihorra-Juan I, Ricos-Tonent JV, et al. Urological complications of pelvic radiotherapy. In: Urological Complications of Pelvic Surgery and Radiotherapy. (Jewett MA, ed.), Isis Medical Media, Oxford, UK, 1995, pp. 51–67.
81. Oesterling JE. Scrotal surgery: a reliable method for the prevention of postoperative hematoma and edema. J Urol 1990; 143: 1201–1202.
82. Manson AL, MacDonald G. "Turban" scrotal dressing. J Urol 1987; 137: 238–239.
83. Haas GP, Melser M, Miles BJ. Method of circumferential pressure dressing of the scrotum following bilateral orchiectomy. Urology 1989; 33: 429–430.
84. Shreedhar R, Duncan T. A technique for preventing post-operative scrotal haematoma. Br J Clin Pract 1984; 38: 93–94.
85. McDougal WS. Scrotal reconstruction using thigh pedicle flaps. J Urol 1983; 129: 757–759.
86. Balakrishnan C. Scrotal avulsion: a new technique of reconstruction by split-thickness graft. Br J Plast Surg 1956; 9: 38–42.
87. McAninch JW. Management of genital skin loss. Urol Clin North Am 1989; 16: 387–397.
88. Still EF, Goodman RC. Total reconstruction of a two-compartment scrotum by tissue expansion. Plast Reconstr Surg 1990; 85: 805–807.
89. Heckler FR. Gracilis muscle and the musculocutaneous flaps to the perineum. In: Grabb's Encyclopedia of Flaps. (Strauch B, Vasconez EJ, Hall-Findlay EJ, eds.), Little, Brown, Boston, MA, 1990, Vol. 3, p. 1446.
90. Tripathi FM, Sinha JK, Choudhury AK, Bhattacharya V. Repair of burns of the scrotum using a gracilis myocutaneous flap. Burns 1989; 15: 181–182.
91. Waguespack RL, Thompson IM, Cioffi WG Jr, et al. Contemporary results of the management of burns of the genitalia and perineum. J Urol 1992; 147: 288A.
92. Gomes CM, Ribeiro-Filho L, Giron AM, Mitre AI, Figueira ERR, Arap S. Genital trauma due to animal bites. J Urol 2000; 165: 80–83.
93. Brakenbury PH, Muwanga C. A comparative double blind study of amoxicillin-clavulanate vs placebo in the prevention of infection after animal bites. Arch Emerg Med 1989; 6: 251–256.

94. Altarac S. Management of 53 cases of testicular trauma. Eur Urol 1994; 25, 119–123.
95. Gross M. Rupture of the testicle: the importance of early surgical treatment. J Urol 1969; 101: 196–197.
96. Bronk WS, Berry JL. Traumatic rupture of the testicle: report of a case and review of the literature. J Urol 1962; 87: 564–566.
97. Schneiderman C. Traumatic rupture of the testicle. J Urol 1957; 78: 54–57.
98. Wasko R, Goldstein AG. Traumatic rupture of the testicles. J Urol 1966; 95: 721–723.
99. McAninch JW, Kahn RI, Jeffrey RB, Laing FC, Krieger MJ. Major traumatic and septic genital injuries. J Trauma 1984; 24: 291–298.
100. Merricks JW, Papierniak FB. Traumatic rupture of the testicle. J Urol 1970; 103: 77–79.
101. Del Villar RG, Ireland GW, Cass AS. Early exploration following trauma to the testicle. J Trauma 1973; 13: 600–601.
102. Cline KJ, Mata JA, Venable DD, Eastham JA. Penetrating trauma to the male external genitalia. J Trauma 1998; 44: 492–494.
103. Campbell MF. Pediatric Urology. Vol. 2. MacMillan, 1937, p. 188.
104. Atwell JD, Ellis H. Rupture of the testis. Br J Surg 1961; 49: 345–346.
105. Brandes SB, Buckman RF, Chelsky MJ, Hanno PM. External genitalia gunshot wounds: a 10-year experience with 56 cases. J Trauma 1995; 39: 266–271.
106. Goulding FJ. Traumatic dislocation of the testis: addition of two cases with a changing etiology. J Trauma 1976; 16: 1000–1002.
107. Nagarajan VP, Pranikoff K, Imahori SC, Rabinowitz R. Traumatic dislocation of testis. Urology 1983; 22: 521–524.
108. Pollen JJ, Funckes C. Traumatic dislocation of the testes. J Trauma 1982; 22: 247–249.
109. Singer AJ, Das S, Gavrell GJ. Traumatic dislocation of the testes. Urology 1994; 35: 310–312.
110. O'Donnell C, Kumar U, Kiely EA. Testicular dislocation after scrotal trauma. Br J Urol 1998; 82: 768.
111. Jordan GH. Lower genitourinary tract trauma and male external genital trauma (nonpenetrating injuries, penetrating injuries, and avulsion injuries) Part II. AUA Update Ser 2000; 19, lesson 11, 80–87.
112. Kukadia AN, Ercole CJ, Gleich P, Hensleigh H, Pryor JL. Testicular trauma: potential impact on reproductive function. J Urol 1996; 156: 1643–1646.
113. Markey CM, Jaquier AM. Dramatic changes in testicular blood flow induced by minor ischemia. Paper presented at annual meeting of American Society of Andrology, Raleigh, NC, March 31–April 4, 1995. Abstract 104.
114. Daugaard G, Petersen HD, Ambildgaard U, et al. Sequelae to genital trauma in torture victims. Arch Androl 1983; 10: 245–248.

6 Blunt and Penetrating Trauma to the Penis

Jack H. Mydlo, MD

CONTENTS

    INTRODUCTION
    CLINICAL FEATURES
    PATHOLOGY
    DIAGNOSTIC IMAGING
    OTHER INJURIES
    TREATMENT
    COMPLICATIONS
    PREVENTION
    SUMMARY
    REFERENCES

INTRODUCTION

Penile fracture, or penile rupture, is the most common blunt injury to the erect penis and is caused by tearing or cracking of the corporal cavernosal bodies. The first documented report of this injury was more than 1000 yr ago. Although the most common etiology is vaginal intercourse, sometimes from hitting the perineum during thrusting, it can happen from any type of blunt trauma affecting the tumescent shaft. This includes masturbation, with or without devices; falling out of bed with an erection; extreme sexual activity, especially during coitus in which the female is on top; forceful correction of a congenital chordee; and even tucking an erect penis into underwear (1). Although injury to the flaccid penis that leads to corporal rupture has been reported from sports accidents and animal and human bites, this is not regarded as penile fracture (2).

CLINICAL FEATURES

This entity is underreported, usually because of the reluctance and shame that victims have to seek treatment (1,2). The patients are usually between 30 and 40 yr of age and may present with the classic "eggplant deformity" of the swollen penis along with ecchymosis confined to Buck's fascia. The patient usually states that he was engaged in sexual activity until he or his partner heard a "snap" and then noticed resolution of his erection along with increased swelling of the shaft. Sometimes, a palpable defect in the

Table 1
Organ Injury Scale for Penile Injury

AAST grade	Penile injury
I	Cutaneous laceration or contusion
II	Laceration of Buck's fascia (cavernosum) without tissue loss
III	Cutaneous avulsion, laceration through glans or meatus, or cavernosal or urethral defect <2 cm
IV	Partial penectomy or cavernosal or urethral defect = 2 cm
V	Total penectomy

AAST, American Association for the Surgery of Trauma. (From ref. 46.)

tunica is present, but other times this is concealed by the hematoma. A butterfly-shape hematoma in the perineum may suggest a urethral injury (3).

Blunt trauma to the penis usually occurs during erections because during the flaccid state the shaft can undergo extremes of torque and bending without damage to the corporal bodies. More than 1300 cases of penile fracture appeared in the medical literature from 1935 to 2001, the majority reported from Mediterranean countries (1). The largest series contained 172 cases from Iran (4).

Those such injuries from the Middle East are mostly caused by masturbation, whereas the majority of the cases from the Western hemisphere are caused by vigorous intercourse, especially when the female is on top (5). Besides excessive force at coitus, other risk factors for penile fracture that have been described include penovaginal disproportion, fellatio, and anal intercourse (1).

Penetrating penile trauma is also rare and usually is caused by animal attacks, military duty, farm machinery accidents, and even zipper injuries (6). With the increase in violence in cities, increased penetrating injuries to the penis have been documented. This is also commonly seen in drug trafficking confrontations. It is also a particularly favorite target for scorned lovers, both male and female (7). Maintenance of function, restoration of urethral integrity, and preservation of cosmetic appearance are the ultimate goals of intervention.

For both blunt and penetrating penile trauma, blood at the meatus usually indicates that there is urethral injury; however, the absence of blood at the meatus does not rule out urethral trauma, and physician discretion is important (8). In penetrating trauma, the trajectory of the missile or the caliber of the bullet may give important insights concerning the extent and path of damage. Retrograde urethrography, as well as cystoscopy, may be helpful (9). However, the surgeon should always be alert for the possibility, although small, of a false-negative urethrogram because of an overlying clot, which prevents extravasation (9). The organ injury scale for penile injury is shown in Table 1.

PATHOLOGY

Fracture of the penis involves disruption of the tunica albuginea and the corpus cavernosum. The tissue thickness of the tunica albuginea, usually 2 mm in the resting state, is much thinner during erection, almost 0.25 mm (10). The rigidity of the tunica albuginea is overwhelmed by the sudden rise in intracorporeal pressure, usually greater than 1500 mmHg, which happens from increased torque during abnormal bending (11). At this thinness and pressure, the tunica becomes vulnerable to rupture.

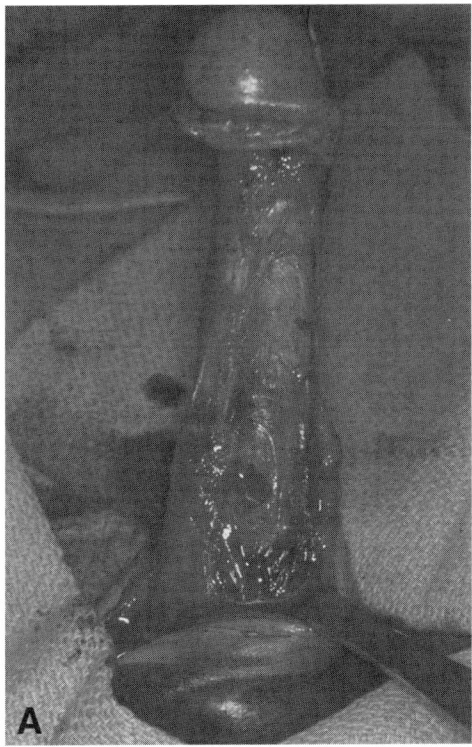 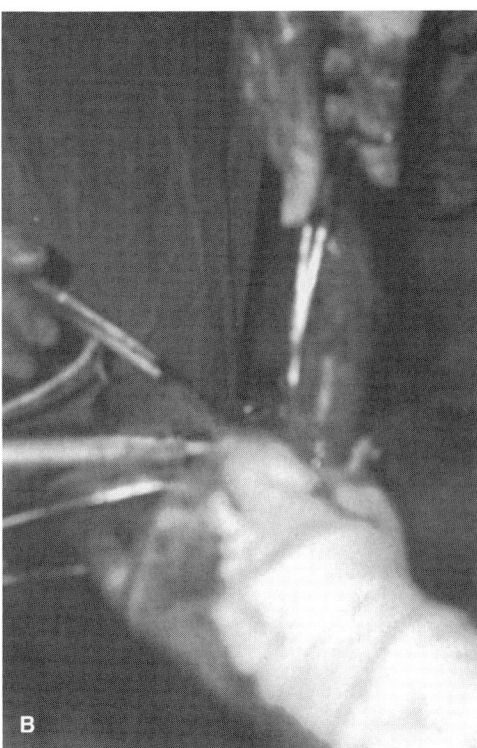

Fig. 1. (A) Unilateral corporal rupture demonstrated after degloving penis. (Photo courtesy of H. Wessells, MD.) (B) Bilateral corporal cavernosal rupture with laceration of urethra (catheter seen in middle). (From ref. *9* with permission; © 1998 Elsevier.)

During coitus, the dorsal penile vessels, hard and engorged, are between the hard corpora cavernosa and the bony structures around the vagina and are prone to traumatic rupture *(12)*. There is also the belief that predisposing factors, such as fibrosclerosis, may affect some patients more than others during intercourse, and that is why a small minority of patients are susceptible to rupture *(13)*. Perhaps with the introduction of pharmacotherapies for erection dysfunction, especially in the older population who have less-pliable tissue, an increase in the incidence of penile fracture may be seen in the elderly *(13)*.

The hematoma, if confined to Buck's fascia, is limited to the penile shaft. If the fascia is disrupted, the hematoma will spread to the scrotum and perineum. Although tears of the corpora are usually transverse and unilateral, reports of bilateral corporal ruptures, with and without urethral injuries, can occur (Fig. 1A,B) *(9)*. Furthermore, the urethra can rupture without rupture of the corpus cavernosa *(14)*.

Ruptures of the dorsal vein and artery may also mimic penile fractures; however, they may be differentiated from penile fracture by cavernosography *(15)*. Rupture of the suspensory ligament may also mimic penile rupture; this is not followed by rapid detumescence, but rather a "flail" penis *(16)*.

DIAGNOSTIC IMAGING

The diagnosis of penile fracture is commonly made based on the usual clinical features and the associated history. Although initially many of our patients had radiographic

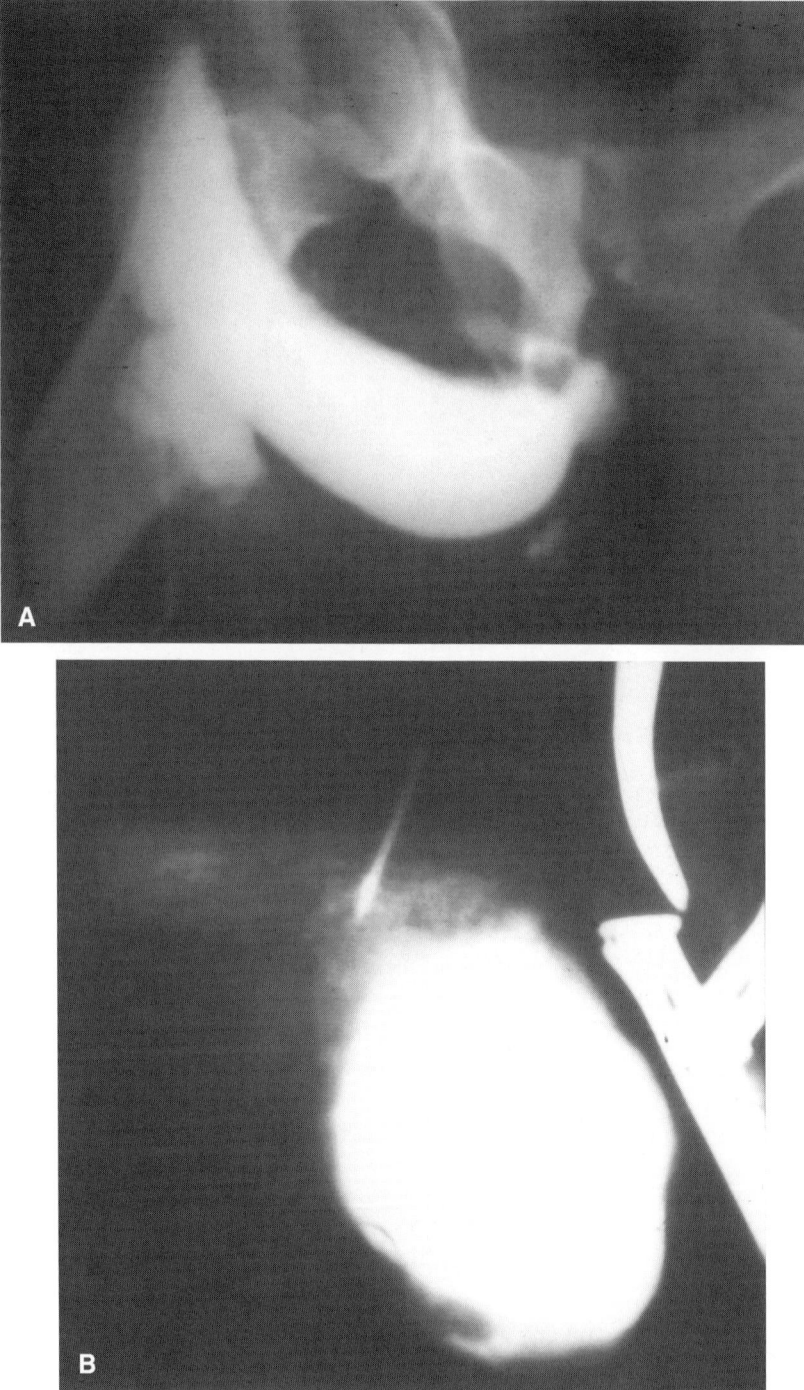

Fig. 2. (A) Cavernosogram reveals small amount of extravasation of contrast consistent with penile fracture. **(B)** Cavernosogram reveals large amount of extravasation from corpora rupture. (From ref. 9 with permission; copyright 1998 Elsevier.)

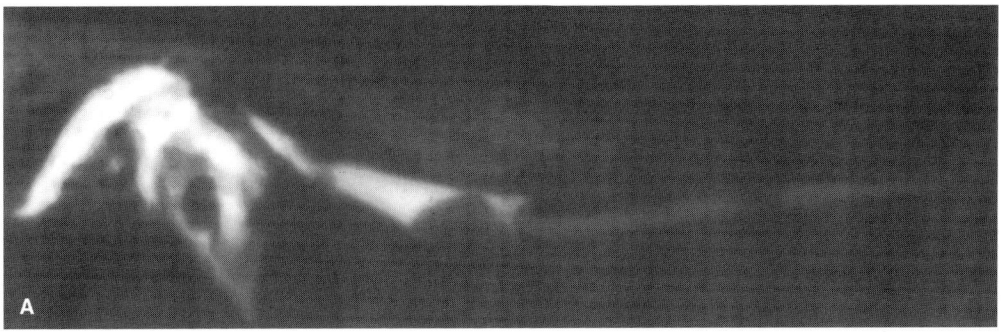
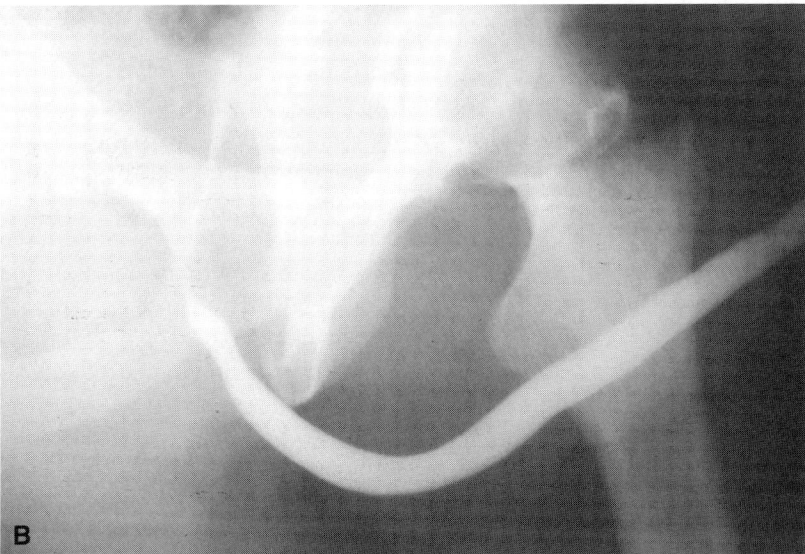

Fig. 3. (A) Extravasation of contrast during urethrogram in patient with penile fracture. (From ref. 9 with permission; copyright 1998 Elsevier.) **(B)** False-negative urethrogram in patient who presented with penile fracture and blood at the meatus. Urethral rupture was confirmed on surgical exploration.

imaging to confirm the diagnosis of penile fracture, such as a cavernosogram (Fig. 2A,B), subsequently we relied on clinical examination alone and corroborated our findings during surgery. Other reported series have also relied on clinical diagnosis alone, and the finding of corporal disruption was only confirmed at exploration (17,18). We also evaluate the corpora and urethra during surgical exploration using an injection of isotonic saline, which may reveal additional sites of disruption.

The classic presentation of penile fracture described in the preceding section usually makes it easy to diagnose. Reports of cavernosography, sonography, and magnetic resonance imaging in the evaluation of these patients sometimes contribute little to the overall assessment (19–21). In fact, there is still a small risk of a false-negative cavernosogram when the rupture site seals early by clot (9). Also, although retrograde urethrography is useful to assess for suspected concomitant urethral disruption (Fig. 3A), we had several false-negative urethrograms caused by either overlying clot or perhaps not enough pressure injected (Fig. 3B) (9). Therefore, during our more recent surgical explorations for penile injury, we simply injected saline into the corpora using a butterfly needle and into the urethra using a 60-cc Toomey syringe. It effectively plugs up the urethra and demonstrates its integrity *(21)*.

Other reports have suggested limited exploration over the palpable defect in an attempt to surgically repair the rupture *(22)*. However, in most centers when the index of suspicion for corporal rupture is high because of the clinical history, early and complete exploration using a degloving procedure is still favored *(23)*.

OTHER INJURIES

Iatrogenic

Crush injuries in the operating room from retractors, especially the large fixed-ring abdominal retractors, can inadvertently occur in the penis during surgery. Although these incidents have been described, not much has been published on their causes, perhaps because of the medical-legal issues involved in such a preventable accident. Similarly, accidental burn injuries from the Bovie coagulator have occurred because of accidental activation while resting on the penis or excessive use during circumcisions or other penile surgeries *(24)*.

When urologists place a penile prosthesis, especially the semirigid models, the process of corporal cavernosal dilation using metal dilators can sometimes perforate the median septum or perforate the urethra *(25)*. We recommend that once one corpora has been dilated, a metal rod or dilator should be left in place while the surgeon dilates the other side so there will be no crossover. Furthermore, after both corpora have been dilated, we irrigate each corpora and check the urethral meatus to make sure there is no extravasation of water, which would indicate urethral violation *(25)*. Moreover, correct measurement of the corporal length is important. If the length of the semirigid prosthesis is too long for the corpora, the tips can induce pressure necrosis of the glans with possible erosion.

Psychological Causes

Insertion of foreign bodies into the urethra, either for sexual gratification or because of psychiatric disturbances, has been reported *(26)*. In our experience, we have seen paper clips, hairpins, and safety pins inserted into the urethra. Cystoscopic removal may be attempted; however, if the sharp edge of the object, like an open safety pin, is facing toward the meatus, we suggest pushing the entire pin into the bladder and then retrieving it after reversing its position. This will cause less urethral or penile abrasion.

Although much has been published about Munchausen's disease, which concerns the desire to have attention by medical staff and others by involving unnecessary procedures, it has been suggested that there may be some sexual gratification when the procedures involve the penis and genitalia *(27)*.

Bicycle Accidents

Much has been reported on the shape of certain bicycle seats as a possible cause of early erectile dysfunction caused by compression of the pudendal arteries *(28)*. However, in the United States, most men's bicycles have a median bar that runs from the seat to the handlebar. This is placed high compared to the lower-set bar on female bicycles. Apparently, the idea for this design dates to the early female bicycle riders. In that era, most female riders wore dresses and therefore would need a lower bar so they could mount the bicycle and still maintain their modesty. Such a reason today is obsolete because most female bicyclists rarely wear dresses while riding.

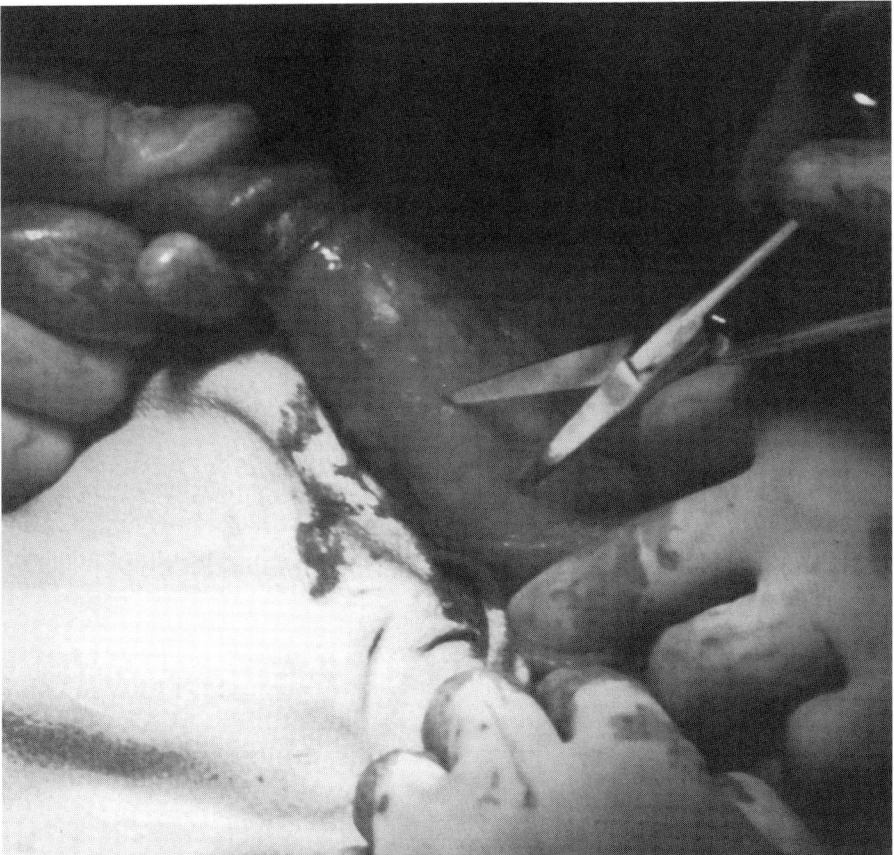

Fig. 4. Complete degloving of penis allows complete inspection of corpora and spongiosum.

However, the higher-mounted bar in men's bicycles has been associated with several crush injuries to the penis during bicycle accidents or short stops in which the rider accelerates forward *(29, 30)*. Although a "female" bicycle may be safer as far as protecting the male genitalia, we assume most men would refuse to ride a "girl's bike"

TREATMENT

Initial reports of treatment for penile fracture discussed splinting, compresses, and a combination of anti-inflammatory and analgesic medications *(31)*. However, long-term results of conservative management demonstrated significant complication rates, such as curved or painful erections, impotence, arteriovenous fistula formation, infection, and plaque formation *(31,32)*.

Once a patient with blunt or deeply penetrating penile trauma presents, we recommend immediate surgical exploration using the degloving technique, either by a circumferential incision 1 cm below the corona or by incising the scrotum and inverting the shaft (Fig. 4). This will allow visual inspection of both corporal bodies and the spongiosum. We prefer to have a urethral catheter in place when exploring the tubular structures because the overlying hematoma may affect the surgeon's orientation *(33)*.

In patients with penetrating injuries such as gunshot wounds, there are usually multiple other organ injuries. A review by Cline et al. found a urethral injury incidence of

22% in their experience of penetrating penile trauma, and 5 to –10% had other organ injuries *(7)*. Therefore, if the patient is hemodynamically unstable because of multiple wounds or other reasons, we recommend initial placement of a urethral catheter after a urethrogram is normal or reveals partial disruption. If there is total disruption or attempted Foley placement is not possible, we recommend suprapubic tube placement and surgical correction later (Fig. 5A). It is important to trace the trajectory of the missile to determine a possible "blast" effect (Fig. 5B). We recommend separating the three corporal bodies for adequate evaluation *(33)*.

Because the diagnosis of penile rupture is fairly clear, some authors have abandoned preoperative radiologic imaging and presently perform immediate surgical exploration *(34)*. Although we advocate a degloving procedure, other surgical incisions include direct longitudinal, inguinoscrotal, and suprapubic. The choice of repair is a matter of custom or preference. A direct longitudinal incision over the site may be simple, but can be associated with poor cosmesis. The inguinal-scrotal incision can be associated with wound infection as well as cause angulation at the base of the penis. Moreover, urethral repair may be difficult from this position. The suprapubic incision is useful for penile vascular surgery *(1)*. The fact that there are many approaches suggests that no one incision is ideal for every case *(1)*.

Although several reports have advocated repairing a penile rupture right over the site of injury, we feel that this is difficult to palpate accurately in the presence of a hematoma. Moreover, other rupture sites may be missed. In one of our cases, a patient was treated surgically at another institution, where he underwent an incision over the presumed site of injury. He presented at our emergency room 24 h after discharge because of repeat swelling and ecchymosis. After degloving, we found another site of corporal injury, separate from the repaired site; we sutured this injury, and the patient did well postoperatively *(21)*.

We prefer absorbable suture after adequate debridement (if it is a penetrating injury) and antibiotic irrigation. The lacerations of the tunica albuginea are usually sutured longitudinally in the axis of the shaft. However, if this will result in narrowing of the shaft, then we advocate transverse repair. As mentioned, postoperatively we also instill saline in the urethra and corpora to assess the integrity of our repair (Fig. 6).

Another variation in the treatment of blunt or penetrating trauma to the penis involves delayed presentation. Some patients do not seek medical attention right away because of embarrassment or other reasons *(35)*. In one case, we had a patient who had a zipper injury to the shaft and became so enraged that he ripped the pants off his body and walked around with the imbedded zipper in his penis for several days (Fig. 7). The resultant swelling of the embedded metal did not allow simple dismemberment of the zipper by breaking the median bar. The skin was excised, debrided, and closed without any complications *(36)*. In other cases, we have seen patients present with presumed histories of penile fracture who apparently reported good erections after the fact *(35,37)*. However, the reported complications of conservative treatment for penile fracture, notably curvature, shortening, and the like, are certainly a risk. Therefore, we advocate surgical exploration even several days or weeks after the event because corporal weakening and scar formation may lead to problems in the future. Many of the younger patients we saw usually refused elective surgical correction after the initial insult, especially if they perceived that that their erections were normal *(35)*.

After surgical repair for both penetrating or blunt trauma, we also use a snug dressing to prevent swelling and hematoma formation, which could compromise wound healing or lead to abscess formation. If the patient's penis was degloved and he was not circumcised, we usually removed the redundant foreskin prior to reapproximation (Fig. 8). This

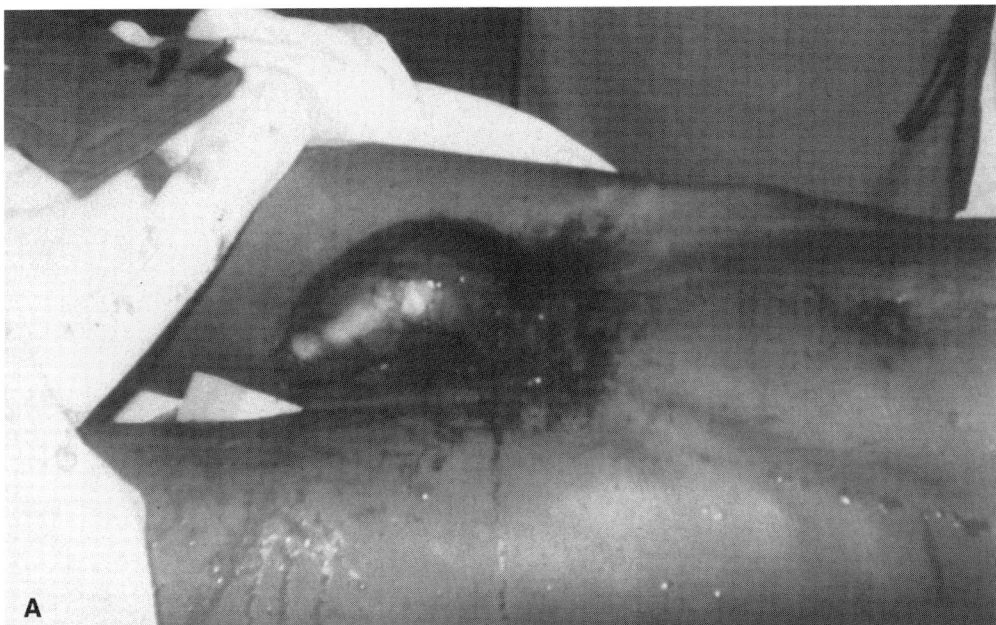

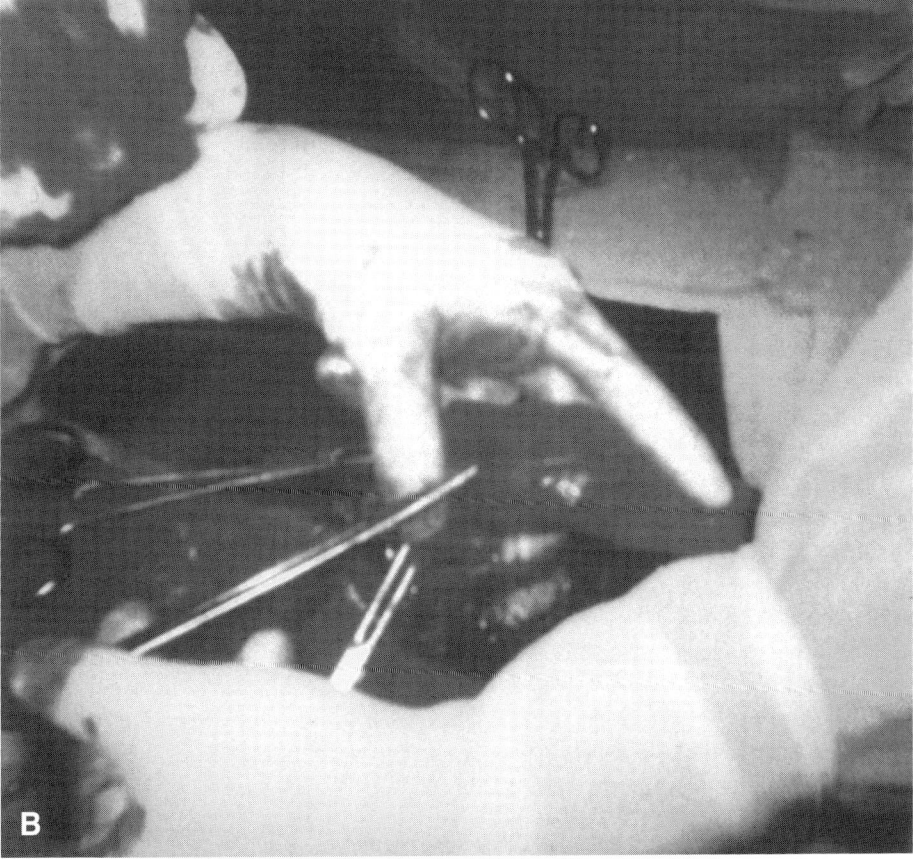

Fig. 5. (A) Gunshot wound to penis. Urethrogram was normal, and urethral catheter was placed. **(B)** Scissors placed in bullet hole demonstrate trajectory. Separation of corporal bodies is important to evaluate integrity fully and determine blast effect and trajectory.

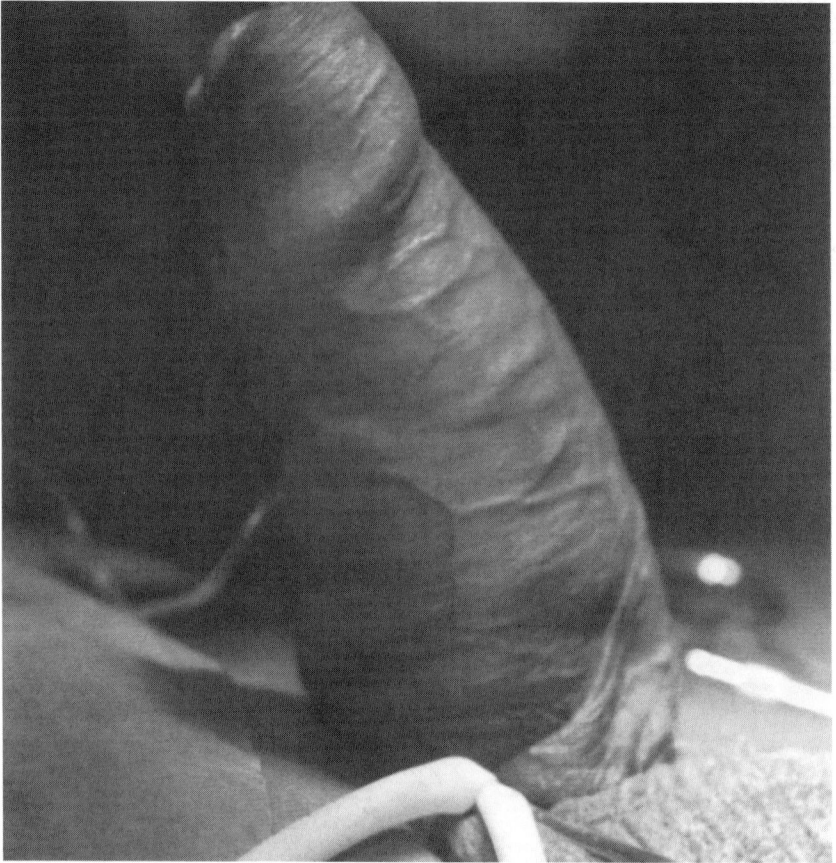

Fig. 6. Artificial erection with tourniquet at the base of penis and instillation of isotonic saline through a butterfly needle can help determine other sites of damage as well as the integrity of the surgical repair.

greatly reduces the amount of postoperative edema and discomfort of the patient. We have kept all patients on 1 mg diethylstilbesterol (DES), daily for 1 to 2 wk, or an injection of an luteinizing hormone-releasing hormone (LHRH) agonist or ketoconazole to prevent erections, which we found to be very effective. We did not have any cases of deep vein thrombosis or other side effects.

In our experience with 53 patients with blunt and penetrating penile injuries, we have had no abscesses, stricture formation, or significant sequelae in the immediate postoperative period. At 1 and 2 yr, 46 of the 53 patients were evaluated with a brief history and physical examination. Each reported erections adequate for intercourse without associated pain. Only 3 patients stated they had mild curvature. However, those three patients did not seek intervention. We did have several urethral strictures that resulted from urethral ruptures from penile fractures. Most responded well to periodic urethral dilations, but 2 required internal optical urethrotomy *(21,33)*.

COMPLICATIONS

Reported complication rates following conservative therapy for penile fracture range from 10 to 53% *(31)*. Although some reports of nonoperative management described

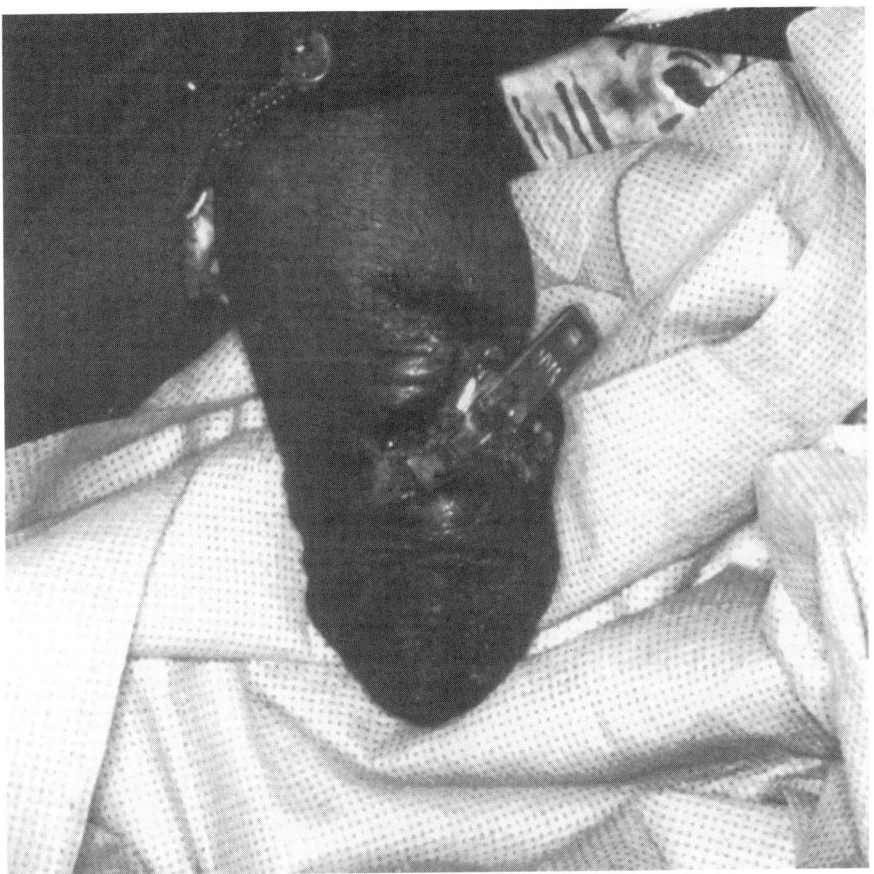

Fig. 7. Embarrassed male came to emergency department 3 d after this zipper injury. (From ref. *36* with permission; copyright 2000 Karger AG.)

residual deformity, not all patients required surgical repair *(37)*. In one report, we discussed five patients with presumed penile fracture who refused surgical exploration as well as diagnostic radiography *(35)*. As mentioned in the Pathology section, there have been isolated reports in the literature of dorsal vein and artery ruptures that have mimicked penile fracture on presentation. It is possible that this could have occurred and may have accounted for the symptoms seen in this group of patients with presumed penile fracture who refused any diagnostic workup or treatment. This may also be the reason why they did not have any serious sequelae regarding erectile function. Despite some penile angulation, patients were able to have adequate erections for intercourse *(35)*.

The embarrassment associated with these injuries often makes patients delay or defer seeking medical care. Thus, the true incidence of this injury may be underestimated. Therefore, a number of patients may go untreated, making it difficult to assess the actual risk of complications in patients managed conservatively because they refuse treatment. It is thought that fibrosis from the rupture results in deviation of the penis, as seen in Peyronie's disease *(38)*. Pseudodiverticula and fistulas may also occur *(39,40)*. Penile refracture, which may occur during coitus shortly after repair, has been reported because of the weakness of the tissue integrity *(13)*. Therefore, it is recommended to wait 6 to 8 wk after the initial injury to engage in sexual activity. Sometimes, patients may have an

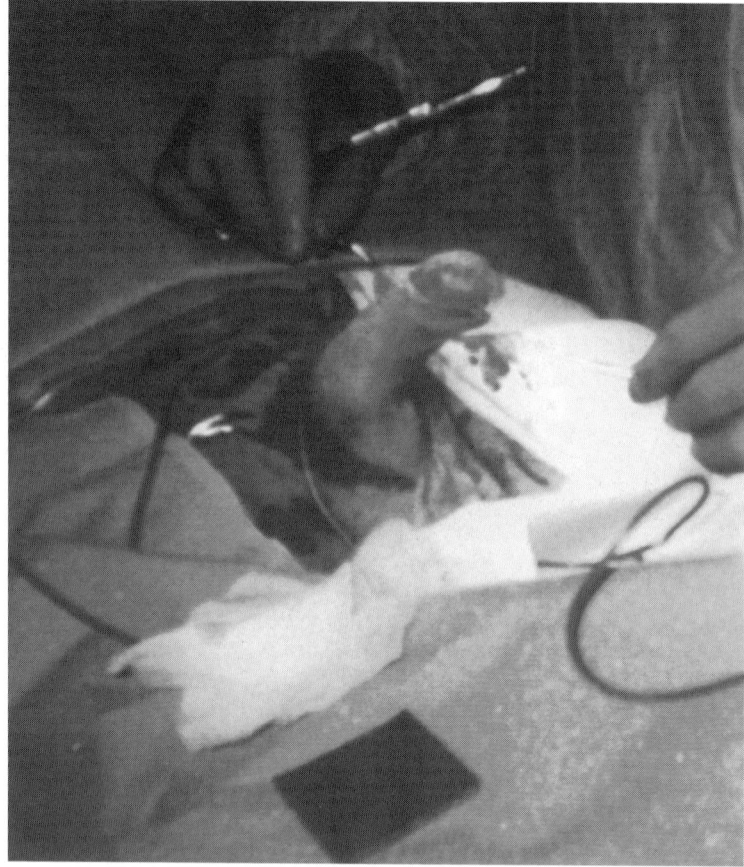

Fig. 8. Removal of foreskin or residual shaft skin after degloving reduces edema after reapproximation.

erection immediately postoperatively, and this may compromise the integrity of the repair, which may lead to another rupture. As mentioned in this section, we found that the use of LHRH analogues, 1 mg DES, or ketoconazol was sufficient to decrease the incidence of spontaneous erections and allow proper healing *(33)*.

Even after proper diagnosis, treatment, and recovery period, there are still patients who will have erectile dysfunction. It has been suggested that weak erections after a routine repair are usually caused by a venous leak into the corpora cavernosum rather than an arteriogenic pathology and may resolve with time *(6,41)*.

In those patients who have penetrating injury to the corporal bodies, one should be aware of the possibility of fistula formation, especially in those cases with blast effect *(39,40)*. Therefore, it is important to debride involved, possibly ischemic, surrounding tissues properly. If not, the initial repair may be effective only transiently. Breakdown of the tissues later could lead to fistula formation. Fortunately, we did not detect this problem in our experience, although longer term follow-up may unmask this potential consequence.

There also may be neurovascular damage or sensory damage to the penis, especially in penetrating wounds to the penis. We have seen erectile dysfunction or sensory damage mostly in those patients with close-range gunshot wounds that resulted in much tissue loss *(33)*.

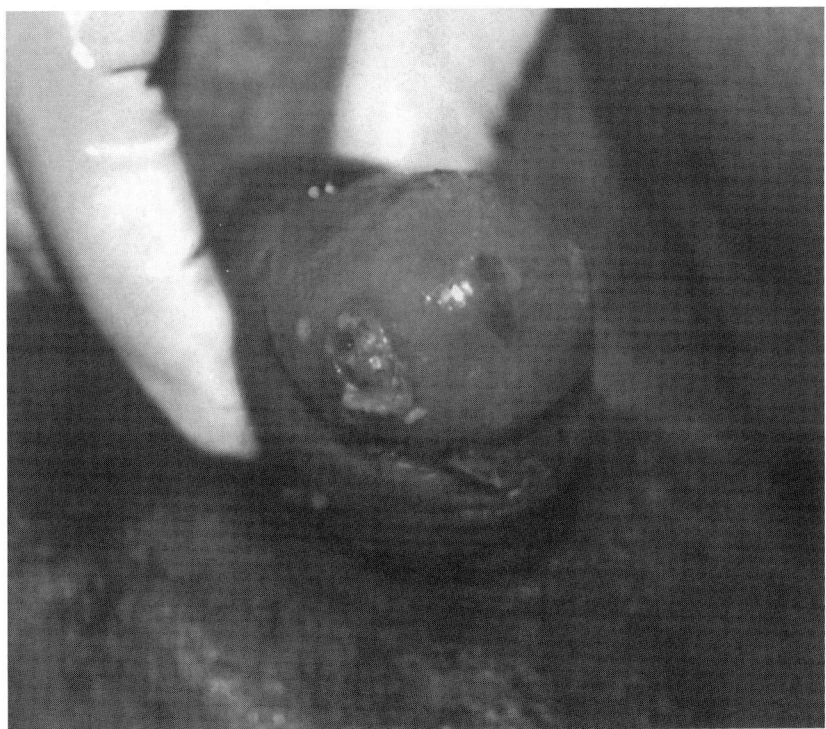

Fig. 9. Human bite to penis resulted in local infection of glans, which eventually resolved with antibiotics.

Some penetrating wounds may appear to be superficial, but may still lead to infections, ischemia, and gangrene. We had two patients with localized glandular ischemia that developed after human and dog bites and who did not have progression of their disease. They were treated with antibiotics and conservative management and did well (Figs. 9 and 10). However, we also had a patient who presented to us 2 d after suffering a human bite to the penis, which became grossly infected, gangrenous, and involved the scrotum. This required significant debridement of both the shaft and the scrotum, with subsequent split-thickness skin grafting. Another patient presented to us with very aggressive verrucous carcinoma of the penis, which 18 mo prior were simple condyloma. He was in urinary retention, and his shaft was ischemic and gangrenous and was about to undergo autonecrosis. In this case, we had to perform a total penectomy.

If penetrating penile injuries lead to ischemia and gangrene, treatment options are twofold: distal amputation or conservative management. The problem with distal amputation in those patients with poor vascular supply is that poor healing of the stump may lead to more complications, especially in diabetics. In addition, in patients who have had either partial or distal penile amputations, higher incidence of suicide has been reported *(42–44)*. Therefore, all attempts to save the penis should be made. Because the experience of hyperbaric oxygen treatment in gangrene is limited, we speculate that it can help distal penile amputation sloughing or poor healing. Like the penetrating penile injuries, gangrene of the glans may lead to cavernosal-spongiosum fistulas, which could later lead to erectile dysfunction *(39)*.

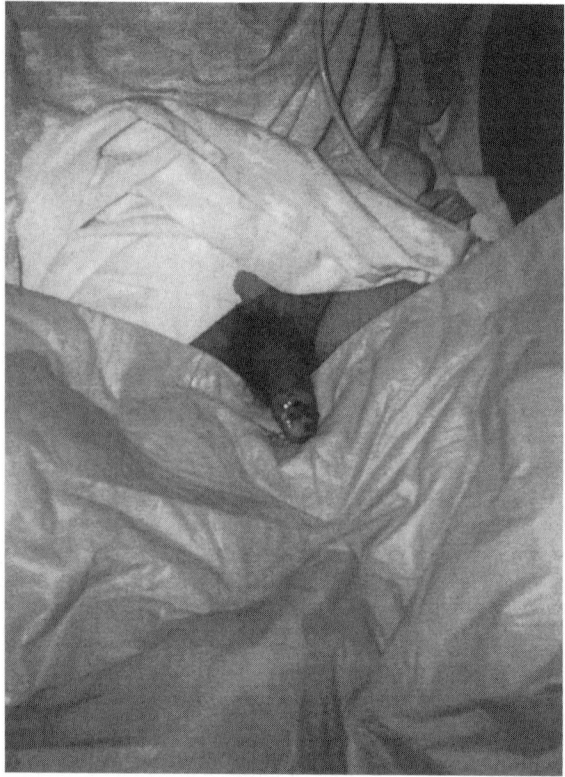

Fig. 10. Man with dog bite to penis was treated with antibiotics, and resulting eschar sloughed off.

Penile amputation has also been reported and is sometimes associated with schizophrenia or romantic upheavals *(44)*. In the pediatric population, it may occur during a circumcision *(45)*. If able to retrieve the transected tip, it is important not to place it in direct contact with ice because this may cause necrosis. Rather, place the tip in a plastic bag filled with cold isotonic saline and then place this bag in a larger bag or container filled with ice *(44)*. If it is the tip of the glans alone that was amputated, generally these can heal well with reattachment because of the great vascularity of the glans. It is important to realign the urethra of the glans to the proximal urethra over a pediatric feeding tube or urethral catheter. Longer amputated segments will require microsurgery (Fig. 11).

PREVENTION

Although there have been no controlled studies, it has been suggested that preventive measures, such as avoiding vigorous sexual intercourse, forceful penile manipulations, and unusual coital positions and postures, be encouraged *(1)*. However, we doubt there will be adherence to these preventive measures. Therefore, we can only prepare for these events with immediate and thorough medical care. After surgical repair, it is also recommended to abstain from sexual activity for 6 to 8 wk. However, abstinence may still not prevent natural nocturnal erections from causing damage to the repair or refracture.

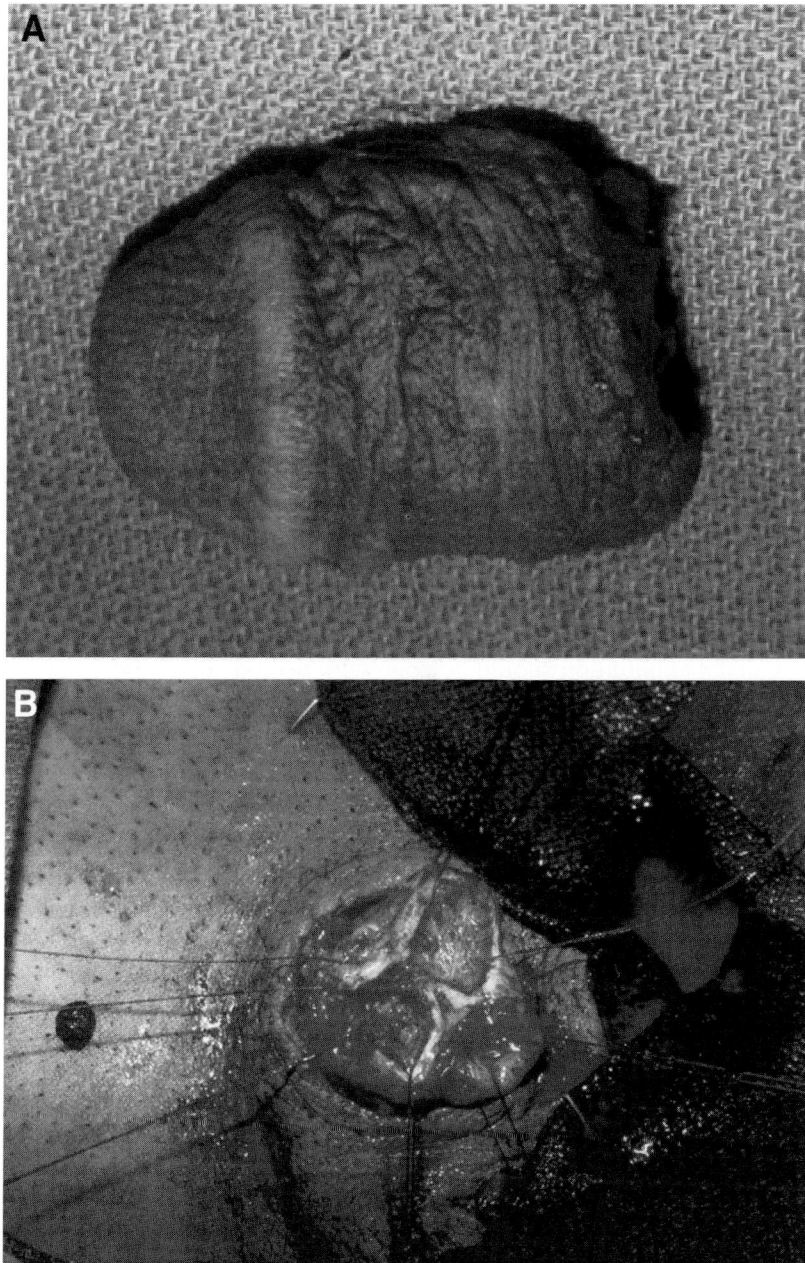

Fig. 11. (**A**) Amputated penis and (**B**) proximal cavernosal bodies prepared for replantation. (Courtesy of J. W. McAninch, MD.)

Last, all procedures involving the penis, especially those that can affect erectile function, are potential sources of litigation. It is of the utmost importance that the patient and his significant other clearly understand the consequences of the injury as well as the treatment, and that this is documented in the chart. It is not unusual, especially in an inner city trauma center, for the patient to blame the doctor for his situation rather than blaming his activity, his attacker, or his own actions. The consequent belligerent or hostile atmosphere that sometimes occurs may hinder the physician from further evaluation or treatment of these patients *(33)*.

SUMMARY

Our diagnostic and surgical treatment has evolved into a systematic approach for blunt and penetrating trauma and possible ischemic injuries. Based on history and physical examination, we feel that the patient can be brought straight to the operating room without imaging studies for blunt and penetrating trauma. We use a degloving approach with a urethral catheter in place, which greatly facilitates orientation. Instillation of saline into the urethra and corporal bodies before and after repair usually detects additional pathology as well as demonstrates the integrity of our repair. We also recommend debridement of the tissues injured by penetration, as well as separation of the corporal bodies from the spongiosum to inspect for other damage or blast effect. The surgeon should also be wary of a potential fistula formation. A snug dressing overnight is used for all injuries to limit dead space and control any potential hematoma or abscess formation. Oral DES or an LHRH agonist is given to prevent erections, which could compromise the surgical repair.

For those patients with localized glandular gangrene, if there is no progression of the ischemia, conservative management may be offered. However, if the gangrene progresses, distal amputation should be done with postoperative hyperbaric oxygen to prevent stump sloughing. These patients need to be followed over the long term to rule out fistula formation between the corporal bodies.

REFERENCES

1. Eke N. Fracture of the penis: a review. Br J Surg 2002; 89(5): 555–565.
2. Fergany AF, Angermeier KW, Montague DK. Review of Cleveland Clinic experience with penile fracture. Urology 1999; 54: 352–355.
3. Taha SA, Sharayah A, Kamal BA, Salem AA, Khwaja S. Fracture of the penis: surgical management. Int Surg 1988; 73: 63–64.
4. Zargooshi J. Penile fracture in Kermanshah, Iran: report of 172 cases. J Urol 2000; 164: 364–366.
5. Eke N. Urologic complications of coitus. BJU Int 2002 89(3): 273–277.
6. Goldman HB, Dmochowski RR, Cox CE. Penetrating trauma to the penis: functional results. J Urol 1996; 155(2): 551–553.
7. Cline KJ, Mata JA, Venable DD, Eastham JA. Penetrating trauma to male external genitalia. J Trauma 1998; 44(3): 492–494.
8. Kowalczyk J, Athens A, Grimaldi A. Penile fracture: an unusual presentation with lacerations of bilateral corpora cavernosa and partial disruption of the urethra. Urology 1994; 44: 599–601.
9. Mydlo JH, Hayyeri M, Macchia RJ. Urethrography and cavernosography imaging in a small series of penile fractures: a comparison with surgical findings. Urology 1998; 51(4): 616.
10. Cendron M, Whitmore KE, Carpiniello V, et al. Traumatic rupture of the corpus cavernosum: evaluation and management. J Urol 1990; 144: 987–991.
11. Karadeniz T, Topsakal M, Ariman A, Erton H, Basak D. Penile fracture: differential diagnosis, management and outcome. Br J Urol 1996; 77: 279–281.
12. Asgari MA, Hosseini SY, Safarinejad MR, Samadzadeh B, Bardideh AR. Penile fractures: evaluation, therapeutic approaches and long term results. J Urol 1996; 155: 148–149.
13. DeRose AF, Giglio M, Carmignani G. Traumatic rupture of the corpora cavernosa: new physiopathic acquisitions. Urology 2001; 57: 319–322.
14. Bertero EB, Campos RS, Mattos D Jr. Penile fracture with urethral injury. Braz J Urol 2000; 26: 295–297.

15. Nicely ER, Constabile RA, Moul JW. Rupture of the deep dorsal vein of the penis during sexual intercourse. J Urol 1992; 147: 150–153.
16. Ruckle HC, Hadley HR, Lui PD. Fracture of the penis: diagnosis and management. Urology 1992; 40(1): 3335.
17. Morris SB, Miller MAW, Anson K. Management of penile fracture. J Royal Soc Med 1998; 91(8): 427–430.
18. Karadeniz T, Topsakal M, Ariman A, Erton H, Basak D. Penile fracture: differential diagnosis, management and outcome. Br J Urol 1996; 77(2): 279–282.
19. Koga S, Saito Y, Arakaki Y, et al. Sonography in fracture of the penis. Br J Urol 1993; 72(2): 228–231.
20. Dincel C, Caskurlu T, Resim S, Bayraktar Z, Tasci AI, Sevin G. Fracture of the penis. Int Urol Nephrol 1998; 30(6): 761–763.
21. Mydlo JH. Surgeon experience with penile fracture. J Urol 2001; 166(2): 526–529.
22. Kalash SS, Young JD Jr. Fracture of penis: controversy of surgical vs conservative management. Urology 1984; 24(1): 21–24.
23. Mansi MK, Emran M, el-Mahrouky A, el-Mateet MS. Experience with penile fractures in Egypt: long-term results of immediate surgical repair. J Trauma 1993; 35: 67–70.
24. Selli C, Scott CA, DeAntoni P, Moro U, Crisci A, Cartei G. Squamous cell carcinoma arising at the base of the penis in a burn scar. Urology 1999; 54(5): 923–925.
25. Szostak MJ, DelPizzo JJ, Sklar GN. The plug and patch: a new technique for repair of corporal perforation during placement of penile prostheses. J Urol 2000; 163(4): 1203–1205.
26. Garcia Riestra V, Vareal Salgado M, Fernandez Garcia L. Urethral foreign bodies: a review. Arch Espan Urol 1999; 52(1): 74–76.
27. Mydlo JH, Macchia RJ, Kanter JL. Munchausen's syndrome: a medico-legal dilemma. Med Sci Law 1997; 37(3): 198–201.
28. Marceau L, Kleinman K, Goldstein I, McKinlay J. Does bicycling contribute to the risk of erectile dysfunction? Results from the Massachusetts Male Aging Study (MMAS). Int J Impot Res 2001; 13(5): 298–302.
29. Sommer F, Konig D, Graft C, et al. Impotence and genital numbness in cyclists. Int J Sports Med 2001; 22(6): 410–413.
30. Schwarzer U, Sommer F, Klotz T, Cremer C, Engelmann U. Cycling and penile oxygen pressure: the type of saddle matters. Eur Urol 2002; 41(2): 139–143.
31. Nicolaisen GS, Melamud A, Williams RD, McAninch JW. Rupture of the corpus cavernosum: surgical management. J Urol 1983; 130: 917–920.
32. Wespes E, Libert M, Simon J, Schulman CC. Fracture of the penis: conservative vs surgical treatment. Eur Urol 1987; 13: 166–168.
33. Mydlo JH, Harris CF, Brown JG. Blunt, penetrating and ischemic injuries to the penis. J Urol 2002; 168: 1433–1435.
34. Waller DA, Britton JP, Ferro MA. Rotational injury of the penis. Br J Urol 1990; 65: 425–428.
35. Mydlo JH, Gershbein AB, Macchia RJ. Non-operative management for presumed penile fracture. J Urol 2001; 16(2): 424.
36. Mydlo JH. Treatment of delayed zipper injury. Urol Int 2000; 64: 45.
37. Cummings JM, Parra RO, Boullier JA. Delayed repair of penile fracture. J Trauma 1998; 45(1): 153.
38. Jarow JP, Lowe FC. Penile trauma: an etiologic factor in Peyronie's disease and erectile dysfunction. J Urol 1997; 158(4), 1388–1390.
39. Motiwala HG. Urethrocavernous fistula following sexual intercourse. J Urol 1993; 149: 371–373.
40. Hargreaves DG, Plail RO. Fracture of the penis causing a corporo-urethral fistula. Br J Urol 1994; 73: 9799.
41. Munarriz RM, Yan QR, Nehra A, Udelson D, Goldstein I. Blunt trauma: the pathophysiology of hemodynamic injury leading to erectile dysfunction. J Urol 1995; 153: 1831–1834.
42. Weiner DM, Lowe FC. Surgical management of ischemic penile gangrene in diabetics with end stage atherosclerosis. J Urol 1996; 155: 926–929.

43. Stein M, Anderson C, Riccardi R, Chamberlain JW, Lerner S, Glicklich. Penile gangrene associated with chronic renal failure: report of 7 cases and a review of the literature. J Urol 1994; 152: 2014–2016.
44. Jezior JR, Brady JD, Schlossberg SM. Management of penile amputation injuries. World J Surg 2001; 25(12): 1602–1609.
45. Aydin A, Aslan A, Tuncer S. Penile amputation due to circumcision and reimplantation. Plast Reconstr Surg 2002; 110(2): 707–708.
46. Moore EE, Malangoni MA, Cogbill TH, et al. Organ injury scaling VII: cervical vascular, peripheral vascular, adrenal, penis, testis, and scrotum. J Trauma 1996; 41: 523.

II INFECTION

7 Infection of the Upper Urinary Tract

Maxwell V. Meng, MD and Jack W. McAninch, MD

CONTENTS

INTRODUCTION
PYELONEPHRITIS
IMAGING FOR PYELONEPHRITIS
RENAL ABSCESS
PERINEPHRIC ABSCESS
PYONEPHROSIS
EMPHYSEMATOUS PYELONEPHRITIS
XANTHOGRANULOMATOUS PYELONEPHRITIS
SUMMARY
REFERENCES

INTRODUCTION

Infections of the urinary tract are a common problem and are associated with significant morbidity and utilization of medical resources. It is estimated that urinary tract infections (UTIs) involving the urethra, bladder, ureters, or kidneys account for 1 million hospitalizations each year *(1)*. The majority of UTIs occur in healthy women and are typically uncomplicated infections of the bladder (cystitis), with management amenable to outpatient oral antibiotics. Nevertheless, up to one-quarter of the hospitalizations for UTI involve infection of the kidney (pyelonephritis)*(2)*. In this chapter, we discuss infection of the upper urinary tract and appropriate evaluation and management of pyelonephritis as well as more serious sequelae, including abscesses and chronic renal infections.

PYELONEPHRITIS

Pyelonephritis is defined as infection, usually bacterial, of the kidney and renal pelvis with resulting tubulointerstitial inflammation of the renal parenchyma. Even in cases of "uncomplicated" pyelonephritis in the woman, pyelonephritis itself is considered a complicated infection of the urinary tract *(3)*. Thus, consideration of an underlying anatomic or functional abnormality of the urinary tract is necessary. This aids in the appropriate utilization of imaging studies, antibiotic therapy, and adjunctive interventions to effect a rapid and effective resolution of the infection with minimal morbidity.

From: *Urological Emergencies: A Practical Guide*
Edited by: H. Wessells and J. W. McAninch © Humana Press Inc., Totowa, NJ

Table 1
Risk Factors for Complicated Upper Urinary Tract Infection

Men
Nosocomial infections
Women
    Anatomic abnormality of urinary tract
    Functional abnormality of urinary tract
    Pregnancy
    Spinal cord injury
    Comorbid diseases (diabetes, sickle cell disease)
    Unresolved UTI
    Persistent UTI
    Infection with urea-splitting organism
    Recurrent febrile UTI as child
    Febrile UTI (>3 days)
    Renal colic
    Gross hematuria

UTI, urinary tract infection.

Pathogenesis and Pathophysiology

Escherichia coli causes 80% of all community-acquired UTIs in healthy individuals and 50% of UTIs in patients in the hospital or with diabetes *(4)*. Similarly, *E. coli* is the most common cause of pyelonephritis. Although all individuals are potentially susceptible to UTI and pyelonephritis, certain characteristics increase the risk of complicated infections. Table 1 summarizes such risk factors. Variables that increase exposure to uropathogens include the presence of foreign body (e.g., catheter) and vaginal intercourse. Variables important in the stratification of risk include gender, age, and underlying conditions that affect the urinary tract, including pregnancy and diabetes *(5,6)*.

Lower UTIs, namely cystitis, rarely progress to pyelonephritis, although the bladder is usually affected during upper UTI. Uropathogenic bacteria that cause pyelonephritis have special characteristics and may be transmitted via the fecal–oral route and person-to-person direct contact, including sexual activity *(7)*. *Escherichia coli* responsible for UTIs exhibit several differences from *E. coli* within the bowel flora. These include P pili, aerobactin, s fimbrial adhesion, and hemolysin *(8)*. The importance of P fimbriated *E. coli* in acute pyelonephritis has been demonstrated in both children and adults, as well as in the monkey *(9–11)*. In addition, an association has been found between renal dysfunction and P fimbria receptors in those with renal scarring *(12)*. The P pili not only cause adherence to the urothelial cells facilitating infection, but also bind to fibronectin in the extracellular matrix. This contributes to the inflammatory response and may be important in the secondary inflammation after epithelial cell injury.

Acute pyelonephritis results in increased interleukin (IL)-6 and IL-8 levels in both the urine and serum *(13)*. This activation of the cytokine pathway is dependent on *E. coli* adhesion to the urothelial cells. The T lymphocytes and polymorphonuclear cells are recruited to the site of infection by the cytokines and then release enzymes that degrade the extracellular matrix. Thus, the inflammatory response and renal damage are mediated by both the local cytokine activation and lymphocyte activation. The combination of multiple virulence factors determines the degree of pathogenicity of the bacteria *(14)*.

Epidemiology

Although UTI in general has been well studied, few reports specifically examined the epidemiology of pyelonephritis. It is estimated that 25 to 50% of patients diagnosed with pyelonephritis in the emergency department are hospitalized *(15,16)*. Nicolle et al. reported that the mean rates of hospitalization for acute pyelonephritis were 10.86 per 10,000 population among women and 3.32 per 10,000 population among men *(17)*. In women, pregnancy was an important variable, and diabetes was a contributor in both men and women. Rates of hospitalization among women aged 20 to 29 yr were similar to that among women 70 yr and older.

In a survey from the United States, similar rates of hospitalization were reported, 11.7 per 10,000 population among women and 2.4 per 10,000 population among men *(18)*. Rates of hospitalization increased with age, but were not associated with diabetes. Men had higher rates of mortality in the hospital compared with women (16.5 vs 7.3 per 1000). Age was the strongest predictor of mortality, with those 60 yr and older at highest risk of death. The mean duration of hospitalization and average number of diagnoses per hospital stay both increased with age. Little variation in mortality was observed among various hospital sizes, ownership, location, and teaching status. These data suggest that patient, rather than hospital, characteristics determined outcome, and that relatively uniform application of care standards occurred.

Diagnosis of Pyelonephritis

Although pyelonephritis is defined as infection within the renal parenchyma, the diagnosis is based on the presence of a UTI with associated clinical features of fever and flank pain. The evaluation for all patients with known or suspected UTI should specifically assess for the presence or absence of fevers, flank pain, prior urinary infection, previous antibiotic use, prior urological procedures and operations, history of nephrolithiasis, gross hematuria, and medical comorbidities (diabetes, sickle cell disease). Many other terms for acute pyelonephritis have been used and may create ambiguity; these include focal pyelonephritis, lobar nephronia, and focal bacterial nephritis. Other terms, also based solely on radiological findings, include renal carbuncle and renal phlegmon.

CLINICAL PRESENTATION

A wide spectrum of clinical findings may be present. Classically, fever and chills are found in conjunction with costovertebral tenderness. Nevertheless, the initial presentation may range from symptoms of cystitis with mild flank pain to frank sepsis *(19)*. Lower urinary tract symptoms of dysuria, frequency, and urgency may also be present. In a study of patients with recurrent UTI, fever and flank pain were no more diagnostic of pyelonephritis than of cystitis. Physical examination should include measurement of vital signs to determine if evidence of sepsis (hypotension, tachycardia) is present. Because of overlap of symptoms (e.g., nausea, abdominal pain), the differential diagnosis should include appendicitis, perforated viscus, cholecystitis, and pelvic inflammatory disease.

Laboratory Findings

The urinalysis usually shows white blood cells, red blood cells, and white blood cell casts. In most patients, the urine culture will demonstrate more than 100,000 colony-forming units of bacteria, typically *E. coli*. However, 20% of patients have cultures with fewer bacteria ($<10^5$) and negative results on Gram staining *(20)*. *E. coli* accounts for more than 80% of cases of acute pyelonephritis. Other members of the Enterobacteriaceae family can be found, including *Klebsiella*, *Proteus*, *Pseudomonas*, *Serratia*, and *Citrobacter*. Gram-positive organisms, such as *Enterobacter faecalis*, *Staphylococcus aureus*, and *Staphylococcus epidermidis*, may also cause pyelonephritis.

Serum laboratory tests may show a leukocytosis, increased erythrocyte sedimentation rate, and elevated C-reactive protein levels. The creatinine level may be elevated, and some patients present with acute renal failure. Blood cultures may be positive, confirming bacteremia.

Invasive tests are the most reliable method of confirming pyelonephritis; however, these are impractical and therefore not routinely used in most patients. Initially described by Stamey in 1963, ureteral catheterization specifically collects multiple urine specimens from both upper urinary tracts to quantitate bacterial counts. The method is well described in detail elsewhere *(21)* and was validated in multiple studies. Subsequently, Fairley described the bladder washout test to help differentiate upper from lower UTI *(22)*. The technique is simpler, with determination of bacterial counts from the urine after washing the bladder with a combination of neomycin and two lytic enzymes. Currently, noninvasive tests to localize infection to the kidneys are not reliable. Documenting true upper UTI is typically reserved for patients with recurrent or persistent infections, for which the information determines subsequent treatment decisions.

Treatment of Pyelonephritis

Despite the recognition of acute pyelonephritis as a significant infection, limited data are available regarding the optimal antimicrobial regimen (Fig. 1). Nevertheless, a shift in the treatment paradigm has been observed, with primary outpatient management using oral antibiotics. This is appropriate in stable patients with uncomplicated acute pyelonephritis. Oral fluoroquinolones are the first-line drugs, with broad-spectrum activity and excellent urinary levels of drug. Table 2 summarizes effective oral regimens for uncomplicated pyelonephritis.

Although previous studies have examined the efficacy of trimethoprim-sulfamethoxazole (TMP-SMX) and ampicillin for pyelonephritis, these should currently not be used alone for empiric therapy unless the causative organism is known to be sensitive; there is a high prevalence of resistance to TMP-SMX among uropathogens *(23)*. Nitrofurantoin should not be used because it does not achieve reliable serum or tissue levels. Many current fluoroquinolones can be used, but the newer moxifloxacin has lower urinary levels and should be avoided for pyelonephritis. If Gram-positive cocci are seen on the Gram stain, amoxicillin or amoxicillin-clavulanic acid should be added or used alone if the culture confirms enterococcus susceptible to ampicillin.

Traditionally, women with pyelonephritis have been treated for up to 6 wk with antibiotics, but several studies have shown that shorter courses are equally efficacious. The IDSA Clinical Practice Guideline Committee analyzed available reports regarding treatment for pyelonephritis *(24)*. TMP-SMX was preferred to ampicillin, and 2 wk of therapy was adequate for most women. In a randomized, prospective trial including

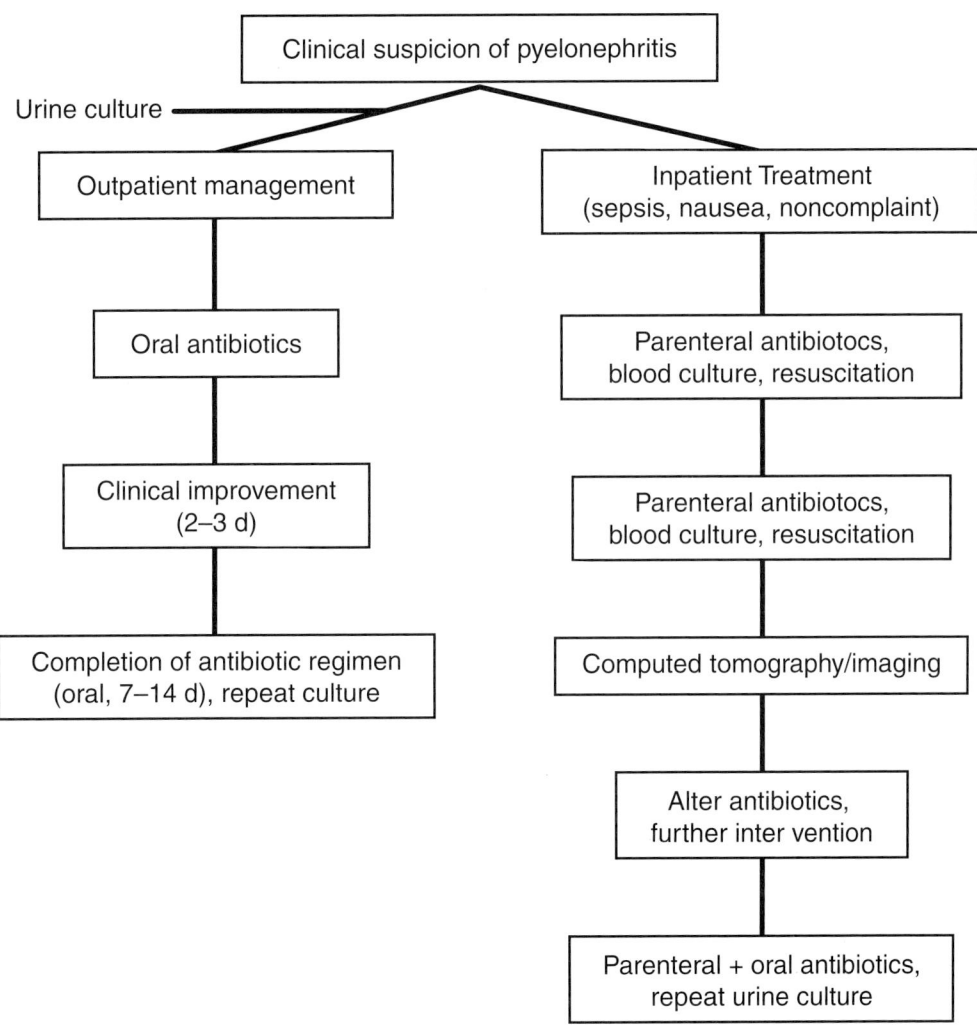

Fig. 1. Treatment algorithm for acute pyelonephritis.

Table 2
Oral Antibiotic Regimens for Acute Pyelonephritis (Uncomplicated)

Drug (dose)	Interval	Duration
Amoxicillin (500 mg)	q8 h	10–14 d
Amoxicillin (875 mg)	q12 h	10–14 d
Amoxicillin-clavulanate (875/125 mg)	q12 h	10–14 d
Ciprofloxacin (500 mg)	q12 h	7–10 d
Gatifloxacin (400 mg)	q24 h	7–10 d
Levofloxacin (250 mg)	q24 h	7–10 d
TMP-SMX (160/800 mg)	q12 h	7–10 d

TMP-SMX, trimethoprim-sulfamethoxazole.

Table 3
Parenteral Antibiotics for Acute Pyelonephritis (Uncomplicated)

Drug (dose)	Interval
Ceftriaxone (1–2 g)	q24 h
Cefepime (1 g)	q12 h
Ciprofloxacin (200–400 mg)	q12 h
Gatifloxacin (400 mg)	q24 h
Levofloxacin (250–500 mg)	q24 h
Gentamicin (3–5 mg/kg)	q24 h
Gentamicin (1 mg/kg)	q8 h
Ampicillin (1 g)	q6 h
TMP-SMX (160/800 mg)	q12 h
Aztreonam (1 g)	q8–12 h
Ampicillin-sulbactam (1.5 g)	q6 h
Piperacillin-tazobactam (3.375 g)	q6–8 h

TMP-SMX, trimethoprim-sulfamethoxazole.

Table 4
Parenteral Antibiotics for Acute Pyelonephritis (Complicated)

Drug (dose)	Interval
Ampicillin (2 g)	q6 h
Gentamicin (1.5 mg/kg)	q8 h
Ciprofloxacin (400 mg)	q12 h
Levofloxacin (500 mg)	q24 h
Ticarcillin-clavulanate (3.1 g)	q8 h
Imipenem-cilastatin (500 mg)	q6–8 h
Aztreonam (1 g)	q8 h

TMP-SMX, 6 wk of therapy were no better than 2 wk and was associated with more side effects *(25)*. Additional studies also suggested that regimens of 10 to 14 d are sufficient *(26)*. Talan et al. compared the efficacy of ciprofloxacin (7 d) with TMP-SMX (14 d) in treating uncomplicated acute pyelonephritis *(27)*. Bacteriological cure rates at 4 to 11 d were 99% for ciprofloxacin and 89% for TMP-SMX ($p = 0.004$); clinical cure rates were 96 and 83%, respectively.

In reliable patients with moderate symptoms (e.g., fever, vomiting), temporary intravenous hydration and parenteral antibiotic dosing (i.e., fluoroquinolone, ceftriaxone, aminoglycoside) can be safely initiated with subsequent outpatient oral antibiotic regimen. In these situations, early follow-up is essential, as is prompt return if symptoms persist or worsen. In all cases of acute pyelonephritis, urine cultures should be checked at 48 h to ensure that the organism is not resistant to the selected antibiotic. Repeat urine cultures are performed 5 to 7 d after starting therapy and 4 to 6 wk after completion of antibiotics to confirm that the infection has resolved. A significant number (10–30%) of patients relapse after 10 to 14 d of adequate antibiotics, and these individuals require a second 14-d course; rarely, 6 wk of antibiotics are necessary to eradicate the renal infection *(28,29)*.

Pyelonephritis Necessitating Hospitalization

As mentioned, a significant minority of patients with pyelonephritis require hospitalization for parenteral antibiotic therapy. Indications for admission in those with uncomplicated pyelonephritis include the inability to maintain oral fluids or medication, uncertain social situation, poor compliance, and uncertain diagnosis. Moreover, those with uncomplicated pyelonephritis and normal urinary tracts but severe infection warrant admission for antibiotic and supportive therapy. Patients with complicated pyelonephritis require hospitalization more often; criteria include infection in men, hospital-acquired infection, urinary tract abnormality, nephrolithiasis, and catheterization or instrumentation. It is generally recommended that pregnant women with pyelonephritis be observed during initiation of antibiotics.

After urinary cultures have been obtained, parenteral therapy is chosen. Tables 3 and 4 summarize appropriate regimens for uncomplicated pyelonephritis in the severely ill patient and complicated pyelonephritis, respectively. Common options include fluoroquinolone, aminoglycoside with or without ampicillin, or extended-spectrum cephalosporin. Complicated infections and those caused by nosocomial pathogens require broad-spectrum coverage, typically an aminoglycoside and ampicillin; consideration must be given to the possibility of Gram-positive organisms. Urine and blood cultures are obtained after initiating therapy, and antimicrobials should be altered based on the results of susceptibility testing.

Patients may have persistent symptoms and fevers despite the initiation of appropriate antibiotic treatment, and observation is warranted for 48 to 72 h. After resolution of symptoms in the absence of bacteremia, conversion to oral antibiotics after 2 to 3 d is indicated to complete 7 to 14 d of therapy. If the blood cultures are positive, parenteral antibiotics should be continued for 7 d, with subsequent completion of oral antibiotics to 7 to 14 d. When clinical improvement does not occur at this point, further evaluation is needed. Imaging, discussed in a separate section, should be obtained to identify potential urinary obstruction or renal and perirenal abscesses. Urinary drainage can be accomplished by placement of either a ureteral stent or a percutaneous nephrostomy tube.

Urosepsis

The incidence of serious infections in hospitalized patient has increased over the past three decades. Gram-negative bacterial infection is the most common cause of sepsis and carries an overall mortality in excess of 10% *(30,31)*. Although bacteremia resulting from UTI and pyelonephritis can be managed with appropriate antibiotic therapy alone, sepsis syndrome and septic shock are dire conditions that necessitate emergent intervention.

Sepsis syndrome is defined as clinical evidence of infection associated with hyper- or hypothermia (>38°C or <36°C), tachycardia (>90 beats/min), tachypnea (>20 breaths/min), and evidence of inadequate organ perfusion *(32)*. *Septic shock* is the sepsis syndrome and hypotension (<90 mmHg) despite adequate volume replacement. The pathophysiology of sepsis has been studied extensively and arises from the vigorous host response to Gram-negative infection *(33)*. The release of proinflammatory cytokine mediators by lipopolysaccharide-responsive cells (macrophages, endothelial cells) is initiated primarily by endotoxin, a lipopolysaccharide component of the bacterial outer membrane. Lipid A, a component of endotoxin, induces release of factors that include tumor necrosis factor-α, IL-1, IL-6, and IL-8. The intravascular activation of the inflammatory pathway via the cytokine overproduction results in the hemodynamic collapse.

After sepsis is diagnosed or suspected, aggressive supportive care is needed. All potential sources of bacteremia must be cultured, and appropriate broad-spectrum antibiotics should be administered. Volume resuscitation, ventilatory support, and hemodynamic monitoring and management may be required. The urinary tract should be studied to determine whether obstruction or stasis is present or whether abscess formation has occurred.

IMAGING FOR PYELONEPHRITIS

Routine upper urinary tract imaging is not indicated in patients with pyelonephritis. However, persistence or worsening of symptoms at 48 to 72 h requires further evaluation. The intravenous urogram (IVU) has limited utility in individuals with pyelonephritis. Generalized or focal renal enlargement may be noted and can mimic a renal mass. Delayed appearance of the nephrogram may result from infection of the renal parenchyma. However, the IVU is negative in up to 75% of patients with pyelonephritis (34). Ureteral obstruction may be evidence on IVU, although dilation of the collecting system, without obstruction, may be seen with acute pyelonephritis.

Although renal ultrasonography is noninvasive and without ionizing radiation, information gained is limited (35). Renal size and shape are apparent, and dilation of the collecting system can be detected. Focal areas of infection, with enlargement or suggestion of a mass, may be evident. Typically, acute pyelonephritis appears as a hypoechoic area, but can appear hyperechoic with or without loss of normal corticomedullary junction differentiation. Echogenic material within the dilated renal pelvis may suggest pyonephrosis, often with a urine-debris level.

Computed tomography (CT) provides the most detailed images of both acute pyelonephritis and associated findings and sequelae, and it is the study of choice for investigation of pyelonephritis (Fig. 2). If the infection is sufficiently severe, global or focal renal enlargement can be visualized. Edema and inflammation may result in decreased attenuation of the affected parenchyma on noncontrast scans. After intravenous contrast administration, wedge-shaped or linear zones of decreased attenuation radiating from the calyces toward the renal capsule are consistent with acute pyelonephritis, the result of tubular obstruction by inflammatory cells and debris, ischemia, and interstitial edema. In diffuse pyelonephritis, poor enhancement of the parenchyma and delayed contrast excretion can be found. Less-common CT signs include thickening of the pelvicalyceal wall, obliteration of the renal sinus and perinephric fat planes, and thickening of Gerota's fascia.

It is important to note that acute pyelonephritis may appear as focal, masslike areas of decreased enhancement on CT. Delayed CT images may help differentiate an inflammatory mass from tumor. In addition, repeat CT after resolution of infection should be performed if the diagnosis of malignancy remains uncertain.

RENAL ABSCESS

A renal abscess is a focal collection of pus confined to the renal parenchyma. Currently, these lesions primarily arise from progression of acute pyelonephritis caused by Gram-negative organisms. Prior to the antimicrobial era, most renal abscesses resulted from hematogenous spread of staphylococci infection (36). These abscesses, or carbuncles, occurred in higher risk patients with dialysis, diabetes, and intravenous drug use. Carbuncles also occurred more frequently in men, typically involving a single unilateral lesion.

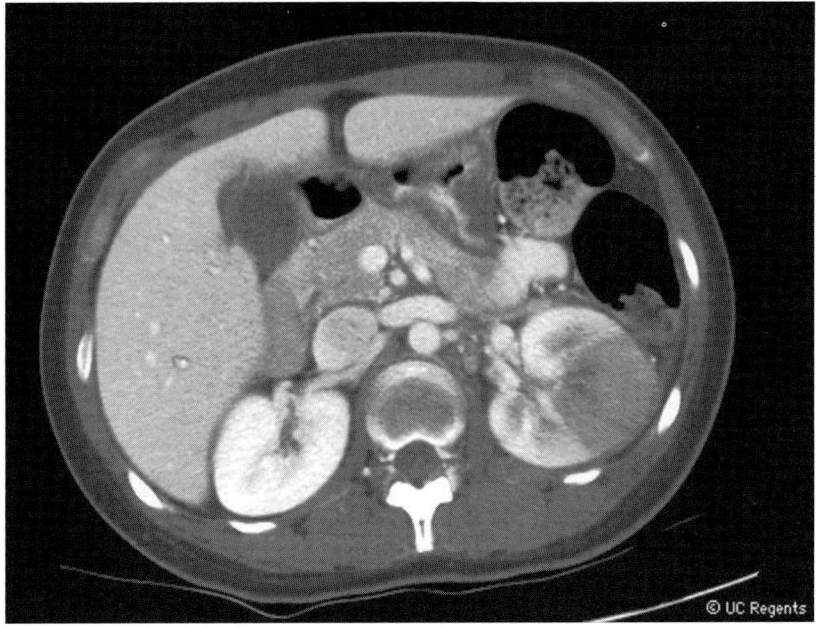

Fig. 2. Contrast-enhanced computed tomography demonstrating evidence of left pyelonephritis. Note the enlarged renal contour, compared to the right side, as well as the wedge-shaped area. (Courtesy of Drs. Benjamin Yeh and Fergus Coakley, Department of Radiology, University of California, San Francisco.)

Presentation and Diagnosis

Most patients present with signs and symptoms consistent with acute pyelonephritis; however, in some patients the symptoms are subtle, and diagnosis may be delayed until surgical intervention. In addition to a history of UTI, abscess formation is associated with urinary stasis, calculi, pregnancy, neurogenic bladder, and diabetes. Evidence of skin infections or intravenous drug use may suggest the dissemination of Gram-positive organisms via the blood stream.

Abscesses appear as hypoechoic or anechoic complex masses with increased through transmission on ultrasonography. Early abscess formation, however, may be difficult to distinguish from acute pyelonephritis. As the abscess encapsulates, the borders become increasingly well defined, and the abscess becomes a distinct mass. Debris within the abscess appears as internal echoes, but the degree of fluid and solid appearance can vary greatly.

CT is the most accurate method of identifying renal abscesses, which appear as a low-density mass *(37,38)* (Figs. 3 and 4). The lesions are apparent on both pre- and post-contrast images, with the pesudocapsule more evident after contrast enhancement; the debris and pus do not enhance. The presence of a chronic abscess leads to obliteration of adjacent tissue planes and thickening of Gerota's fascia.

Treatment

In the past, surgical drainage and debridement, and occasionally nephrectomy, were required for renal abscesses. Contemporary management of renal abscesses begins with parenteral antibiotics and close observation. If a urinary source is suspected, then anti-

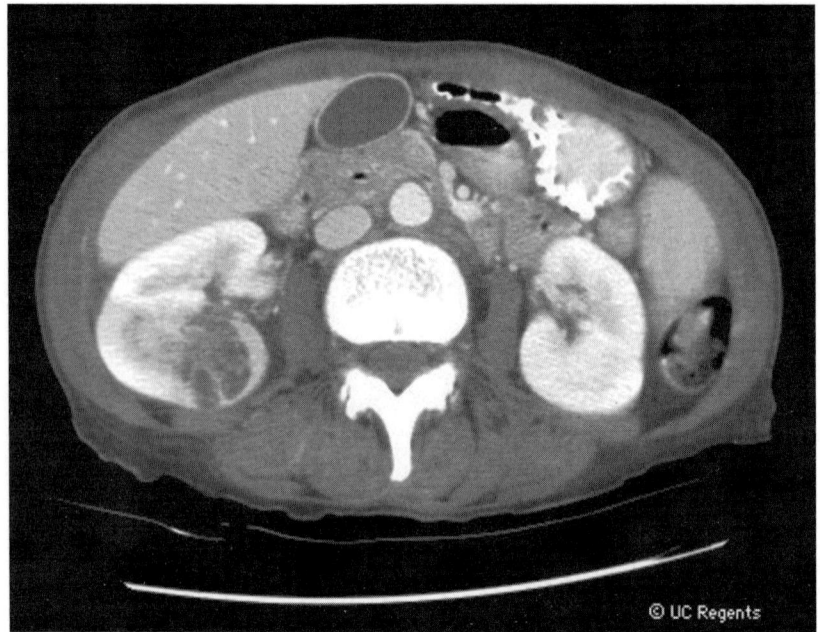

Fig. 3. Contrast-enhanced computed tomography demonstrating evidence of right pyelonephritis and abscess formation. Note the posterior region of reduced attenuation, consistent with pyelonephritis, and the multiple septae within the abscess. (Courtesy of Drs. Benjamin Yeh and Fergus Coakley, Department of Radiology, University of California, San Francisco.)

biotic selection is as described for Gram-negative organisms. If hematogenous spread from the skin is possible, coverage of *Staphylococcus* with a penicillinase-resistant penicillin, cephalosporin, or vancomycin is necessary. CT is crucial in identifying the lesion and its size. Abscesses smaller than 3 cm are usually amenable to intravenous antibiotics alone *(39)*.

After clinical improvement, intravenous antibiotics should be continued for 24 to 48 h. Subsequently, an additional 2 wk of oral antibiotic therapy should be completed, with radiographic confirmation of cure. In the immunocompromised patient, early consideration of percutaneous aspiration or drainage may hasten resolution of infection and recovery. Abscesses of 3 to 5 cm are amenable to percutaneous, image-guided drainage *(40,41)*.

Dalla Palma et al. recently described successful medical treatment of renal abscesses smaller than 5 cm, without evidence of complications *(42)*. Antibiotic therapy was continued for at least 4 wk, and follow-up CT was important. Traditionally, larger abscesses (>5 cm) required open surgical drainage and, potentially, nephrectomy. The improvements in interventional radiological techniques may permit the percutaneous management in many of these patients, with decrease in morbidity. This must be balanced against the potential for prolonged hospitalization, multiple procedures, and unknown long-term sequelae.

PERINEPHRIC ABSCESS

Suppurative infections surrounding the kidney, within the perinephric space, are difficult to diagnose and treat. Most perinephric abscesses result from an underlying

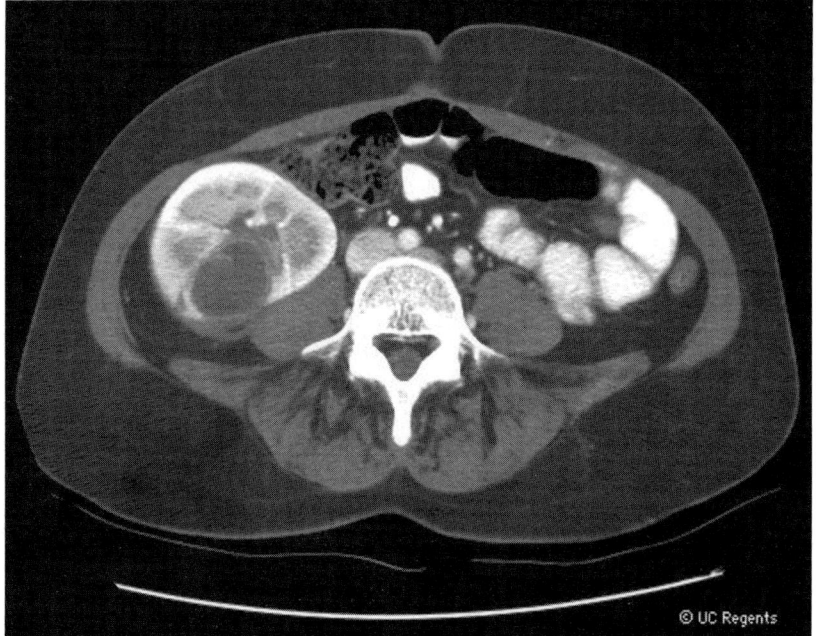

Fig. 4. Contrast-enhanced computed tomography with right renal abscess. Note the appearance of the pseudocapsule of the abscess cavity. (Courtesy of Drs. Benjamin Yeh and Fergus Coakley, Department of Radiology, University of California, San Francisco.)

renal infection, with abscess development and rupture within Gerota's fascia; subsequent breach of Gerota's fascia and spread lead to paranephric abscesses. These purulent collections surrounding the kidney may also arise from a hematogenous source or primarily from an adjacent organ, such as the bowel, pancreas, pleural space, and gallbladder *(36)*.

A variety of bacterial organisms can lead to perinephric abscess formation. Similar to renal abscesses, early studies documented a significant number of staphylococcal infections, with modern series reporting a greater number of infections attributable to *E. coli* and *Proteus*. Urine culture most reliably detects the organism, with blood and abscess fluid only 50% sensitive *(43,44)*. Risk factors for development of perinephric infection include nephrolithiasis, prior UTI, diabetes, immunocompromised state, and abnormal urinary tract. Despite modern medicine, the natural history and outcome of perinephric abscesses have not changed significantly. Overall, nephrectomy is performed in up to 20% of patients, and mortality approaches 15% *(44–46)*.

Diagnosis and Treatment

The traditionally poor outcome of perinephric abscesses has been partially attributed to significant delays in diagnosis. Most patients have prolonged symptoms, longer than 14 d. Common signs and symptoms included fever, abdominal pain, and dysuria. A review of 25 patients confirmed these earlier reports *(44)*. Despite 40% of patients having multiple predisposing conditions, only 33% were correctly diagnosed as the time of hospitalization. The mean time to diagnosis after hospitalization was 3.4 d. Although

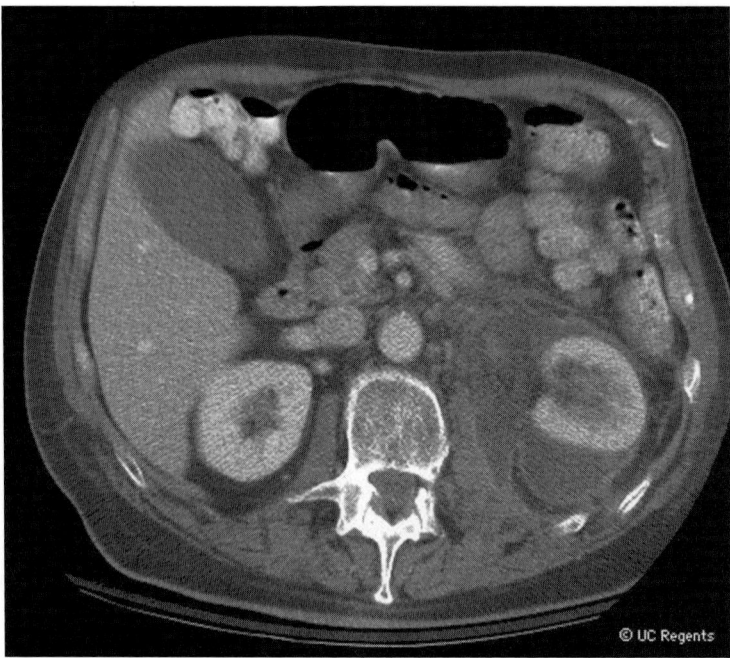

Fig. 5. Computed tomography demonstrating perinephric abscess around the left kidney. Note the pus surrounding the kidney, confined within Gerota's fascia, and normal appearance of the renal parenchyma. (Courtesy of Drs. Benjamin Yeh and Fergus Coakley, Department of Radiology, University of California, San Francisco.)

plain abdominal radiography and IVU can provide information such as identification of stones, air, and urinary obstruction, these findings are nonspecific. Ultrasonography can show a sonolucent mass adjacent or displacing the kidney; nevertheless, the sensitivity may be as low as 64% when compared to CT. Therefore, abdominal CT is the preferred imaging study when perinephric abscess is suspected. CT provides excellent anatomic details, with clear definition of the size and extent of the abscess and relationship to other organs (Fig. 5).

After identification of the perinephric abscess, treatment has typically consisted of parenteral antibiotics and drainage. In earlier reports, medical therapy was associated with high rates of mortality despite treatment (65%), likely because of delayed surgical intervention *(46)*. Thus, drainage of perinephric abscesses has been an important principle and an integral part of management. Advances in imaging techniques, combined with the ability for adequate percutaneous drainage of abscesses, have suggested that open surgical drainage or nephrectomy can be avoided. The decision is based on the size of the lesion and degree of illness. Small abscesses (<3 cm) generally resolve with antibiotic treatment alone.

In our series, the eight patients successfully managed with antibiotics had a mean abscess size of 1.8 cm, and all abscesses were less than 3 cm *(44)*. Conversely, two patients with unrecognized abscesses died despite intravenous antibiotics. Thus, the early identification of perinephric abscesses is crucial, and the decision to treat using antibiotics alone requires consideration of associated conditions and accurate staging of the abscess (Fig. 6).

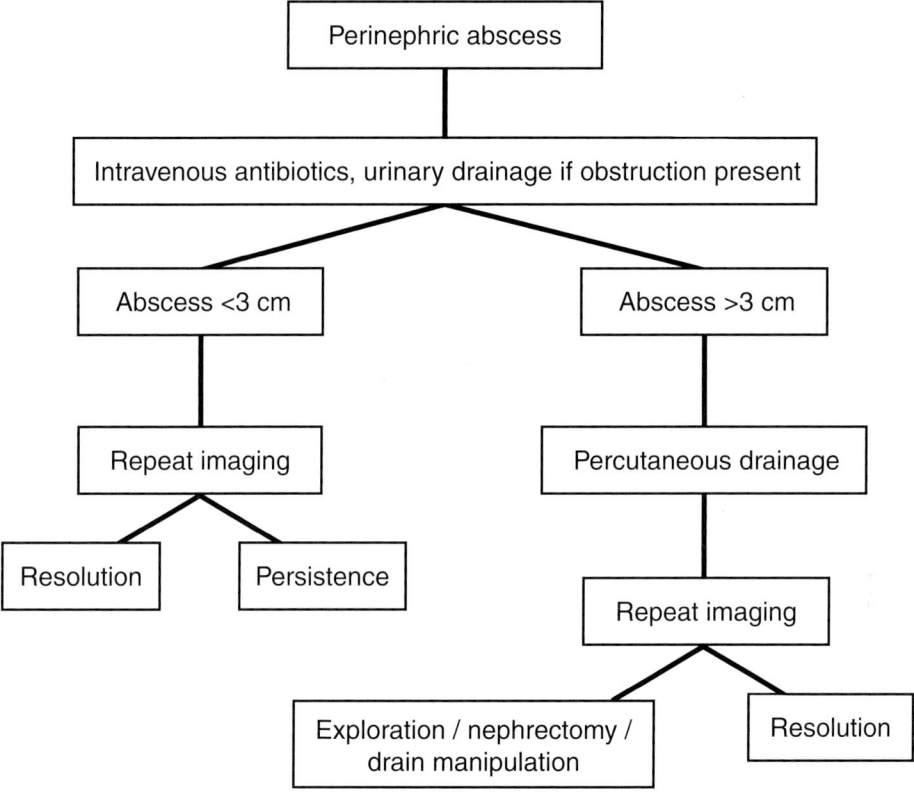

Fig. 6. Treatment algorithm for perinephric abscess.

Large abscesses (>5 cm) can be cured with antibiotics in conjunction with percutaneous catheter drainage. In 11 patients managed using this strategy, there was no mortality; however, longer hospitalization and prolonged catheter placement were necessary. Moreover, one-third of patients ultimately required nephrectomy for persistent infection in the nonfunctional kidney. Thus, percutaneous drainage is likely safe and reasonable for most abscesses, including those larger than 3 cm, but it must be realized that repeated or more aggressive intervention is often necessary. In addition, the perinephric abscess associated with a poorly functioning kidney may benefit from early nephrectomy.

PYONEPHROSIS

Pyonephrosis describes a suppurative infection in a hydronephrotic renal unit. In many cases, it is associated with destruction of the kidney and minimal renal function. In general, patients are ill with sepsis syndrome or shock. The diagnosis is similar to acute pyelonephritis, although urinalysis and urine culture may not reveal bacteriuria if the system is completely obstructed.

Imaging and Treatment

Renal ultrasonography may show echogenic material within a dilated collecting system or a urine-debris level; in some cases, findings may be suggestive only for hydronephrosis.

CT can also identify hydronephrosis and the level of obstruction; however, pyonephrosis may be indistinguishable from simple, uninfected hydronephrosis. Findings that suggest pyonephrosis include delayed nephrogram, fluid-fluid level, and gas within the collecting system. Retrograde pyelography can identify ureteral obstruction, filling defects from pus or stone, and permit collection of material for culture.

The obstructed and infected urinary system requires prompt drainage and antibiotic therapy. Options include a ureteral stent and percutaneous nephrostomy tube. In stable patients with anatomy amenable to retrograde instrumentation, cystoscopy and ureteral stent placement are indicated. In extremely ill patients, a percutaneous approach may be the most rapid means of renal decompression. Watson et al. reported excellent outcome in 315 patients requiring percutaneous nephrostomy drainage for pyonephrosis *(47)*. Direct renal access provided not only effective drainage, but also additional information regarding uropathogens in 37%. Subsequently, after resolution of the acute infection, definitive management of the cause of obstruction can be performed.

EMPHYSEMATOUS PYELONEPHRITIS

Emphysematous pyelonephritis is a potentially life-threatening necrotizing infection of the renal parenchyma *(48)*. Historically, management has involved aggressive surgical intervention because of the severity of infection and significant mortality. Similar to perinephric abscesses, however, there has been a significant shift in the modern management paradigm.

Pathophysiology

The acute necrotizing nature of emphysematous pyelonephritis results from the synergism of gas-forming bacteria, high tissue glucose, poor tissue perfusion, and susceptible host (e.g., diabetes, urinary obstruction) *(49)*. Bacterial pathways that result in gas formation include mixed acid fermentation by Enterobacteriaceae (e.g., *E. coli, Klebsiella pneumoniae, Proteus*) and butyric fermentation (*Clostridium*). The primary components of the gas are H_2 and CO_2; trace amounts of ammonia and methane may be detected.

Diagnosis and Treatment

Adults are exclusively at risk for emphysematous pyelonephritis, with women affected more often than men. Signs and symptoms are consistent with acute pyelonephritis that precedes frank necrosis, but do not improve despite antibiotics. The finding of intraparenchymal gas is pathomnemonic for emphysematous pyelonephritis; this produces a mottled shadow overlying the kidney as well as crescent configuration around the renal contour. Plain abdominal radiography, IVU, or ultrasonography can detect parenchymal gas. This should be distinguished from air within the collecting system, which is a less-serious condition responsive to antibiotics alone. CT provides details regarding the gas pattern and anatomic extent of infection (Fig. 7). Several authors have proposed schemes based on extent of infection and gas for classification of emphysematous pyelonephritis (Table 5) *(49,50)*.

No uniform management strategy exists for emphysematous pyelonephritis. In addition to antibiotics and supportive care, relief of urinary obstruction in the affected kidney is indicated if present. Conservative management, with antibiotics alone or in conjunction with percutaneous catheter drainage, is increasingly utilized with good outcomes

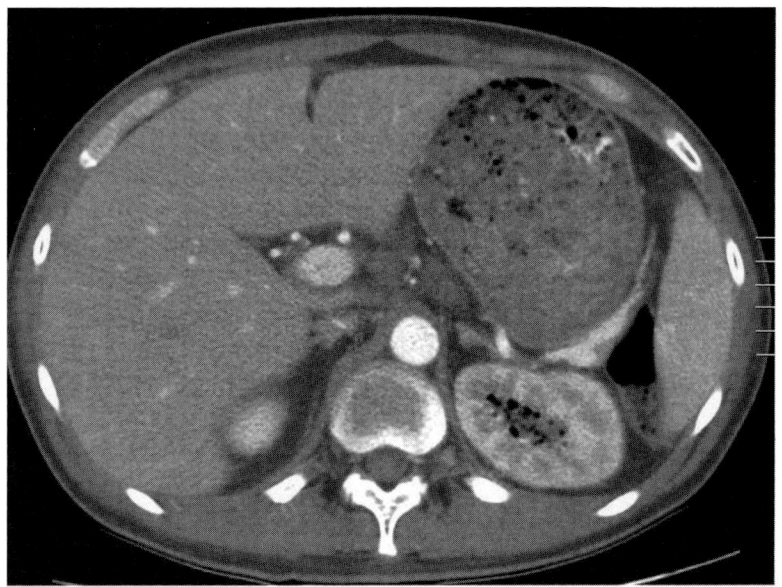

Fig. 7. Computed tomography demonstrating gas within the left kidney. This diabetic patient had evidence of fungal pyelonephritis. (Courtesy of Drs. Benjamin Yeh and Fergus Coakley, Department of Radiology, University of California, San Francisco.)

Table 5
Classification Systems for Emphysematous Pyelonephritis

Stage	Characteristics
I	Gas within parenchyma or perinephric tissue
II	Gas in kidney and surroundings
III	Extension of gas through Gerota's fascia
	Bilateral involvement

Class	Characteristics
1	Emphysematous pyelitis
2	Parenchymal gas confined to kidney
3A	Extension of gas or abscess to perinephric area
3B	Extension to pararenal space
4	Bilateral involvement or infection of solitary kidney

(49,51,52). Accurate assessment of extent and nature of infection is vital to the decision process. Huang et al. proposed that localized (classes 1 and 2) infections can be treated with percutaneous drainage; this approach is also feasible for more extensive (classes 3 and 4) cases without systemic manifestations. Fulminant infection may be best managed with initial nephrectomy. Best et al. reported complete resolution of infection in five patients with antibiotics alone; however, they differentiated between gas-forming renal abscess characterized by large gas lesion, as in their series, and true diffuse necrotizing infection with multiple small bubbles *(52)*. Surgical drainage or nephrectomy is indicated if the infection persists or progresses.

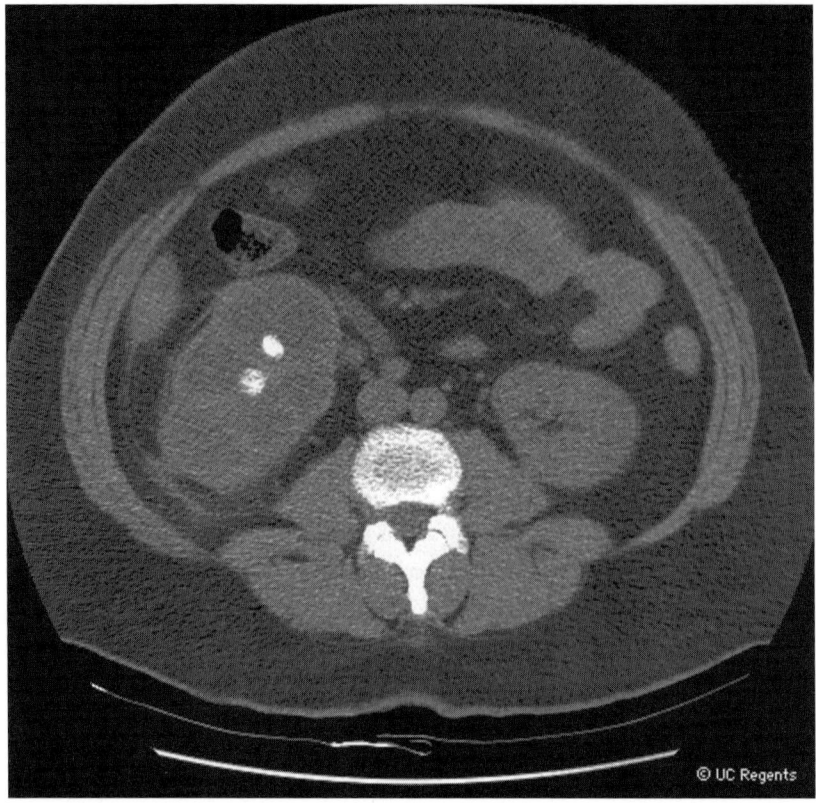

Fig. 8. Noncontrast computed tomography in a patient with right xanthogranulomatous pyelonephritis. Note the calcifications, enlarged renal form, and areas of reduced attenuation, potentially representing pus, dilated calyces, or inflammatory tissue. (Courtesy of Drs. Benjamin Yeh and Fergus Coakley, Department of Radiology, University of California, San Francisco.)

XANTHOGRANULOMATOUS PYELONEPHRITIS

Xanthogranulomatous pyelonephritis (XGP) is the end result of severe, chronic infection of the kidney. It is relatively uncommon (0.6–1.4% of renal inflammation evaluated pathologically), but typically is unilateral; it develops in the presence of urinary obstruction and nephrolithiasis *(53,54)*.

Pathogenesis

The combination of urinary obstruction, nephrolithiasis, and UTI are important elements in the development of XGP *(55)*. Nephrolithiasis is noted in nearly 90% of patients, with many having staghorn calculi. Infection is usually secondary to either *E. coli* or *Proteus mirabilis*; other uropathogens include *Klebsiella*, *Pseudomonas*, and *Enterobacter*. Progressive destruction of the renal parenchyma occurs, with impairment in renal function. Histologically, XGP is characterized by sheets of lipid-laden macrophages (xanthoma cells) around abscesses within the parenchyma, admixed with lymphocytes, giant cells, and plasma cells. The kidney grossly is enlarged, with destruction and replacement of the parenchyma by yellow nodules and pericalyceal granulation.

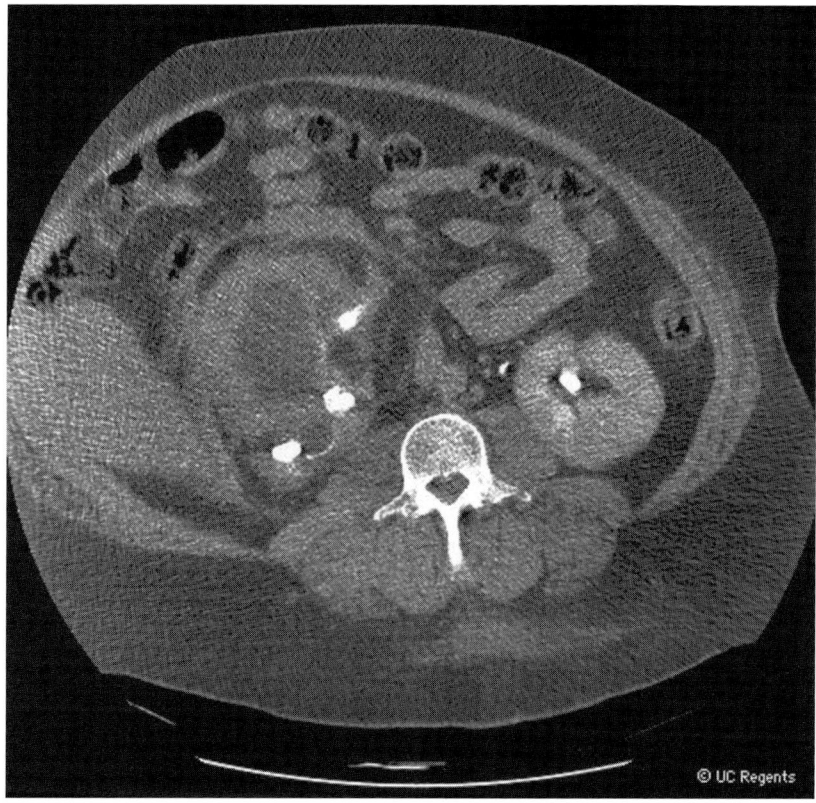

Fig. 9. Delayed computed tomography demonstrating right xanthogranulomatous pyelonephritis. Note the multiple calcifications as well as nearly absent renal parenchyma and evidence of inflammation within Gerota's fascia. (Courtesy of Drs. Benjamin Yeh and Fergus Coakley, Department of Radiology, University of California, San Francisco.)

Diagnosis and Treatment

Most patients present with typical evidence of upper urinary tract infection: flank pain, fever, and bacteriuria. Although the diagnosis of XGP relies on a pathological diagnosis, some have suggested that urinary cytology can accurately predict XGP in 80% of cases *(56)*. Nevertheless, XGP can be suggested by the combination of enlarged kidney, presence of calculi, and poorly functioning kidney *(57)*. IVU may detect all of these features, although with less sensitivity than CT. Ultrasound can be useful in noting renal enlargement, stones, and multiple hypoechoic foci corresponding to xanthoma granulomas.

CT is the preferred modality in the evaluation of XGP (Figs. 8 and 9). Characteristic features include a large, reniform mass with poor function. Nonenhanced images demonstrate a central calcification, typically without pelvic dilation. The renal parenchyma is usually thin and contains multiple round hypodense masses that represent dilated calyces, abscesses, or inflammatory tissue. CT also depicts the degree of perinephric and pararenal involvement, with frequent extension into the psoas, back, or abdominal wall muscles. Cutaneous and renocolic fistulas may be visualized, as well as reactive lymphadenopathy. Precise identification of these features is important for planning surgical intervention.

The appropriate management of XGP is often unclear given the diagnostic uncertainty in many cases. The radiographic appearance may mimic other renal diseases, including malakoplakia, lymphoma, urothelial carcinoma, and renal carcinoma. Antimicrobial therapy should be initiated, and long-term treatment can eradicate the infection. If symptoms or UTI persists or if underlying malignancy cannot be excluded, then nephrectomy is warranted. An attempt should be made to excise the kidney and surrounding inflammatory tissue completely; these operations are often challenging and associated with significant morbidity. Only recently have reports documented the utility of laparoscopy in removing XGP kidneys, with moderate success and limited complications *(58)*.

SUMMARY

Infection of the upper urinary tract is relatively common and associated with potentially serious sequelae. Both uncomplicated pyelonephritis and purulent renal infections can be difficult to diagnose and require a high index of suspicion. Accurate identification of the causative organism allows the tailored use of antibiotic therapy, and careful follow-up and subsequent specimen culture help ensure adequate treatment of the infection.

Utilization of radiographic studies, primarily computed tomography, is warranted when the clinical picture is either unclear or deteriorates. Aggressive resuscitation and management may be necessary when systemic manifestation or sepsis results. The early identification of more severe complications of renal infection is crucial for prompt intervention, which is indicated by the severity of infection and size of abscess. The evolution of minimally invasive techniques of abscess (renal and perinephric) drainage has reduced patient morbidity; however, inadequate drainage may result in significant morbidity and mortality and open surgical drainage and/or nephrectomy may still be required.

REFERENCES

1. Patton JP, Nash DB, Abrutyn E. Urinary tract infection: economic considerations. Med Clin North Am 1991; 75: 495–513.
2. Jacobson SH, Hylander B, Wretlind B, Brauner A. Interleukin-6 and interleukin-8 in serum and urine in patients with acute pyelonephritis in relation to bacterial-virulence-associated traits and renal function. Nephron 1994; 67: 172–179.
3. Schaeffer A. Infections of the urinary tract. In: Campbell's Urology, 8th ed. (Walsh PC, Wein AJ, Vaughan ED Jr, Retik AB, eds.), Saunders, Philadelphia, PA, 2002, p. 515.
4. Ronald A. The etiology of urinary tract infection: traditional and emerging pathogens. Am J Med 2002; 113: 14s–19s.
5. Rubenstein JN, Schaeffer AJ. Managing complicated urinary tract infections: the urologic view. Infect Dis Clin North Am 2003; 17: 333–351.
6. Foxman B, Brown P. Epidemiology of urinary tract infections: transmission and risk factors, incidence, and costs. Infect Dis North Am 2003; 17: 227–241.
7. Zhang L, Foxman B. Molecular epidemiology of *Escherichia coli* mediated urinary tract infection. Front Biosci 2003; 8: e235–244.
8. Marrs CF, Zhang L, Tallman P, et al. Variations in 10 putative uropathogen virulence genes among urinary, fecal and periurethral *Escherichia coli*. J Med Microbiol 2002; 51: 138–142.
9. Elo J, Tallgren LG, Vaisanen V, Korhonen TK, Svenson SB, Makela PH. Association of P and other fibriae with clinical pyelonephritis in children. Scand J Urol Nephrol 1985; 19: 281–284.
10. Latham R, Stamm W. Role of fibriated *Escherichia coli* in urinary tract infections in adult women: correlation with localization studies. J Infect Dis 1984; 149: 835–840.

11. Roberts JA, Marklund BI, Ilver D, et al. The Gal α(1-4)Gal-specific tip adhesion of *Escherichia coli* P-fibriae is needed for pyelonephritis to occur in the normal urinary tract. Proc Natl Acad Sci USA 1994; 91:11,889–893.
12. Svenson SB, Kallenius G. Density and localization of P-fibriae-specific receptors of mammalian cells: fluorescence-activated cell analysis. Infection 1983; 1: 6–12.
13. Svanborg C, Godaly G. Bacterial virulence in urinary tract infections in adults. Infect Dis Clin North Am 1997; 11:513–529.
14. Roberts JA. Management of pyelonephritis and upper urinary tract infections. Urol Clin North Am 1999; 26:753–763.
15. Pinson AG, Philbrick JT, Lindbeck GH, Schorling JB. ED management of acute pyelonephritis in women: a cohort study. Am J Emerg Med 1994; 12: 271–278.
16. Safrin S, Siegal D, Black D. Pyelonephritis in adult women: inpatient vs outpatient therapy. Am J Med 1988; 85: 793–798.
17. Nicolle LE, Friesen D, Harding GKM, Roos LL. Hospitalization for acute pyelonephritis in Manitoba, Canada, during the period from 1989 to 1992: impact of diabetes, pregnancy, and aboriginal origin. Clin Infect Dis 1996; 22: 1051–1056.
18. Foxman B, Klemstine KL, Brown PD. Acute pyelonephritis in US hospitals in 1997: hospitalization and in-hospital mortality. Ann Epidemiol 2003; 13: 144–150.
19. Stamm WE, Hooton TM. Management of urinary tract infections in adults. N Engl J Med 1993; 329: 1328–1334.
20. Rubin RH, Beam TR, Stamm WE. An approach to evaluating antibacterial agents in the treatment of urinary tract infections. Clin Infect Dis 1992; 14: S246–251.
21. Stamey TA. Pathogenesis and Treatment of Urinary Tract Infections. Williams and Wilkins, Baltimore, MD, 1980.
22. Fairley KF, Bond AG, Brown RB, Habersberge EB. Simple test to determine one site of urinary tract infection. Lancet 1967; 2: 427–428.
23. Hooton TM. The current management strategies for community-acquired urinary tract infection. Infect Dis Clin North Am 2003; 17: 303–332.
24. Warren JW, Abrutyn E, Hebel JR, Johnson JR, Schaeffer AJ, Stamm WE. Guidelines for antimicrobial treatment of uncomplicated acute bacterial cystitis and acute pyelonephritis in women. Clin Infect Dis 1999; 29: 745–758.
25. Stamm WE, McKevitt M, Counts GW. Acute renal infection in women: treatment with trimethoprim-sulfamethoxazole or ampicillin for 2 or 6 weeks. A randomized trial. Ann Intern Med 1987; 106: 341–345.
26. Hooton TM, Stamm WE. Diagnosis and treatment of uncomplicated urinary tract infection. Infect Dis Clin North Am 1997; 11: 551–581.
27. Talan DA, Stamm WE, Hooton TM, et al. Comparison of ciprofloxacin (7 days) and trimethoprim-sulfamethoxazole (14 days) for acute uncomplicated pyelonephritis in women: a randomized trial. JAMA 2000; 283: 1583–1590.
28. Tolkoff-Rubin NE, Wilson ME, Zuromskis BP, Jacoby I, Martin AR, Rubin RH. Single dose amoxicillin therapy of acute uncomplicated urinary tract infections in women. Antimicrob Agents Chemother 1984; 25: 626–629.
29. Johnson JR, Stamm WE. Diagnosis and treatment of acute urinary tract infections. Infect Dis Clin North Am 1987; 1: 773–791.
30. Peters KD, Kochanek KD, Murphy SL. Deatus: final data for 1996. Natl Vital Stat Rep 1998; 47: 1–100.
31. Bone R. Gram-negative sepsis: a dilemma of modern medicine. Clin Microbiol Rev 1993; 6: 57–68.
32. Bone R, Balk RA, Cerra FB, et al. Definition for sepsis and organ failure and guidelines for the use of innovative therapies in sepsis. Chest 1992; 101: 1644–1655.
33. Glauser MP, Heumann D, Baumgartner JD, Cohen J. Pathogenesis and potential strategies for prevention and treatment of septic shock: an update. Clin Infect Dis 1994; 18: S205–216.
34. Kanel KT, Kroboth FJ, Schwentker FN, Lecky JW. The intravenous pyelogram in acute pyelonephritis. Arch Intern Med 1988; 148: 2144–2148.

35. Kawashima A, LeRoy AJ. Radiologic evaluation of patients with renal infections. Infect Dis Clin North Am 2003; 17: 433–456.
36. Dembry L-M, Andriole VT. Renal and perirenal abscesses. Infect Dis Clin North Am 1997; 11: 663–680.
37. Hoddick W, Jeffrey RB, Goldberg HI, Federle MP, Laing FC. CT and sonography of severe renal and perirenal infections. AJR Am J Roentgenol 1983; 140: 517–520.
38. Soulen MC, Fishman EK, Goldman SM, Gatewood OM. Bacterial renal infection: role of CT. Radiology 1989; 171: 703–707.
39. Hoverman IV, Gentry LO, Jones DW, Guerriero WG. Intrarenal abscess: report of 14 cases. Arch Intern Med 1980; 140: 914–916.
40. Siegel JF, Smith A, Moldwin R. Minimally invasive treatment of renal abscess. J Urol 1996; 155: 52–55.
41. Fowler JE, Perkins T. Presentation, diagnosis and treatment of renal abscesses: 1972–1988. J Urol 1994; 151: 847–851.
42. Dalla Palma L, Pozzi-Mucelli F, Ene V. Medical treatment of renal and perirenal abscesses: CT evaluation. Clin Radiol 1999; 54: 792–797.
43. Edelstein H, McCabe RE. Perinephric abscess. Modern diagnosis and treatment in 47 cases. Medicine (Baltomore) 1988; 67: 118–131.
44. Meng MV, Mario LA, McAninch JW. Current treatment and outcomes of perinephric abscesses. J Urol 2002; 168: 1337–1340.
45. Salvatierra O Jr, Bucklew WB, Morrow JW. Perinephric abscess: a report of 71 cases. J Urol 1967; 98: 296–302.
46. Thorley JD, Jones SR, Sanford JP. Perinephric abscess. Medicine 1974; 53: 441–451.
47. Watson RA, Esposito M, Richter F, Irwin RJ Jr, Lang EK. Percutaneous nephrostomy as adjunct management in advanced upper urinary tract infection. Urology 1999; 54: 234–239.
48. Ahlering TE, Boyd SD, Hamilton CL, et al. Emphysematous pyelonephritis: a 5-year experience with 13 patients. J Urol 1985; 134: 1086–1088.
49. Huang JJ, Tseng CC. Emphysematous pyelonephritis: clinicoradiological classification, management, prognosis, and pathogenesis. Arch Intern Med 2000; 160: 797–805.
50. Michaeli J, Mogle P, Perlberg S, Hemiman S, Caine M. Emphysematous pyelonephritis. J Urol 1984; 131: 203–208.
51. Chen MT, Huang CN, Chou YH, Huang CH, Chiang CP, Liu GC. Percutaneous drainage in the treatment of emphysematous pyelonephritis: 10-year experience. J Urol 1997; 157: 1569–1573.
52. Best CD, Terris MK, Tacker JR, Reese JH. Clinical and radiological findings in patients with gas forming renal abscess treated conservatively. J Urol 1999; 162: 1273–1276.
53. Malek RS. Xanthogranulomatous pyelonephritis: a great imitator. In: Journal of Continuing Education in Urology. (Stamey TA, ed.), Medical Digest, Northfield, 1978, p. 17.
54. Ghosh H. Chronic pyelonephritis with xanthogranulomatous change: a report of three cases. Am J Clin Pathol 1955; 25: 1043–1049.
55. Malek RS, Elder JS. Xanthogranulomatous pyelonephritis: a critical analysis of 26 cases and of the literature. J Urol 1978; 119: 589–593.
56. Ballesteros JJ, Faus R, Gironella J. Preoperative diagnosis of renal xanthogranulomatosis by serial urine cytology: preliminary report. J Urol 1980; 124: 9–11.
57. Goldman SM, Hartman DS, Fishman EK, Finizio JP, Gatewood OM, Siegelman SS. CT of xanthogranulomatous pyelonephritis: radiologic-pathologic correlation. AJR Am J Roentgenol 1984; 141: 963–969.
58. Shekarriz B, Meng MV, Lu H-F, Yamada H, Duh Q-Y, Stoller ML. Laparoscopic nephrectomy for inflammatory renal conditions. J Urol 2001; 166: 2091–2094.

8 Genital and Infectious Emergencies
Prostatitis, Urethritis, and Epididymo-Orchitis

Khoa B. Tran, MD and Hunter Wessells, MD, FACS

CONTENTS
INTRODUCTION
ACUTE BACTERIAL PROSTATITIS
PROSTATIC ABSCESS
URETHRITIS
EPIDIDYMITIS AND ORCHITIS
SUMMARY
REFERENCES

INTRODUCTION

The management of acute genitourinary tract infections has dramatically changed because of advances in diagnostic testing and antibiotic availability. In the past, the ability to recognize and treat lower urinary tract and genital infections required diagnostic acumen, mostly based on physical findings. Now, sophisticated molecular and radiological tests facilitate the recognition of acute prostatitis, urethritis, and epididymo-orchitis. These entities usually involve common pathogenic organisms and high-risk patient populations. However, each disease entity has a distinct pathology, necessitating individual evaluation and management. This chapter is limited in scope to the acute bacterial infections of the prostate, urethra, and male reproductive organs.

ACUTE BACTERIAL PROSTATITIS

Definition and Presentation

In 1995, the National Institute of Diabetes and Digestive and Kidney Diseases convened a workshop on prostatitis to create a classification system for prostatitis syndromes (1). Acute bacterial prostatitis (acute infection of the prostate) was designated in this schema as category I. Chronic bacterial, chronic nonbacterial, and asymptomatic prostatitis were assigned categories II, III, and IV, respectively. Acute prostatitis is rare and accounts for less than 5% of all prostatitis syndromes *(2)*. Acute prostatitis is characterized by rapid onset of fever, chills, low back and perineal/rectal pain, urinary frequency, urgency, nocturia, hesitancy, or sensation of incomplete bladder emptying *(3)*. Generalized symptoms, such as malaise, arthralgia, and myalgia, may also accompany urological symptoms. Past medical history may be significant for a prior history of urinary tract infection, indwelling or intermittent urethral catheterization, urethral instrumentation, diabetes, chronic renal insufficiency, and other immunocompromised states.

Physical Examination

Patients may have elevation in temperature and appear clinically ill. The abdominal examination may reveal bladder distension, and the genitalia may show an associated urethritis or epididymitis. Rectal examination usually reveals an exquisitely tender swollen prostate gland. The consistency of the gland has been described as boggy, irregular, partially or totally firm, or warm to the touch. Aggressive rectal examination or massage is not recommended because of the risk of severe pain or bacteremia *(4)*.

Laboratory

Urinalysis is almost invariably abnormal with acute prostatitis. Bacteriuria, pyuria, and hematuria are common. The midstream urine should be cultured, and antibiotic sensitivity should be tested. Other laboratory studies may be indicated, including complete blood count with differential, blood cultures (if the patient is febrile), and chemistry studies.

Microbiology

Microbial pathogens associated with acute prostatitis and prostatic abscess include *Escherichia coli*, other Enterobacteriaceae, *Staphylococcus*, *Enterococcus*, *Neisseria gonorrhoeae*, and *Chlamydia trachomatis* *(3)*.

Treatment

Acute bacterial prostatitis (National Institutes of Health [NIH] category I) should be treated promptly with oral fluoroquinolones or sulfanomides. For severe symptoms, patients should be hospitalized and treated with parenteral antibiotics. Recommended doses of fluoroquinolones are as follows: 500 mg ciprofloxacin twice daily; 600 mg levofloxacin daily; or 400 mg norfloxacin twice daily. Alternatively, acute prostatitis can be treated with oral trimethoprim-sulfamethoxazole (TMP-SMX; 160 mg TMP and 800 mg SMX). With associated urosepsis, intravenous antibiotics are indicated (2 g ampicillin intravenously every 6 h and 5 mg gentamicin/kg/d) *(2)*.

From the results of susceptibility testing from urine culture, appropriate changes in antimicrobial therapy should be made. Incomplete patient response may indicate the need to alter antibiotic therapy or the presence of prostatic abscess. Oral therapy should be continued for a total of at least 4 wk after the diagnosis of acute bacterial prostatitis to prevent the development of chronic bacterial prostatitis *(5)*. Additional general supportive measures, including hydration, analgesics, stool softeners, antipyretics, and bed rest, have also been employed *(5)*.

Related Urological Problems

Acute urinary retention caused by acute prostatitis (or prostatic abscess) traditionally has been managed with suprapubic cystostomy tube placement. Anecdotal reports of complications related to urethral catheterization exist *(6)*, but no prospective studies or large case series have shown a clear relationship between transurethral catheterization and worse outcomes of acute bacterial prostatitis.

PROSTATIC ABSCESS

Presentation

Prostatic abscess may be evident at the time of presentation of a patient with acute prostatitis. It may also develop after a course of oral antimicrobial therapy and have a more indolent presentation. Clinical signs of prostatic abscess are variable and include urinary retention, fever, dysuria, frequency, and perineal pain. Presentations can be similar to those for acute prostatitis. Tenderness and fluctuance are unreliable indicators *(7)*. Patients with diabetes mellitus and acute prostatitis signs/symptoms are predisposed to prostatic abscess formation *(8)*.

Radiological Evaluation

Computed tomography or transrectal ultrasonography is important for the prompt and accurate diagnosis of prostatic abscess (Figs. 1 and 2). Transrectal ultrasonography also may be useful for abscess fluid aspiration (perineally or transrectally) for diagnostic or therapeutic purposes.

Treatment

Urgent urological consultation is imperative to ensure prompt drainage of the abscess. In combination with appropriate antimicrobial therapy, incision and drainage will lead to the resolution of most prostatic abscesses. Transurethral, perineal, and transrectal drainage of prostatic abscesses have been described *(9–12)*. Ultrasound-guided transurethral incision or resection is now the most common treatment strategy for prostatic abscess *(10,13)*.

URETHRITIS

Presentation

Acute urethritis in the male is commonly caused by sexually transmitted diseases (STDs; gonorrhea or chlamydia) and rarely caused by *Ureaplasma ureolyticum (14,15)*. Classic gonococcal urethritis produces a profuse, purulent urethral discharge with dysuria. Although gonococcal urethritis can present with scant or absent discharge, this scenario is more likely to occur with nongonoccal urethritis. In all cases, laboratory diagnosis is essential for accurate diagnosis.

Microbiology

Neisseria gonorrhoeae (the most common cause of urethritis) has an incubation period of 1 to 9 d. *Chlamydia trachomatis* is responsible for most cases of nongonococcal urethritis in the male and has an incubation period of 7 to 21 d. Coinfection with gonococcal organisms is found in up to 40% of patients with *C. trachomatis (16)*.

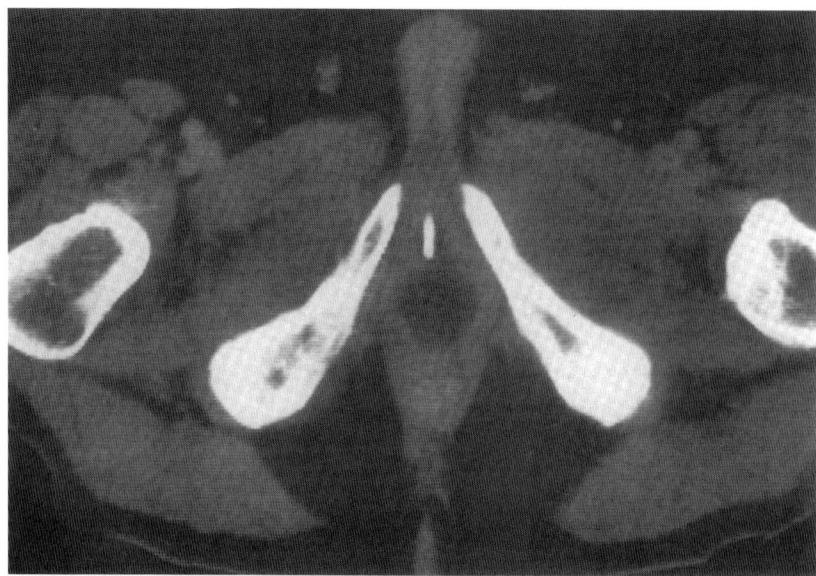

Fig. 1. Computed tomographic scan of prostatic abscess demonstrating low-density collection within prostatic apex close to urethral catheter. (From ref. *38.*)

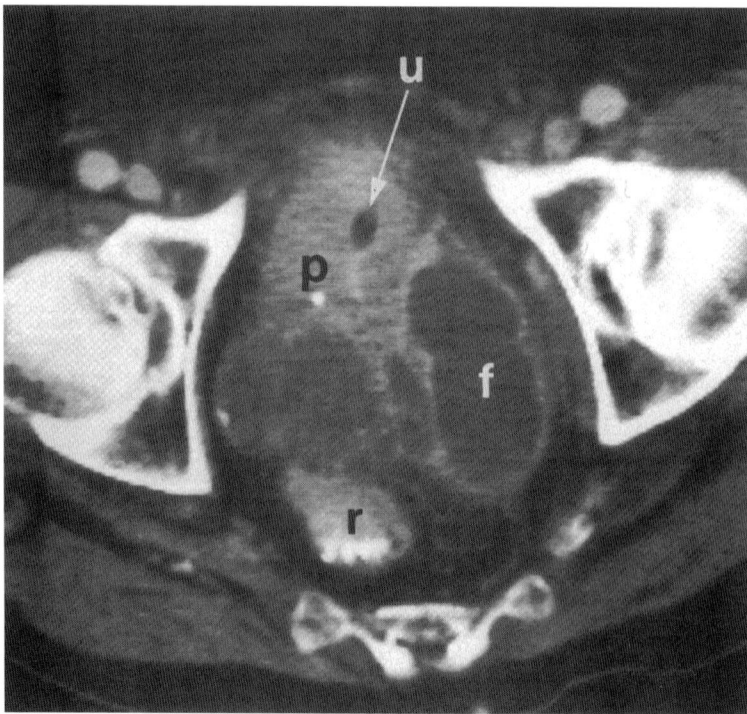

Fig. 2. Computed tomographic scan of prostatic abscess showing multiple low-density fluid collections (f), within the prostate (p), urethra (u), and rectum (r). (From ref. *38.*)

Diagnostic Testing

Standard cell culture techniques remain sensitive and specific for gonococcal and chlamydial urethritis *(17,18)*. A urethral specimen collected with a calcium alginate urethrogenital swab is preferred for inoculation of culture medium and Gram staining. The Gram stain remains highly sensitive and specific (intracellular Gram-negative diplococci) for *N. gonorrhoeae (17)*, but not for *C. trachomatis*. Urethral inflammation, as determined by a Gram stain from a urethral swab specimen, in the absence of *N. gonorrhoeae* is suggestive of nongonococcal urethritis *(19)*. The use of ligase chain reaction nucleic acid amplification strategies has enhanced the specificity and sensitivity of testing for *C. trachomatis*, especially when the high coinfection rate with *N. gonorrhoeae* is considered *(20)*.

Treatment

Recommended treatments for gonococcal and nongonoccal urethritis in men are listed respectively in Tables 1 and 2 based on data from the Centers for Disease Control and Prevention. Sexual partners of patients infected with *N. gonorrhoeae* or *C. trachomatis* should be treated on the basis of contact *(21)*.

EPIDIDYMITIS AND ORCHITIS

Etiology

The causes of epididymo-orchitis reflect common causes of genitourinary infection in men based on particular age groups. In children and older men (>35 yr), the most common cause of epididymitis is coliform organisms that result in bacteriuria. In contrast, the organisms that cause urethritis or STD are the common etiologies of epididymitis and orchitis in young adult men (<35 yr) *(22)*.

Presentation and Differential Diagnoses

The clinical syndrome of acute epididymitis (or epididymo-orchitis) results from infection and inflammation of the epididymis or testis. It is usually caused by the spread of infection from the urethra or bladder and characterized by progressive increase in pain and swelling of one epididymis or testis. It may be associated with fever, lower urinary tract symptoms, and the sensation of a mass in the scrotum *(23)*. Pertinent information from the history of present illness includes duration, acuity of onset, location, radiation, associated symptoms, and ameliorating factors. These factors may help distinguish between epididymo-orchitis and testicular torsion. Epididymo-orchitis usually has a 2- to 3-d period of progressive increase in scrotal discomfort before severe pain is noted. The pain is localized to the scrotum and does not radiate. Nausea and vomiting are absent. In contrast, testicular torsion has a very acute onset, with pain in the testicle possibly radiating into the lower abdominal quadrants. It is usually associated with anorexia, nausea, or vomiting.

The past medical history of a patient with epididymo-orchitis may be entirely unremarkable or indicate conditions predisposing to chronic bacteriuria with coliform organisms. These conditions include congenital urological anomalies (hypospadias, neurogenic bladder, ectopic ureteroceles), practice of anal intercourse, and acquired obstructive urinary diseases (benign prostatic hyperplasia, prostate cancer, urethral strictures) in older men *(24–26)*.

Table 1
Treatment of Patients With Uncomplicated Gonococcal Infections of the Urethra and Rectum

Recommended regimens	
Cefixime	400 mg orally in a single dose
	Or
Ceftriaxone	125 mg im in a single dose
	Or
Ciprofloxacin[a]	500 mg orally in a single dose
	Or
Ofloxacin[a]	400 mg orally in a single dose
	Or
Levofloxacin[a]	250 mg orally in a single dose
Plus, if chlamydial infection is not ruled out	
Azithromycin	1 g orally in a single dose
	Or
Doxycycline	100 mg orally twice a day for 7 d

[a] Not advised for infection acquired in Asia, the Pacific, Hawaii, and probably California. Adapted from CDC Sexually Transmitted Diseases Treatment Guidelines 2002. MMWR 2002; 51 (No. RR–6).

Table 2
Treatment of Patients With Nongonococcal Urethritis

Recommended regimens	
Azithromycin	1 g orally in a single dose
	Or
Doxycycline	100 mg orally twice a day for 7 d
Alternative Regimens	
Erythromycin base	500 mg orally four times a day for 7 d
	Or
Erythromycin ethylsuccinate	800 mg orally four times a day for 7 d
	Or
Ofloxacin	300 mg twice a day for 7 d
	Or
Levofloxacin	500 mg once daily for 7 d

Adapted from CDC Sexually Transmitted Diseases Treatment Guidelines 2002. MMWR 2002; 51 (No. RR–6).

Physical Examination

The physical exam should be focused to differentiate epididymo-orchitis from other urological and nonurological conditions. Vital signs are usually normal, but if the temperature is elevated in the patient with possible epididymitis, a severe infection or associated abscess should be suspected. The abdomen is examined to exclude other intraabdominal processes (renal colic, appendicitis, hernia) that cause radiation to the groin. The penis and urethral meatus are inspected for signs of urethritis, and the scrotum is carefully examined with the patient in the supine position. The overlying scrotal skin is inspected for erythema, fixation, or fluctuance that indicates abscess. The palpation of scrotal contents is directed first to the contralateral uninvolved side and subsequently to the ipsilateral affected side. The presence of an ipsilateral cremasteric reflex is a useful adjunctive sign (Rabinowitz's sign) in indicating epididymis rather than torsion *(27)*. With the epididymis, the head or tail may be enlarged and tender with or without involvement of the testis or surrounding structures.

The position of the testis may be helpful in differentiating torsion and infection. Epididymo-orchitis is associated with normal lie of the testis and relief of pain with scrotal elevation (Prehn's sign). Torsion may be associated with a high horizontal lie of the testis. However, this sign is not uniformly present. With epididymitis, the spermatic cord may be tender and swollen, possibly extending into the groin. Importantly, the prostate should be examined to exclude concurrent prostatitis.

Diagnostic Testing

Urinalysis or urethral smear can usually determine the microbial cause of epididymitis *(23)*. For suspected cases of STD (especially in men younger than 35 yr), Gram stain of the urethral smear is advisable. A midstream urine specimen should be performed in all patients and examined for the presence of Gram-negative bacteria. In less-obvious cases of testicular pain without clear evidence of abnormalities on physical exam, the presence of blood on urinalysis should raise the possibility of renal colic, masquerading as torsion or epididymitis, with radiation of pain to the scrotum.

Microbiology

In men under 35 yr of age, the most common bacteria that causes epididymo-orchitis are STD organisms. The percentage of men in this age group with *E. coli* infection ranges from 0 to 24%, most commonly caused by anal intercourse *(25)*. In men over the age of 35 yr, the majority of pathogenic bacteria are *E. coli*, although STD organisms may still cause a substantial amount of epididymo-orchitis *(22)*. Other rare pathogenic bacteria include *Haemophilus influenzae (28)*. Rare systemic infections that cause epididymitis include tuberculosis, atypical microbacteria, cryptococcus, brucellosis, and schistosomiasis *(29–31)*.

Radiological Evaluation

Color duplex scrotal ultrasonography can help to visualize the epididymis, testis, and surrounding tissues to distinguish epididymitis from torsion *(32)*. Sonographic features of acute epididymitis include enlargement of the epididymitis and a primarily inhomogeneous echogenic texture (Fig. 3). Echogenic areas within the swollen epididymis and a reactive hydrocele may be present. Usually, the visualized testis is normal, although

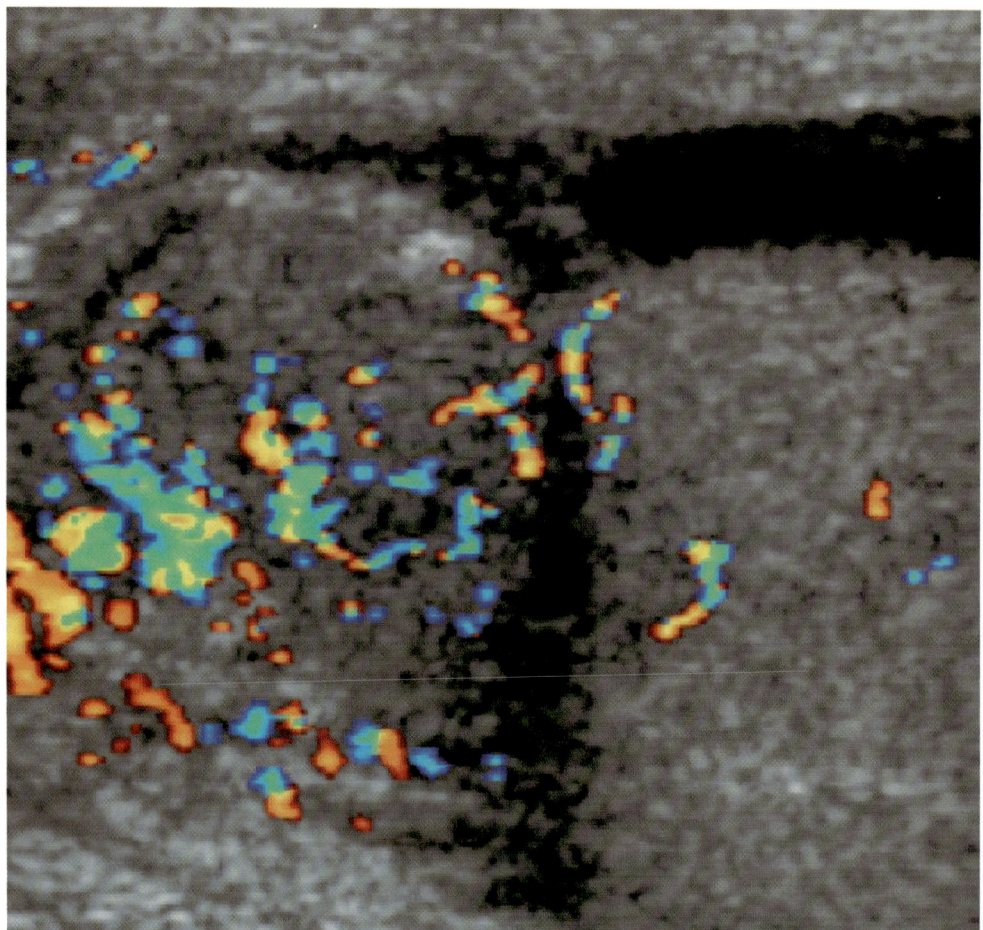

Fig. 3. Acute epididymitis. Note that the epididymis (left-sided structure demonstrating increased color flow on Doppler) is equal in size to the adjacent testis. (Photograph courtesy of T. Dubinsky, MD.)

with orchitis the testis may have increased blood flow with color Doppler (Fig. 4) or a diffusely abnormal echogenicity with no residual normal tissue (Fig. 5).

A helpful finding in inflammation of the scrotal contents is thickening of the superficial skin overlying the testis or epididymis, which is useful in differentiating a very extensive orchitis from neoplasm. Diffuse inflammation of the testis usually causes mild-to-moderate enlargement with preservation of the normal oval shape and smooth contour of the testis. Focal inflammation of the epididymis can also be delineated on ultrasonography. A localized lesion (enlarged and hypoechoic or with mixed echogenicity) may be compared with the normal contralateral epididymitis. Focal orchitis may show localized areas of decreased echogenicity secondary to the proximity of the inflamed epididymis *(33)*.

Associated Testicular Infarction

Testicular infarction (caused by compromise of testicular blood flow from edema and swelling) may occur secondary to epididymo-orchitis *(34–36)*. The infarction secondary

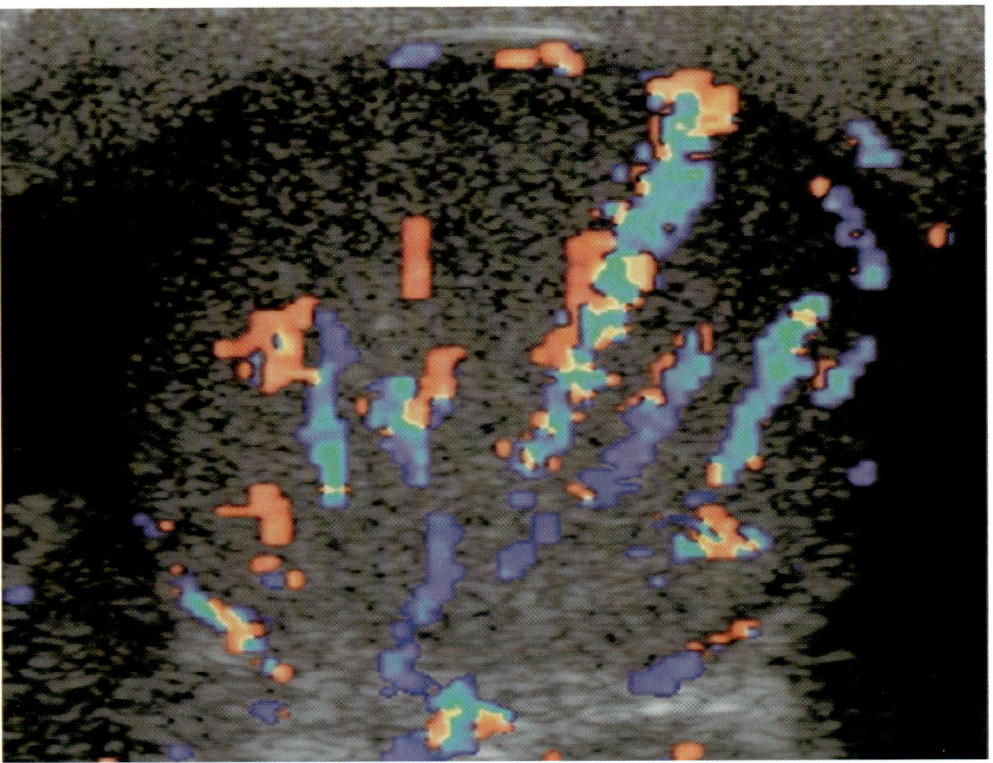

Fig. 4. Orchitis. The testis is enlarged and has increased blood flow visible on color Doppler scanning. (Photograph courtesy of T. Dubinsky, MD.)

to acute inflammation may be difficult to differentiate from torsion and requires exploration and orchiectomy *(37)*.

Associated Abscesses

Abscesses of the epididymis, testis, or scrotum related to acute bacterial or mycobacterial infection are easily detected on ultrasonography. Focal hypoechoic or anechoic regions in the epididymis or testis with involvement of the overlying scrotal soft tissue and skin can usually be differentiated from simple reactive hydroceles.

Treatment

Appropriate antimicrobial therapy for acute epididymitis is based on history, physical examination, and findings from urinalysis or urethral smear. Antimicrobial therapy should be instituted empirically, and follow-up adjustment based on culture and sensitivities is indicated. For mild-to-moderate epididymo-orchitis caused by bacteriuria, a 14-d course of broad-spectrum antibiotics, such as fluoroquinolone or TMP-SMX, is recommended. In severe epididymo-orchitis associated with systemic illness, a combination of intravenous β-lactam and aminoglycoside antibiotics is indicated. For epididymo-orchitis caused by STD organisms, treatment should include single-dose therapy to cover *N. gonorrhoeae* and a 10- to 14-d course of therapy for nongonococcal urethritis (*see* Tables 1 and 2). In all cases of acute epididymo-orchitis, supportive

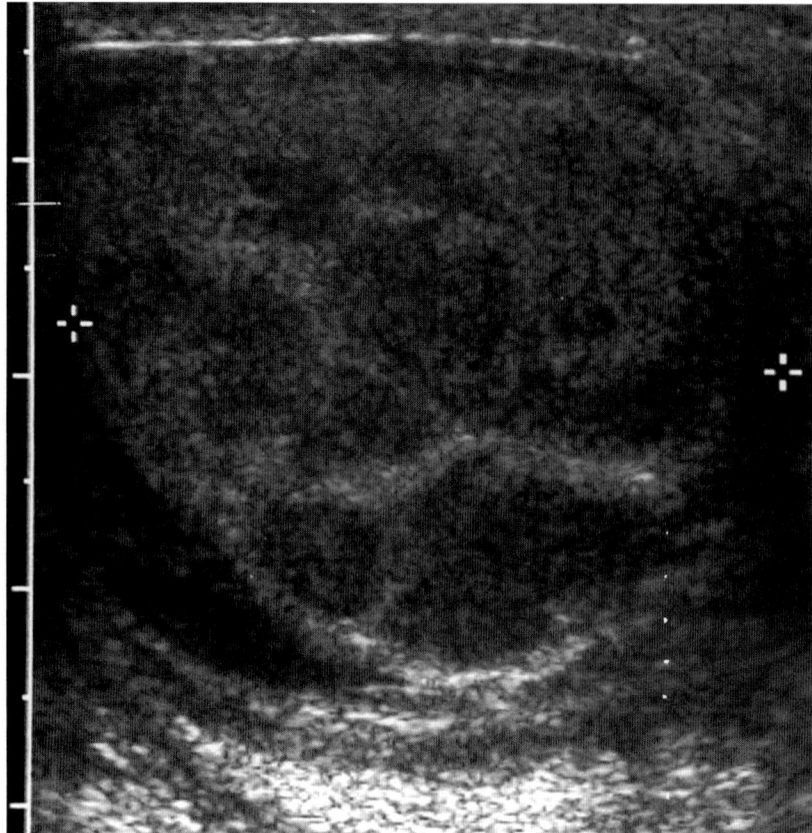

Fig. 5. Orchitis with intratesticular abscess formation. Note marked inhomogeneity of testicular parenchyma. (Photograph courtesy of T. Dubinsky, MD.)

measures, including bed rest, scrotal elevation, nonsteroidal anti-inflammatory drugs, or local spermatic cord block, may be helpful *(23)*.

Indications for Scrotal Exploration, Drainage of Abscess, or Orchiectomy

Antibiotic therapy and supportive measures will allow most cases of epididymo-orchitis to resolve without need for surgical intervention. However, scrotal exploration/drainage or orchiectomy may be indicated for abscesses or an infarcted testis secondary to severe infection, respectively. The ultrasonographic presence of fluid adjacent to the testis does not necessitate incision and drainage in all cases. Systemic illness; obvious fluctuance; significant inflammatory changes of the scrotum, spermatic cord, or perineum; or obvious abscess formation with echogenic material indicates the need for scrotal exploration and drainage. A decision regarding orchiectomy can be difficult. However, in many cases, the testis will be extensively involved in inflammatory and infectious processes and require removal. Abscesses arising solely from an acutely inflamed and infected epididymis may be drained and debrided without the need for orchiectomy. If exploration and drainage are not elected, hospitalization with broad-spectrum intravenous antibiotics, frequent physical examination, and repeat imaging of the scrotum and testicle is advised.

SUMMARY

The persistence of unprotected sexual exposures in the United States and other developed and developing countries will ensure the continued need to identify and treat urethritis, prostatitis, and epididymitis. Nucleic acid amplification and high-resolution scrotal ultrasonography will ensure appropriate diagnosis and treatment of cases related to STDs. For men with prostatitis, the diagnosis rests on accurate history and detailed physical examination. Appropriate use of antimicrobial agents is critical to avoid progressively increasing rates of bacterial resistance.

REFERENCES

1. Krieger JN, Nyberg L Jr, Nickel JC. NIH consensus definition and classification of prostatitis. JAMA 1999; 282: 236–237.
2. Lipsky BA. Prostatitis and urinary tract infection in men: what's new; what's true? Am J Med 1999; 106: 327–334.
3. Roberts RO, Lieber MM, Bostwick DG, Jacobsen SJ. A review of clinical and pathological prostatitis syndromes. Urology 1997; 49: 809–821.
4. Krieger JN. Prostatitis syndromes: pathophysiology, differential diagnosis, and treatment. Sex Transm Dis 1984; 11: 100–112.
5. Meares EM Jr. Prostatitis syndromes: new perspectives about old woes. J Urol 1980; 123: 141–147.
6. Pfau A. Prostatitis. A continuing enigma. Urol Clin North Am 1986; 13: 695–715.
7. Weinberger M, Cytron S, Servadio C, Block C, Rosenfeld JB, Pitlik SD. Prostatic abscess in the antibiotic era. Rev Infect Dis 1988; 10: 239–249.
8. Dajani AM, O'Flynn JD. Prostatic abscess. A report of 25 cases. Br J Urol 1968; 40: 736–739.
9. Barozzi L, Pavlica P, Menchi I, De Matteis M, Canepari M. Prostatic abscess: diagnosis and treatment. AJR Am J Roentgenol 1998; 170: 753–757.
10. Meares EM Jr. Prostatic abscess. J Urol 1986; 136: 1281–1282.
11. Kadmon D, Ling D, Lee JK. Percutaneous drainage of prostatic abscesses. J Urol 1986; 135: 1259–1260.
12. Cytron S, Weinberger M, Pitlik SD, Servadio C. Value of transrectal ultrasonography for diagnosis and treatment of prostatic abscess. Urology 1988; 32: 454–458.
13. Trauzzi SJ, Kay CJ, Kaufman DG, Lowe FC. Management of prostatic abscess in patients with human immunodeficiency syndrome. Urology 1994; 43: 629–633.
14. Harrison WO. Gonococcal urethritis. Urol Clin North Am 1984; 11: 45–53.
15. Bowie WR. Nongonococcal urethritis. Urol Clin North Am 1984; 11: 55–64.
16. Lin JS, Donegan SP, Heeren TC, et al. Transmission of *Chlamydia trachomatis* and *Neisseria gonorrhoeae* among men with urethritis and their female sex partners. J Infect Dis 1998; 178: 1707–1712.
17. Manavi K, Young H, Clutterbuck D. Sensitivity of microscopy for the rapid diagnosis of gonorrhoea in men and women and the role of gonorrhoea serovars. Int J STD AIDS 2003; 14: 390–394.
18. Jensen IP, Fogh H, Prag J. Diagnosis of *Chlamydia trachomatis* infections in a sexually transmitted disease clinic: evaluation of a urine sample tested by enzyme immunoassay and polymerase chain reaction in comparison with a cervical and/or a urethral swab tested by culture and polymerase chain reaction. Clin Microbiol Infect 2003; 9: 194–201.
19. Chernesky MA, Jang D, Lee H, et al. Diagnosis of *Chlamydia trachomatis* infections in men and women by testing first-void urine by ligase chain reaction. J Clin Microbiol 1994; 32: 2682–2685.
20. Taylor-Robinson D. Tests for infection with *Chlamydia trachomatis*. Int J STD AIDS 1996; 7: 19–25.
21. Orr DP, Johnston K, Brizendine E, Katz B, Fortenberry JD. Subsequent sexually transmitted infection in urban adolescents and young adults. Arch Pediatr Adolesc Med 2001; 155: 947–953.
22. Berger RE, Alexander ER, Harnisch JP, et al. Etiology, manifestations and therapy of acute epididymitis: prospective study of 50 cases. J Urol 1979; 121: 750–754.
23. Luzzi GA, O'Brien TS. Acute epididymitis. BJU Int 2001; 87: 747–755.

24. Mittemeyer BT, Lennox KW, Borski AA. Epididymitis: a review of 610 cases. J Urol 1966; 95: 390–392.
25. Berger RE, Kessler D, Holmes KK. Etiology and manifestations of epididymitis in young men: correlations with sexual orientation. J Infect Dis 1987; 155: 1341–1343.
26. Hoppner W, Strohmeyer T, Hartmann M, Lopez-Gamarra D, Dreikorn K. Surgical treatment of acute epididymitis and its underlying diseases. Eur Urol 1992; 22: 218–221.
27. Rabinowitz R. The importance of the cremasteric reflex in acute scrotal swelling in children. J Urol 1984; 132: 89–90.
28. Thomas D, Simpson K, Ostojic H, Kaul A. Bacteremic epididymo-orchitis due to *Hemophilus influenzae* type B. J Urol 1981; 126: 832–833.
29. Skoutelis A, Marangos M, Petsas T, Chionis I, Barbalias G, Bassaris H. Serious complications of tuberculous epididymitis. Infection 2000; 28: 193–195.
30. Mitchell CJ, Huins TJ. Letter: Acute brucellosis presenting as epididymo-orchitis. Br Med J 1974; 2: 557–558.
31. Kazzaz BA, Salmo NA. Epididymitis due to *Schistosoma haematobium* infection. Trop Geogr Med 1974; 26: 333–336.
32. Hendrikx AJ, Dang CL, Vroegindeweij D, Korte JH. B-mode and colour-flow duplex ultrasonography: a useful adjunct in diagnosing scrotal diseases? Br J Urol 1997; 79: 58–65.
33. Herbener TE. Ultrasound in the assessment of the acute scrotum. J Clin Ultrasound 1996; 24: 405–421.
34. Sue SR, Pelucio M, Gibbs M. Testicular infarction in a patient with epididymitis. Acad Emerg Med. 1998; 5: 1128–1130.
35. Desai KM, Gingell JC, Haworth JM. Fate of the testis following epididymitis: a clinical and ultrasound study. J R Soc Med 1986; 79: 515–519.
36. Kirk D, Gingell JC, Feneley RC. Infarction of the testis: a complication of epididymitis. Br J Urol 1982; 54: 311–312.
37. Vordermark JS, Favila MQ. Testicular necrosis: a preventable complication of epididymitis. J Urol 1982; 128: 1322–1324.
38. Rifkin MD. Inflammation of the lower urinary tract: the prostate, seminal vesicles, and scrotum. In: Clinical Urography. (Pollack HM, ed.), Saunders, Philadelphia, PA, 1990, pp. 940–960.

9 Penile Prosthesis Infection

Dominick J. Carbone, Jr., MD

CONTENTS

    INTRODUCTION
    INCIDENCE, RISK FACTORS, AND PROPHYLAXIS
    PATHOPHYSIOLOGY AND PATHOGENIC ORGANISMS
    CLINICAL PRESENTATION
    MANAGEMENT OF PENILE PROSTHESIS INFECTION
    NEW DEVELOPMENTS IN PERIPROSTHETIC INFECTION
    SUMMARY
    REFERENCES

INTRODUCTION

Depending on the specific nature of the presentation, penile prosthesis infection can represent a true urological emergency. Certainly, infection is the most disastrous and feared complication of penile prosthesis surgery and is often associated with significant functional, cosmetic, and psychological sequelae. Penile prosthesis infection can result in removal of the device, with a substantial degree of accompanying morbidity, including patient disability, loss of penile length, and extreme difficulty in the insertion of another device.

Although advances in the formulation of biocompatible materials have improved results with surgery over the last three decades, implant infection can still produce catastrophic results, such as subsequent genital gangrene *(1,2)* with extensive tissue loss and life-threatening sepsis. Moreover, in this age of economic consciousness, it should be noted that the cost of preventing penile prosthesis infection is quite minimal; the cost of treating the patient with an infected penile prosthesis is generally quite substantial. For all of these reasons, urologists need to be familiar with the presentation and management of penile prosthesis infections.

INCIDENCE, RISK FACTORS, AND PROPHYLAXIS

Incidence

Given that 10 to 30 million men in the United States suffer from erectile dysfunction *(3)* and that approx 20,000 men *(4)* are treated with penile prosthesis implantation

From: *Urological Emergencies: A Practical Guide*
Edited by: H. Wessells and J. W. McAninch © Humana Press Inc., Totowa, NJ

annually, the incidence of periprosthetic infection is fortunately rather rare. Most series report an incidence of 2.3% *(5,6)*, although a single article did report an infectious complication rate as high as 8.3% *(7)*.

Risk Factors

A number of significant risk factors for periprosthetic infection have been reported. Although most are related to patient characteristics, a few are under the surgeon's direct control. Perhaps the most important among these, as Jarow noted, is increased duration of surgery *(8)*. In fact, in his study, operative time was the only finding correlated with an increased risk of infection. Exposure of the wound to the operating environment for a longer period of time, and hence an increased propensity for bacterial colonization, appeared to be the reason for the higher incidence of infection noted in the group with prolonged operative times.

Another factor that increases the risk of infection that lies under the surgeon's direct control is the performance of multiple surgical procedures at the time of implantation. For example, Fallon and Ghanem noted that circumcision performed simultaneously with penile prosthesis implantation markedly increased the risk of infection in their series *(9)*, and most textbook authors suggested that multiple procedures should not be performed at the time of penile prosthesis surgery *(10)*.

Finally, prolonged hospitalization, because it promotes skin flora changes, is thought to increase the risk of infection. Thus, short hospital stays are recommended for decreasing wound infections *(4)*.

Most risk factors for infection, however, have to do with patient characteristics. Certain of these are well established and agreed on generally. For example, placement of a penile prosthesis next to another foreign body clearly increases the risk of infection. Carson showed an incontrovertible increase in infection risk when using additional foreign bodies such as Gore-Tex or Dacron in association with penile prosthesis implantation *(11)*. In addition, Radomski and Herschorn noted that preexisting urinary tract infection is a clear risk factor for periprosthetic infection *(12)*. Obviously, it is incumbent on the operating surgeon to document the presence of sterile urine preoperatively.

On the other hand, some risk factors are more controversial. One of the most controversial is diabetes mellitus. Some authors have reported that diabetes is associated with infection; others have not. For example, in the study by Jarow *(8)*, the presence of diabetes did not correlate with an increased risk of infection. Similarly, an article by Montague and associates failed to reveal an association between diabetes and increased infection risk *(13)*. Conversely, in the study by Fallon and Ghanem, diabetes did correlate with an increased infection risk *(9)*. In a retrospective review conducted by Wilson and coworkers of 1337 patients, infection rates were higher in diabetics for both virgin and revision cases *(14)*. The findings, however, were not statistically significant.

Even more controversial than the effect of diabetes itself is whether glycosylated hemoglobin can be used as a preoperative marker for potential infection in diabetic patients. Bishop et al. *(15)* suggested that altered defense mechanisms typical of poorly controlled diabetic patients will tend to increase the risk of infection, and they sought to determine whether glycosylated hemoglobin, a marker of glucose control, could be used to predict the risk of infection. In their study, 31% of the poorly controlled diabetics developed infection following implantation; only 5% of the adequately controlled patients suffered this complication. They suggested that patients with a glycosylated hemoglobin level of 11.5% should be more optimally controlled prior to prosthesis surgery. However, their study included only 90 patients. Conversely, a larger prospective study of 114 diabetics conducted by Wilson and coworkers *(16)* showed no statically significant increase in infection risk with increased levels of glycosylated hemoglobin A1C. They suggested that glycosylated hemoglobin is not a good predictor of postoperative penile prosthesis infection.

Another somewhat controversial risk factor for periprosthetic infection is spinal cord injury and other neurological deficits. Gross and colleagues noted a jump in postoperative infection rates from 8 to 33% after implantation in men with spinal cord injury *(17)*. Similarly, in the review of 1337 patients by Wilson et al. *(12)*, the 9% rate of infection in men with spinal cord injury was significantly higher than the index 1% infection rate. In contrast, Diokno and Sunda *(18)* reported that as long as men with spinal cord injury and neurogenic bladder continue to practice safe, intermittent self-catheterization, no increased risk of infection following penile implantation surgery was noted.

Perhaps the most plausible explanation for these apparent discrepancies is that the overall risk of postsurgical infection is quite small; thus, host factors such as diabetes and spinal cord injury do not in and of themselves represent strict contraindications to penile implant surgery. Rather, the presence of risk factors in the patient should make the surgeon even more vigilant regarding the principles of infection prevention.

Prophylaxis

Certain principles of infection prevention in penile prosthesis implantation have universal agreement. First and foremost, frequent and copious mechanical antibiotic irrigation throughout the procedure minimizes bacterial adherence and reduces infection *(19)*. In the same vein, patient shaving is generally carried out immediately before the procedure, and a 10-min scrub is performed to reduce the presence of skin flora that can produce infection *(20)*. Interestingly, Garber and Marcus *(21)* demonstrated that there is no difference in infection rate between scrotal and infrapubic approaches when a preoperative scrub is performed. Obviously, limiting operating room traffic, minimizing tissue devitalization, and performing adequate wound closure are also effective steps in reducing perioperative infections. Finally, as noted in the information on risk factors, short hospital stays can contribute to reduced infection. Ghanem et al. *(22)* suggested that performing the surgery in an outpatient setting may help minimize risk.

Although well established, the use of perioperative prophylactic antibiotics to reduce the risk of periprosthetic infection is not without controversy. Many surgeons favor second- or third-generation cephalosporins or more expensive agents, such as vancomycin. Although the use of vancomycin as a prophylactic antibiotic for periprosthetic surgery is sometimes criticized in the infectious disease literature, the urological literature in fact supports the practice.

In a comparison of vancomycin, gentamicin, and aztreonam, Walters et al. *(23)* demonstrated a significantly elevated cavernous tissue antibiotic level for vancomycin compared to the other two agents. On the basis of this finding, the authors concluded that intravenous vancomycin may represent an optimal prophylactic antibiotic for penile prosthesis surgery.

At the other end of the spectrum, the literature also supports oral prophylaxis. Schwartz and colleagues *(24)* examined antibiotic tissue levels in the corpus cavernosa of patients undergoing penile implant surgery, and they showed that oral fluoroquinolone prophylaxis was just as effective in obtaining high tissue levels in the corpus cavernosum as a gentamicin-cefazolin combination. These authors therefore concluded that outpatient oral prophylaxis with fluoroquinolones prior to penile prosthesis surgery is feasible; moreover, they suggested that a total cost savings of $36 million could be realized if this approach was universally adopted.

Review of the literature demonstrated that a large number of specific agents have been effective prophylaxis for penile implant surgery, and the operating surgeon must tailor the choice on a rational consideration of cost and patient risk factors. Ultimately, because most organisms that infect penile prostheses are indigenous to the patient's skin and are not of hospital origin, a variety of antibiotics will be effective in achieving prophylaxis.

Perhaps even more important than the specific agent chosen is the timing of antibiotic administration. Classen and colleagues (25) showed that prophylactic antibiotics are most effective if administered during the 2-h window prior to incision, and that infection rates will increase substantially if antibiosis is given more than 2 h preoperatively or in the postoperative period.

PATHOPHYSIOLOGY AND PATHOGENIC ORGANISMS

Pathophysiology

To understand the pathophysiology of penile prosthesis infection, one must understand the normal reaction of human tissue to placement of a foreign body. When a device is placed within the body, a complex response follows. This response is characterized by inflammation, fibrosis, and scar tissue formation, resulting in production of a pseudocapsule surrounding the device *(26–28)*. This pseudocapsule contains proteinaceous molecules that play active roles in bacterial adhesion *(29,30)*. Moreover, this propensity to bacterial adherence has been documented both with silicone elastomer used in the prostheses of American Medical Systems (Minnetonka, MN) as well as the bioflex material utilized in Mentor penile prosthesis *(31,32)*. The bacteria then produce a mucopolysaccharide matrix that protects them from both cellular- and noncellular-mediated immune defense mechanisms *(4)*.

Taken together, these three layers—the pseudocapsule attached to the surface of the foreign body, the base film of microorganisms, and the surface film produced by the bacteria themselves—form the biofilm *(33,34)*. It is on the surface of the biofilm that periprosthetic infection can arise and spread, and the biofilm makes eradication by antibiotic administration extremely unlikely.

Pathogenic Organisms

The most common organism in penile prosthesis infection is *Staphylococcus epidermidis (35)*. In fact, Licht and coworkers found *S. epidermidis* in implants removed strictly for mechanical malfunction in patients with no clinical evidence of infection *(36)*. It has been shown that *S. epidermidis* and other staphylococcal species have an increased ability to produce the very biofilm that enhances their infectious potential *(31,37)*.

Gram-negative enteric bacteria may also be responsible for prosthetic infections. In the article by Mulcahy's group *(7)*, Gram-negative organisms such as *Proteus mirabilis, Pseudomonas aeruginosa, Escherichia coli*, and *Serratia marcescens* were noted. Similarly, in the report from Montague *(6)*, Gram-negative organisms accounted for 20% of all penile prosthesis infections in the series. These infections tended to occur earlier than those noted in patients infected with staphylococcal organisms. Most important, these Gram-negative infections can occasionally combine with anaerobic organisms such as *Bacteroides* to produce the genital gangrene that is the most feared complication of penile prosthesis surgery *(1,2)*.

CLINICAL PRESENTATION

Generally, penile prosthesis infections follow one of two patterns: clinically evident or subclinical. Of the two, the former pattern may represent a true urological emergency. Although clinically evident penile prosthesis infections ultimately tend to make themselves rather obvious, the initial presentation may be somewhat more insidious. Early infections that occur less than 3 weeks from the time of device insertion will tend to be more aggressive. These complications may manifest themselves as frank pus draining from the wound with significant erosion of components, as well as fever, leukocytosis, toxicity, and eschar formation. These early infections are often the result of Gram-negative colonization, as noted in the preceding section.

Clinically evident infections that occur more than 3 wk from the time of device insertion are more commonly caused by staphylococcal organisms. The onset of symptoms in these cases may be more gradual, and the clinical manifestation of infection may be somewhat subtler. In these patients, presentations may include skin fixation of device components (particularly the scrotal pump), a small area of tubing erosion, the presence of a sinus tract, fluctuance in the region of prosthetic components, and generalized swelling of the penis. In addition, purulent drainage may be evident, although it should be cautioned that pus emanating from a small portion of the wound could well represent a superficial wound infection from a source such as a stitch abscess. If compression of the device itself results in increased purulent drainage, periprosthetic infection is usually present. In these patients, findings such as fever, leukocytosis, and toxicity will generally be absent, although the patient will usually complain of significant pain. A fairly high degree of suspicion is necessary to diagnose these somewhat indolent infections; thus, these presentations do not generally constitute a urological emergency.

The final pattern, subclinical infection, does not represent a urological emergency and can be extremely difficult to diagnose. These infections also tend to occur more frequently than their clinically evident counterparts and are generally the result of *S. epidermidis* infection *(38)*. Subclinical infections usually are suspected when the patient has chronic pain for more than 3 mo following device insertion or pain that is temporarily improved by the administration of oral antibiotics. Device migration can also be a sign of subclinical infection. It should be cautioned, however, that patients usually report a fairly high degree of pain associated with the initial device insertion, and that the perioperative pain may take some weeks to resolve despite the absence of any infection.

MANAGEMENT OF PENILE PROSTHESIS INFECTION

Generally, when infection of a penile prosthesis is confirmed or highly suspected, surgical intervention is appropriate. Anecdotal evidence suggests that patients with subclinical infection may occasionally be successfully treated with 3 d of intravenous vancomycin followed by 1 mo of oral trimethoprim-sulfamethoxazole or rifampin *(34)*, but no clinical studies exist to substantiate the efficacy of this approach. Theoretically, if the antibiotics are administered before the biofilm is mature, eradication is possible.

Deroue al. *(39)* suggested a regimen by which patients with penile prosthesis infection are treated with a daily povidone bath, daily expressions of pus, irrigation with clindamycin, and oral clindamycin therapy. They reported favorable results, with eradication of infection and prosthesis retention in a small series of three patients; larger studies are lacking.

If an infection is found, one of two approaches is generally taken. Clearly, the most conservative approach is to remove the device, irrigate and debride the wound, place drains, and allow the infectious process to heal. In patients with significant tissue necrosis, diabetics with significant purulence, or rapidly developing infections with cylinder erosion (as would be likely in a true urological emergency), this conservative approach is favored by most surgeons *(40)*. After 3 to 6 mo, a subsequent attempt at prosthesis placement may be considered if the patient desires. Drawbacks of this approach can include fibrosis, penile shortening, and occasional technical difficulty associated with placement of a penile prosthesis in fibrotic corporeal tissue. This difficulty can usually be overcome if a downsized device with a diameter of 10 mm or less is utilized. In a series from the Cleveland Clinic, the authors reported an overall success rate of 92% with insertion of a downsized device in cases of corporeal fibrosis primarily caused by previous infection *(41)*.

Salvage procedures have been developed by which the entire prosthesis and all foreign parts are removed, the wound is thoroughly cleansed, and then a new prosthesis is reinserted at the same sitting. For the properly selected patient, salvage surgery appears to be the most effective surgical alternative. Specifically, patients infected with virulent organisms associated with cellulitis shortly after original implant surgery are not thought to be good candidates for salvage procedures *(41)*. The patient presenting with the classic, gradual, indolent onset typical of staphylococcal infections as described in the Clinical Presentation section appears to be the optimal candidate for the salvage procedure.

A number of salvage techniques have been described. Furlow and Goldwasser *(43)* reported on 22 men with device erosion caused by infection and treated with removal and replacement of the device followed by postoperative irrigation through a small Jackson-Pratt drain for 3 to 5 d following the procedure. Overall, 116 cases were managed successfully. Similarly, Teloken et al. *(44)* reported on a "rescue procedure" by which a new penile prosthesis was placed after 72 h of continuous irrigation of the corpora cavernosa with rifamycin. Fishman and colleagues *(45)* successfully salvaged infected penile implants in 84% of 44 patients; the average follow-up was 4 yr.

Many urologists involved in implant surgery are following the technique described by Mulcahy's group *(46)* in performing salvage procedures for infected penile prostheses. First, complete removal of all components of the prosthesis is performed. This includes any permanent foreign materials such as suture or polytetrafluoroethylene; complete removal of all foreign bodies is critical for procedure success. Next, irrigation is carried out in a stepwise fashion utilizing kanamycin and bacitracin, hydrogen peroxide, a povidone-iodine solution, and pressure irrigation with saline containing vancomycin and gentamicin; the order is then reversed and repeated. A red rubber catheter is used to direct the irrigating solutions throughout the corporeal bodies. After the washout, gloves and instruments are changed, new drapes are placed over the old drapes, and a new prosthesis is inserted in the standard fashion.

In the original report, salvage was successful in 91% of cases; in the more recent follow-up of 55 patients followed 6 to 93 mo, overall success rate was 82% *(42)*. Success of the procedure appears to be because removal of the infected device and subsequent washout result in removal of the biofilm layer of well-encapsulated infecting organisms, allowing infection-free insertion of another device. The procedure is based on similar experience with salvage therapies for foreign bodies in the vascular, orthopedic, and cardiac surgery literature *(47–49)*.

NEW DEVELOPMENTS IN PERIPROSTHETIC INFECTION

Obviously, the optimal therapeutic strategy for penile prosthesis infection is prevention. As outlined in this chapter, virtually all authors agreed that short hospital stays, attention to skin preparation, meticulous dissection that minimizes tissue injury, strict intraoperative sterile technique, and minimization of the duration of the procedure itself can all help reduce the incidence of postoperative infection.

Two new approaches to the prevention of penile prosthesis infection have been studied. Although somewhat different, both of these approaches involve alteration of the surface of the penile prosthesis. Recall that infection occurs in the biofilm surrounding the device; thus, it has been theorized that alteration of the prosthetic surface may alter the local milieu involved in the development of infection. Although both approaches are preliminary and require further study, they both have shown some promise in reducing the incidence of this feared complication.

In the first approach, silicone utilized in the production of penile prostheses is impregnated with minocycline/rifampin. The concept behind this novel approach is that antimicrobial impregnation of penile prostheses could potentially prevent bacterial colonization of the prosthesis, the first step in implant infection.

In an animal study, Darouiche et a1. *(50)* inoculated minocycline/rifampin-impregnated and control silicone pump bulb sections with 10^3 to 10^4 colony-forming units of *Staphylococcus aureus*. After preparation, the devices were implanted in the backs of rabbits. In vitro zones of inhibition against *S. aureus* by the minocycline/rifampin-impregnated and control devices were determined. All six of the tested antimicrobial-impregnated devices but none of the control devices produced zones of inhibition against *S. aureus*, with the mean zone of inhibition 23 mm. Potentially, this could reduce bacterial colonization of the penile prosthesis at the time of surgery.

Clinical studies of this new device have been carried out and have been published in abstract form. In a preliminary report, Carson *(51)* noted encouraging results with minocycline- and rifampin-impregnated penile implants. In his abstract, the antibiotic-coated devices had reduced infection rates at 6 mo follow-up ($p < 0.0049$). Wilson and coworkers *(52)* have reported particularly promising results with the antibiotic-coated devices in salvage procedures.

Obviously, minocycline and rifampin were chosen because they target staphylococci, the most common pathogen in penile implant infection. One theoretical drawback of antibiotic-coated devices is their potential implantation in patients with unrecognized allergies to minocycline or rifampin. Clearly, larger studies with longer follow-up times are needed to assess the ultimate impact of these promising devices.

Another approach that has been utilized in an attempt to reduce the rate of periprosthetic infection is to create a hydrophilic polyvinylpyrrolidone coating designed to inhibit bacterial adherence while simultaneously prolonging the effect of antibiotics utilized intraoperatively. In this case, the device would not be precoated with the antibiotics themselves; rather, the coating would supposedly enhance the effect of antibiotics chosen at the time of operation.

In an animal study published in abstract form, Hellstrom and coworkers *(53)* reported on the efficacy of coating. Disks with and without the coating were soaked in an aqueous solution of gentamicin and bacitracin; following implantation of devices into rabbits, the zone of inhibition surrounding the disks was investigated. Hellstrom et al. reported that the coated disks demonstrated a sustained antibiotic activity, especially against *S. epidermidis*, for at least 3 d. It was speculated that this effect, along with the antiadherence properties of the hydrophilic polyvinylpyrrolidone coating, could potentially reduce the chance of prosthetic infection.

Li and colleagues *(54)* also demonstrated that the polyvinylpyrrolidone coating decreased bacterial adherence of *S. epidermidis* compared with uncoated bioflex. Specifically, they reported a decrease in adherence of *S. epidermidis* to the coated Bioflex® by 41% compared to the uncoated bioflex ($p < 0.05$). Obviously, the hope is that if bacterial adherence is reduced, the incidence of penile prosthesis infection will ultimately follow suit.

It should be stressed that these studies are all preliminary, and as of this writing, a randomized, double-blind study demonstrated a reduced infection rate in patients implanted with either device has not been published in a peer-reviewed journal. Nevertheless, these specialized coatings do show some promise in potentially reducing the incidence of the devastating complication of periprosthetic infection.

SUMMARY

Occasionally, penile prosthesis infection can represent a true urological emergency. In this instance, the presentation will be obvious. The patient will have significant tissue necrosis, marked purulence, or rapidly developing infection with cylinder erosion. A conservative approach involving removal of all prosthesis components is indicated. In the more common, indolent presentation secondary to *S. epidermidis* infection, surgical therapy with immediate salvage insertion of a new device represents the current optimal surgical alternative.

REFERENCES

1. Dardar AH, Pettersson BA. Penile gangrene: a complication of penile prosthesis. Scand J Urol Nephrol 1995; 19: 355–356.
2. Walther PJ, Andriani RT, Maggio MI, Carson CC. Fournier's gangrene: a complication of penile prosthetic implantation in a renal transplant patient. J Urol 1987; 137: 299–300.
3. Carbone DJ, Seftel AD. Erectile dysfunction. Diagnosis and treatment in older men. Geriatrics 2002; 57(9): 18–24.
4. Carson CC. Management of prosthesis infections in urologic surgery. Infect Urol 1999; 26: 829–839.
5. Kabalin JN, Kessler R. Infectious complications of penile prosthesis surgery. J Urol 1988; 139: 953–955.
6. Montague DK. Periprosthetic infections. J Urol 1987; 138: 68–69.
7. Thomalla JV, Thompson ST, Rowland RG, Mulcahy JJ. Infectious complications of penile prosthetic implants. J Urol 1987; 138: 65–67.
8. Jarow JP. Risk factors for penile prosthetic infection. J Urol 1996; 156: 402–404.
9. Fallon B, Ghanem H. Infected penile prosthesis: incidence and outcomes. Int J Impot Res 1999; 1: 175–188.
10. Mulcahy JJ. The complex penile prosthesis. In: Male infertility and sexual dysfunction. (Hellstrom WJG, ed.), Springer-Verlag, New York, NY, 1997, pp. 549–562.

11. Carson CC. Increased infection risk with corpus cavernosum reconstruction and penile prosthesis implantation. Int J Impot Res 1996; 8: 155.
12. Radomski SB, Herschorn S. Risk factors associated with penile prosthesis infection. 1992; 147: 383–385.
13. Montague DK, Angermeier KW, Lakin MM. Penile prosthesis infections. Int J Impot Res 2001; 14: 326–328.
14. Wilson SK, Delk JR. Inflatable penile implant infection: predisposing factors and treatment suggestions. J Urol 1995; 153(3): 659–661.
15. Bishop JR, Moul JW, Sihelnik SA, et al. Use of glycosylated hemoglobin to identify diabetics at high risk for penile periprosthetic infections. J Urol 1992; 147: 386–388.
16. Wilson SK, Carson CC, Cleves MA, Delk JR. Quantifying risk of penile prosthesis infection with elevated glycosylated hemoglobin. J Urol 1998; 159(5): 1537–1539.
17. Gross AJ, Sauerwein DH, Kutzenberter J, et al. Penile prostheses in paraplegic men. Br J Urol 1996; 78: 262–264.
18. Diokno AC, Sonda LP. Compatibility of genitourinary prostheses and intermittent self-catheterization: J Urol 1981; 125: 659–667.
19. Acar O, Mutlu B, Cimen K, et al. The role of intraoperative antibiotic irrigation and postoperative antibiotic therapy for contaminated implantable prosthesis: in a rat model in vivo. Int J Impot Res 2000; 12: 285–288.
20. Lynch MJ, Scott GM, Inglis JA, Pryor JP. Reducing the loss of implants following penile prosthetic surgery. Br J Urol 1994; 73: 423–427.
21. Garber BB, Marcus SM. Does surgical approach affect the incidence of inflatable penile prosthesis infection? Urology 1998; 52(2): 291–293.
22. Ghanem HM, Fahmy I, Fallon B. Infection control in outpatient unicomponent penile prosthesis surgery. Int J Impot Res 1999; 11: 25–27.
23. Walters FP, Neal DE, Rege AB, et al. Cavernous tissue antibiotic levels in penile prosthesis surgery. J Urol 1992; 147: 1282–1284.
24. Schwartz BF, Swanzy S, Thrasher BJ. A randomized prospective comparison of antibiotic tissue levels in the corpora cavernosa of patients undergoing penile prosthesis implantation using gentamicin plus cefazolin vs an oral fluoroquinolone for prophylaxis. J Urol 1996; 156(3): 991–994.
25. Classen DC, Evans RS, Pestotink SL, et al. Timing of prophylactic administration of antibiotics and the risk of surgical wound infection. N Engl J Med 1992; 326: 281–286.
26. Gristina AG. Biomaterial centered infection: microbial adhesion vs tissue integration. Science 1987; 237: 588–595.
27. Reid G, Tieszer C, Foerch R, et al. The binding of urinary components and uropathogens to a silicone latex urethral catheter. Cells Mater 1992; 2: 253–160.
28. Reid G, Davidson R, Denstedt JD. XPS, SEM and EDX analysis of conditioning film deposition onto ureteral stents. Surf Interface Anal 1994; 21: 581–586.
29. Wadstrom T. Molecular aspects of bacterial adhesion, colonization, and development of infections associated with biomaterials. J Invest Surg 1989; 2: 253–160.
30. Brokke P, Dankert J, Carballo J, Feijen J. Adherence of coagulase negative staphylococci onto polyethylene catheters in vitro and in vivo, a study on the influence of various plasma proteins. J Biomater Appl 1991; 5: 204–226.
31. Nickel JC, Heaton J, Morales A, et al. Bacterial biofilm in persistent penile prostheses associated infections. J Urol 1986; 135: 586–595.
32. Roberts JA, Fussell EN, Lewis RW. Bacterial adherence to penile prosthesis. Int J Impot Res 1989; 1: 167–178.
33. Reid G, Busscher HJ. Microbial biofilms and urinary tract infections. In: Urinary Tract Infections. (Brumfitt W, Hamilton Miller T, Bailey RR, eds.), Chapman and Hall, London, 1998, pp. 111–118.
34. Busseher HJ, Bos R, van der Mei HC. Initial microbial adhesion is a determinant for the strength of biofilm adhesion. FEMS Microbiol Lett 1995; 128: 229–234.
35. Wilson SK. Delk JR II. Inflatable penile implant infections: predisposing factors and treatment suggestions. J Urol 1995; 153: 659–661.

36. Licht MR, Montague DK, Angermeier KW, et al. Cultures from genitourinary prostheses at reoperation: Questioning the role of *Staphylococcus epidermidis* in periprosthetic infection. J Urol 1995; 154: 387–390.
37. Moul JW, Carson CC. Infectious complications of penile prostheses. Infect Urol 1989; 1: 97–108.
38. Parsons CL, Stein PC, Dobke MK, et al. Diagnosis and therapy of subclinically infected prostheses. Surg Gynecol Obstet 1993; 177: 504–506.
39. Deroue H, Uder M, Freyfogle FB, Stoeckle M. Successful conservative treatment of infected penile prostheses. Eur Urol 2002; 41: 66–70.
40. Carson CC. Penile prosthesis implantation and infection for Sexual Medicine Society of North America. Int J Imp Res 2001; 13(suppl 5): S35–S38.
41. Carbone DJ, Daitch JA, Angermeier KW, Lakin MM, Montague DK. Management of severe corporeal fibrosis with implantation of prosthesis via a transverse scrotal approach. J Urol 1997; 159: 125–127.
42. Mulcahy JJ. Long-term experience with salvage of infected penile implants. J Urol 1999; 163: 481–482.
43. Furlow WL, Goldwasser B. Salvage of the eroded inflatable penile prosthesis: a new concept. J Urol 1987; 138: 312–314.
44. Teloken C, Souto JC, Da Ros C, Thorel E, Souto C. Prosthetic penile infection: "rescue procedure" with rifamycin. J Urol 1992; 148: 1905–1906.
45. Fishman IJ, Scott FB, Selim AM. Rescue procedure: an alternative to complete removal for treatment of infected penile prostheses. J Urol 1987; 137: 202A.
46. Brant MD, Ludlow JK, Mulcahy JM. The prosthesis salvage operation: immediate replacement of the infected penile prosthesis. J Urol 1996; 155: 155–157.
47. Bandyk DF, Bergamini TM, Kinney BV, Seabrook GR, Towne JB. *In situ* replacement of vascular prostheses infected by bacterial biofilms. J Vasc Surg 1992; 13: 575.
48. Karchmer AW, Archer GL, Dismukes WE. *Staphylococcus epidermidis* causing prosthetic valve endocarditis: microbiologic and clinical observations as guides to therapy. Ann Intern Med 1983; 98: 447.
49. Carlsson AS, Josefsson G, Lindberg L. Revision with gentamicin-impregnated cement for deep infections in total hip arthroplasties. J Bone Joint Surg 1978; 60: 1059.
50. Darouiche RO, Mansouri MD, Raad II. Efficacy of antimicrobial-impregnated silicone sections from penile implants in preventing device colonization in an animal model. Urology 2002; 59: 303–307.
51. Carson CC. Efficacy of antibiotic impregnation of inflatable penile prosthesis in decreasing infection in original implants. J Urol 2004; 171(4): 1611–1614.
52. Wilson SK, Henry GD, Delk JR, Cleves MA. Prevention of infection in revision of penile prostheses by using antibiotic coated prosthesis and Mulcahy salvage protocol. J Urol 2003; 169: 1264A.
53. Hellstrom WG, Hyun JS, Sanabria J, et al. Assessment of in-vivo performance of anti-microbial-soaked, bioflex-coated resist. J Urol 2002; 167: 599a.
54. Li H, Rajpurkar AD, Fairfax MR, Dhabuwala CB. Comparison of bacterial adherence in polyvinylpyrrolidone coated bioflex and plain bioflex. J Urol 2003; 169: 1311a.

10 Fournier's Gangrene

Peter C. Black, MD and Hunter Wessells, MD, FACS

CONTENTS

INTRODUCTION
ETIOLOGY AND PATHOGENESIS
PRESENTATION AND DIAGNOSIS
MANAGEMENT
COVERAGE
PROGNOSIS
SUMMARY
REFERENCES

INTRODUCTION

Fournier's gangrene is a necrotizing infection of the skin, subcutaneous fat, and superficial fascia of the external genitalia and perineum. It was first described as an idiopathic and fulminant disease in young men *(1)*, but has since been recognized to follow a more indolent course in certain cases, to involve all ages and both genders *(2–5)*, and to be related to an identifiable source in most cases *(2,5–10)*. It remains, however, a life-threatening disease that requires rapid diagnosis and immediate surgical management. Mortality rates appear to have been reduced with appropriate surgical and medical intervention, but in selected patients may still be as high as 50%.

ETIOLOGY AND PATHOGENESIS

Fournier's gangrene is a synergistic infection with multiple aerobic and anaerobic bacteria *(5,11)*. These include *Escherichia coli*, *Bacteroides species*, staphylococci, *Proteus*, streptococci, *Pseudomonas*, enterococci, and *Clostridium perfringens (6–8,11,12)*.

Multiple comorbid conditions have been associated with Fournier's gangrene. Between 32 and 77% of patients have diabetes mellitus *(2–4,6,7,9,13–15)*. Alcoholism, immunosuppression (including acquired immunodeficiency syndrome [AIDS]) *(16)*, malignancy, obesity, malnutrition, and intravenous drug use predispose to necrotizing genital infections *(2–4,7,9,15,17)*. Local trauma and surgery to the external genitalia are further risk factors *(5,9,17)*.

From: *Urological Emergencies: A Practical Guide*
Edited by: H. Wessells and J. W. McAninch © Humana Press Inc., Totowa, NJ

The source of infection is identifiable in more than 75% of cases *(2,5–10)*. Perirectal and perianal abscesses are both the most common and most moribund causes *(2,5–8,10,13,18)*. Periurethral infection resulting from stricture disease or instrumentation with urinary extravasation is identified in approx 20–30% of cases *(5,10,17,18)*. A scrotal abscess, epididymitis, or skin lesions, such as suprainfected sebaceous cysts, can also progress to Fournier's gangrene *(5,10)*.

The route of rapid spread of necrotizing infection is determined by the contiguous fascial anatomy of the external genitalia, perineum, and abdomen. Bacterial infection can spread along the dartos fascia of the scrotum and penis, Colles' fascia of the perineum, the fascia lata onto the thigh, and Scarpa's fascia of the anterior abdominal wall up as high as the axillae. Histological characterization shows dermal and subcutaneous necrosis covered by intact epidermis *(19)*. The primary pathophysiological mechanism of the superficial necrosis is via thrombosis of small subcutaneous arterioles in their investing fascia, which leads to ischemia, allowing aerobic bacterial growth and contributing to rapid extension of infection *(7,20,21)*.

PRESENTATION AND DIAGNOSIS

The findings on exam of a patient with Fournier's exam are characteristic; the history and secondary signs and symptoms will give clues on the source of the infection. The infection commonly starts as cellulitis adjacent to the portal of entry. Genital pain, swelling, and erythema are the most prominent symptoms *(3)*. Fournier's gangrene can be distinguished from acute cellulitis by the concomitant signs of systemic toxicity, including fever, mental status changes, tachypnea, and tachycardia *(22)*. On the other hand, physical findings may underrepresent the true extent of the disease. Marked progression may occur within hours, leading to crepitus and dark purple discoloration of the tissue (Fig. 1), followed later by sloughing, drainage, and demarcation of dead tissue.

A history of local trauma, obstructive voiding symptoms, recent instrumentation, or urethral stricture will direct further evaluation. Perirectal pain, rectal bleeding, and a history of anal fissures are suggestive of perianal or rectal sources. If the infection originates in the scrotal skin, the palpation of the scrotal contents should be normal; secondary involvement of the scrotal skin caused by an intrascrotal process should reveal abnormal intrascrotal findings on physical exam.

Laboratory analysis will often show leukocytosis and anemia as well as an elevated serum creatinine, hyponatremia, hypocalcemia, and hypoalbuminemia *(20)*.

Radiographic studies can be useful when the physical exam does not allow definitive diagnosis of Fournier's gangrene. Scrotal ultrasonography is useful to delineate an intrascrotal process if physical exam is indeterminate. Scrotal and perineal ultrasound *(23)* as well as plain radiographs or computed tomography *(24)* may reveal the presence of gas in the soft tissue, a hallmark of gangrene (Fig. 2). The identification of subcutaneous or deep tissue gas should prompt immediate surgical exploration. Some abscesses will produce gas in the absence of necrotizing fasciitis, but these patients will still require drainage of the collection. It is likely that, left untreated, such collections could progress to Fournier's gangrene.

Retrograde urethrography is indicated when a urethral injury or urinary extravasation is suspected. This may assist in deciding whether to place a suprapubic cystostomy tube *(22)*.

Chapter 10 / Fournier's Gangrene 159

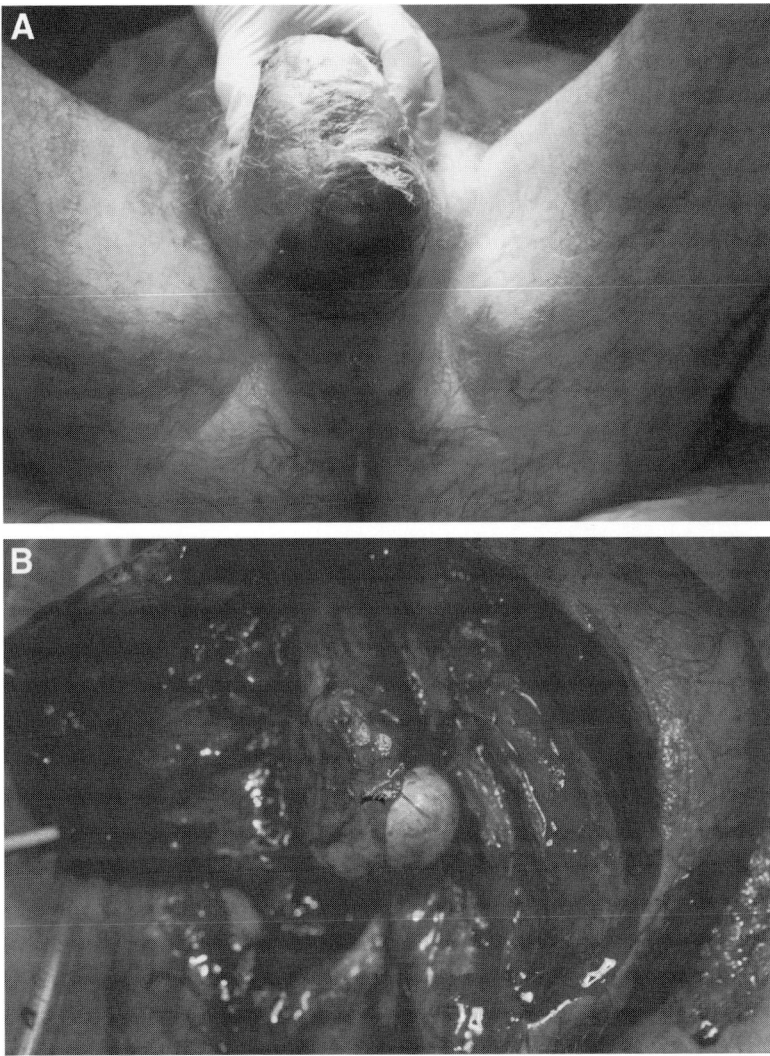

Fig. 1. Appearance of genitalia in a patient with acute necrotizing infection of scrotal skin.

MANAGEMENT

Emergent Management

The treatment of Fournier's gangrene depends on rapid recognition, radical debridement of necrotic tissue, and broad spectrum antibiotics. Intravenous hydration is initiated immediately, and the intravenous antibiotics are started, including penicillin for Gram-positive organisms, a third-generation cephalosporin or aminoglycoside for Gram-negative organisms, and metronidazole or clindamycin for anaerobic organisms (4,11). The critically ill patient may need correction of electrolytes, ventilatory support, and vasopressors. Purulent discharge is sent for culture from the emergency room or at the time of incision in the operating room.

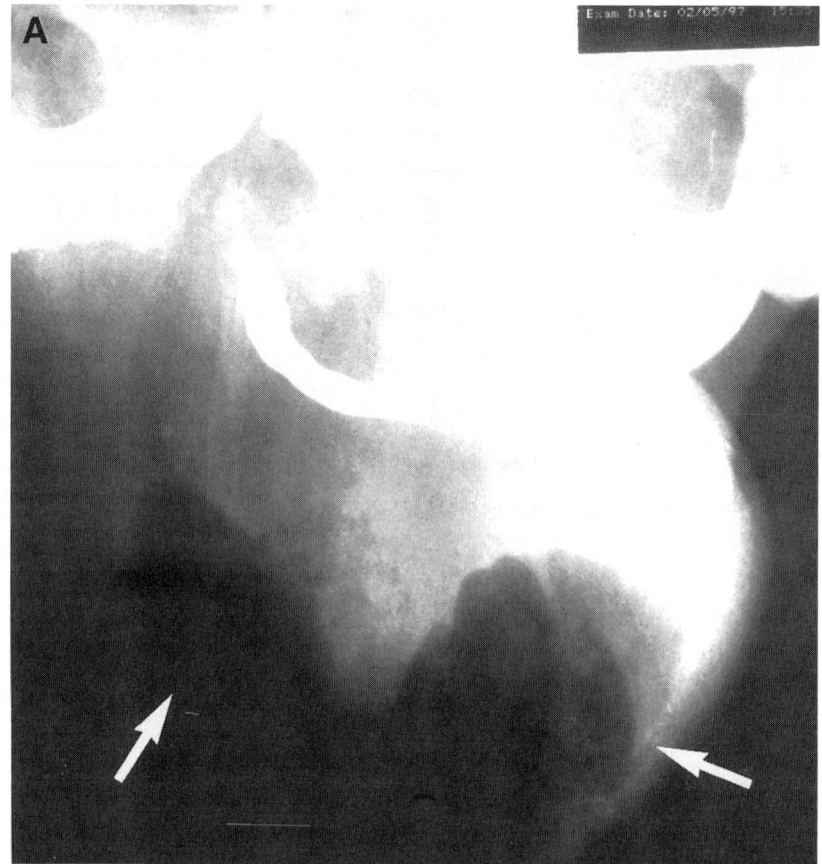
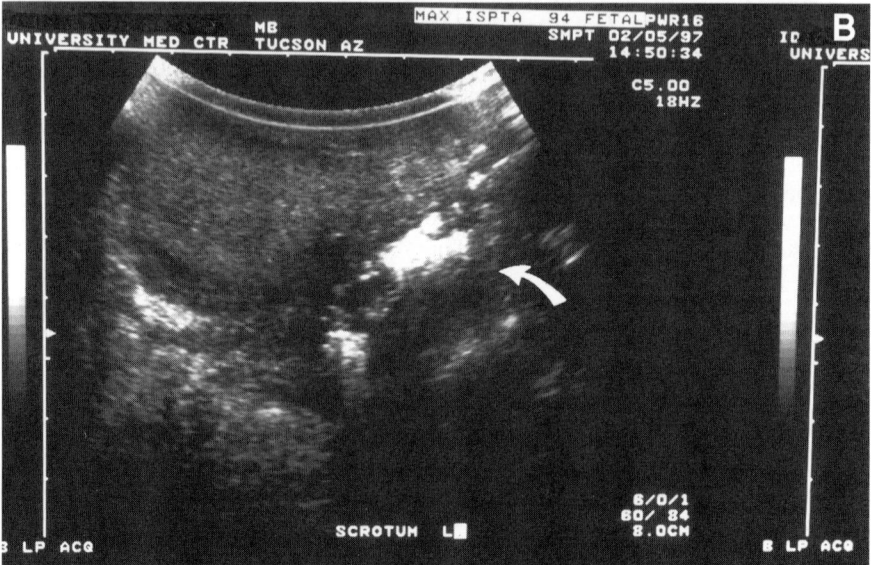

Fig. 2. Radiographic appearance of gas in soft tissues. (**A**) Plain radiograph of scrotum showing air (arrow). (**B**) Sonographic characteristic of gas is high echogenicity (arrow).

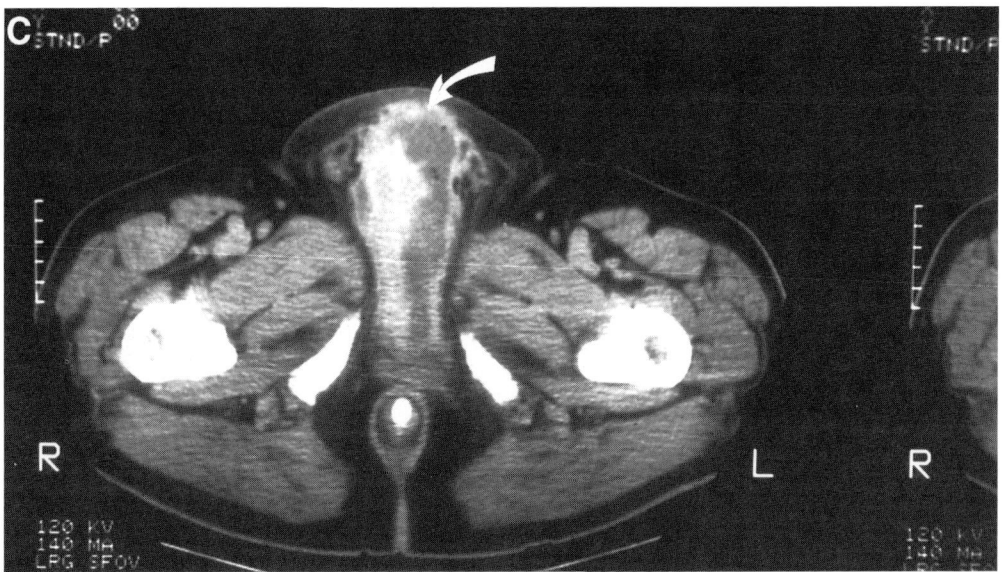

Fig. 2. *(Continued)* **(C)** Computed tomography clearly demonstrates an abscess with air (arrow).

Even with the advent of antibiotics, Fournier's gangrene remains a surgical emergency. Aggressive, sharp excision of all devitalized skin, subcutaneous tissue, and fascia is performed expeditiously. Debridement is extended into vital tissue at all margins. The glans penis, corpus spongiosum, corpora cavernosa, and testes are almost always preserved because of their deep blood supply, which is independent of the compromised fascial and subcutaneous circulation. The perineal artery, a branch of the internal pudendal artery, supplies the skin and superficial fascial planes of the perineum and posterior scrotum. The blood supply to the skin and dartos fascia of the anterior scrotum and penis is derived from the external pudendal branches of the femoral artery.

Buck's fascia on the penile shaft and the corpora are uninvolved by the necrotizing process because they receive blood from the dorsal, cavernosal, and bulbar arteries, which are further branches of the internal pudendal artery. The spermatic fascia, tunica vaginalis, and testes are supplied by the cremasteric, vasal, and testicular arteries, respectively, and are generally spared from necrotizing gangrene. These structures rarely require debridement and should be preserved. Once the tunica vaginalis has been violated, superinfection of the testis is more likely and may necessitate secondary orchiectomy (Fig. 3). Primary orchiectomy should be performed at the time of debridement if the etiology of the necrotizing infection is epididymo-orchitis or scrotal abscess *(17)*.

We perform debridement with scalpel, scissors, and 0 chromic suture ligatures rather than electrocautery, which is more time consuming. Significant hemorrhage may occur and necessitates careful hemostasis. Pressure irrigation is used to reduce bacterial load on the wound bed prior to dressing application. Intraoperative proctoscopy and cystoscopy are performed when indicated for suspected rectal or urethral sources of infection *(22)*.

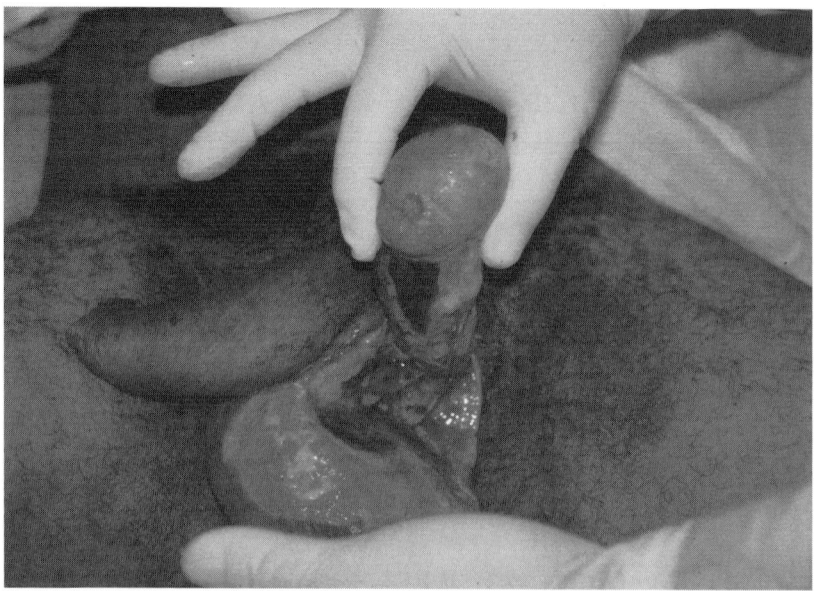

Fig. 3. Suprainfection of exposed tunica albuginea of testis that required orchiectomy.

Large complex wounds with massive contamination and simultaneous colorectal or urinary tract disease may necessitate fecal or urinary diversion. Fecal diversion is achieved with end colostomy, and suprapubic cystostomy is preferred for urinary diversion *(9,10,13,25)*. Our experience has been that few patients require colostomy, and Foley catheter drainage is sufficient in the absence of urethral stricture of fistula.

Repeat inspection and debridement should be scheduled within 24 h; two to four surgeries are commonly required for each patient *(4,10,14)*. It remains controversial whether the denuded testes should be placed in thigh pouches (Fig. 4) or kept free and wrapped in moist gauze dressings. Until the wound bed is free of gross contamination, the testes should be kept in standard dressings. Once the wound becomes clean, the thigh pouch offers the advantage of easier dressing changes and less patient discomfort. In cases of isolated scrotal gangrene, placement of the testes in thigh pouches may allow primary closure of the perineum and more rapid discharge of the patient. Scrotal reconstruction can then be planned electively. It is important to place the testes anteriorly to avoid compression and pain with adduction. The rare patient may prefer to leave the testes in thigh pouches.

The majority of patients will have additional areas of skin loss of the penis, perineum, thighs, or lower abdominal wall (Fig. 5). In such cases, we leave the testes exposed: Delayed scrotal reconstruction with skin grafts at the time of coverage of other reconstruction makes sense (*see* Coverage section).

Postoperative Management

Debrided wounds are left open, and aggressive wound care is initiated postoperatively with saline gauze dressings, whirlpool or waterpick therapy, and repeat debridement. This prepares the wounds for secondary coverage. Intravenous antibiotics are stopped when the wound is clean. Quantitative cultures are sometimes used to estimate the degree

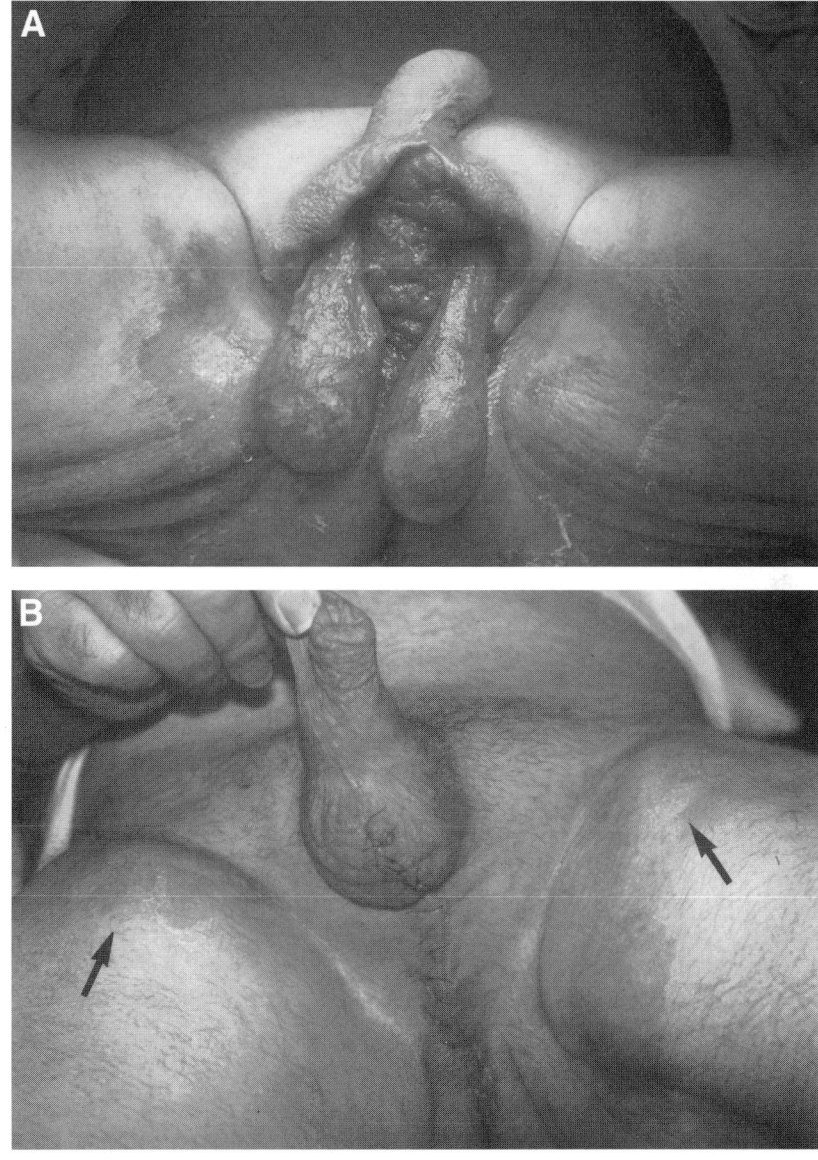

Fig. 4. Primary closure of scrotal defect by placement of testes in thigh pouches.

of contamination prior to reconstruction, although in our experience these do not correlate with outcomes of coverage procedures (Walsh T and Wessells H, unpublished data, 2004). Important postoperative concerns include the careful control of diabetes and sufficient caloric and protein intake to allow adequate wound healing.

Hyperbaric oxygen therapy is used increasingly as an adjunct after rapid debridement *(5,15,17,22)*. High oxygen tension is thought to improve wound healing and mitigate ongoing necrosis in the hypoxic tissues at the margins of the debrided field. Mechanisms include stimulation of leukocyte function, enhanced neovascularization, and inhibited toxin formation by anaerobic bacteria *(17,26)*. A decrease in patient mortality was

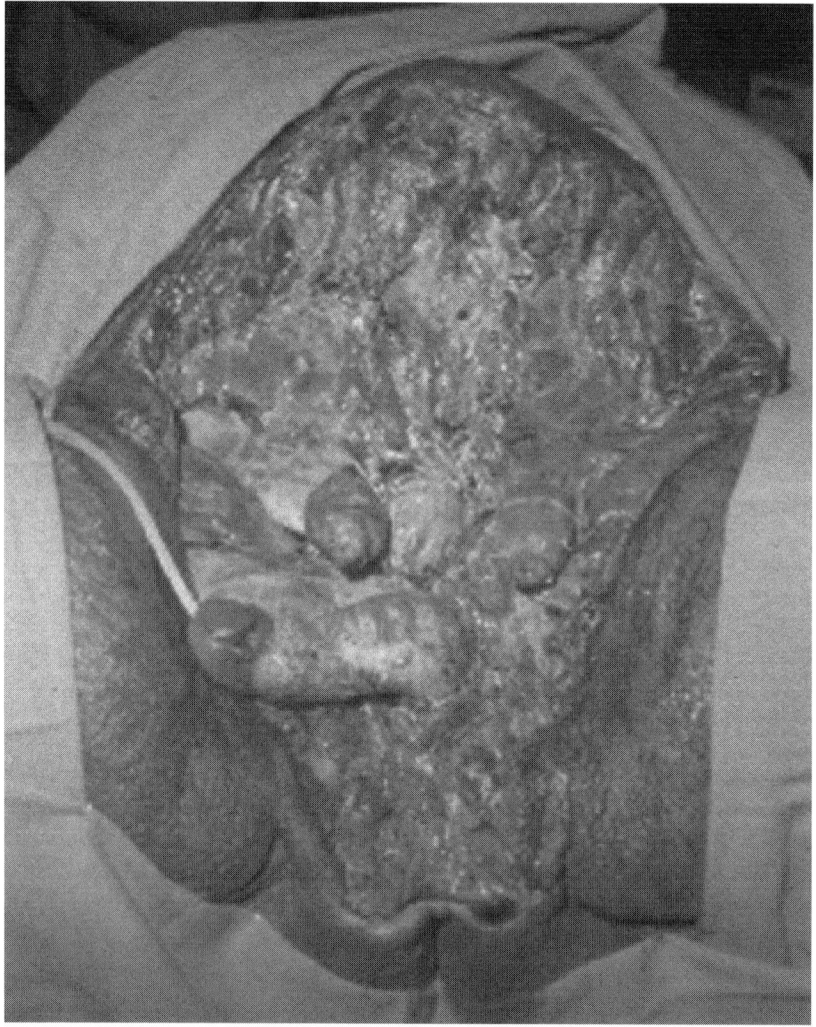

Fig. 5. Massive lower abdominal and genital skin loss.

detected with hyperbaric oxygen treatment in one study *(17)*. Therapy is started as soon after debridement as possible with three dives within the first 24 h *(17)*. This is followed by two dives per day for an additional 7 d and once-daily dives thereafter until 5 d after surgical closure of the wounds. If infection is controlled rapidly and completely with conventional treatment, hyperbaric oxygen may be unnecessary.

The topical application of honey is a novel treatment that has been advocated when hyperbaric oxygen is not accessible *(9,27,28)*. Unprocessed honey has a pH of 3.6 and is thought to contain enzymes that promote digestion of necrotic tissue. It also has topical antibacterial activity and increases local oxygenation *(9)*.

COVERAGE

Once the wound bed is clean and clear of infection, reconstruction is based on the size of the defect, presence or absence of the testes, sexual function, remaining transferable genital skin, and overall patient status. Such secondary reconstruction is planned once the wounds are clean and granulating, usually 7 to 21 d after initial debridement. Patients with limited skin loss can perform dressing changes at home while waiting for elective reconstruction.

Remnant foreskin *(29)* and scrotal skin *(30,31)* have been used for penile skin coverage, but most authors prefer split-thickness skin grafting (STSG) for its ease of use, versatility, and good take *(32,33)*. STSG is preferable to full-thickness grafting in the contaminated wounds found with Fournier's gangrene *(34)*. Meshed grafts allow better drainage of the wound bed and have the potential advantage of better take on contaminated wounds in debilitated patients. McAninch used meshed STSG in impotent men, for whom graft contraction is not a concern *(32)*. In potent men, unmeshed STSG sheets are used. We used unexpanded meshed STSG in nine patients regardless of sexual function and with penile skin loss of different etiologies; we showed excellent graft take with no functional impairment *(35)*.

Reconstruction of total scrotal skin loss is more challenging. Tissue expanders have been used to reconstruct a two-compartment scrotum when there is at least a small remnant of scrotal skin *(36)*. When primary closure is impossible because of the extent of skin loss, scrotal coverage is usually achieved with flaps or meshed STSG. After prior placement of the testes in thigh pouches, the patient can undergo a subsequent staged closure with rotational thigh flaps or grafting. Flaps are preferred by some for purported improvement in functional outcome, with a resultant sensate and hair-bearing scrotum *(37)*.

In Fournier's gangrene, flaps are often unavailable, and STSG may already be required for abdominal wall or penile wounds. We prefer meshed STSG for the scrotal reconstruction because of its availability and excellent take (Fig. 6). Perineal defects provide a suboptimal graft bed, and as a result we reapproximate any remnant scrotum or medial thigh skin over Penrose drains whenever possible. Modest defects in the perineum, groin, and adjacent areas may be allowed to close by secondary intention and reepithelialization.

PROGNOSIS

Despite maximal medical and surgical treatment, Fournier's gangrene remains a potentially lethal disease. In recent series, the associated mortality rate varied widely, between 4 *(10)* and 38% *(20)*, but is approx 20 to 30% on average *(5,8,13,15)*. The lower mortality rates *(9,10,17,26)* reported in some series raise the question whether necrotizing fasciitis was indeed present in all cases.

Advanced age *(7,8,20,38)* and more extensive disease predict a poor outcome *(8,15,38)*. A colorectal or perianal source also appears to confer a worse prognosis *(5)*, which may be related to delay in diagnosis and more extensive disease.

Eke et al. reported in their review of 1726 cases that patient condition at the time of presentation is predictive of outcome *(5)*. Although there is little evidence that specific comorbidities are predictive *(38)*, renal insufficiency *(20,38)* and hepatic dysfunction at the time of presentation adversely affected survival *(38)*. In addition, Fournier's gangrene may take a fulminant course in the immunocompromised patient *(15)*, although some reports indicated no worse prognosis in human immunodeficiency virus (HIV)/AIDS *(7,8,12)*. Diabetes has not been predictive of a poor outcome because of its high prevalence in this patient population.

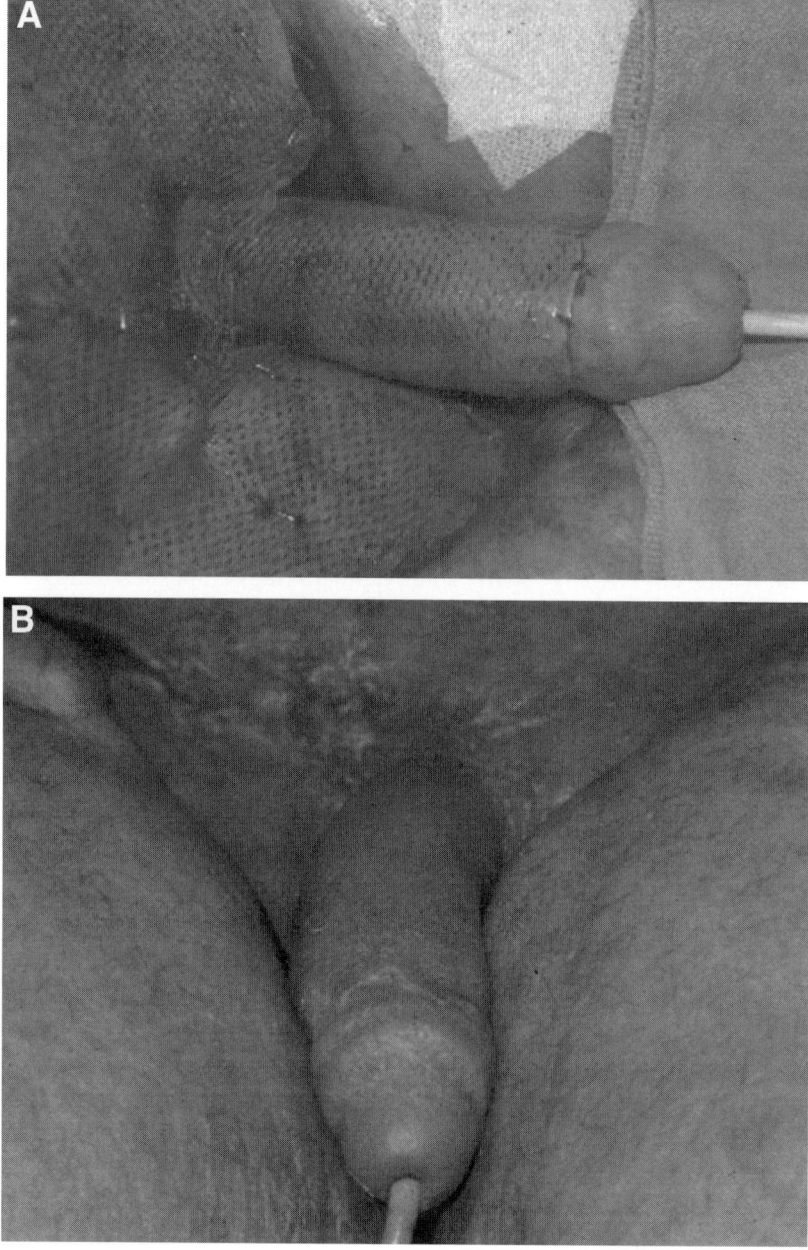

Fig. 6. Split-thickness skin graft coverage of penis and scrotum.

The Acute Physiology and Chronic Health Evaluation II classification system has been employed to develop a severity index for Fournier's gangrene *(38)*. The index consists of admission vital signs (temperature, heart rate, respiratory rate) and laboratory values (hematocrit, white blood count, serum sodium, potassium, creatinine, and bicarbonate). The index predicted mortality accurately in one series *(38)* and appears promising for future clinical and research use. It will need validation in a prospective series of patients.

SUMMARY

Fournier's gangrene is a necrotizing infection by multiple synergistic bacteria of the superficial soft tissue of the external genitalia. An origin of the disease is usually identifiable and is most often a perirectal or periurethral infection or a superficial process of the perineal or scrotal skin. Many patients also have clear risk factors such as diabetes mellitus. The superficial spread of disease in the fascial planes of the penis, scrotum, perineum, and anterior abdominal wall is predictable based on the blood supply and fascial anatomy. The key to management of this urological emergency remains rapid diagnosis and emergent surgical debridement along with medical resuscitation and antibiotics. Hyperbaric oxygen treatment is now used as an adjunct in select patients. After debridement, prolonged dressing care is necessary to prepare the wound bed for autografting or other skin coverage. Despite optimal medical and surgical care, Fournier's gangrene remains a potentially lethal disease.

REFERENCES

1. Fournier J. Gangrëne-foudroyante de la verge. Semaine Med 1883; 3: 345–348.
2. Yaghan RJ, Al-Jaberi TM, Bani-Hani I. Fournier's gangrene: changing face of the disease. Dis Colon Rectum 2000; 43: 1300–1308.
3. Smith GL, Bunker CB, Dinneen MD. Fournier's gangrene. Br J Urol 1998; 81: 347–355.
4. Norton KS, Johnson LW, Perry T, Perry KH, Sehon JK, Zibari GB. Management of Fournier's gangrene: an 11 year retrospective analysis of early recognition, diagnosis, and treatment. Am Surg 2002; 68: 709–713.
5. Eke N. Fournier's gangrene: a review of 1726 cases. Br J Surg 2000; 87: 718–728.
6. Baskin LS, Carroll PR, Cattolica EV, McAninch JW. Necrotising soft tissue infections of the perineum and genitalia. Bacteriology, treatment and risk assessment. Br J Urol 1990; 65: 524–529.
7. Clayton MD, Fowler JE Jr, Sharifi R, Pearl RK. Causes, presentation and survival of 57 patients with necrotizing fasciitis of the male genitalia. Surg Gynecol Obstet 1990; 170: 49–55.
8. Benizri E, Fabiani P, Migliori G, et al. Gangrene of the perineum. Urology 1996; 47: 935–939.
9. Hejase MJ, Simonin JE, Bihrle R, Coogan CL. Genital Fournier's gangrene: experience with 38 patients. Urology 1996; 47: 734–739.
10. Corman JM, Moody JA, Aronson WJ. Fournier's gangrene in a modern surgical setting: improved survival with aggressive management. BJU Int 1999; 84: 85–88.
11. Vick R, Carson CC 3rd. Fournier's disease. Urol Clin North Am 1999; 26: 841–849.
12. Basoglu M, Gul O, Yildirgan I, Balik AA, Ozbey I, Oren D. Fournier's gangrene: review of 15 cases. Am Surg 1997; 63: 1019–1021.
13. Villanueva-Saenz E, Martinez Hernandez-Magro P, Valdes Ovalle M, Montes Vega J, Alvarez-Tostado FJ. Experience in management of Fournier's gangrene. Tech Coloproctol 2002; 6: 5–10; discussion 11–13.
14. Nisbet AA, Thompson IM. Impact of diabetes mellitus on the presentation and outcomes of Fournier's gangrene. Urology 2002; 60: 775–779.
15. Dahm P, Roland FH, Vaslef SN, et al. Outcome analysis in patients with primary necrotizing fasciitis of the male genitalia. Urology 2000; 56: 31–35; discussion 35–36.
16. Elem B, Ranjan P. Impact of immunodeficiency virus (HIV) on Fournier's gangrene: observations in Zambia. Ann R Coll Surg Engl 1995; 77: 283–286.
17. Hollabaugh RS Jr, Dmochowski RR, Hickerson WL, Cox CE. Fournier's gangrene: therapeutic impact of hyperbaric oxygen. Plast Reconstr Surg 1998; 101: 94–100.
18. Asci R, Sarikaya S, Buyukalpelli R, Yilmaz AF, Yildiz S. Fournier's gangrene: risk assessment and enzymatic debridement with lyophilized collagenase application. Eur Urol 1998; 34: 411–418.
19. Stamenkovic I, Lew PD. Early recognition of potentially fatal necrotizing fasciitis. The use of frozen-section biopsy. N Engl J Med 1984; 310: 1689–1693.

20. Olsofka JN, Carrillo EH, Spain DA, Polk HC Jr. The continuing challenge of Fournier's gangrene in the 1990s. Am Surg 1999; 65: 1156–1159.
21. Baskin LS, Dixon C, Stoller ML, Carroll PR. Pyoderma gangrenosum presenting as Fournier's gangrene. J Urol 1990; 144: 984–986.
22. Paty R, Smith AD. Gangrene and Fournier's gangrene. Urol Clin North Am 1992; 19: 149–162.
23. Kane CJ, Nash P, McAninch JW. Ultrasonographic appearance of necrotizing gangrene: aid in early diagnosis. Urology 1996; 48: 142–144.
24. Wessells H. Genital skin loss: unified reconstructive approach to a heterogeneous entity. World J Urol 1999; 17: 107–114.
25. Nathan B. Fournier's gangrene: a historical vignette. Can J Surg 1998; 41: 72.
26. Pizzorno R, Bonini F, Donelli A, Stubinski R, Medica M, Carmignani G. Hyperbaric oxygen therapy in the treatment of Fournier's disease in 11 male patients. J Urol 1997; 158: 837–840.
27. Efem SE. Recent advances in the management of Fournier's gangrene: preliminary observations. Surgery 1993; 113: 200–204.
28. Bergman A, Yanai J, Weiss J, Bell D, David MP. Acceleration of wound healing by topical application of honey. An animal model. Am J Surg 1983; 145: 374–376.
29. Parkash S, Gajendran V. Surgical reconstruction of the sequelae of penile and scrotal gangrene: a plea for simplicity. Br J Plast Surg 1984; 37: 354–357.
30. Castanares S, Belt E. Surgical reconstruction of the penis in skin losses, using scrotum skin. Br J Plast Surg 1968; 21: 253–257.
31. Gomez R. Genital skin loss: reconstructive techniques. Probl Urol 1994; 8: 290–301.
32. McAninch JW. Management of genital skin loss. Urol Clin North Am 1989; 16: 387–397.
33. Dandapat MC, Mohapatro SK, Patro SK. Elephantiasis of the penis and scrotum. A review of 350 cases. Am J Surg 1985; 149: 686–690.
34. Vincent MP, Horton CE, Devine CJ Jr. An evaluation of skin grafts for reconstruction of the penis and scrotum. Clin Plast Surg 1988; 15: 411–424.
35. Black PC, Friedrich J, Engrav L, Wessells H. Meshed unexpanded split-thickness skin grafting for reconstruction of penile skin loss. J Urol 2004; 172: 976–999.
36. Still EF 2nd, Goodman RC. Total reconstruction of a two-compartment scrotum by tissue expansion. Plast Reconstr Surg 1990; 85: 805–807; discussion 808.
37. McDougal WS. Scrotal reconstruction using thigh pedicle flaps. J Urol 1983; 129: 757–759.
38. Laor E, Palmer LS, Tolia BM, Reid RE, Winter HI. Outcome prediction in patients with Fournier's gangrene. J Urol 1995; 154: 89–92.

III Vascular and Hemorrhagic Emergencies

11 Renal Artery Embolism and Renal Vein Thrombosis

Edward J. Yun, MD and Christopher J. Kane, MD

CONTENTS

INTRODUCTION
RENAL ARTERY EMBOLISM AND INFARCTION
RENAL VEIN THROMBOSIS
SUMMARY
REFERENCES

INTRODUCTION

In this chapter, we explore two categories of emergencies involving the major renal vasculature: renal infarction and renal vein thrombosis (RVT). Although both conditions ultimately cause renal ischemia, the etiologies, presentation, treatment strategies, and ultimate prognoses of occlusion of the renal artery and vein are quite different. We review the current literature with an emphasis on the optimal evaluation and treatment of patients with renal artery infarction and RVT.

RENAL ARTERY EMBOLISM AND INFARCTION

Renal artery thrombosis was first described by Von Recklinghausen in 1861 *(1)*. The first successful revascularization was performed by Rohl in 1971 *(2)*. With the advent of diagnostic modalities such as spiral computed tomography (CT) and magnetic resonance imaging, as well as the development of thrombolytics and percutaneous methods of embolectomy, the clinical approach to this condition has changed significantly over the past 30 yr. Although prospective studies are lacking because of the relative rarity of this condition, an accumulation of retrospective data on treatment and outcomes exists and can provide some guidance toward optimal therapy.

Renal artery occlusion has many etiologies, some of which are listed in Table 1. In general, these can be divided into spontaneous, traumatic, and iatrogenic causes, which present differently and have varying approaches to management. We therefore discuss each of these categories of renal infarction separately.

From: *Urological Emergencies: A Practical Guide*
Edited by: H. Wessells and J. W. McAninch © Humana Press Inc., Totowa, NJ

Table 1
Etiologies of Renal Infarction

Spontaneous renal infarction
    Cardiovascular
        Atrial fibrillation
        Ischemic heart disease
        Mitral stenosis
        Endocarditis
        Atherosclerosis
        Hypertension
    Autoimmune
        Polyarteritis nodosa
        Systemic lupus erythematosis
        Fibromuscular dysplasia
        Behcet's disease
        Henoch-Schonlein purpura
    Other
        Drug abuse
        Hypercoagulable states
        Malignancy (e.g., bronchial cancer)
        Chagas disease
        Polycythemia vera
Acquired renal infarction
    Trauma
        Blunt injury
        Penetrating injury
    Surgical procedures
        Renal transplantation
        Cardiac valve repair
        Endovascular stenting
        Angiography
        Interventional polymers

Spontaneous Renal Infarction

In a review, Domanovits et al. identified cardiovascular disease as the most common predisposing condition leading to spontaneous renal infarction *(3)*. They found that 65% of affected patients had a history of atrial fibrillation, 53% had hypertension, and 41% had evidence of ischemic heart disease. Other medical conditions that increase the risk of spontaneous renal artery embolism and infarction include hypercoagulable states, renal artery aneurysm, and inflammatory disorders, such as polyarteritis and fibromuscular dysplasia. Interventional radiological procedures, such as endovascular stenting, have also led to renal embolic events. In a review of complications related to renal artery stenting for renal artery stenosis, Ivanovic et al. found that 2.6% of patients undergoing these procedures suffered from renal artery thrombosis in the postoperative period *(4)*.

INCIDENCE AND PRESENTATION

The true incidence of spontaneous renal infarction is unknown. Autopsy studies have found an incidence of 1.4% *(5)*, with most of these cases not identified antemortem. This is thought to be because an acute renal artery embolic event can be asymptomatic or may mimic many other medical conditions. Common presenting symptoms in patients with renal artery thrombosis include abdominal or back pain, costovertebral angle tenderness, and hypertension. The most common symptom is flank pain, found in 65 to 77% of cases *(3,6)*. These symptoms may masquerade as renal colic, pyelonephritis, cholelithiasis, lower back disease, and myocardial infarction, and often an embolic event to the kidney is not suspected.

Laboratory investigation plays a limited role in the diagnosis of renal infarction. Microscopic hematuria has been reported in 60 to 80% of cases and pyuria less frequently. Leukocytosis has been reported in 71% of identifiable cases *(6)*. Most patients at presentation have or will develop an elevated serum lactate dehydrogenase as renal tissue becomes nonviable. Other laboratory parameters that have been reported to be abnormal in renal infarction include aspartase aminotransferase, alkaline phosphatase, C-reactive protein, and fibrinogen.

DIAGNOSIS

Renal artery occlusion should be suspected when a patient with a history of increased risk for thromboembolism presents with the aforementioned signs and symptoms. Diagnostic confirmation can be achieved using arteriography, intravenous pyelography, nuclear medicine scanning, or ultrasound, but the most commonly utilized mode of reliable, rapid identification of arterial occlusion has been CT *(6)*. Typical radiological findings include a filling defect in the renal artery and lack of enhancement of the affected kidney. In some cases, an abrupt cutoff of an enhancing renal artery may be seen in the presence of normal renal contour and a central renal hematoma *(7)*. Spontaneous renal emboli appear to involve the left kidney more frequently, which is thought to be because of the more acute angle of the left renal artery off the aorta.

TREATMENT

Intervention in renal infarction has consisted of both nonsurgical and surgical options. Outcome studies in the literature have been limited to case reports and retrospective reviews, and controversy still exists regarding the optimal choice and timing of treatment. Typically, medical management has been elected in spontaneous, unilateral cases of thrombosis, whereas surgical or percutaneous interventions have been described in cases of a solitary kidney, bilateral involvement, and situations of failed medical therapy.

Nonoperative management for spontaneous renal infarction includes anticoagulation and fibrinolytics. Therapy can be given systemically or locally with selective catheterization. Typical local thrombolytic therapy involves continuous infusion of an agent such as streptokinase, urokinase, or tissue plasminogen activator over a period of 4 to 24 h into the affected artery *(8,9)*. Although restoration of blood flow to the affected kidney is achieved in many instances, return of renal function is often not seen with long-term follow-up *(10)*.

Surgical repair in cases of renal infarction with a normal contralateral kidney remains controversial. Those supporting immediate surgical correction via open thromboembolectomy or bypass grafting argue that renal salvageability cannot accurately be assessed, and thus all efforts should be made for immediate restoration of blood supply *(11)*. Surgical techniques that have been described include thrombectomy with end-to-end reanastamosis, autotransplantation, or aortorenal saphenous vein bypass graft, among others. Some investigators have suggested that attempt at surgical revascularization should be made if the presumed warm ischemia time is less than 5 h.

Spirnak et al. reviewed reports of 35 patients who had undergone attempted revascularization for unilateral renal artery thrombosis and a normal contralateral kidney. They found that true success, defined as arterial patency, normal renal function, and no hypertension at long-term follow-up, occurred in only 2 patients, and both had undergone surgery within 4 h of the occlusive episode *(10)*. Successful revascularizations may be achieved following longer periods of ischemia in patients with spontaneous renal artery embolism and no associated injuries.

In cases of bilateral renal artery occlusion or renal infarction in a solitary kidney, attempt at surgical or thrombolytic revascularization is indicated regardless of ischemia time. With success defined as renal function able to sustain life without dialysis, Lohse et al. reported that successful surgical revascularizations were performed in 4 of 10 patients with bilateral renal artery thromboses *(12)*. Similarly, there have been reports of restoration of renal function in bilateral renal artery thrombosis using thrombolytic therapy *(8,9)*.

Because many patients with renal artery embolus present late or have a delay in diagnosis, the issue of whether to attempt revascularization several days or weeks following the initial episode is raised. It is generally accepted that, under physiological temperatures, a kidney becomes nonviable following 60–90 min of total circulatory arrest *(13)*. Both animal studies and human retrospective reviews, however, have shown persistent renal function in longer intervals of occlusion. This variability is thought to be because of the frequent presence of collateral circulation. Indeed, distal renal artery reconstitution or the presence of collateral circulation via the suprarenal, inferior phrenic, lumbar, genital, and ureteric arteries can provide for continued but suboptimal renal perfusion following an embolic event. Most reports of successful delayed repair have acknowledged the presence of collateral circulation *(14)*.

Percutaneous thromboembolectomy has emerged as a viable option for renal artery thrombosis. Successful rheolytic aspiration via hydrodynamic catheterization has been described for renal artery and other visceral emboli *(15,16)*. This and other minimally invasive, mechanical techniques hold promise and may replace surgical embolectomy in select patients.

Acquired Renal Artery Infarction

Renal Infarction in the Setting of Trauma

Renal infarction secondary to trauma can result from either penetrating or blunt injury. Although the mechanism of injury is clear for penetrating wounds, the etiology of renal occlusion in blunt trauma is not completely understood. Most investigators believe that rapid deceleration leads to stretching and subsequent disruption of the intimal layer of the renal artery, with resultant thrombosis. This thought is supported by findings that the left kidney, which is less supported by surrounding organs and thus more susceptible to stretch injury and intimal tearing, is more frequently involved than the right *(17)*. Others suggest that direct trauma to the artery accounts for the thrombotic event.

There are several considerations to be made specific to cases of renal infarction caused by trauma. First, there is the emergent need to exclude a main renal artery laceration and other intraabdominal injuries that may indicate immediate exploratory laparotomy. Thus, in a patient stable to undergo imaging, spiral CT is preferred over possibly more time-consuming studies such as arteriography. If an occlusion is discovered, the decision for immediate vs delayed operative intervention may be obviated by a concomitant intraabdominal injury for which the general surgeons will explore the patient.

When exploring trauma patients with suspected renal vascular injuries, early vascular control is imperative. McAninch and Carroll found that early vascular control during explorations for renal trauma reduced nephrectomy rates from 56 to 18% *(18)*. Specific techniques that may be required for renal arterial injuries include direct repair or resection with end-to-end anastomosis or bypass grafting using vein or synthetic material *(19)*.

Renal Infarction Caused by Surgical Procedures

Renal transplantation and other procedures involving vascular anastomoses predispose patients to the risk of renal artery occlusion. In a review of complications of more than 1200 renal transplants, Osman et al. found that 0.4% of transplants are complicated by arterial thrombosis, and that ischemia and complications of treatment can lead to transplant loss *(20)*.

The diagnosis of vascular occlusion can be challenging. Late renal artery stenosis presents with worsening hypertension and decreased renal function. Early arterial occlusion typically presents with acute oliguria, with Doppler ultrasound images suggestive of poor perfusion. In this setting, the differential diagnosis includes acute rejection, acute tubular necrosis, cyclosporine toxicity, and RVT *(21)*. Diagnosis is confirmed with arteriography, and interventional techniques can be employed acutely.

Renal artery complications after transplant can also be managed with open revision. Takahashi et al. recently reviewed the diagnosis and management of renal allograft perfusion failure caused by dissection *(22)*. The authors believe interventional techniques such as stenting are superior to open revision because of decreased treatment-related complications and less chance for graft loss.

RENAL VEIN THROMBOSIS

RVT predominantly affects two subpopulations: neonates with risk factors for clotting abnormalities and adults with nephrotic syndrome. We consider the diagnosis and treatment options of these two populations separately, discussing the disease process in adults first.

Etiology

The most common medical cause of RVT in adults is nephrotic syndrome. This association was identified as early as 1840, when Rayer described thrombosis of the renal veins and inferior vena cava in a patient with proteinuria *(23)*. In nephrotic patients, the combination of low serum albumin, high fibrinogen levels, low antithrombin III levels, and hypovolemia predispose for the development of thrombotic disease *(24)*. Other hematological abnormalities that have been inconsistently described include platelet hyperaggregability, thrombocytosis, and elevations of proteins C and S. Membranous glomerulonephritis has been identified as the most common nephrotic state resulting in RVT, accounting for nearly 70% of cases *(25)*.

Presentation

Like renal artery occlusion, the diagnosis of RVT is commonly missed, especially in the presence of a normally functioning contralateral kidney. The finding is usually made

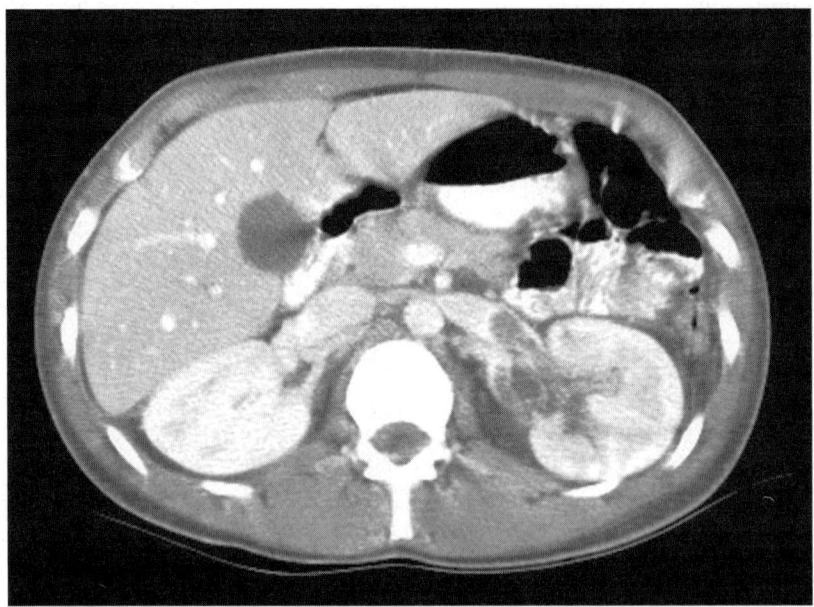

Fig. 1. Left main renal vein thrombus in a 27-yr-old woman with the nephrotic syndrome.

when a patient with clotting abnormalities presents with worsening renal function, flank pain, or peripheral edema. In some occasions, patients are not identified until they present with complications of the renal thrombus and hypercoagulable state, such as pulmonary embolism.

It should be noted that symptoms of flank pain, costovertebral angle tenderness, and hematuria may be absent in the majority of cases. McCarthy et al. found that local symptoms were present in only 34% of patients with RVT *(26)*. More commonly, the presentation is related to the nephrotic syndrome, with progressive ankle swelling and mild-to-moderate deterioration in renal function. In a prospective screening evaluation of 151 nephrotic patients, 33 had RVTs, and 29 of these patients had peripheral edema only, suggesting that the majority of cases go undiagnosed or are diagnosed at a later time *(27)*.

Diagnosis

In adults, intravenous pyelogram has been used in the past to identify abnormalities in renal size and calyceal appearance. However, Llach et al. found that intravenous pyelogram is commonly nondiagnostic in cases of more chronic thrombosis *(27)*. Venous thrombus can be more readily identified via CT, magnetic resonance imaging, ultrasound, or venography. Thrombus location and size can be estimated accurately on contrast CT imaging (Fig. 1). If an interventional radiological procedure is elected, renal venography remains the gold standard for optimal visualization of the thrombus.

Therapy

The rationale for immediate intervention in RVT in adults is to prevent further thromboembolic events and to maintain renal function. Anticoagulation with systemic

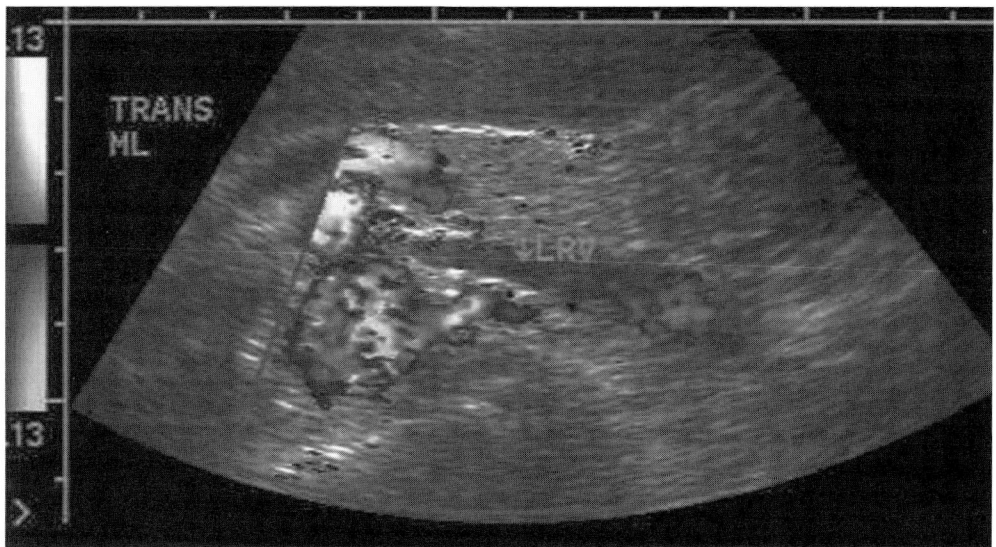

Fig. 2. Doppler ultrasound image of an infant with left renal vein thrombosis.

unfractionated heparin followed by outpatient management with warfarin has been the standard treatment to prevent propagation of the thrombus *(28)*. The use of low-molecular-weight heparins also has been described, with the advantage of increased bioavailability, longer half-life, and potentially fewer drug interactions compared to warfarin *(29)*. A disadvantage of low-molecular-weight heparin is the difficulty in reversing anticoagulation should complications caused by therapy arise.

Thrombolytic therapy has been reported, but is controversial, with several deaths resulting from bleeding complications. Surgical thrombectomy is rarely indicated because, in most cases, intrarenal thrombosis has already occurred by the time of diagnosis. Operative intervention should only be considered in cases refractory to medical intervention, with bilateral renal vein involvement, or in the case of a solitary kidney.

A relatively new, less-invasive mode of therapy for acute RVT is percutaneous mechanical thrombectomy. Via sheath access of the femoral vein, a thrombectomy device is passed multiple times through the thrombus under fluoroscopic guidance. In isolated cases, visual evidence of antegrade venous flow and return of normal renal function with this technique have been reported *(30)*.

Prognosis

The prognosis of RVT in adults has been dependent on several factors, including the presence of preexisting renal insufficiency and type of nephropathy. In a review of 27 nephrotic patients with RVT, Laville et al. found that patients with normal renal function at presentation had a significantly lower mortality rate (1/12) than those with renal impairment (10/15) during the first 6 mo *(25)*. Mortality in patients with RVT was most commonly caused by pulmonary embolism, hemorrhagic complications, or the patient's underlying disease process. This study also confirmed increased survival in patients with membranous glomerulonephritis compared to those with other forms of the nephrotic syndrome, such as minimal change disease and focal segmental glomerulosclerosis.

Renal Vein Thrombosis in Children

ETIOLOGY

In the pediatric population, RVT is primarily a disease of infancy. A review found that 83% of cases in children occur within the first month of life *(31)*. The pathophysiology is assumed to be decreased renal blood flow in a child with preexisting risk factors for thrombus formation. These include severe dehydration, hypotension, cardiac disease, polycythemia, protein C deficiency, and factor V Leiden heterozygosity. Additional prenatal and perinatal risk factors include preeclampsia, maternal diabetes, traumatic birth, and fetal distress.

PRESENTATION

In infants, RVT has been described to present with the "diagnostic triad" of palpable abdominal mass, gross hematuria, and thrombocytopenia. In a review of 23 cases over a 10-yr period, however, Zigman et al. found this to be true in only 13% cases *(31)*. Considered separately, palpable mass (39%) was found with similar frequency as gross hematuria and thrombocytopenia (35% each). Clinical suspicion should thus also include maternal and infant risk factors, and the presence of a combination of these should warrant an investigation for RVT.

DIAGNOSIS

Once clinical suspicion is established, the diagnosis of RVT in children is best achieved using Doppler ultrasound (Fig. 2). This modality is highly sensitive in infants, detecting 22 out of 23 cases in a modern study *(31)*. If nondiagnostic, a CT scan may be utilized. The radiological appearance of neonatal RVT includes renal enlargement and ischemia and can be confused with other causes of renal enlargement such as Wilms' tumor, pyelonephritis, and renal abscess. Also, the radiological appearance depends on the acuity of the radiological study as neonatal RVT evolves in appearance. Early, the kidney swells and appears echogenic on ultrasound; later, the appearance becomes more heterogeneous, with a loss of corticomedullary differentiation *(32)*.

TREATMENT

Like adults, children with RVT have also been treated successfully with anticoagulation. The use of a thrombolytic agent such as recombinant tissue-type plasminogen activator has been reported in the literature *(33)*. It should be noted, however, that intraventricular hemorrhage is a significant risk in this population, especially in the case of premature infants, and deaths have been reported *(34)*.

With routine use of anticoagulation to treat RVT, outcomes in children have improved dramatically over the past 30 yr. A retrospective review found that, in a cohort of 23 children with a mean follow-up of 42 mo, all patients not treated with anticoagulation developed renal function impairment; reduced renal function was seen in only 33% of those who had received heparin *(31)*. Despite resolution of clot and maintenance of renal function, long-term hypertension is found in 17% of patients, affirming the need for close surveillance of children with RVT.

In summary, RVT should be suspected in neonates who have either maternal or fetal risk factors with associated abdominal mass, hematuria, or thrombocytopenia. It should also be considered in adults with nephrotic syndrome who present with symptoms of colic, especially in those with membranous nephropathy. Treatment centers on anticoagulation, with consideration of thrombolytics or percutaneous aspiration in select cases. With this regimen, mortality and morbidity of this condition can be minimized.

SUMMARY

Renal artery embolism or thrombosis should be considered in the differential diagnosis of a patient with acute flank pain; particularly patients with risk factors such as atrial fibrillation or autoimmune disorders. Clinical suspicion is the key to prompt diagnosis and appropriate therapy, usually with anticoagulation or directed thrombolysis.

Acquired renal artery infarction can occur from trauma or from surgical procedures such as renal transplant or vascular procedures. The specific treatment depends on the clinical situation and may be anticoagulation, endovascular procedures, or open declotting or revision.

Renal vein thrombosis occurs primarily in two populations: adults with nephrotic syndrome and infants with hypercoaguable conditions. Adults with nephrotic syndrome may present with flank pain or worsening renal function and edema. Diagnosis is usually by CT with or without contrast depending on renal function. Therapy is usually with systemic anticoagulation. The prognosis depends on a patient's renal function and whether other thrombotic complications can be avoided.

Pediatric renal vein thrombosis occurs most commonly in newborns of diabetic mothers or with risk factors for thrombosis such as dehydration, polycythemia or protein c deficiency. The presentation is clasically from hematuria, palpable abdominal mass, and thrombocytopenia. The diagnosis is usually established with renal Doppler ultrasound. Treatment is anticoagulation or directed thrombolysis although the risk of cerebral hemorrhage is present, particularly in premature infants.

Through clinical suspicion, appropriate diagnostic testing, and prompt therapy, the late sequela of renal vascular emergencies can be minimized.

REFERENCES

1. Von Recklinghausen F. Haemorrhagische niereninfarktr. Virchos Arch Pathol Anat Physiol 1861; 20: 205–207.
2. Rohl L. Vascular surgery in urology. Proc R Soc Med 1971; 64: 589–594.
3. Domanovits H, Paulis M, Nikfardtam M, et al. Acute renal infarction. Medicine 1999; 78: 386–394.
4. Ivanovic V, McKusick MA, Johnson CM 3rd, et al. Renal artery stent placement: complications at a single tertiary care center. J Vasc Interv Radiol 2003; 14(2): 217–225.
5. Hoxie H, Coggin C. Renal infarction. Arch Intern Med 1940; 65: 587–594.
6. Ouriel K, Andrus CH, Ricotta JJ, DeWeese JA, Green RM. Acute renal artery occlusion: when is revascularization justified? J Vasc Surg 1987; 5: 348–353.
7. Sclafani S, Goldstein A, Panetta T, et al. CT diagnosis of renal pedicle injury. Urol Radiol 1985; 7: 63.
8. Pilmore HL, Walker RJ, Solomon C, Packer S, Wood D. Acute bilateral renal artery occlusion: successful revascularization with streptokinase. Am J Nephrol 1995; 15: 90–91.
9. Takeda M, Katayama Y, Takahashi H, et al. Transarterial fibrinolysis using tissue plasminogen activator in a patient with acute renal failure due to acute thrombosis of bilateral renal arteries. Nephron 1994; 66: 240–241.
10. Spirnak JP, Resnick MI. Revascularization of traumatic thrombosis of the renal artery. Gynecol Obstet 1987; 164: 22–26.
11. Lacombe M. Acute non-traumatic obstructions of the renal artery. J Cardiovasc Surg 1992; 33: 163–168.
12. Lohse JR, Botham RJ, Waters RF. Traumatic bilateral renal artery thrombosis: case report and review of the literature. J Urol 1982; 127: 522–525.

13. Leary FJ, Utz DC, Wakim KG. Effects of continuous and intermittent renal ischemia on renal function. Surg Gynecol Obstet 1963; 116: 311–317.
14. Pontremoli R, Rampoldi V, Morbidelli A, Fiorini F, Ranise A, Garibotto G. Acute renal failure due to acute bilateral renal artery thrombosis: successful surgical revascularization after prolonged anuria. Nephron 1990; 56: 322–324.
15. Wagner HJ, Meuller-Hulsbeck S, Pitton MB, Weiss W, Wess M. Rapid thrombectomy with a hydrodynamic catheter: results from a prospective, multicenter trial. Radiology 1997; 205: 675–681.
16. Sternbergh WC, Ramee SR, DeVun DA, Money SR. Endovascular treatment of multiple visceral artery paradoxical emboli with mechanical and pharmacological thrombolysis. J Endovasc Ther 2000; 7: 155–160.
17. Carroll PR, McAninch JW. Renovascular trauma: risk assessment, surgical management, and outcome. J Trauma 1990; 30: 547–554.
18. McAninch JW, Carroll PR. Renal trauma: kidney preservation through improved vascular control—a refined approach. J Trauma 1982; 22: 285–290.
19. Haas CA, Spirnak JP. Traumatic renal artery occlusion: a review of the literature. Tech Urol 1998; 4(1): 1–11.
20. Osman Y, Shokeir A, Ali-el-Dein B, et al. Vascular complications after live donor renal transplantation: study of risk factors and effects on graft and patient survival. J Urol 2003; 169: 859–862.
21. Rerolle JP, Antoine C, Raynaud A, et al. Successful endoluminal thrombo-aspiration of renal graft venous thrombosis. Transpl Int 2000; 13: 82–86.
22. Takahashi M, Humke U, Girnat M, Kramann B, Uder M. Early posttransplantation renal allograft perfusion failure due to dissection: diagnosis and interventional treatment. Am J Roentgenol 2003; 180: 759–763.
23. Rayer P. Traite des maladies des reins et des alterations de la secretion urinaire. JB Baillere 1840; 2: 590–599.
24. Jackson CA, Greaves M, Patterson AD, Brown CB, Preston FE. Relationship between platelet aggregation, thromboxane synthesis and albumin concentration in the nephrotic syndrome. Br J Haematol 1982; 52: 69–77.
25. Laville M, Aguilera P, Maillet PJ, Labeeuw M, Madonna O, Zech P. The prognosis of renal vein thrombosis: a re-evaluation of 27 cases. Nephrol Dial Transplant 1988; 3: 247–256.
26. McCarthy LJ, Titus JL, Daugherty GW. Bilateral renal vein thrombosis and the nephrotic syndrome in adults. Ann Intern Med 1963; 58: 837.
27. Llach F, Papper S, Massry SG. The clinical spectrum of renal vein thrombosis: acute and chronic. Am J Med 1980; 69: 819–827.
28. Llach F, Nikakhtar B. Renal thromboembolism, atheroembolism, and renal vein thrombosis. In: Diseases of the Kidney, 6th ed. (Schrier RW, Gottschalk CW, eds.), Little, Brown, and Company, Boston, MA, 1997, Vol. 2, pp. 1893–1918.
29. Yang SH, Lee CH, Ko SF, Chen JB, Chung FR, HSU KT. The successful treatment of renal-vein thrombosis by low-molecular-weight heparin in a steroid-sensitive nephrotic patient. Nephrol Dial Transplant 2002; 17: 2017–2019.
30. Jaar BG, Kim HS, Samaniego MD, Lund GB, Atta MG. Percutaneous mechanical thrombectomy: a new approach in the treatment of acute renal vein thrombosis. Nephrol Dial Transplant 2002; 17: 1122–1125.
31. Zigman A, Yazbeck S, Emil S, Nguyen L. Renal vein thrombosis: a 10-year review. J Pediatr Surg 2000; 35: 1540–1542.
32. Hibbert J, Howlett DC, Greenwood KL, MacDonald LM, Saunders AJ. The ultrasound appearance of neonatal renal vein thrombosis. Br J Radiol 1997; 70: 1191–1194.
33. Chalmers EA, Gibson BES. Thrombolytic therapy in the management of pediatric thromboembolic disease. Br J Haematol 1999; 104: 14–21.
34. Weinschenk N, Pelidis M, Fiascone J. Combination thrombolytic and anticoagulant therapy for bilateral renal vein thrombosis in a premature infant. Am J Perinatol 2001; 18: 293–297.

12 Retroperitoneal and Upper Tract Hemorrhage

Atul D. Rajpurkar, MD
and Richard A. Santucci, MD

CONTENTS

> INTRODUCTION
> ETIOLOGY
> CLINICAL PRESENTATION
> DIAGNOSTIC INVESTIGATIONS
> MANAGEMENT
> SUMMARY
> REFERENCES

INTRODUCTION

Massive bleeding from the upper urinary tract (kidney and ureter) can present as either retroperitoneal hematoma or brisk hematuria. Retroperitoneal hemorrhage (RPH) secondary to a urological condition is an uncommon entity that can result from a variety of causes. It may result from local pathology involving either the kidney or adrenal or may be secondary to a bleeding disorder or systemic illness. RPH can present acutely or may have an insidious course. Because of its varying presentation and etiology, RPH represents a diagnostic challenge and may be associated with significant morbidity and mortality. Therefore, it is essential for the urologist to be aware of the common etiologies and diagnoses and treat them promptly to ensure a successful outcome.

Brisk hematuria from an upper tract source can also be diagnostically challenging because successful treatment will rely on accurate determination of the cause of bleeding. Most of the renal lesions that present with RPH can also present with hematuria if the lesion ruptures into the renal calyces. The resulting hematuria is rarely life threatening in the acute situation. Brisk hematuria can also result from a fistulous connection between the ureter and iliac artery or aorta, which is uncommon, but potentially fatal.

From: *Urological Emergencies: A Practical Guide*
Edited by: H. Wessells and J. W. McAninch © Humana Press Inc., Totowa, NJ

ETIOLOGY

Retroperitoneal Hemorrhage

RPH can arise from either the kidney or the adrenal gland, although ruptured abdominal aortic aneurysm is the most common cause of retroperitoneal hematoma and should be ruled out (Fig. 1). It may occur because of specific renal disorders such as tumors and cysts or systemic causes such as bleeding disorders, anticoagulant therapy, and polyarteritis nodosa.

RENAL CAUSES OF RPH

Neoplastic

Malignant. Tumors of the kidney are the most common cause for spontaneous retroperitoneal bleeding, accounting for 57 to 63% of all renal bleeds *(1–3)*. Of these, malignant lesions account for 30 to 34% and benign for 24 to 33% of cases. Although cancer of the kidney rarely ruptures spontaneously, it is the most common tumor to present with RPH because of its relatively common occurrence. Of note, data seem to suggest that the risk of spontaneous renal bleed is independent of the size of the tumor *(3)*. Other malignant lesions, such as transitional cell carcinoma *(4)*, Wilms' tumor *(5)*, sarcoma *(6)*, and metastatic lesions *(7)*, have also been reported to present with retroperitoneal bleed.

Benign. Of the benign tumors, almost all cases of retroperitoneal bleed are caused by angiomyolipomas (AMLs) (Fig. 2A,B) *(1–3)*. These benign tumors consist of smooth muscle, blood vessels, and fatty tissue in varying proportions and can occur either sporadically (80%) or as a part of tuberous sclerosis (TS) complex (20%). TS complex is an autosomal dominant disorder with incomplete penetrance, characterized by mental retardation, epilepsy, and adenoma sebaceum *(8,9)*. When AMLs are associated with TS, they commonly present earlier (mean age 30 yr), occur with less predilection for the female gender (only twice as common in females compared to males), and are multicentric, larger, more likely to grow, and more prone to rupture (10% of cases) *(9)*.

The rate of reported bleeding with AML ranges widely. Mouded et al. described a 15% incidence of rupture in 97 patients with AMLs *(10)*. However, Oesterling and others have shown that 82% of AMLs larger than 4 cm on computed tomography (CT) are symptomatic and present with RPH in 51% of cases *(11)*. Rarely, these tumors have been reported to undergo malignant transformation *(12,13)*. Other benign lesions such as adenomas and oncocytomas have also been described to present with retroperitoneal bleed in rare case reports.

Vascular. Vascular causes account for 17 to 26% of renal causes of RPH *(1–3)*. Of these, rupture of renal artery aneurysm is the most serious and can occur at any age, with the preponderance in the fifth to seventh decades of life *(14)*. Although angiographic studies suggested a 0.3 to 1% incidence of renal artery aneurysm *(15)*, spontaneous rupture is uncommon. However, noncalcified saccular aneurysms *(16)* and the presence of pregnancy and hypertension *(17–19)* are believed to increase the risk of spontaneous rupture. When rupture is associated with pregnancy, a mortality rate of 80% has been reported *(14)*.

Polyarteritis nodosa is a systemic condition characterized by deposition of immune complexes within the media of small- and medium-size arteries that leads to progressive weakness of the arterial wall and resultant aneurysm formation. Rupture of these aneurysms is responsible for approx 12% of RPHs in some series *(1–3)*.

I. RENAL CAUSES:
A. Systemic:
1. Use of anticoagulants
2. Bleeding disorders such as leukemias, hemophilias etc
3. Polyarteritis nodosa

B. Local:
1. Neoplastic
   - Benign: such as angiomyolipoma, adenoma
   - Malignant
     - Primary
       - renal cell Ca
       - Wiln's tumor
       - Transitional cell Ca
       - Sarcoma
     - Metastatic
2. Vascular
   - renal artery aneurysm
   - renal vein thrombosis
   - arteriovenous malformation and fistula
     - Spontaneous
     - Acquired
   - polyarteritis nodosa
3. Inflammatory
   - Cortical abscess
   - Nephritis
4. Cysts
   - Adult polycystic
   - Other cystic lesions

C. Idiopathic

II. ADRENAL CAUSES:
A. Local:
1. Neoplastic:
   - Pheochromocytoma
   - Adenoma
   - Neuroblastoma
   - Metastases
2. Cystic lesions

B. Systemic:
1. Medical causes:
   - Severe sepsis
   - Acute myocardial infarction
2. Surgical causes:
   - Burns
   - Surgery ex. major abdominal or CABG
3. Obstetric etiology: Pre-eclampsia
4. Drug-induced:
   - ACTH therapy for^flammatoryJBowel
   - Anticoagulation
5. Coagulopathy:
   - Thrombocytopenia
   - Post-surgery
6. Thrombo-embolic diathesis: Antiphospholipid antibody syndrome

Fig. 1. Common causes of retroperitoneal hemorrhage arising from the kidney or adrenal gland. ACTH, adrenocorticotropic hormone; Ca, cancer; CABG, coronary artery bypass grafting.

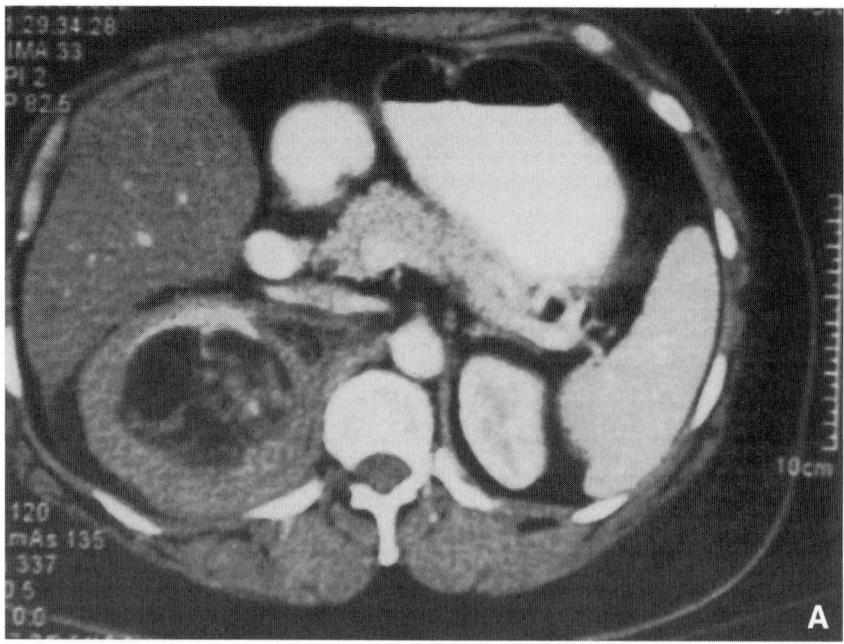

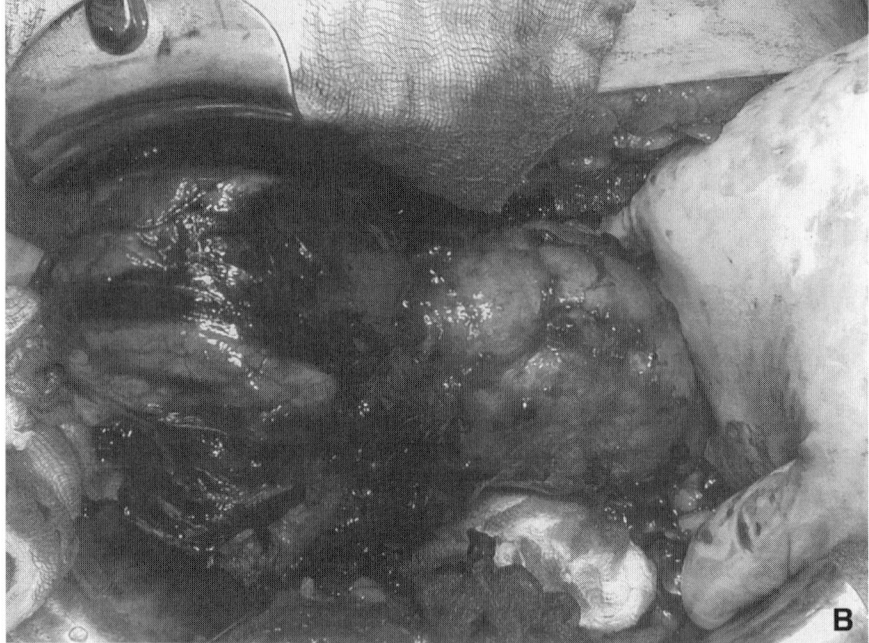

Fig. 2. (A) CT scan shows large angiomyolipoma of the right kidney with associated perirenal hematoma. **(B)** Intraoperative appearance of same angiomyolipoma showing upper pole lesion with hemorrhage.

Other vascular causes such as renal infarction, renal vein thrombosis, and congenital arteriovenous malformations (AVMs) have also been described to present with RPH *(20)*.

Inflammatory/Infectious. Inflammatory lesions such as severe pyelonephritis, cortical abscesses, and xanthogranulomatous pyelonephritis can also present with RPH and account for 2.4 to 10% of cases *(3,21)*.

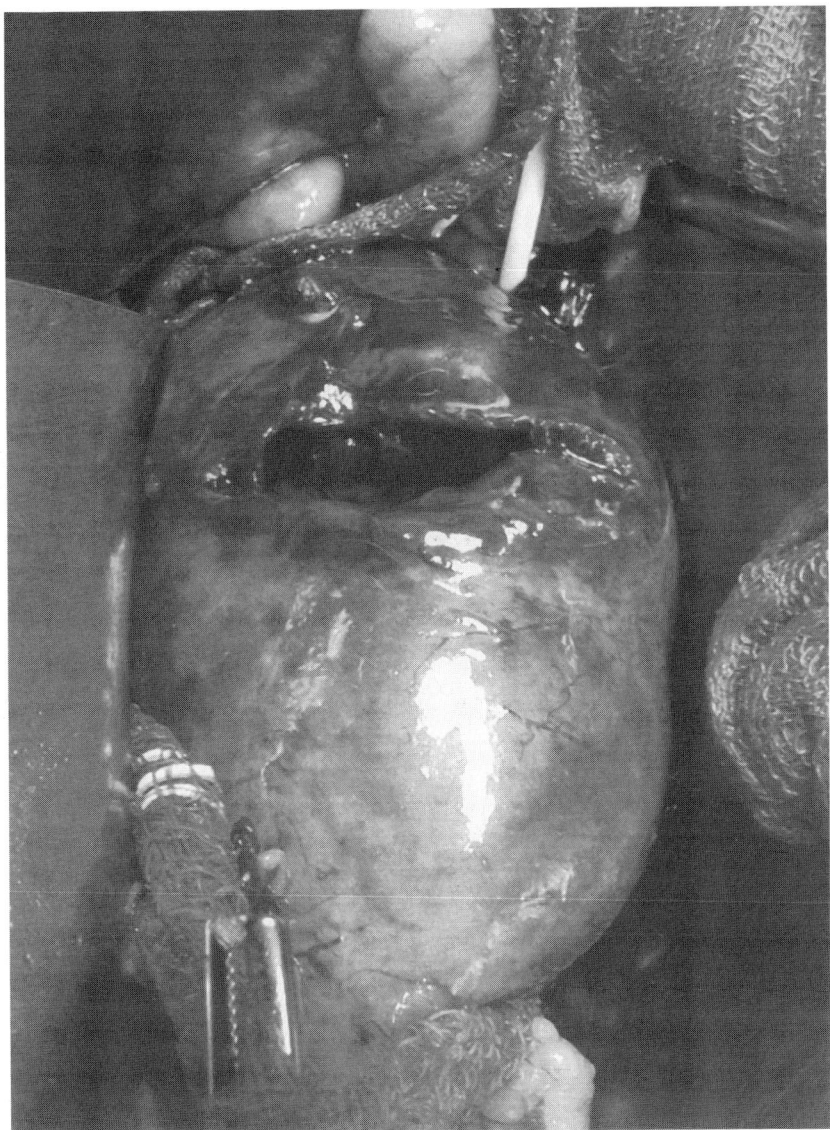

Fig. 3. Intraoperative appearance of a ruptured renal cyst.

Cystic. Hemorrhagic rupture of cysts has been reported in autosomal dominant polycystic kidney disease as well as the acquired cysts of end-stage renal disease (2–3% of reported cysts) (22,23). Hypertension, bleeding tendency of uremia, and use of anticoagulants during hemodialysis predispose to the development of RPH in these cases (23–25). Bleeding into a simple renal cyst with rupture has also been described and is commonly secondary to a coagulation defect, a ruptured cyst wall (26), or trauma (Fig. 3).

Bleeding Disorders. Bleeding disorders such as hemophilia and leukemias can also present with bleeding into the retroperitoneal space, and it is essential to rule out these conditions in any case of RPH. Although the history of hemophilia is usually known by the patient, diligence in diagnosing other causes of bleeding diathesis may be required. Systemic sequelae of generalized bleeding and history of petechiae, easy bruisability, hemarthrosis, or other signs of inappropriate bleeding may be elucidated in these patients.

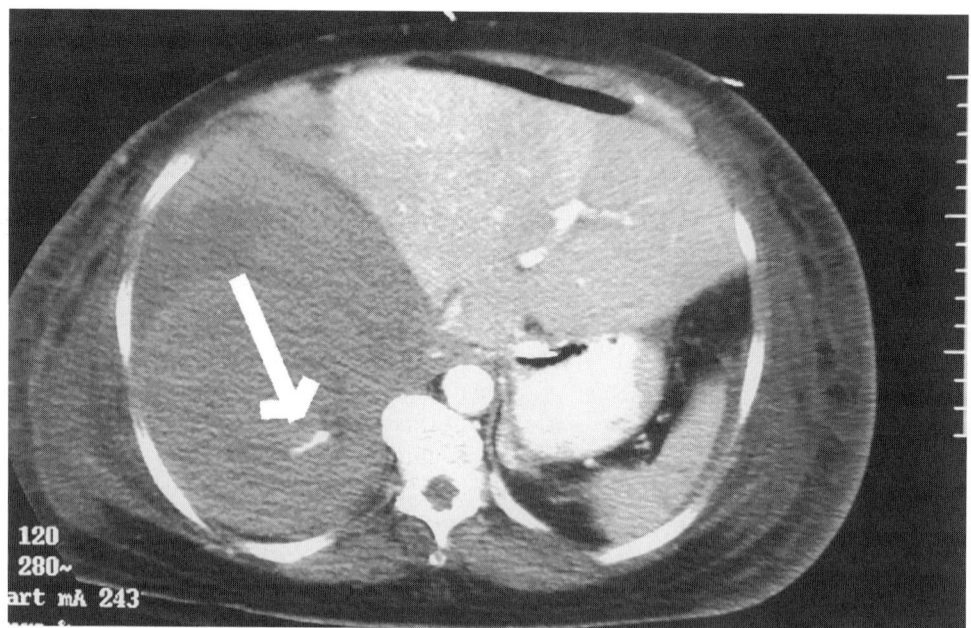

Fig. 4. Computed tomography scan appearance of retroperitoneal hemorrhage following biopsy of the kidney. Note acute extravasation of the contrast, which denotes brisk bleeding.

In addition, patients on anticoagulants or acquired bleeding diathesis may also present with RPH, with an incidence of 4.3 to 6.6% for heparin and 0.1 to 0.6% for warfarin (27–30).

Other. Perirenal hematomas have also been described following renal biopsies (Fig. 4) (60–85% incidence demonstrated in follow-up CT scan) (31,32) and occur independent of presence of coagulopathy, clinical signs of bleeding, fall in hemoglobin levels, or performance of the procedure by an experienced person (31). Follow-up CT scans in these patients, however, have shown a spontaneous resolution in the hematomas in the majority of instances.

Idiopathic. Uncommonly, in 6.7% of cases, no cause for RPH is identifiable in the kidney (3).

ADRENAL CAUSES OF RPH

Adrenal hemorrhage is a heterogeneous entity that occurs in a wide variety of clinical conditions and is infrequently diagnosed when the patient is alive. It has been reported in 0.14 to 1.8% of autopsy studies, although the incidence is higher in critically sick patients (33). The exact mechanism of adrenal hemorrhage in a stressed adrenal is not known, but interplay of various factors may be responsible. Of these, increased adrenocorticotropic hormone secretion with an increase in adrenal vascularity and adrenal cortical necrosis, adrenal venoconstriction with resultant stasis and possible adrenal venous thrombosis, and associated coagulopathy may play a role in its development. The common causes for hemorrhage in a stressed adrenal are listed in Fig. 1.

Systemic Causes

These conditions commonly lead to bilateral massive adrenal hemorrhage caused by an overworked stressed adrenal. As shown in Fig. 1, they can result from a variety of causes, ranging from severe sepsis and acute myocardial infarction to burns, trauma, and obstetric causes.

Neoplastic

Neoplasm of the adrenal gland is the most common cause of unilateral adrenal hemorrhage. Pheochromocytoma is the most common adrenal tumor to present with RPH. Other causes, such as adrenal adenoma (20), adrenal cyst (34), adrenal myelolipoma (35–37), adrenocortical adenoma (37,38), and adrenal gland metastases (39), have also been described in the literature.

Pheochromocytomas are catecholamine-producing tumors of neuroectodermal origin that are extraadrenal in 10%, are malignant in 10%, occur in children in 10%, and are inherited as autosomal dominant in 10% of cases. They may be either familial or sporadic. The familial group may be a part of multiple endocrine neoplasia type 2 or 3 (40–42), or neuroectodermal dysplasias (consisting of von Hippel-Lindau disease, TS, Sturge-Weber syndrome, and von Recklinghausen's syndrome). Pheochromocytomas rarely present with retroperitoneal rupture and have a high mortality if the condition is not diagnosed preoperatively because of the development of either precipitous hypertension from the release of catecholamines or severe hypotension from blood loss and contracted blood volume secondary to chronically elevated catecholamines. The hemorrhage may be precipitated by indiscriminate use of α-blockers, which can cause vasoconstriction with resultant necrosis of the gland and hemorrhage.

Adrenal myelolipoma is a benign tumor that consists of a mixture of fatty tissue, myeloid elements, and lymphocytes and has a strong association with hypertension, obesity, and chronic disease. Rupture is rare and is described only in case reports (35–37).

Brisk Hematuria

Brisk hematuria can result from rapid and extensive blood loss into the upper urinary tract. All the lesions described in the preceding sections can lead to hematuria if the lesion communicates with the renal calyces, although this is generally uncommon. Here, we describe two rare but clinically important causes of brisk hematuria.

URETEROARTERIAL FISTULA

Ureteroarterial fistulas are an uncommon, but potentially lethal, cause of brisk hematuria, with a reported mortality of approx 34 to 40% (43–46). Often, the diagnosis is made at postmortem examination. Fistulous communication commonly occurs in the region where the ureter crosses the iliac artery at the pelvic brim (47). The kidney and ureter proximal to the fistula are commonly obstructed (with resultant hydroureter and hydronephrosis) because of fibrosis of the ureter in the region of the fistula.

Predisposing factors are many. Among them, prior, long-standing ureteral stents account for 65% of cases. The advent of softer stents has led to a decrease in stent erosion, although coincident factors such as prior surgery, irradiation, or arterial pathology such as mycotic aneurysm may still lead to pressure necrosis of the ureter from chronic indwelling stents. Another cause of ureteroarterial fistula is presence of vascular disease or vascular graft surgery (38% of cases). Spontaneous rupture of iliac artery aneurysms into the ureter has been reported, probably secondary to pressure necrosis of the adherent, fixed ureter (to the aneurysm) from the chronic pulsations of the aneurysm (48–50). Similarly, the combination of a vascularly compromised ureteric wall (resulting from dissection during arterial graft surgery) and fixation of the ureter to the site of the arterial graft can predispose to pressure necrosis of the ureter and subsequent fistula formation (51). Finally, prior genitourinary/pelvic surgery and radiation account for 68 to 46% of cases of ureteroarterial fistulas reported in the literature.

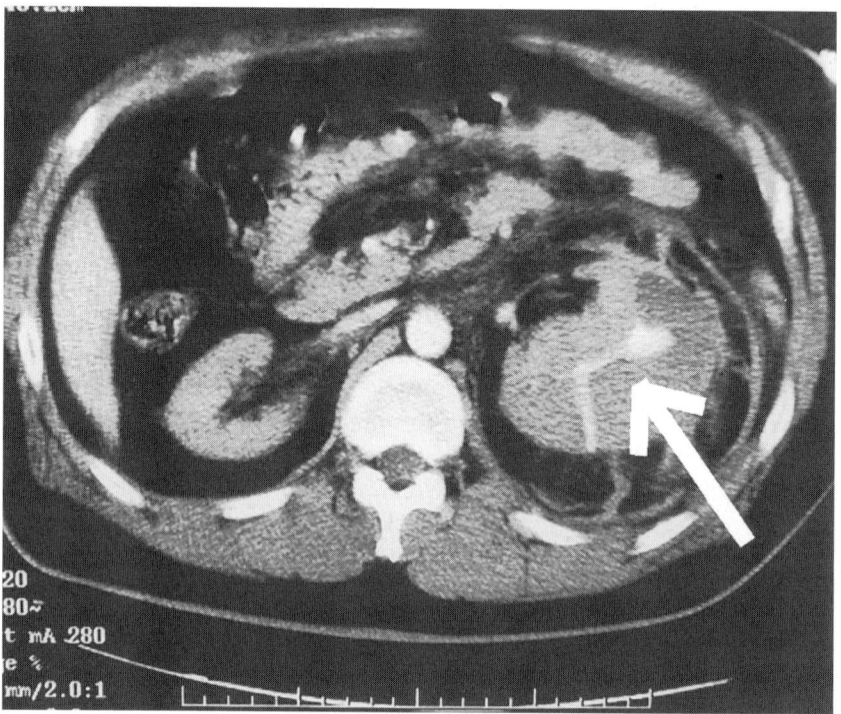

Fig. 5. Computed tomography scan showing renal arteriovenous malformation (AVM) secondary to renal biopsy.

ARTERIOVENOUS MALFORMATION AND FISTULA

Rarely, AVMs of the kidney may present with massive hematuria. Etiologically, these lesions are of two types: spontaneous or acquired. Acquired arteriovenous fistulas (AVFs) are more common, may be secondary to surgery (partial or total nephrectomy, percutaneous renal surgery) *(52–54)*, renal biopsy (Fig. 5) *(55–58)*, trauma *(59,60)*, renal tumors, or inflammatory renal pathology and may present from 3 wk to 26 yr following the original injury.

Spontaneous AVFs are rarer (only 110 cases have been described in the literature) *(61)* and are of two types, congenital and idiopathic, based on their appearance. Congenital AVFs are classically cirsoid in appearance (a tangle of small-diameter tortuous vessels with multiple variceal AV communications). The subepithelial location of these lesions accounts for a common presentation of hematuria in these patients (75%). On the other hand, idiopathic AVMs are characterized by one or more large AV communication, leading to an aneurysmal appearance on pathology. Hematuria occurs in about 35% of these patients, and hypertension and congestive cardiac failure are more common presentations caused by renal ischemia and circulatory overload (secondary to the larger size of the AVF) *(61)*.

CLINICAL PRESENTATION

Retroperitoneal Hemorrhage

Establishment of a preoperative diagnosis of RPH is a diagnostic challenge as it has variable etiologies and may often present with nonspecific signs and symptoms that are difficult to interpret clinically. Therefore, a high index of clinical suspicion is required to diagnose this condition and treat it aggressively.

The presentation is usually acute, although delayed presentation has been described. Commonly, patients present with acute-onset pain in the flank or in the general abdomen; the pain is continuous, of increasing severity, and may be associated with nausea and vomiting. There may also be a history of hematuria if the renal parenchyma has ruptured. Examination may reveal signs of hypovolemia such as pallor, tachycardia, and in extreme cases, signs of circulatory collapse with cold clammy skin, thready pulse, and hypotension.

Abdominal examination may reveal bruising in the loin, abdomen, or groin. There may be associated abdominal tenderness, guarding, distension, and hypoactive bowel sounds. An abdominal mass may also be palpable on occasion. Rarely, patients with RPH have presented with femoral/lumbar/obturator neuropathy caused by the expanding hematoma (62–65). Occasionally, this condition may present in pregnant patients and is caused either by rupture of renal angiolipoma or renal artery aneurysm or by adrenal hemorrhage secondary to preeclampsia.

Patients with AML may have stigmata of TS complex, whereas patients with polyarteritis nodosa may have a history of myalgia, gastrointestinal complaints, low-grade fever, and weight loss. Patients with inflammatory conditions (such as renal abscess/ nephritis) may be febrile and demonstrate signs of underlying disease. Patients with cystic disease may present with a diagnosis of the condition (e.g., history of autosomal dominant polycystic kidney disease or renal failure on dialysis).

Patients with adrenal hemorrhage from systemic causes are difficult to diagnose as they may present with nonspecific signs, and the clinical picture is obscured by other coexisting conditions in a critically ill patient. These patients may present with minimal abdominal signs and symptoms, but may occasionally complain of abdominal pain and backache. Usually, adrenal hemorrhage is associated with adrenal insufficiency characterized by altered sensorium, fever, lethargy, hypotension unresponsive to routine fluid resuscitation, leukocytosis, hyponatremia, hyperkalemia, and increased serum urea nitrogen with a normal creatinine.

Patients with pheochromocytoma may occasionally present with a history of headaches and hypertension and other signs such as café-au-lait spots or subcutaneous nodules of von Recklinghausen's syndrome. The majority of patients with pheochromocytomas have also been reported to present with pulmonary edema and respiratory distress. Patients with functioning adrenocortical adenomas may have evidence of Cushing's syndrome (20).

Because patients taking anticoagulants or with bleeding disorders can present with RPH, it is important to rule out these conditions in the evaluation of the patient with retroperitoneal bleeding. Laboratory evaluation of routine blood tests may warn the physician of ongoing blood loss with falling hemoglobin and hematocrit, leukocytosis, and a rising serum urea nitrogen. Urine analysis may show evidence of hematuria.

Brisk Hematuria

Ureteroarterial Fistula

Patients with ureteroarterial fistulas may present with a history of prior radiation, pelvic or vascular surgery, or long-standing indwelling stents. As these conditions are very uncommon, they are rarely considered in the differential diagnosis of hematuria. Often, there may be a history of mild hematuria ranging from 3 wk to 3 mo that precedes the onset of massive hematuria *(48)*. A high index of clinical suspicion combined with a history of predisposing factors should alert the physician of this potentially lethal condition.

ARTERIOVENOUS MALFORMATION

Patients with AVM/AVF may have a history of prior renal biopsy (Fig. 5), renal surgery, or trauma. Depending on severity of bleeding and size of the AVM, these patients present with recurrent hematuria, lumbar pain caused by clot colic, severe anemia, hypertension, and cardiac failure. Abdominal examination may reveal an abdominal bruit or thrill.

In both RPH and brisk hematuria, laboratory evaluation of routine blood tests may warn the physician of ongoing blood loss with falling hemoglobin and hematocrit, leukocytosis, rising serum urea nitrogen. Urine analysis may show evidence of hematuria.

Sequelae of RPH

If RPH is not diagnosed and treated promptly, it can lead to serious early consequences, such as hypovolemic shock, multisystem organ failure, coagulopathy, and death. Potential late complications include retroperitoneal fibrosis and Page kidney. Originally described by Page in 1939, Page kidney consists of development of hypertension secondary to the formation of thick dense scar tissue around the kidney *(66)*. Rarely, this condition has been described secondary to perirenal hematomas following renal surgery or trauma *(67)*. Transient perirenal hematomas that produce hypertension have also been described *(68)*. Given the great number of renal surgeries performed, this form of hypertension should be considered a rare phenomenon and has been mentioned to make the urologist aware of this possibility.

DIAGNOSTIC INVESTIGATIONS

Retroperitoneal Hemorrhage

The aim of diagnostic investigations is to diagnose RPH, to evaluate severity, and to determine the probable cause of the condition.

IMAGING STUDIES

CT scan of the abdomen is the investigation of choice to diagnose or rule out RPH. A meta-analysis of patients with RPH demonstrated that CT scan is 100% sensitive in diagnosing this entity *(3,48)*. Although the specificity for detecting an underlying renal mass is only moderate (0.56), it has a higher sensitivity and specificity compared to an abdominal ultrasound. To maximize the diagnostic accuracy of CT scan, Bosniak recommended scanning before and after intravenous contrast and taking 5 mm thick sections. As described in the Management section, Bosniak, Belville, and coworkers recommend serial CT scans for evaluating an indeterminate cause of RPH if the patient's condition is stable *(69,70)*. This approach yields a diagnostic accuracy of 92%.

CT is also useful in detecting and differentiating renal cell carcinoma from other causes, such as AML, transitional cell carcinoma, adrenal hemorrhage, bleeding because of anticoagulants, and bleeding from cysts *(69,70)*. Besides, it is easily available at most centers, is quick, is noninvasive, and gives additional helpful diagnostic information. Lesions such as angiolipomas will be suggested by the presence of fat within the lesion (Hounsfield units ≤ 40), oncocytomas may have the central stellate scar, renal cell carcinoma can be staged, and metastases can be diagnosed. CT scan has also been useful in determining the size of the hematoma, which some preliminary studies indicates may be useful in estimating blood loss *(71)*.

Magnetic resonance imaging (MRI) is indicated if CT scan is unavailable or CT scan findings are equivocal (e.g., to differentiate AML from renal cell cancer). MRI can also be used for planning the appropriate surgical approach for some renal lesions or for managing pregnant patients.

Angiography is not a primary diagnostic modality for RPH. However, it is useful for the diagnosis of vascular diseases associated with spontaneous renal hemorrhage, such as polyarteritis nodosa, AVM, and renal artery aneurysm, and when emergency embolization is planned.

OTHER STUDIES

Plain X-ray of the abdomen is commonly used to assess a patient for acute abdomen, but is not sensitive in diagnosing RPH. However, it may provide indirect clues to the diagnosis, such as loss of psoas shadow, calcification over the kidney (suggestive of renal mass), or enlarged or abnormal contour of the renal shadow.

Once the diagnosis of RPH has been established, it may be necessary to differentiate various etiologies as this may decide the further course of action, (e.g., surgical vs nonsurgical, type of surgical procedure, etc). Other studies may be indicated to help diagnose conditions such as pheochromocytomas, Cushing's syndrome, or bleeding disorders.

Brisk Hematuria

INVESTIGATIONS FOR URETEROARTERIAL FISTULAS

Often, patients with ureteroarterial fistulas will have undergone investigations such as cystoscopy or intravenous pyelogram to evaluate hematuria. If clinical suspicion suggests this etiology, arteriography and retrograde ureterography are the most sensitive investigations to diagnose ureteroarterial fistula. However, they are successful in diagnosing the condition in only 41 *(43,46,72)* and 45% *(46,72)* of cases, respectively. CT scan of the abdomen may demonstrate the presence of hydronephrosis and probable hematoma in the region of the ureter.

Vandersteen et al. used provoked arteriography to establish the diagnosis of ureteroarterial fistula *(43)*. They performed an initial standard arteriogram, and if that was inconclusive, the indwelling ureteral stent was removed over a guide wire (if the ureter was previously unstented, it was accessed either in an antegrade or retrograde manner with a guide wire). If no bleeding occurred, a deflated angioplasty balloon was introduced over the guide wire and alternately advanced and withdrawn within the ureter to provoke the hemorrhage. An arteriogram was then performed to demonstrate the ureteroarterial fistula. The authors claimed 100% sensitivity in diagnosing the condition with this approach. The additional advantage of this approach is that a definitive arteriographic embolization can be attempted if the diagnosis is established. It is important to keep the operating room available and ready in case these measures are not successful in controlling the hemorrhage.

INVESTIGATIONS FOR AVM AND AVF

As with ureteroarterial fistula, often patients with AVM/AVF will have undergone investigations for hematuria. Findings on intravenous pyelogram such as an irregular filling defect or compression of the renal pelvis by dilated vessels may serve to warn of an underlying AVM and should warrant further investigations.

Duplex and color ultrasound has also been useful in diagnosing the condition *(73–75)*. AVMs have also been demonstrated after postinjection CT scans of contrast, which show the vascular luminal nature of the fistula, dilation of the renal vein, and early opacification of the inferior vena cava. MRI has also been used to demonstrate these lesions *(76–78)*.

However, angiography is the diagnostic procedure of choice as it helps define the type and anatomy (site and blood supply) of AVF. In the cirsoid type, the presence of tortuous, dilated, and multichanel vessels is associated with early filling of the renal veins, whereas the idiopathic type is characterized by aneurysmal dilation of the artery and vein and early passage of the contrast medium into the renal vein, inferior vena cava, or even the ovarian/gonadal vein *(61,79)*. The arteriographic appearance in the acquired AVM/AVF is similar to that of the idiopathic AVM/AVF.

MANAGEMENT

Principles of management are predicated on resuscitation of the patient, establishment of the diagnosis if possible, and definitive treatment.

Resuscitation of the Patient

Depending on the severity and acuity of bleeding, patients may present with hemorrhagic shock caused by the depletion of intravascular volume. Therefore, it is important to initiate resuscitative measures immediately. Restoration of intravascular volume can be achieved by administration of intravenous fluids (crystalloids/colloids) by a large-bore intravenous cannula. Blood transfusion for correction of anemia may also be needed. As resuscitative measures are initiated, baseline laboratory tests need to be performed to determine severity of hemorrhage (hemoglobin, hematocrit), determine renal function (serum urea nitrogen, serum creatinine), rule out bleeding diathesis (bleeding and clotting times, prothrombin time, international normalized ratio [INR], activated partial thromboplastin time, platelet count, etc.), and crossmatch blood.

Establishment of Diagnosis

Once the patient is adequately resuscitated, an attempt must be made to establish the diagnosis of RPH and determine the etiology of RPH. If the patient continues to have signs of exsanguinating hemorrhage despite resuscitative measures, it may not be possible to spend time trying to establish the diagnosis; the patient may need surgical or angiographic intervention (Fig. 6) urgently to try to control the bleeding surgically.

CT scan of the abdomen is the investigation of choice to diagnose RPH rapidly and with a high level of accuracy in those stable enough to undergo it. Further investigations may be indicated if the diagnosis is uncertain and the patient is stable enough.

Definitive Treatment

RETROPERITONEAL HEMORRHAGE

Definitive treatment is determined by the underlying cause of RPH, the patient's general condition, and the urgency of the situation. Conservative management is indicated when the cause of RPH is determined to be secondary to the presence of a bleeding diathesis. Use of fresh frozen plasma, clotting factors, platelets, and protamine may be indicated to correct the underlying abnormality.

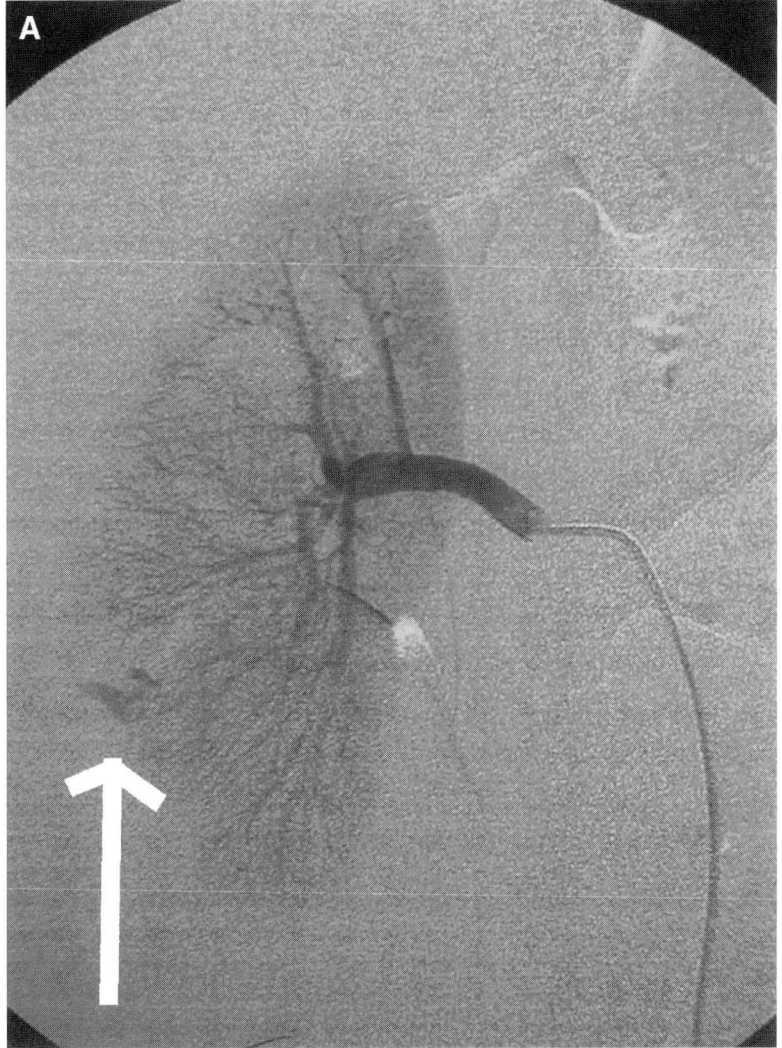

Fig. 6. (A) Angiogram showing active bleeding with upper pole "blush" of escaping blood/contrast. **(B)** Angiogram of the arteriovenous malformation after coil embolization.

If the bleeding is suspected as caused by adrenal crisis in a critically ill patient, prompt initiation of steroid therapy may be indicated even prior to confirmation of the diagnosis. In such cases, the bleeding is commonly bilateral, and aggressive supportive therapy along with steroid replacement and correction of the underlying cause of the condition may help salvage the patient.

On the other hand, unilateral adrenal hemorrhage may be secondary to an adrenal tumor. Because pheochromocytoma is the most common cause of adrenal tumor and is associated with a high intraoperative mortality if undiagnosed prior to surgery, it is imperative to diagnose it and initiate appropriate measures preoperatively. Aggressive fluid resuscitation and blood pressure management are necessary in these patients.

When the cause of RPH is secondary to a renal tumor, it is essential to differentiate AML from other malignant tumors. CT scan is useful in diagnosing the lesion preoperatively, but in the presence of uncertainty, it may be necessary to supplement CT with MRI

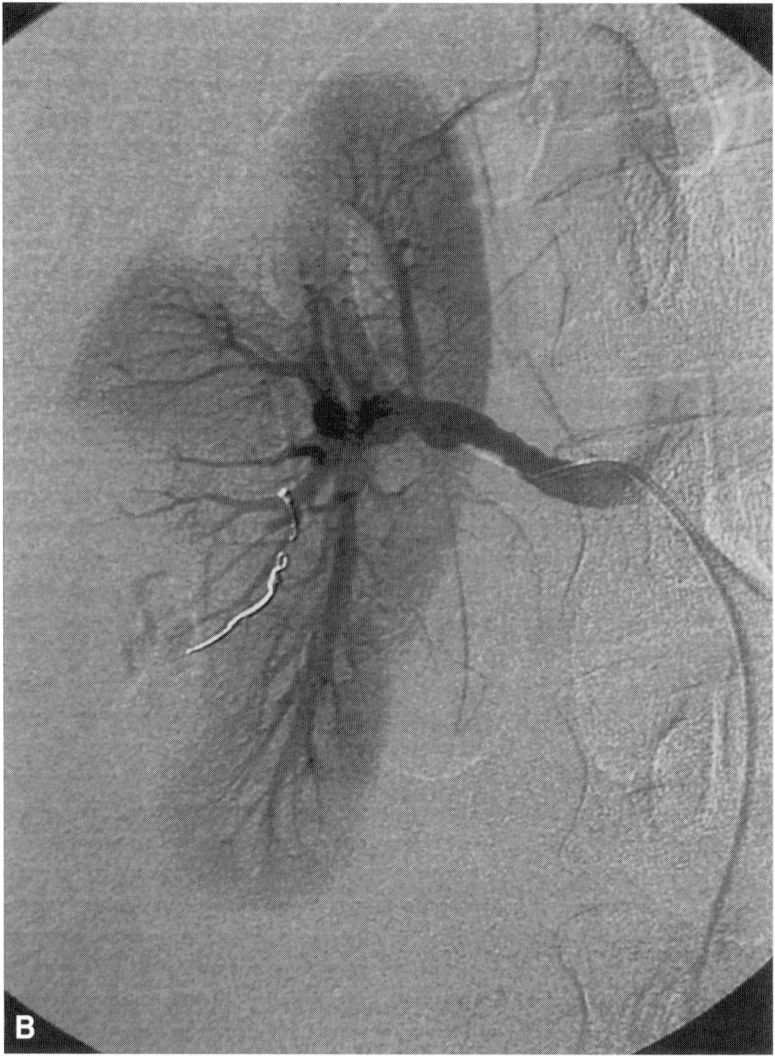

Fig. 6. *Continued*

or even intraoperative biopsy of the lesion. Preserving renal function is an important consideration in these patients, especially in the presence of the TS complex, for which the tumors may be multiple and bilateral.

Angiographic embolization may be an option in the management of renal bleeding, especially for patients with poor renal reserve and who are poor surgical candidates. The advantages of angiographic embolization of AMLs, for example, include the preservation of renal parenchyma, ability to embolize bleeding vessels selectively, and to circumvent the need for surgery.

Nelson and Sanda *(80)* summarized the results of angiographic embolization of angiolipomas in 76 patients and showed a 10% incidence of complications (5% abscesses, 3% pleural effusion), 17% incidence of recurrent symptoms or hemorrhage, 14% incidence of repeat embolization, and 16% incidence of surgery. Of the patients, 85% experienced a postembolization syndrome consisting of flank pain, fever, leucocytosis, and nausea. Treatment consisted of administration of antipyretics, antiemetics, and analgesics, and most patients recovered in 2 to 5 d *(81)*.

Surgical options include enucleation of the tumor, partial nephrectomy, and complete nephrectomy. Complete nephrectomy is usually indicated for a tumor located near the hilum, a tumor sufficiently large to cause a greater risk for partial than total nephrectomy, suspicion of malignancy, associated renal cell carcinoma, or inability to control bleeding by less-conservative means *(80)*.

When the cause is secondary to a ruptured renal artery aneurysm, emergency nephrectomy is usually required as a renal artery aneurysm commonly extends into the renal hilum, making conservative surgery impractical. Rarely, renal arterial bleeding may be secondary to a congenital AVM or from aneurysm of a segmental artery, in which case angiographic embolization/partial nephrectomy is an option *(14)*.

RPH secondary to polyarteritis nodosa should be managed by conservative means whenever possible as often this condition is associated with renal dysfunction. Treatment options include corticosteroid and immunosuppressive therapy *(82)*, selective arterial embolization *(83)*, and partial nephrectomy. Spontaneous rupture of renal cysts is rare, although it may occur after trauma. Treatment is conservative or operative just as in other cases of RPH secondary to a renal etiology.

In a small percentage of cases, it is not possible to demonstrate the exact cause of RPH in the kidney despite thorough investigation. Kendall et al. needed to perform nephrectomy in seven patients with an inconclusive preoperative diagnosis *(84)*. They were able to demonstrate a small carcinoma in five of the seven cases and concluded that imaging studies may not demonstrate smaller cancerous lesions within the kidney. Bosniak, Belville, and coworkers *(69,70)* recommended detailed evaluation of the imaging studies and serial scanning to help identify the cause of RPH in these patients. They suggested that this approach did not increase the risk to the patient and avoided unnecessary removal of normal kidneys. When RPH is present but the kidney appears largely normal, it may also be necessary to rule out other nonurological causes of RPH (e.g., acute pancreatitis).

BRISK HEMATURIA

Ureteroarterial Fistula

Because the cause of the ureteroarterial fistula is connection between the ureter and the iliac artery, the definitive management should be directed toward management of both the ureteric as well as the arterial lesion. The most common urological procedures performed in the past are nephrectomy and ureteral ligation *(46,85,86)*, followed by autotransplantation, renal embolization, or renal irradiation *(86,87)*. The disadvantages of these approaches are that they do not address the underlying ureteric pathology and are associated with an increased morbidity. It is not surprising, therefore, that some of these procedures have been associated with massive bleeding from the ureteral stump in the postoperative period *(44,86)*.

No consensus exists on the vascular management; the most common vascular interventions include primary vascular repair *(49,88)* and iliac artery ligation *(89–91)* with or without femoral bypass and placement of interposition graft. Complications such as distal limb gangrene requiring amputation and operative death have been reported following these procedures.

A review of the literature showed that an aggressive multidisciplinary approach involving urology, radiology, and vascular surgery can successfully bring down the mortality of ureteroarterial fistula from 63 to 31% *(48)*. Vandersteen et al. were able to salvage all renal units successfully and achieved 0% mortality in four patients with five ureteroarterial fistulas with such an approach *(43)*. Based on their experience, they recommended provocative angiography to diagnose the fistula. In the presence of ureteroarterial fistula, they utilized arterial embolization to control the hemorrhage. Following the control of arterial bleeding, ureteral stents may be routinely and successfully replaced to manage the ureteral obstruction. In the event the patients developed distal limb ischemia, they recommended extra-anatomic bypass (femoro-femoral) to correct the problem.

When embolization is unsuccessful in controlling the hemorrhage, or if the patient undergoes surgery as the primary approach (severe shock or condition diagnosed on the operating table), ligation of the iliac artery is a suitable way of controlling the arterial hemorrhage. This approach is usually well tolerated without further reconstruction if there is no distal arterial disease. In the event the patient has distal arterial disease, an extra-anatomic bypass is the fastest and the safest operative procedure to correct it. Direct *in situ* arterial repair locally (at the site of fistula) is generally not recommended because of associated local sepsis and contamination, as well as the potential for vessel weakness secondary to irradiation, aneurysmal dilation, or mycotic aneurysm *(48)*.

The aim of urological management is to try to salvage renal function whenever possible. Once arterial control is obtained, attention is focused toward correction of the urological lesion. Various treatment options described include "no further treatment" *(92,93)*, nephrectomy and/or nephroureterectomies (in the presence of nonfunctioning kidneys), and procedures to divert urine flow away from the fistula (transureteroureterostomy, ureteroureterostomy, percutaneous nephrostomy, and ligation of the ureter) *(50,94,95)*.

Arteriovenous Malformation/Fistula

Several case reports described nonoperative observation of AVMs because some AVMs are known to disappear over a period of time. For example, although 1 to 18% of patients have been reported to develop an AVM following renal biopsy, nearly 80% of these disappeared over a period of many months *(96)*. Observation is justified in asymptomatic or peripherally located small AVMs or when symptoms are adequately controlled by medical means. In the presence of significant symptoms, however, treatment is indicated.

The aim of treatment is to salvage renal function. Treatment options include arteriographic embolization *(97–100)*, excision of the lesion, partial or total nephrectomy *(79)*, ligation of fistula *(101)*, alcohol injection of the fistula *(102)*, endofistulorrhaphy *(103)*, and endovascular management of the fistula *(104,105)*.

SUMMARY

Spontaneous RPH has multiple etiologies, may be life threatening, and requires a high index of clinical suspicion to diagnose it. CT scan is an accurate and sensitive investigation to diagnose the condition. If CT scan fails to determine the cause of the hemorrhage, additional investigations, such as MRI and angiography, may help clinch the diagnosis in patients who are stable. It is equally important to identify medical causes for RPH, such as bleeding disorders (iatrogenic or pathological) or adrenal crisis in the appropriate patients. If no cause of RPH is detectable in spite of various investigative procedures, serial CT scans in a stable patient are a safe and viable approach to ensure that a small RCC or other important deseases not missed.

REFERENCES

1. McDougal WS, Kursh ED, Persky L. Spontaneous rupture of the kidney with perirenal hematoma. J Urol 1975; 114: 181–184.
2. Cinman AC, Farrer J, Kaufman JJ. Spontaneous perinephric hemorrhage in a 65-year-old man. J Urol 1985; 133: 829–832.
3. Zhang JQ, Fielding JR, Zou KH. Etiology of spontaneous perirenal hemorrhage: a meta-analysis. J Urol 2002; 167: 1593–1596.
4. Nguyen HT, Wolf JS Jr, Nash PA, Hovey RM, McAninch JW. Acute retroperitoneal hemorrhage due to transitional cell carcinoma of the renal pelvis. J Urol 153: 140–141.
5. Heyns CF, Rossouw DJ. Spontaneous rupture of adult Wilms' tumor. Cancer 1989; 64: 173–177.
6. Aragona F, Pegoraro V, Artibani W, et al. Sarcomatous carcinoma of the kidney presenting as spontaneous retroperitoneal hemorrhage. Report of a case with immunocytochemical study. Eur Urol 1988; 14: 417–421.
7. Mastrodomenico L, Korobkin M, Silverman PM, Dunnick NR. Perinephric hemorrhage from metastatic carcinoma to the kidney. J Comput Assist Tomogr 1983; 7: 727–729.
8. Eble JN. Angiomyolipoma of kidney. Semin Diagn Pathol 1998; 15: 21–40.
9. Neumann HP, Schwarzkopf G, Henske EP. Renal angiomyolipomas, cysts, and cancer in tuberous sclerosis complex. Semin Pediatr Neurol 1998; 5: 269–275.
10. Mouded IM, Tolia BM, Bernie JE, Newman HR. Symptomatic renal angiomyolipoma: report of 8 cases, 2 with spontaneous rupture. J Urol 1978; 119: 684–688.
11. Oesterling JE, Fishman EK, Goldman SM, Marshall FF. The management of renal angiomyolipoma. J Urol 1986; 135: 1121–1124.
12. Christiano AP, Yang X, Gerber GS. Malignant transformation of renal angiomyolipoma. J Urol 1999; 161: 1900–1901.
13. Ferry JA, Malt RA, Young RH. Renal angiomyolipoma with sarcomatous transformation and pulmonary metastases. Am J Surg Pathol 1991; 15: 1083–1088.
14. Pode D, Caine M. Spontaneous retroperitoneal hemorrhage. J Urol 1992; 147: 311–318.
15. Tham G, Ekelund L, Herrlin K, Lindstedt EL, Olin T, Bergentz SE. Renal artery aneurysms. Natural history and prognosis. Ann Surg 1983; 197: 348–352.
16. Harrow BR, Sloane JA. Aneurysm of the renal: report of five cases. J Urol 1959; 81: 35.
17. Burt RL, Johnston FR, Silverthorne RG, Lock FR, Dickerson AJ. Ruptured renal artery aneurysm in pregnancy. Obstet Gynecol 1956; 7: 229.
18. Cohen SG, Cashdan A, Burger R. Spontaneous rupture of a renal artery aneurysm during pregnancy. Obstet Gynecol 1972; 39: 897–901.
19. Chamblin WD, Marine WC. Massive retroperitoneal hemorrhage complicating pregnancy: case report. Am J Obstet Gynecol 1956; 72: 680.
20. Saito T, Kurumada S, Kawakami Y, Go H. Uchiyama T, Ueki K. Spontaneous hemorrhage of an adrenal cortical adenoma causing Cushing's syndrome. Urol Int 1996; 56: 105–106.
21. Murray HW, Soave R, Collins MH. Fatal retroperitoneal hemorrhage. An unusual complication of renal cortical abscess. JAMA 1979; 241: 1823–1824.
22. Soffer O, Miller LR, Lichtman JB. CT findings in complications of acquired renal cystic disease. J Comput Assist Tomogr 1987; 11: 905–908.
23. Levine E, Grantham JJ, MacDougall ML. Spontaneous subcapsular and perinephric hemorrhage in end-stage kidney disease: clinical and CT findings. AJR Am J Roentgenol 1987; 148: 755–758.
24. Balci NC, Sirvanci M, Tufek I, Onat L, Duran C. Spontaneous retroperitoneal hemorrhage secondary to subcapsular renal hematoma: MRI findings. Magn Reson Imaging 2001; 19: 1145–1148.
25. Milutinovich J, Follette WC, Scribner BH. Spontaneous retroperitoneal bleeding in patients on chronic hemodialysis. Ann Intern Med 1977; 86: 189–192.
26. Papanicolaou N, Pfister RC, Yoder IC. Spontaneous and traumatic rupture of renal cysts: diagnosis and outcome. Radiology 1986; 160: 99–103.
27. Sagel SS, Siegel MJ, Stanley RJ, Jost RG. Detection of retroperitoneal hemorrhage by computed tomography. AJR Am J Roentgenol 1977; 129: 403–407.
28. Scott WW Jr, Fishman EK, Siegelman SS. Anticoagulants and abdominal pain. The role of computed tomography. JAMA 1984; 252: 2053–2056.

29. Lowe GD, McKillop JH, Prentice AG. Fatal retroperitoneal haemorrhage complicating anticoagulant therapy. Postgrad Med J 1979; 55: 18–21.
30. Mant MJ, O'Brien BD, Thong KL, Hammond GW, Birtwhistle RV, Grace MG. Haemorrhagic complications of heparin therapy. Lancet 1977; 1: 1133–1135.
31. Ginsburg JC, Fransman SL, Singer MA, Cohanim M, Morrin PA. Use of computerized tomography to evaluate bleeding after renal biopsy. Nephron 1980; 26: 240–243.
32. Rosenbaum R, Hoffsten PE, Stanley RJ, Klahr S. Use of computerized tomography to diagnose complications of percutaneous renal biopsy. Kidney Int 1978; 14: 87–92.
33. Rao RH. Bilateral massive adrenal hemorrhage. Med Clin North Am 1995; 79: 107–129.
34. Pasciak RM, Cook WA. Massive retroperitoneal hemorrhage owing to a ruptured adrenal cyst. J Urol 1988; 139: 98–100.
35. Goldman HB, Howard RC, Patterson AL. Spontaneous retroperitoneal hemorrhage from a giant adrenal myelolipoma. J Urol 1996; 155: 639.
36. Catalano O. Retroperitoneal hemorrhage due to a ruptured adrenal myelolipoma. A case report. Acta Radiol 1996; 37: 688–690.
37. Hoeffel C, Chelle C, Clement A, Hoeffel JC. Spontaneous retroperitoneal hemorrhage from a giant adrenal myelolipoma. J Urol 1997; 158: 2251.
38. O'Kane HF, Duggan B, Lennon G, Russell C. Spontaneous rupture of adrenocortical carcinoma. J Urol 2002; 168: 2530.
39. Yamada AH, Sherrod AE, Boswell W, Skinner DG. Massive retroperitoneal hemorrhage from adrenal gland metastasis. Urology 1992; 40: 59–62.
40. Manger WM, Gifford RW Jr. Pheochromocytoma: current diagnosis and management. Cleve Clin J Med 1993; 60: 365–378.
41. Raue F, Frank K, Meybier H, Ziegler R. Pheochromocytoma in multiple endocrine neoplasia. Cardiology 1985; 72: 147–149.
42. Larsson C, Nordenskjold M, Raue F, Frank K, Meybier H, Ziegler R. Multiple endocrine neoplasia. Pheochromocytoma in multiple endocrine neoplasia. Cancer Surv 1990; 9: 703–723.
43. Vandersteen DR, Saxon RR, Fuchs E, Keller FS, Taylor LM Jr, Barry JM. Diagnosis and management of ureteroiliac artery fistula: value of provocative arteriography followed by common iliac artery embolization and extraanatomic arterial bypass grafting. J Urol 1997; 158: 754–758.
44. Cass AS, Odland M. Ureteroarterial fistula: case report and review of literature. J Urol 1990; 143: 582–583.
45. Dervanian P, Castaigne D, Travagli JP, et al. Arterioureteral fistula after extended resection of pelvic tumors: report of three cases and review of the literature. Ann Vasc Surg 1992; 6: 362–369.
46. Minamide M, Okano T, Isaka S, Yasuda K, Shimazaki J. [Fistula between iliac artery aneurysm and ureter: a case report and review of the literature]. Hinyokika Kiyo 1993; 39: 1163–1166.
47. Gelder MS, Alvarez RD, Partridge EE. Ureteroarterial fistulae in exenteration patients with indwelling ureteral stents. Gynecol Oncol 1993; 50: 365–370.
48. Batter SJ, McGovern FJ, Cambria RP. Ureteroarterial fistula: case report and review of the literature. Urology 1996; 48: 481–489.
49. Rennick JM, Link DP, Palmer JM. Spontaneous rupture of an iliac artery aneurysm into a ureter: a case report and review of the literature. J Urol 1976; 116: 111–113.
50. Grime PD, Wilmshurst CC, Clyne CA. Spontaneous iliac artery aneurysm-ureteric fistula. Eur J Vasc Surg 1989; 3: 455–456.
51. Schapira HE, Li R, Gribetz M, Wulfsohn MA, Brendler H. Ureteral injuries during vascular surgery. J Urol 1981; 125: 293–297.
52. Lalude AO, Martin DC. Renal arteriovenous fistula: a complication of anatrophic nephrolithotomy. J Urol 1983; 130: 754–756.
53. Lee WJ, Smith AD, Cubelli V, et al. Complications of percutaneous nephrolithotomy. AJR Am J Roentgenol 1987; 148: 177–180.
54. Segura JW, Patterson DE, LeRoy AJ, et al. Percutaneous removal of kidney stones: review of 1000 cases. J Urol 1985; 134: 1077–1081.
55. Gainza FJ, Minguela I, Lopez-Vidaur I, Ruiz LM, Lampreabe I. Evaluation of complications due to percutaneous renal biopsy in allografts and native kidneys with color-coded Doppler sonography. Clin Nephrol 1995; 43: 303–308.

56. deSouza NM, Reidy JF, Koffman CG. Arteriovenous fistulas complicating biopsy of renal allografts: treatment of bleeding with superselective embolization. AJR Am J Roentgenol 1991; 156: 507–510.
57. Matsell DG, Jones DP, Boulden TF, Burton EM, Baum SL, Tonkin IL. Arteriovenous fistula after biopsy of renal transplant kidney: diagnosis and treatment. Pediatr Nephrol 1992; 6: 562–564.
58. Merkus JW, Barendregt WB, van Asten WN, van Langen H, Hoitsma AJ, van der Vliet JA. Changes in venous hemodynamics after renal transplantation. Transpl Int 1998; 11: 284–287.
59. McAlhany JC Jr, Black HC Jr, Hanback LD Jr, Yarbrough DR 3rd. Renal arteriovenous fistula as a cause of hypertension. Am J Surg 1971; 122: 117–120.
60. Messing E, Kessler R, Kavaney PB. Renal arteriovenous fistulas. Urology 1976; 8: 101–107.
61. Fogazzi GB, Moriggi M, Fontanella U. Spontaneous renal arteriovenous fistula as a cause of haematuria. Nephrol Dial Transplant 1997; 12: 350–356.
62. Cianci PE, Piscatelli RL. Femoral neuropathy secondary to retroperitoneal hemorrhage. JAMA 1969; 210: 1100–1101.
63. Rajashekhar RP, Herbison GJ. Lumbosacral plexopathy caused by retroperitoneal hemorrhage, report of two cases. Arch Phys Med Rehabil 1974; 55: 91–93.
64. Lazaro RP, Brinker RA, Weiss JJ, Olejniczak S. Femoral and obturator neuropathy secondary to retroperitoneal hemorrhage: the value of the CT scan. Comput Tomogr 1981; 5: 221–224.
65. Mastroianni PP, Roberts MP. Femoral neuropathy and retroperitoneal hemorrhage. Neurosurgery 1983; 13: 44–47.
66. Page IH. Production of persistent arterial hypertension by cellophane perinephritis. JAMA 1939; 113: 246–248.
67. Sterns RH, Rabinowitz R, Segal AJ, Spitzer RM. "Page kidney." Hypertension caused by chronic subcapsular hematoma. Arch Intern Med 1985; 145: 169–171.
68. Killian ST, Calvin JK. Renal hypertension in children; clinicopathologic studies. Am J Dis Child 1941; 62: 1242.
69. Belville JS, Morgentaler A, Loughlin KR, Tumeh SS. Spontaneous perinephric and subcapsular renal hemorrhage: evaluation with CT, US, and angiography. Radiology 1989; 172: 733–738.
70. Bosniak MA. Spontaneous subcapsular and perirenal hematomas. Radiology 1989; 172: 601–602.
71. Tong YC, Chun JS, Tsai HM, Yu CY, Lin JS. Use of hematoma size on computerized tomography and calculated average bleeding rate as indications for immediate surgical intervention in blunt renal trauma. J Urol 1992; 147: 984–986.
72. Jafri SZ, Farah J, Hollander JB, Diokno AC. Urographic and computed tomographic demonstration of ureteroarterial fistula. Urol Radiol 1987; 9: 47–49.
73. Macpherson RI, Fyfe D, Aaronson IA. Congenital renal arteriovenous malformations in infancy. The imaging features in two infants with hypertension. Pediatr Radiol 1991; 21: 108–110.
74. Middleton WD, Kellman GM, Melson GL, Madrazo BL. Postbiopsy renal transplant arteriovenous fistulas: color Doppler US characteristics. Radiology 1989; 171: 253–257.
75. Rollino C, Garofalo G, Roccatello D, et al. Colour-coded Doppler sonography in monitoring native kidney biopsies. Nephrol Dial Transplant 1994; 9: 1260–1263.
76. Amparo EG, Higgins CB, Hricak H. Primary diagnosis of abdominal arteriovenous fistula by MR imaging. J Comput Assist Tomogr 1984; 8: 1140–1142.
77. Beauchamp N, Kuhlman JE. MR features of bleeding renal arteriovenous fistulae. J Comput Assist Tomogr 1993; 17: 297–299.
78. Develing L, Leiner T, Kitslaar PJ. Magnetic resonance angiography for postnephrectomy arteriovenous fistula. Eur J Vasc Endovasc Surg 2002; 23: 178–179.
79. Crotty KL, Orihuela E, Warren MM. Recent advances in the diagnosis and treatment of renal arteriovenous malformations and fistulas. J Urol 1993; 150: 1355–1359.
80. Nelson CP, Sanda MG. Contemporary diagnosis and management of renal angiomyolipoma. J Urol 2002; 168: 1315–1325.
81. Soulen MC, Faykus MH Jr, Shlansky-Goldberg RD, Wein AJ, Cope C. Elective embolization for prevention of hemorrhage from renal angiomyolipomas. J Vasc Interv Radiol 1994; 5: 587–591.
82. Leib ES, Restivo C, Paulus HE. Immunosuppressive and corticosteroid therapy of polyarteritis nodosa. Am J Med 1979; 67: 941–947.

83. Smith DL, Wernick R. Spontaneous rupture of a renal artery aneurysm in polyarteritis nodosa: critical review of the literature and report of a case. Am J Med 1989; 87: 464–467.
84. Kendall AR, Senay BA, Coll ME. Spontaneous subcapsular renal hematoma: diagnosis and management. J Urol 1988; 139: 246–250.
85. Dyke CM, Fortenberry F, Katz PG, Sobel M. Arterial-ureteral fistula: case study with review of published reports. Ann Vasc Surg 1991; 5: 282–285.
86. Keller FS, Barton RE, Routh WD, Gross GM. Gross hematuria in two patients with ureteral-ileal conduits and double-J stents. J Vasc Interv Radiol 1990; 1: 69–77; discussion 77–69.
87. Bullock A, Andriole GL, Neuman N, Sicard G. Renal autotransplantation in the management of a ureteroarterial fistula: a case report and review of the literature. J Vasc Surg 1992; 15: 436–441.
88. Reiner RJ, Conway GF, Threlkeld R. Ureteroarterial fistula. J Urol 1975; 113: 24–25.
89. Quillin SP, Darcy MD, Picus D. Angiographic evaluation and therapy of ureteroarterial fistulas. AJR Am J Roentgenol 1994; 162: 873–878.
90. Ahlborn TN, Birkhoff JD, Nowygrod R. Common iliac artery-ureteral fistula: case report and literature review. J Vasc Surg 1986; 3: 155–158.
91. Bodak A, Levot E, Schut A, Vincent JP, Lagneau P. [A case of artero-ureteral fistula. Review of the literature]. J Urol (Paris) 1990; 96: 55–59.
92. Dauplat J, Piollet H, Condat P, Glanddier G, Giraud B. [Two cases of uretero-arterial fistula]. J Urol 1985; 91: 457–461.
93. Toolin E, Pollack HM, McLean GK, Banner MP, Wein AJ. Ureteroarterial fistula: a case report. J Urol 1984; 132: 553–554.
94. Kar A, Angwafo FF, Jhunjhunwala JS. Ureteroarterial and ureterosigmoid fistula associated with polyethylene indwelling ureteral stents. J Urol 1984; 132: 755–757.
95. Smith, RB. Ureteral common iliac artery fistula: a complication of internal double-J ureteral stent. J Urol 1984; 132: 113.
96. Parrish AE. Complications of percutaneous renal biopsy: a review of 37 years' experience. Clin Nephrol 1992; 38: 135–141.
97. Cho KJ, Stanley JC. Non-neoplastic congenital and acquired renal arteriovenous malformations and fistulas. Radiology 1978; 129: 333–343.
98. Wallace S, Schwarten DE, Smith DC, Gerson LP, Davis LJ. Intrarenal arteriovenous fistulas: transcatheter steel coil occlusion. J Urol 1978; 120: 282–286.
99. Subramanyam BR, Lefleur RS, Bosniak MA. Renal arteriovenous fistulas and aneurysm: sonographic findings. Radiology 1983; 149: 261–263.
100. Kearse WS Jr, Joseph AE, Sabanegh ES Jr. Transcatheter embolization of large idiopathic renal arteriovenous fistula. J Urol 1994; 151: 967–969.
101. Merkel FK, Sako Y. Surgical treatment for traumatic arteriovenous fistula. Arch Surg 1975; 101: 438–441.
102. Takebayashi S, Hosaka M, Ishizuka E, Hirokawa M, Matsui K. Arteriovenous malformations of the kidneys: ablation with alcohol. AJR Am J Roentgenol 1988; 150: 587–590.
103. Ehrlich RM. Renal arteriovenous fistula treated by endofistulorrhaphy. Arch Surg 1975; 110: 1195–1198.
104. Bilge I, Rozanes I, Acunas B, et al. Endovascular treatment of arteriovenous fistulas complicating percutaneous renal biopsy in three paediatric cases. Nephrol Dial Transplant 1999; 14: 2726–2730.
105. Feuer DS, Ciocca RG, Nackman GB, Siegel RL, Graham AM. Endovascular management of ureteroarterial fistula. J Vasc Surg 1999; 30: 1146–1149.

13 Hemorrhagic Cystitis

*Kian Tai Chong, MBBS, MRCSEd
and John M. Corman, MD*

CONTENTS
    INTRODUCTION
    ETIOLOGY AND RISK FACTORS
    PATHOLOGY
    CLINICAL PRESENTATION
    INVESTIGATIONS
    PROPHYLAXIS
    MANAGEMENT
    EMERGENCY OPTIONS
    POTENTIAL FUTURE THERAPIES/RESEARCH
    SUMMARY
    REFERENCES

INTRODUCTION

Hemorrhagic cystitis (HC) is a common urological disorder, presenting in 6.5% of patients following pelvic radiation therapy and up to 25% of patients receiving alkylating chemotherapeutic agents. HC can be devastating, with high morbidity and mortality despite aggressive interventions [1]. Massive urothelial hemorrhage may involve both upper and lower urinary tracts [2], leading to acute renal failure that requires emergent urological interventions.

Several authors segregated the severity of HC into five grades [3]:

Grade 1	Single minor bleeding
Grade 2	Repeated minor bleeding
Grade 3	Inpatient medical treatment needed
Grade 4	Inpatient surgical treatment needed
Grade 5	Death

The classification scale is relatively arbitrary as the disease does not proceed in a stepwise fashion. Although most patients present with minor bleeding episodes, the initial presentation may be massive macroscopic hematuria with clot retention that requires emergency clot evacuation and blood transfusion.

From: *Urological Emergencies: A Practical Guide*
Edited by: H. Wessells and J. W. McAninch © Humana Press Inc., Totowa, NJ

Table 1:
Classification Adapted From RTOG Scoring Criteria (Acute Radiation Genitourinary Morbidity) And RTOG/EORTC Late Radiation Morbidity Scheme
(Late Radiation Bladder Morbidity)[a]

	Grade 1	Grade 2	Grade 3	Grade 4	Grade 5
Acute morbidity (RTOG)	Frequency and nocturia twice pretreatment habit. Dysuria and urgency without need for medication.	Frequency and nocturia less than once per hour. Dysuria, urgency, and bladder spasm requiring local anesthetic	Frequency and nocturia at least once per hour. Dysuria, pelvic pain, and bladder spasm requiring regular, frequent narcotics. Gross hematuria with or without clot passage.	Hematuria requiring transfusion. Acute bladder outlet obstruction not owing to clot passage, ulceration, or necrosis.	Death from uncontrolled toxicity.
Late morbidity (RTOG/ EORTC)	Slight epithelial atrophy. Minor telangiectasia. Microscopic hematuria.	Generalized telangiectasia. Moderate frequency. Intermittent macroscopic hematuria.	Severe generalized telangiectasia and petechiae. Severe frequency, dysuria. Frequent hematuria. Bladder capacity <150 cc.	Bladder necrosis. Bladder capacity <100 cc. Severe hemorrhagic cystitis.	Death from uncontrolled hematuria.

[a] Grade 0 refers to no treatment-related morbidity. RTOG, Radiation Therapy Oncology Group; EORTC, European Organisation for Research and Treatment of Cancer.

For clinical trials data analysis, the Radiation Therapy Oncology Group (RTOG) based in the United States and the European Organisation for Research and Treatment of Cancer (EORTC) based in Belgium have classified radiation treatment-related genitourinary morbidity. Table 1 summarizes the RTOG morbidity scoring scheme for acute radiation genitourinary morbidity and RTOG/EORTC morbidity scoring scheme for late radiation bladder complications. Acute morbidity criteria are used grade radiation treatment-related toxicity from the first day of radiation therapy for a total of 90 d. Any radiation treatment-related morbidity that occurs after the initial 90 d will be scored using the RTOG/EORTC criteria.

ETIOLOGY AND RISK FACTORS

Among the risk factors for HC presented in Table 2, previous pelvic irradiation and chemotherapeutic drugs like cyclophosphamide are the most common causes of HC. In a randomized Danish study, up to 25% of 118 patients with early ovarian cancer developed HC after external beam radiation and cyclophosphamide treatment *(4)*.

Radiation-Induced HC

Radiation therapy causes chronic fibrosis and progressive endarteritis. When the urothelium is within the radiation field, the end result of the chronic scarring is urothelial sloughing and bleeding. In treatment of prostatic, bladder, or cervical cancer, the bladder mucosa is primarily at risk. The onset of radiation effects may appear more than 10 yr following pelvic irradiation *(5)*. Patients who are at high risk include those with wide radiation fields and a higher total radiation dose. There is no reliable method to predict which patient will be affected or when the episodes of HC will occur.

Table 2
Common Causes of Hemorrhagic Cystitis

Pelvic irradiation	External beam pelvic radiation
	Interstitial radioactive seed implantation for prostate cancer
Chemotherapeutic agents	Cyclophosphamide
	Ifosfamide
	Busulfan
Viral infections	BK virus
	Adenovirus
	Cytomegalovirus

With conformal radiation techniques and interstitial therapy, the incidence of radiation-induced HC is expected to decline.

Chemotherapeutic Agent-Induced HC

HC is commonly associated with the use of chemotherapeutic agents in both cancer and non-neoplastic diseases. Most published literature on HC and its prevention focuses on transplantation. The most common causative factor is the alkylating oxazaphosphorine agents like cyclophosphamide *(6–8)* and ifosfamide *(9,10)*. Bladder mucosal hemorrhage is caused by acrolein, the toxic metabolite of the alkylating agents. Acrolein toxicity may result in life-threatening exsanguination and disseminated intravascular coagulopathy *(11)*.

A retrospective review of complications in 447 bone marrow transplant patients demonstrated that bleeding episodes are associated with prolonged thrombocytopenia, graft-vs-host disease, and cyclophosphamide regimes *(12)*. The effects of these agents are dose-dependent but independent of patients' age *(10,13)*.

Other cyclophosphamide-induced HC occurs in the treatment of Wegener's granulomatosis *(14)*, Ewing's sarcoma *(15)*, advanced non-small cell lung cancer *(16)*, paratesticular rhabdomyosarcoma *(17)*, and malignant brain tumors *(18)*.

Contemporary chemotherapeutic agents such as busulfan *(19)* and temozolomide *(20)* have a lower incidence of HC.

Viral Infection-Induced HC

In immunocompromised hosts after bone marrow or solid organ transplantations, superimposed infections often complicate clinical outcome. Although viral-associated HC was uncommon in the past, the emerging frequency of viral causes from BK virus *(21–23)*, cytomegalovirus *(24)*, and adenovirus *(25,26)* is a cause for concern.

BK virus is a human polyomavirus related to the papovavirus family. After primary infection, the BK virus stays dormant in renal parenchyma until reactivation in immunocompromised hosts *(27)*. This is one of the most common causes of viral-associated HC after bone marrow and renal transplantations.

Using real-time quantitative polymerase chain reaction, BK viruria is related to the occurrence and severity of HC after bone marrow transplantation, without detectable increase in BK viremia *(28)*. Italian researchers using deoxyribonucleic acid (DNA) hybridization assay and polymerase chain reaction analysis also found concurrent urinary shedding of BK virus in prospective cases *(29)* of HC. This indicates a possible adverse role of direct viral contact on urothelium with resultant HC.

Although less common, adenoviral infection (subtypes 11 and 35) occurs in postrenal transplant recipients *(30)*. Adenoviral-associated HC is usually self-limiting and resolves with adequate hydration within 2 wk.

BK virus-associated HC has also been reported in non-transplant patients with human immunodeficiency virus *(31)*.

Miscellaneous Causes of HC

Esoteric causes of HC include ischemic necrosis from bladder overdistension in neurogenic bladder *(32)* and Boon's disease with massive apoptosis and exfoliation of urothelium caused by hypovolemia *(33)*.

PATHOLOGY

In HC, mucosal hyperemia is associated with neutrophilic infiltration of the lamina propria, endarteritis, and fibroblastic reactions seen in chronic fibrosis. Nonneoplastic variants may include squamous metaplasia (without cellular atypia or keratinization), cystitis cystica (with eosinophilic liquefaction of benign urothelium in lamina propria, almost similar to von Brunn's nests), cystitis follicularis (with submucosal lymphoid follicles reacting to chronic bacterial infection), or inverted papilloma *(34)*.

Because severe dysplasia, carcinoma *in situ*, and transitional or squamous cell carcinoma may present with macroscopic hematuria, it is important to exclude malignancies when diagnosing HC. Risk factors for HC like external beam radiation or cyclophosphamide contribute to a higher risk of bladder cancer development *(35)*.

CLINICAL PRESENTATION

In adult and pediatric patients, most cases of HC occur in immunosuppressed, oncological, and autoimmune patients. Among transplants, bone marrow transplantation *(36,37)* is the most significant contributor.

An initial herald bleed may signify mucosal hemorrhage and warrants further investigations to exclude common causes of hematuria. Quantity and frequency of hematuria are unpredictable. Independent of age, most patients present with single-episode or recurrent minor bleeding.

Patients develop clot retention caused by either continuous profuse bleeding or prior bladder outlet obstruction. In elderly males with enlarged prostate, higher urinary outflow resistance contributes to reduced clot clearance, resulting in the vicious cycle of increased intravesical blood clot formation.

Less commonly, patients may present with chronic fatigue, syncope, or unexplained anemia. Rarely, hypotension and hypovolemic shock may occur with uncontrolled hematuria.

INVESTIGATIONS

Although HC presents with macroscopic hematuria, there are several more common causes of hematuria that must be excluded. These include urinary tract infection with inflammatory cystitis, urolithiasis, benign prostatic hypertrophy, transitional cell carcinoma, and aspirin or coumadin ingestion. First-line investigations to be done are plain X-rays to exclude urolithiasis, urinary bacterial cultures, hematocrit level, and serum coagulation profile if indicated.

Cystoscopy

Cystoscopy under anesthesia is indicated if the patient has uncontrollable bleeding requiring blood transfusion, persistent clot retention despite bladder irrigation, or repeated episodes of HC. Although it is a minimally invasive procedure, bladder perforation is a potential complication caused by friable bladder tissues. This is especially true in a scarred, contracted irradiated bladder with little compliance to saline distension and instrument manipulation.

As both a diagnostic and therapeutic tool, cystoscopy is used for clot evacuation, bladder cauterization, and bladder biopsy to rule out transitional cell carcinoma. Note that even in patients who receive excessive anticoagulants, up to 18% of patients were diagnosed with concurrent urinary malignancies *(38)*. After cystoscopic clot evacuation, continuous bladder irrigation is maintained to ensure clearance of residual clots.

Radiological Imaging

Imaging studies concentrate on exclusion of urinary tract malignancies. Traditionally, intravenous urography is used to exclude urothelial tumors, although its sensitivity in assessing the lower urinary tract is inadequate. Intravenous urography should not be used in patients with poor renal function because of potential worsening of renal dysfunction from contrast nephropathy. In renal dysfunction, other imaging modalities like noncontrast helical computed tomographic studies (CT-KUB) or magnetic resonance imaging *(39)* should be utilized.

A small Italian report of 12 patients used ultrasonography features to describe three different types of bladder abnormalities after bone marrow transplantation. These types are circumscribed thickening of bladder wall, diffuse thickening of the bladder wall, and intraluminal lobulated bulky mass *(40)*. Median bleeding duration was longer in patients with intraluminal lobulated bulky mass at 90 d. Although premature, this technique may be a useful non-invasive imaging modality to screen patients for potential future bleeding episodes.

PROPHYLAXIS

Prevention of hemorrhagic episodes in high-risk patients is the most important strategy. Common methods used include intravenous hyperhydration, continuous bladder irrigation, use of mesna (sodium-2-mercaptoethansulfonate), or modification of the chemotherapeutic conditioning regime.

Mesna is a sulfhydryl compound that binds to acrolein metabolites in the urinary tract. It is administered through intravenous or subcutaneous routes and had raised initial interest in potential applications *(41–44)*. However, mesna and its metabolites may cause significant vasculitic side effects like erythroderma, bullous skin lesions, myalgia, fever, and perimyocarditis *(45)*. Hence, its routine use is superceded by other alternatives like forced diuresis and bladder irrigation.

During high-dose cyclophosphamide treatment for 303 patients, aggressive hyperhydration with intravenous fluid to maintain urine output above 200 mL/h coupled with continuous bladder irrigation showed impressive results with no macroscopic hematuria *(46)*. Using less-stringent requirements for forced diuresis, hyperhydration and mesna were equally effective in randomized trials *(47)*.

The most important factor in preventive measures is the dilution or rapid excretion of the chemotherapeutic metabolites toxic to the urothelium. Hyperhydration with intravenous crystalloids and furosemide to maintain hourly urine output of more than 150 mL is recommended as it is efficacious and cost-effective and has few side effects when *(48)* compared to other alternatives.

MANAGEMENT

Management of patients depends on the clinical presentation, severity of bleeding, and medical resources available. It is uncommon to see an actively bleeding patient with hemorrhagic shock who requires emergency surgical intervention. Be wary, however, of patients with syncope and with blood clots in the urine. The volume of blood contained in a distended bladder is often underestimated by less-experienced physicians. Most patients with mild symptoms are managed in the following first-line and second-line therapies.

First-Line Therapy

Minor bleeding usually resolves spontaneously. No medical treatment is needed other than investigations to exclude common causes of hematuria. If bleeding is persistent with clot formation, causing patient distress with urinary retention, immediate clot evacuation and bladder irrigation is done through a large-bore transurethral urinary catheter. In pediatric boys, suprapubic cystostomy is recommended because of narrow urethra lumen. This is followed by continuous bladder saline irrigation with a three-way urinary catheter is done for at least 24 h to ensure removal of residual clot fragments and termination of hematuria.

If bleeding persists despite conservative management, cystoscopic, clot evacuation, and bladder cauterization are performed. Bladder biopsies should be done concurrently in postradiation patients and in cases of recurrent hematuria of unknown etiology.

Second-Line Therapy

Second-line therapies are indicated for patients with recurrent HC without life-threatening or unstoppable hematuria. Several options are discussed and used depending on resource availability.

Hyperbaric Oxygen Therapy

With more than 200 monoplace and 20 multiplace hyperbaric chambers throughout North America *(49)*, hyperbaric oxygen (HBO_2) therapy is emerging as an important option for early intervention of HC. By definition, a patient who receives hyperbaric oxygen therapy must receive oxygen within an enclosed chamber with pressurization of 1.4 atmosphere absolute (atm abs) or higher. Currently, established clinical uses of HBO_2 include air embolism, carbon monoxide poisoning, decompression sickness, diabetic foot ulcers, postradiation tissue injuries, and soft tissue necrotizing fasciitis *(50)*.

When placed in an enclosed chamber (Fig. 1), pressurized oxygen delivery results in the plasma hypersaturation of dissolved oxygen. Excess plasma oxygenation improves local and regional tissue oxygen supply in tissues with poor oxygenation caused by previous radiation or mechanical or chemical injuries *(51)*. This is achieved by the creation of a steep oxygen gradient between the end arterioles and capillaries and the hypoxic tissues that require treatment.

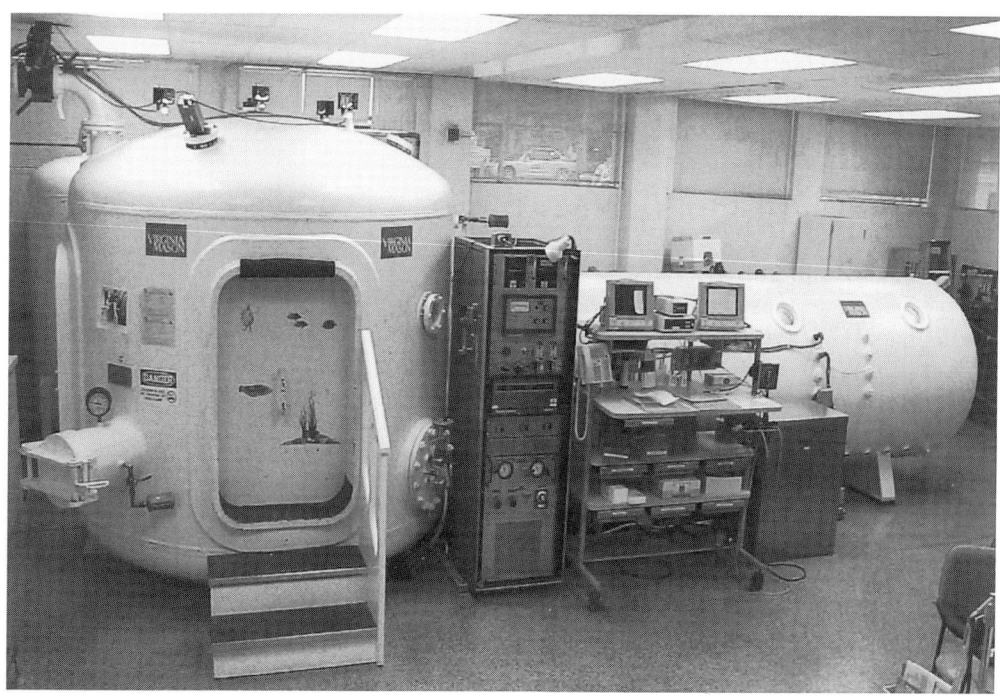

Fig. 1. Hyperbaric oxygen chamber.

Dissolved oxygen in the plasma diffuses across the capillary bed to improve local tissue oxygenation. Adequate tissue oxygenation will ensure efficient production of adenosine triphosphates (ATPs), as well as other components essential for normal cellular function, resulting in primary angiogenesis. Neovascularization occurs with capillary ingrowth into hypoxic tissues.

Compared to normobaric oxygen, hyperbaric oxygen provides an eight- to ninefold increase in vascular density in an irradiated rabbit model *(52)*. In a mouse model, neovascularization can be seen 5 d after initiation of HBO_2 therapy, even in tissues like nonvascularized fat *(53)*. In irradiated human oral tissues treated for mandibular osteoradionecrosis, HBO_2 therapy resulted in significant increase of transmucosal oxygen tension after only five treatments *(54)*. It is the synergistic effect of greater molecular oxygen supply and increased vascular density in the hypoxic tissue that allows adequate collagen synthesis and wound repair to occur.

Hyperbaric oxygen therapy successfully resolves hematuria in most postradiation HC *(55–60)*. HBO_2 is also the only form of therapy that truly promotes tissue healing. Most hyperbaric oxygen therapy sessions are 90 min. A typical treatment course is at least 30 daily sessions at 2.36 atm abs pressure. Absolute contraindications for hyperbaric therapy include presence of emphysema, otitis media or middle ear dysfunction, congestive heart failure, untreated pneumothorax, and concurrent treatment with cisplatinum, doxorubicin, bleomycin, disulfiram, and mafenide acetate *(61)*.

Potential complications include claustrophobia, otalgia, barotraumas, and seizures from central nervous system toxicity. To reduce central nervous system toxicity, at least three to four "air breaks" are given during each session. Air breaks are 5 to 10 min each of normal air breathing. If seizures occur during treatment, conversion to normal air breathing resolves the symptoms.

Traditionally, hyperbaric oxygen therapy has been employed after failure to respond to other treatments. Despite that, meta-analysis of hyperbaric oxygen in managing 190 patients with HC gave impressive results of 76.3% improvement or resolution of hematuria *(62)*. Between 1988 and 2001, we had 86% of 57 patients with complete resolution or marked reduction in hematuria episodes *(63)*.

We strongly recommend hyperbaric oxygen as an early intervention to manage non-life-threatening HC.

INTRAVESICAL THERAPIES

Most second-line therapies are intravesical instillations with variable efficacy and side effect profiles. They generally cause mucosal fibrosis and scarring, working as local astringents as a form of chemical coagulation.

Alum

Intravesical 1% alum solution requires no anesthesia. It usually well tolerated by continuous bladder instillation and irrigation. Potential side effects include suprapubic pain, aluminium toxicity, and renal dysfunction. Isolated reports of treating alum toxicity include using intravenous feroxamine *(64)*.

Formalin

Intravesical 1% formalin (with 0.37% formaldehyde gas in solution) instillation for 30 min induces bladder mucosal fibrosis. Potential problems include intense ureteral edema and fibrosis *(65)*. To prevent upper urinary tract damage and obstruction, vesicoureteric reflux must be excluded by routine cystography, especially in pediatric patients. Fogarty catheters may be placed in the distal ureters to prevent formalin reflux. Up to 10% formalin has been used as intravesical instillation, but the severe bladder irritation necessitates regional or general anesthesia before the procedure.

Patients undergoing formalin instillation often emerge with a contracted poorly compliant bladder that ultimately requires urinary diversion.

Miscellaneous

Other intravesical options include ε-aminocaproic acid, which works by inhibiting formation of stable plasmin. Fibrin degradation cannot occur effectively, and stable blood clots are formed to stop further bleeding. Short-term results appear favorable *(66)*.

Intravesical prostaglandins E_1, E_2, and $F_{2\alpha}$ (Carboprost®) have been tried with varying success *(67–69)*. Silver nitrate has also been applied successfully on isolated bleeding bladder mucosa.

EMERGENCY OPTIONS

Urinary Diversion

When uncontrolled bleeding is apparent, urinary diversion may be performed to reduce distress from clot retention. Suprapubic cystostomy or bilateral percutaneous nephrostomy tube placement *(1)* can slow bleeding while more invasive surgery is contemplated.

Embolization or Surgical Ligation of Internal Iliac Vessels

Transfemoral hypogastric artery embolization is an option to stop hemorrhage. Failure in minimally invasive procedures will usually result in open surgical procedures.

Open Vesicostomy/Subtotal or Total Cystectomy

Exploratory laparotomy is the most aggressive and last resort. Attempts at ligating internal iliac arteries may stop the hemorrhage, and open vesicostomy may control bleeding.

In uncontrolled bleeding, subtotal cystectomy with two-layer repair using absorbable sutures may be adequate for single or clusters of persistent bleeding spots in proximity. However, this treatment is not appropriate therapy for trigonal bleeding, for which cystectomy *(70)* is usually indicated.

POTENTIAL FUTURE THERAPIES/RESEARCH

Antiviral Therapies

Intravenous ribavirin *(71)* is an antiviral agent that can suppress infections of adenovirus subtypes 11 and 35, thereby reducing infections in individuals immunocompromised from bone marrow or renal transplantations. Another option is intravenous or intramuscular vidarabine *(72)*.

Miscellaneous

Other reported treatment options include use of oral conjugated estrogens *(73)*, intravenous factor XIII concentrate *(74)*, and intravesical recombinant human granulocyte-macrophage colony-stimulating factor *(75)*.

SUMMARY

HC is a common problem with potentially devastating effects. With all available resources, clinicians and patients can make informed choices in managing this challenging disease.

REFERENCES

1. Cheng C, Foo KT. Management of severe chronic radiation cystitis. Ann Acad Med Singapore 1992; 21(3): 368–371.
2. Wong TM, Yeo W, Chan LW, Mok TS. Hemorrhagic pyelitis, ureteritis and cystitis secondary to cyclophosphamide: case report and review of literature. Gynecol Oncol 2000; 76(2): 223–225.
3. Levenback C, Eifel PJ, Burke TW, Morris M, Gershenson DM. Hemorrhagic cystitis following radiotherapy for stage Ib cancer of the cervix. Gynecol Oncol 1994; 55(2): 206–210.
4. Sell A, Bertelsen K, Andersen JE, Stroyer I, Panduro J. Randomized study of whole-abdomen irradiation vs pelvic irradiation plus cyclophosphamide in treatment of early ovarian cancer. Gynecol Oncol 1990; 37(3): 367–373.
5. deVries CR, Freiha FS. Hemorrhagic cystitis: a review. J Urol 1990; 143(1): 1–9.
6. Sencer SF, Haake RJ, Weisdorf DJ. Hemorrhagic cystitis after bone marrow transplantation. Risk factors and complications. Transplantation 1993; 56(4): 875–879.
7. Stillwell TJ, Benson RC Jr. Cyclophosphamide-induced hemorrhagic cystitis. A review of 100 patients. Cancer 1988; 61(3): 451–457.
8. Brugieres L, Hartmann O, Travagli JP, et al. Hemorrhagic cystitis following high-dose chemotherapy and bone marrow transplantation in children with malignancies: incidence, clinical course, and outcome. J Clin Oncol 1989; 7(2): 194–199.
9. Mahjoubi M, Azab M, Ghosn M, Theodore C, Droz JP. Phase II trial of ifosfamide in the treatment of metastatic hormone-refractory patients with prostatic cancer. Cancer Invest 1990; 8(5): 477–481.

10. Sarosy G. Ifosfamide—pharmacologic overview. Semin Oncol 1989; 16(1, suppl 3): 2–8.
11. Shanholtz C. Acute life-threatening toxicity of cancer treatment. Crit Care Clin 2001; 17(3): 483–502.
12. Pihusch R, Salat C, Schmidt E, et al. Hemostatic complications in bone marrow transplantation: a retrospective analysis of 447 patients. Transplantation 2002; 74(9): 1303–1309.
13. Hong WK, Nicaise C, Lawson R, et al. Etoposide combined with cyclophosphamide plus vincristine compared with doxorubicin plus cyclophosphamide plus vincristine and with high-dose cyclophosphamide plus vincristine in the treatment of small-cell carcinoma of the lung: a randomized trial of the Bristol Lung Cancer Study Group. J Clin Oncol 1989; 7(4): 450–456.
14. Stillwell TJ, Benson RC Jr, DeRemee RA, McDonald TJ, Weiland LH. Cyclophosphamide-induced bladder toxicity in Wegener's granulomatosis. Arthritis Rheum 1988; 31(4): 465–470.
15. Stillwell TJ, Benson RC Jr, Burgert EO Jr. Cyclophosphamide-induced hemorrhagic cystitis in Ewing's sarcoma. J Clin Oncol 1988; 6(1): 76–82.
16. Williams SF, Bitran JD, Hoffman PC, et al. High-dose, multi-alkylator chemotherapy with autologous bone marrow reinfusion in patients with advanced non-small cell lung cancer. Cancer 1989; 63(2): 238–242.
17. Heyn R, Raney RB Jr, Hays DM, Tefft M, Gehan E, Webber B, Maurer HM. Late effects of therapy in patients with paratesticular rhabdomyosarcoma. Intergroup Rhabdomyosarcoma Study Committee. J Clin Oncol 1992; 10(4): 614–623.
18. Allen JC. Complications of chemotherapy in patients with brain and spinal cord tumors. Pediatr Neurosurg 1991; 17(4): 218–224.
19. Crilley P, Topolsky D, Bulova S, Bigler R, Brodsky I. Bone marrow transplantation following busulfan and cyclophosphamide for acute myelogenous leukemia. Bone Marrow Transplant 1990; 5(3): 187–191.
20. Islam R, Isaacson BJ, Zickerman PM, Ratanawong C, Tipping SJ. Hemorrhagic cystitis as an unexpected adverse reaction to temozolomide: case report. Am J Clin Oncol 2002; 25(5): 513–514.
21. Mylonakis E, Goes N, Rubin RH, Cosimi AB, Colvin RB, Fishman JA. BK virus in solid organ transplant recipients: an emerging syndrome. Transplantation 2001; 72(10): 1587–1592.
22. Reploeg MD, Storch GA, Clifford DB. BK virus: a clinical review. Clin Infect Dis 2001; 33(2): 191–202.
23. Iwamoto S, Azuma E, Hori H, et al. BK virus-associated fatal renal failure following late-onset hemorrhagic cystitis in an unrelated bone marrow transplantation. Pediatr Hematol Oncol 2002; 19(4): 255–261.
24. Bielorai B, Shulman LM, Rechavi G, Toren A. CMV reactivation induced BK virus-associated late onset hemorrhagic cystitis after peripheral blood stem cell transplantation. Bone Marrow Transplant 2001; 28(6): 613–614.
25. Akiyama H, Kurosu T, Sakashita C, et al. Adenovirus is a key pathogen in hemorrhagic cystitis associated with bone marrow transplantation. Clin Infect Dis 2001; 32(9): 1325–1330.
26. Echavarria MS, Ray SC, Ambinder R, Dumler JS, Charache P. PCR detection of adenovirus in a bone marrow transplant recipient: hemorrhagic cystitis as a presenting manifestation of disseminated disease. J Clin Microbiol 1999; 37(3): 686–689.
27. Boubenider S, Hiesse C, Marchand S, Hafi A, Kriaa F, Charpentier B. Post-transplantation polyomavirus infections. J Nephrol 1999; 12(1): 24–29.
28. Leung AY, Suen CK, Lie AK, Liang RH, Yuen KY, Kwong YL. Quantification of polyoma BK viruria in hemorrhagic cystitis complicating bone marrow transplantation. Blood 2001; 98(6): 1971–1978.
29. Azzi A, Fanci R, Bosi A, et al. Monitoring of polyomavirus BK viruria in bone marrow transplantation patients by DNA hybridization assay and by polymerase chain reaction: an approach to assess the relationship between BK viruria and hemorrhagic cystitis. Bone Marrow Transplant 1994; 14(2): 235–240.
30. Londergan TA, Walzak MP. Hemorrhagic cystitis due to adenovirus infection following bone marrow transplantation. J Urol 1994; 151(4): 1013–1014.
31. Barouch DH, Faquin WC, Chen Y, Koralnik IK, Robbins GK, Davis BT. BK virus-associated hemorrhagic cystitis in a human immunodeficiency virus-infected patient. Clin Infect Dis 2002; 35(3): 326–329.

32. Lopez AE, Rodriguez S, Flores I. Management of ischemic hemorrhagic cystitis with hyperbaric oxygen therapy. Undersea Hyperb Med 2001; 28(1): 35–36.
33. Koh LP. Boon's disease: hemorrhagic cystitis in conjunction with massive exfoliation of degenerated urothelial cells (apoptosis?) during intercontinental flights in an otherwise healthy person. Diagn Cytopathol 2001; 25(6): 361–364.
34. Messing EM, Catalona W. Urothelial tumors of the urinary tract. In: *Campbell's Urology*, 7th ed. (Walsh PC, Retik AB, Vaughan ED Jr, Wein AJ, eds.), Saunders, Philadelphia, PA, 1998, Vol. 3, pp. 2327–2410.
35. Pedersen-Bjergaard J, Ersboll J, Hansen VL, et al. Carcinoma of the urinary bladder after treatment with cyclophosphamide for non-Hodgkin's lymphoma. N Engl J Med 1988; 318(16): 1028–1032.
36. Kondo M, Kojima S, Kato K, Matsuyama T. Late-onset hemorrhagic cystitis after hemotopoietic stem cell transplantation in children. Bone Marrow Transplant 1998; 22(10): 995–998.
37. Nevo S, Swan V, Enger C, et al. Acute bleeding after bone marrow transplantation (BMT)—incidence and effect on survival. A quantitative analysis in 1402 patients. Blood 1998; 91(4): 1469–1477.
38. Avidor Y, Nadu A, Matzkin H. Clinical significance of gross hematuria and its evaluation in patients receiving anticoagulant and aspirin treatment. Urology 2000; 55(1): 22–24.
39. Worawattanakul S, Semelka RC, Kelekis NL. Post radiation hemorrhagic cystitis: MR findings. Magn Reson Imaging 1997; 15(9): 1103–1106.
40. Cartoni C, Arcese W, Avvisati G, Corinto L, Capua A, Meloni G. Role of ultrasonography in the diagnosis and follow-up of hemorrhagic cystitis after bone marrow transplantation. Bone Marrow Transplant 1993; 12(5): 463–467.
41. Katz A, Epelman S, Anelli A, et al. A prospective randomized evaluation of three schedules of mesna administration in patients receiving an ifosfamide-containing chemotherapy regime: sustained efficiency and simplified administration. J Cancer Res Clin Oncol 1995; 121(2): 128–131.
42. Meisenberg B, Lassiter M, Hussein A, Ross M, Vredenburgh JJ, Peters WP. Prevention of hemorrhagic cystitis after high-dose alkylating agent chemotherapy and autologous bone marrow support. Bone Marrow Transplant 1994; 14(2): 287–291.
43. Luce JK, Simons JA. Efficacy of mesna in preventing further cyclophosphamide-induced hemorrhagic cystitis. Med Pediatr Oncol 1988; 16(6): 372–374.
44. Haselberger MB, Schwinghammer TL. Efficacy of mesna for prevention of hemorrhagic cystitis after high-dose cyclophosphamide therapy. Ann Pharmacother 1995; 29(9): 918–921.
45. Reinhold-Keller E, Mohr J, Christophers E, Nordmann K, Gross WL. Mesna side effects which imitate vasculitis. Clin Investig 1992; 70(8): 698–704.
46. Vose JM, Reed EC, Pippert GC, et al. Mesna compared with continuous bladder irrigation as uroprotection during high-dose chemotherapy and transplantation: a randomized trial. J Clin Oncol 1993; 11(7): 1306–1310.
47. Shepherd JD, Pringle LE, Barnett MJ, Klingemann HG, Reece DE, Phillips GL. Mesna vs hyperhydration for the prevention of cyclophosphamide-induced hemorrhagic cystitis in bone marrow transplantation. J Clin Oncol 1991; 9(11): 2016–2020.
48. Ballen KK, Becker P, Levebvre K, et al. Safety and cost of hyperhydration for the prevention of hemorrhagic cystitis in bone marrow transplant recipients. Oncology 1999; 57(4): 287–292.
49. Moon RE, Camporesi EM. Hyperbaric oxygen therapy: from the 19th to the 21st century. Respir Care Clin N Am 199; 5(1): 1–5.
50. Hampson NB, chair and ed. *Hyperbaric Oxygen Therapy: 1999 Committee Report*. Undersea and Hyperbaric Medical Society, Kensington, MD, 1999.
51. Robertson PW, Hart BB. Assessment of tissue oxygenation. Resp Care Clin N Am 1999; 5(2): 221–263.
52. Marx RE, Ehler WJ, Tayapongsak P, et al. Relationship of oxygen dose to angiogenesis induction in irradiated tissue. Am J Surg 1990; 160(5): 519–524.
53. Shoshani O, Shupak A, Ullmann Y, et al. The effect of hyperbaric oxygenation on the viability of human fat injected into nude mice. Plas Reconstr Surg 2000; 106(6): 1390–1396.

54. Thorn JJ, Kallehave F, Westergaard P, et al. The effect of hyperbaric oxygen on irradiated oral tissues: transmucosal oxygen tension measurements. J Oral Maxillofac Surg 1997; 55(10): 1103–1107.
55. Matthew R, Rajan N, Josefson L, et al. Hyperbaric oxygen therapy for radiation induced hemorrhagic cystitis. J Urol 1999; 161(2): 435–437.
56. Bevers RF, Bakker DJ, Kurth KH. Hyperbaric oxygen treatment for hemorrhagic radiation cystitis. Lancet 1995; 346(8978): 803–805.
57. Norkool DM, Hampson NB, Gibbons RP, et al. Hyperbaric oxygen therapy for radiation-induced hemorrhagic cystitis. J Urol 1993; 150(2 Pt 1): 332–334.
58. Weiss JP, Mattei DM, Neville EC, et al. Primary treatment of radiation-induced cystitis with hyperbaric oxygen: 10-year experience. J Urol 1994; 151(6): 1514–1517.
59. Crew JP, Jephcott CR, Reynard JM. Radiation-induced hemorrhagic cystitis. Eur Urol 2002; 40(2): 111–123.
60. Ennis RD. Hyperbaric oxygen for the treatment of radiation cystitis and proctitis. Curr Urol Rep 2000; 3(3): 229–231.
61. O'Reilly KJ, Hampson NB, Corman JM. *Hyperbaric Oxygen in Urology*. AUA Update Series Lesson 4, Vol. 21. American Urological Association, Houston, TX, 2002, pp. 26–31.
62. Feldmeier JJ, Hampson NB. A systematic review of the literature reporting the application of hyperbaric oxygen prevention and treatment of delayed radiation injuries: an evidence based approach. Undersea Hyperb Med 2002; 29(1): 4–30.
63. Corman JM, McClure RD, Pritchett TR, Kozlowski P, Hampson NB. Treatment of radiation-induced hemorrhagic cystitis with hyperbaric oxygen. J Urol 2003; 169: 2200–2202.
64. Kanwar VS, Jenkins JJ, Mandrell BN. Aluminium toxicity following intravesical alum irrigation for hemorrhagic cystitis. Med Pediatr Oncol 1996; 27(1): 64–67.
65. Sarnak MJ, Long J, King AJ. Intravesicular formaldehyde instillation and renal complications. Clin Nephrol 1999; 51(2): 122–125.
66. Stefanini M, English HA, Taylor AE. Safe and effective, prolonged administration of epsilon-aminocaproic acid in bleeding from the urinary tract. J Urol 1990; 143(3): 559–561.
67. Ippoliti C, Przepiorka D, Mehra R, et al. Intravesical Carboprost for the treatment of hemorrhagic cystitis after marrow transplantation. Urology 1995; 46(6): 811–815.
68. Laszlo D, Bosi A, Guidi S, et al. Prostaglandin E_2 bladder instillation for the treatment of hemorrhagic cystitis after allogenic bone marrow transplantation. Haematologica 1995; 80(5): 421–425.
69. Trigg ME, O'Reilly J, Rumelhart S, Morgan D, Holida M, de Alarcon P. Prostaglandin E_1 bladder instillations to control severe hemorrhagic cystitis. J Urol 1990; 143(1): 92–94.
70. Koc S, Hagglund H, Ireton RC, Perez-Simon JA, Collins SJ, Appelbaum FR. Successful treatment of severe hemorrhagic cystitis with cystectomy following matched donor allogenic hematopoietic cell transplantation. Bone Marrow Transplant 2000; 26(8): 899–901.
71. Miyamura K, Hamaguchi M, Taji H, et al. Successful ribavirin therapy for severe adenovirus hemorrhagic cystitis after allogenic marrow transplant from close HLA donors rather than distant donors. Bone Marrow Transplant 2000; 25(5): 545–548.
72. Seabra C, Perez-Simon JA, Sierra M, et al. Intramuscular vidarabine therapy for polyomavirus-associated hemorrhagic cystitis following allogenic hemopoietic stem cell transplantation. Bone Marrow Transplant 2000; 26(11): 1229–1230.
73. Miller J, Burfield GD, Moretti KL. Oral conjugated estrogen therapy for treatment of hemorrhagic cystitis. J Urol 1994; 151(5): 1348–1350.
74. Demesmay K, Tissot E, Bulabois CE, et al. Factor XIII replacement in stem-cell transplant recipients with severe hemorrhagic cystitis: a report of four cases. Transplantation, 2002; 74(8): 1190–1192.
75. Vela-Ojeda J, Tripp-Villanueva F, Sanchez-Cortes E, et al. Intravesical rhGM-CSF for the treatment of late onset hemorrhagic cystitis after bone marrow transplant. Bone Marrow Transplant 1999; 24(12): 1307–1310.

14 Priapism

Ricardo Munarriz, MD, Noel N. Kim, MD, Abdul Traish, MD, and Irwin Goldstein, MD

CONTENTS

> INTRODUCTION
> INCIDENCE
> ETIOLOGY OF ISCHEMIC PRIAPISM (VENO-OCCLUSIVE)
> PATHOPHYSIOLOGY OF ISCHEMIC PRIAPISM
> NONISCHEMIC ARTERIAL PRIAPISM
> MANAGEMENT
> SUMMARY
> REFERENCES

INTRODUCTION

The term *priapism* is derived from the Greek god Priapus, the god of seduction, fertility, and sexual love, also known for his giant phallus *(1)*. Since the first reported case of priapism in 1824 by Callaway *(2)*, limited attention has been placed on the study of the incidence, etiology, pathophysiology, diagnosis, and timely treatment of priapism. Therefore, priapism is associated partly with less-than-ideal patient outcomes, including permanent and irreversible erectile dysfunction and the associated devastating psychosocial consequences.

The Thought Leader Panel on Evaluation and Treatment of Priapism developed under the auspices of the American Foundation of Urologic Diseases, with input from a multidisciplinary panel that included experts in pediatrics, hematology-oncology, psychiatry, and urology, defined priapism as a pathological condition of a penile erection that persists beyond or is unrelated to sexual stimulation *(3)*. The Thought Leader Panel also classified priapism into the following types:

1. *Ischemic priapism (veno-occlusive)* is the most common form of priapism; it is usually a painful, rigid erection characterized clinically by absent cavernous blood flow. Ischemic priapism beyond 4 h is a compartment syndrome that requires emergent medical intervention. Potential consequences are irreversible corporal fibrosis and permanent erectile dysfunction.

From: *Urological Emergencies: A Practical Guide*
Edited by: H. Wessells and J. W. McAninch © Humana Press Inc., Totowa, NJ

2. *Nonischemic (arterial) priapism* is a less-common form of priapism caused by unregulated cavernous inflow. The erection is usually painless and not fully rigid. Nonischemic priapism requires evaluation, but is neither a compartment syndrome nor a medical emergency.

INCIDENCE

Well-designed, community-based epidemiological studies investigating the prevalence or incidence of priapism are limited. Current data reveal that the incidence of priapism in the general population is low. A Finnish study, based on hospital discharge data, established the incidence of priapism as between 0.3 and 0.5 cases per 100,000 person-years, with a peak incidence of 1.1 cases per 100,000 person-years in the final years of the study. This was attributed to the new use of intracavernosal vasoactive agents introduced for the treatment of erectile dysfunction *(4)*.

Eland et al. conducted a population-based retrospective cohort study using the Integrated Primary Care Information database, a longitudinal computer-based record of all patients seen by general practitioners in the Netherlands *(5)*. This study demonstrated a slightly higher incidence of noniatrogenic priapism (0.9 cases per 100,000 person-years) and a similar incidence of iatrogenic priapism.

The incidence of priapism in the United States and countries where hemoglobinopathies such as sickle cell sickle are prevalent may be higher than in other countries. A questionnaire-based study in five centers in the United Kingdom and Nigeria of 130 patients with sickle cell anemia reported that the prevalence of priapism was 35% *(6)*.

ETIOLOGY OF ISCHEMIC PRIAPISM (VENO-OCCLUSIVE)

Drugs, Toxins, Hormones, and Parenteral Hyperalimentation

Drugs are responsible for up to 80% of cases of ischemic priapism *(7)*. Intracavernosal injection of vasoactive drugs for the management of erectile dysfunction has become the most common cause of drug-induced priapism *(8)*. The risk of priapism after intracavernosal injection of vasoactive agents such as papaverine and prostaglandin E_1 or a combination of those agents is higher in men with psychogenic, neurogenic, or pure cavernosal arterial insufficiency.

Antihypertensive drugs (phenoxybenzamine *[9]*, labetalol *[10]*, prazosin *[11,12]*) are thought to induce priapism through their α-adrenergic-blocking activity, preventing or delaying physiological detumescence, or by direct relaxation of the smooth muscle of the corpus cavernosum *(13)*.

Duggan and Morgan first reported the association between heparin and priapism after four patients developed ischemic priapism while on heparin for the management of myocardial infarction *(14)*. This association was further studied by Singhal et al., who found 17 of 3337 hemodialysis patients who received heparin experienced an episode of priapism during or shortly after hemodialysis *(15)*. Although the mechanism by which heparin induces priapism is unclear, it is hypothesized that a relatively hypercoagulable state may developed after heparin therapy is discontinued *(16)*. In addition, hemodialysis patients may have a defect of von Willebrand's factor, a platelet adherence molecule, leading to a hypercoagulable state. Thus, they may be more susceptible to priapism. Warfarin has also been associated with priapism *(17)*.

Although tricyclic antidepressants have rarely been associated with priapism, trazadone, a widely used antidepressant and hypnotic, is commonly associated with prolonged erections and priapism *(18–22)*. The most likely mechanism is thought to be mediated by α-adrenergic blockade, which interferes with the normal detumescence mechanism *(23,24)*. Antipsychotic drugs such as phenothiazides have also been associated with ischemic priapism, most likely by blocking dopamine D_1 receptors and to a lesser degree by their antihistamine, antiserotonergic, anticholinergic, and α-blocker properties *(25,26)*.

Cocaine, by either intranasal or topical *(27,28)* administration, has become a common cause of ischemic priapism. The pathophysiological mechanism is complex and multifactorial. On one hand, cocaine is a potent norepinephrine reuptake inhibitor, which may deplete neuronal norepinephrine stores and prevent detumescence *(29)*. On the other hand, cocaine is a potent serotonin reuptake inhibitor that may cause central nervous system stimulation and peripheral vasodilation *(30,31)*. Marijuana has also been associated with priapism *(32,33)*.

In the past, when parenteral hyperalimentation contained high-fat emulsions, ischemic priapism was frequently reported. Several pathophysiological mechanisms, such as hypercoagulability, fat embolism, capillary thrombosis, and decreased capillary blood flow, have been hypothesized as responsible for the development of parenteral hyperalimentation-induced ischemic priapism *(34–36)*.

Finally, toxins (e.g., from a black widow spider) *(37)*, over-the-counter preparations containing ephedra *(29)*, and the administration of several hormones (e.g., testosterone) *(38–40)* or antiestrogens (tamoxifen) *(41)* have been associated with ischemic priapism.

Hematological Disorders

Hematological disorders, particularly hemoglobinopathies, are the most common cause of priapism in the pediatric population *(42)*. The incidence of sickle cell disease in African Americans is estimated as 8.2% *(43)*, and approx 10 to 89% of patients with sickle cell disease will experience priapism *(44,45)*. The majority of sickle cell priapisms occur during nocturnal erections. It is possible that the combination of erythrocyte functional and structural abnormalities, low oxygen tension, and decreased corporal pH during prolonged nocturnal erections may induce the formation of irreversible sickled cell erythrocytes that prevent venous outflow and normal penile detumescence. Sickle cell is probably the most common cause of stuttering priapism, a rare and poorly described syndrome characterized by multiple or recurrent episodes of ischemic priapism.

Other hemoglobinopathies (thalassemia) *(46)* and hyperviscosity states such as leukemia and polycythemia have also been associated with priapism *(47,48)*. The pathophysiology is probably similar to that of sickle cell anemia *(47,48)*.

Metabolic, Neurological, and Malignant Disorders

Metabolic disorders such as amyloidosis *(49)* and Fabry's disease *(50)* are rare causes of priapism, and the literature is limited to single-case reports. The most likely pathophysiological mechanism is caused by the obstruction of the outflow pathway.

Spinal cord injury *(51)*, spinal stenosis *(52)*, and autonomic neuropathy are rare causes of priapism and generally resolve spontaneously or require minimal intervention.

Table 1
Etiology of Priapism

Ischemic priapism
  Drugs
    Intracavernosal agents: papaverine, prostaglandin E_1, phentolamine
    Oral agents: trazadone, benzodiazepines, phenothiazines, Prazosin, phenoxybenzamine,
      labetalol, calcium channel blockers, β-blockers, hydralazine
    Anticoagulants: Heparin, warfarin
    Hormonal agents: testosterone, gonadotropin-releasing hormone, antiestrogens
      (tamoxifen)
    Illegal drugs: cocaine and marijuana
    Parenteral nutrition
    Others: carbon monoxide, black widow spider venom, alcohol
  Hematological disorders
    Hyperviscosity states: polycythemia
    Hemoglobinopathies: sickle cell anemia, thallasemia
    Immunological disorders: lupus, protein C deficiency
  Metabolic disorders: gout, diabetes, nephritic syndrome, renal failure, amyloidosis,
    Fabry's disease
  Neurological disorders: spinal cord lesions, autonomic neuropathy, spinal stenosis
  Malignancies: leukemia, multiple myeloma, prostate, bladder, urethral cancer, renal
    and colorectal cancer
  Idiopathic

Nonischemic priapism
  Blunt perineal trauma
  Penetrating perineal trauma (cavernosal artery laceration/intracavernosal administration
    of vasoactive agents)
  Idiopathic: unrecognized trauma

Malignant priapism is rare nevertheless *(53–55)*; the most common primary tumors responsible for this presentation are those of the bladder, prostate, rectosigmoid colon, and kidney (30, 30, 16, and 11%, respectively) *(56)*. The physiopathological mechanisms by which malignant tumor may lead to priapism probably are obstruction of venous drainage or partial replacement of the sinusoids, which might promote stasis and thrombosis.

Idiopathic

The etiology of ischemic priapism is unknown in approx 30 to 50% of cases *(57)*. A comprehensive and extensive evaluation is mandatory to exclude reversible or life-threatening causes. Other causes associated with priapism such as hypertriglyceridemia *(58)*, corporal abscesses *(59)*, and infectious diseases (tularemia, congenital syphilis, parotitis) *(60)* are listed in Table 1.

PATHOPHYSIOLOGY OF ISCHEMIC PRIAPISM

Ischemic priapism results from an imbalance of the vasoconstrictive and vasorelaxatory mechanisms, leading to a penile closed compartment syndrome biochemically characterized by hypoxia, hypercapnia, and acidosis. Prolonged corporal

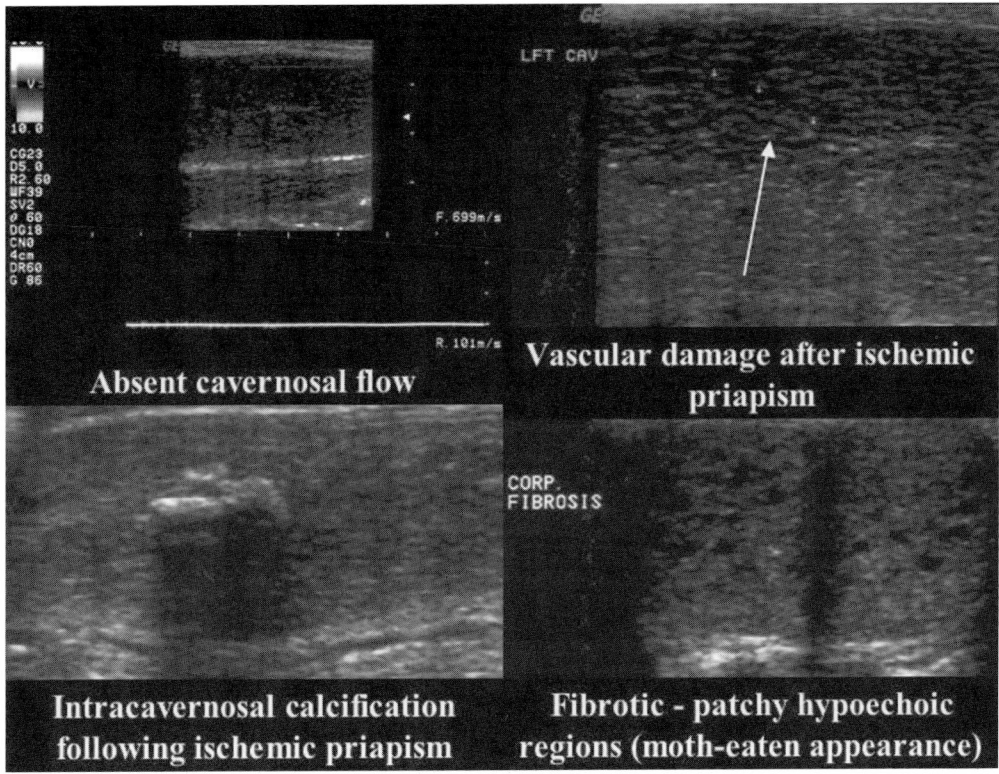

Fig. 1. Penile duplex Doppler ultrasound showing absent cavernosal blood flow in a patient with ischemic priapism; vascular injury after 36-h episode of ischemic priapism; intracavernosal calcification after 48-h episode of ischemic priapism; and corporal fibrosis after priapism (moth-eaten appearance).

smooth muscle exposure to these conditions results in irreversible damage to erectile tissue with subsequent corporal fibrosis (Fig. 1). Acidosis attenuates trabecular smooth muscle contractility to α-adrenergic agonist *(61)*. As a consequence, higher doses of adrenergic agonists may be required to overcome the decreased receptor affinity to achieve detumescence *(62)*.

In addition, hypoxemia activates endothelial cells, leading to a cascade of reactions characterized by increased neutrophil adhesion, decreased mitochondrial respiratory chain activity, and an increase in intracellular calcium.

Reestablishing corporal blood flow during the management of ischemic priapism is associated with reperfusion of ischemic tissues. This drastic increase in corporal oxygen tension generates reactive oxygen species (ROS) that may cause tissue damage. Based on the cardiac reperfusion model described by Goldhaber and Weiss *(63)*, we suggested that several events take place during penile ischemia and reperfusion in the management of priapism: (1) Endogenous scavengers of oxygen free radicals may decrease during ischemia, resulting in reduced levels of antioxidant effects; (2) decreased mitochondrial aerobic metabolism results in the production of ROS; (3) increased adenosine triphosphate hydrolysis results in the accumulation of hypoxanthine, which is subsequently converted to uric acid, another source of ROS; (4) the nitric oxide pathway generates peroxynitrite, peroxynitrite anion, and hydroxyl radical (free radicals); (5) lipid peroxidation and infiltration of the vasculature with neutrophils produces several oxygen free radicals (oxygen free radicals, hydrogen peroxide, hydroxyl radical, and hypochlorous anion), which are released in response to ischemia/reperfusion *(64)*.

NONISCHEMIC ARTERIAL PRIAPISM

High-flow priapism results from unregulated cavernous arterial flow caused by an acute perineal trauma, which leads to the formation of an arterial-lacunar fistula *(65,66)*. Turbulent arterial flow into the fistula causes unregulated release of endothelial nitric oxide, a potent vasodilator and anticoagulant that prevents penile detumescence and clotting of the arterial-lacunar fistula. Arterial priapism is characterized by a permanent, painless, partial erection with almost always normal penile axial rigidity during sexual activity. If arterial priapism is associated with persistent inadequate penile erection during intercourse, it must be suspected that the traumatic event, which resulted in a lacerated cavernosal artery, was also severe enough to cause endothelial injury, leading to arterial obstructive pathology.

Alternatively, the traumatic event may also cause corporal tissue injury that results in corporal veno-occlusive dysfunction. In such cases, vascular testing (duplex Doppler ultrasound and dynamic infusion cavernosometry and cavernosography) is indicated to differentiate cavernosal artery insufficiency from venous leak and to determine if vascular reconstruction is appropriate to reestablish potency.

MANAGEMENT

Ischemic Priapism (Compartment Syndrome of the Corpora Cavernosa)

The diagnosis of priapism is usually made by history and physical examination, but some general diagnostic tests (complete blood count, platelets, differential, reticulocyte count, hemoglobin electrophoresis, urine analysis, urine screening for metabolites of cocaine or for psychoactive drugs) should be considered in an attempt to identify the etiological factor. Prostate-specific antigen is also recommended to rule out the possibility of invasive prostate cancer into the cavernosal bodies. Assessment of corporal blood flow status *must* be carried out in *all patients* by either corporal aspirate (color, consistency, corporal blood gas) or penile duplex Doppler ultrasound (Fig. 2) and repeated after treatment has been performed to assess the status of cavernosal arterial blood inflow continuously.

Should ischemic priapism be diagnosed and treatment initiated to reestablish cavernosal arterial blood flow, the following may be performed. Penile anesthesia (dorsal nerve, subcutaneous local penile shaft block, or circumferential penile block) or systemic analgesia should be considered before therapeutic efforts are carried out to minimize patient suffering and to maximize the efficacy of invasive therapeutic efforts that are sometimes very painful and distressing.

Pharmacological agent administration with or without corporal aspiration, with cardiopulmonary monitoring if needed, is simple and in many cases effective. Phenylephrine has been suggested as the drug of choice because of its pure α_1-agonist and low β_1 activity *(67)*. The recommended dose is 300 to 500 µg intracavernosally every 5 to 10 min up to a maximal dose of 1.5 mg of phenylephrine. McAuley et al., to overcome the decreased affinity of α-adrenergic receptors observed in the presence of the acidosis in ischemic priapism, successfully used high-dose phenylephrine (1000 µg/mL every 10

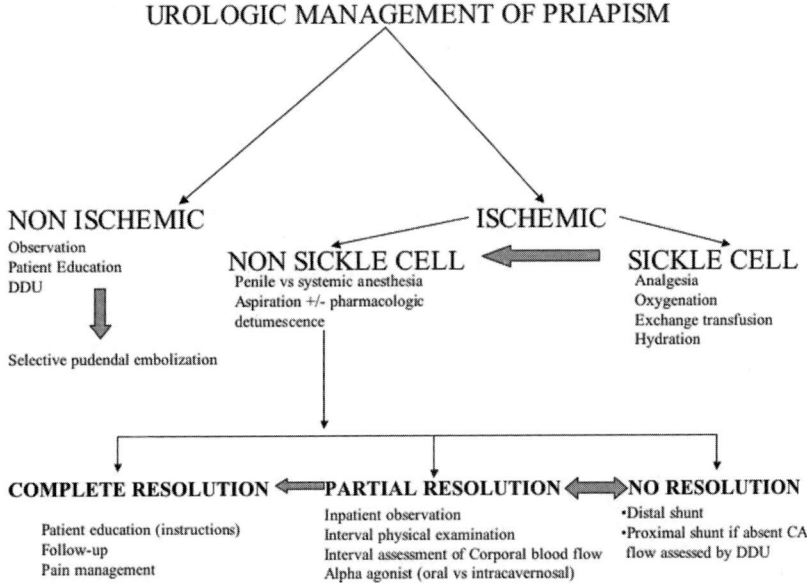

Fig. 2. Algorithm for the management of priapism. DDU, doplex Doppler ultrasound. (Adapted from ref. *3*.)

Table 2
Adrenergic Agents Used in the Treatment of Ischemic Priapism

	α	β$_1$	β$_2$
Ephedrine	+	++	++
Epinephrine	+++	+++	+++
Norepinephrine	+++	++	++
Phenylephrine	+++	Minimal or non	Minimal or non

+, mild; ++, moderate; +++, significant effect/interaction.

min as needed for 7–10 doses) without significant complications *(62)*. Other adrenergic agents may also be used (Table 2).

If pharmacological agent administration fails, corporal irrigation with saline with or without pharmacological agents to induce detumescence should be the next logical step. In addition, appropriate analgesia, hydration, and oxygenation with or without exchange transfusion are indicated for the sickle cell patient.

Successful treatment outcome should be assessed by physical examination of the penis, and in cases of partial resolution, interval assessment of corporal blood flow status by corporal aspirate or penile duplex Doppler ultrasound is mandatory. If the episode of priapism has been successfully resolved, the patient may be discharged home with detailed instructions, follow-up, and oral analgesics.

In the case of partial resolution or because of ischemic edema, persistent partial erection, or persistent pain, inpatient observation is recommended. Interval physical examination of the penis or interval assessment of corporal blood flow status by corporal aspirate or penile duplex Doppler ultrasound is mandatory. Adrenergic

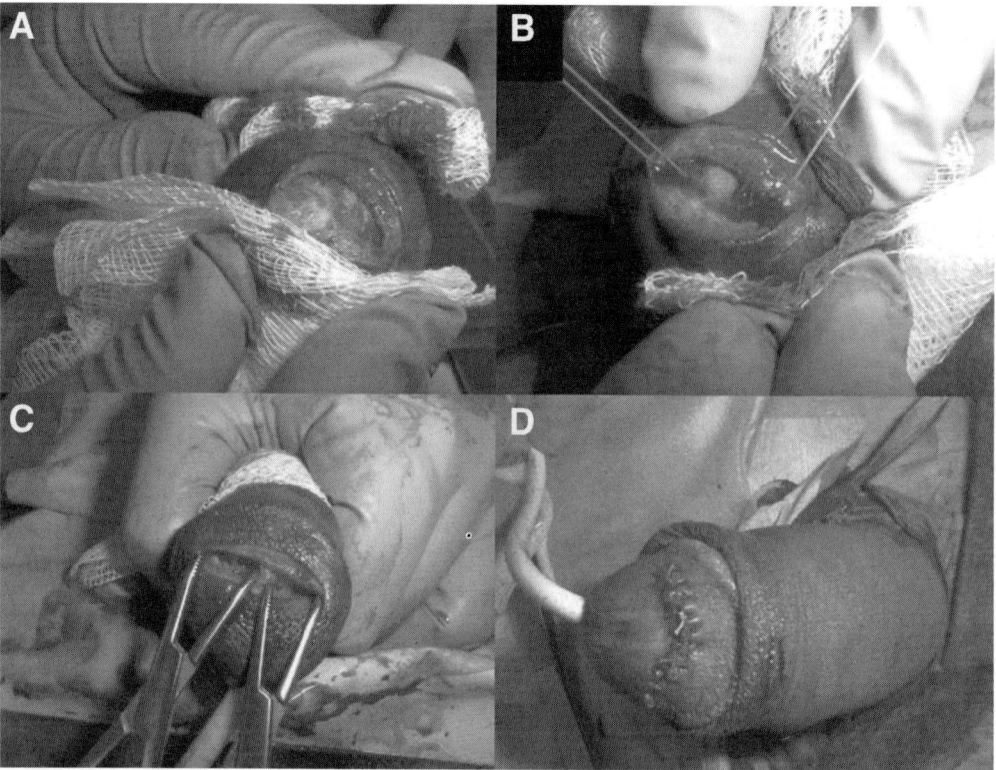

Fig. 3. Al Ghorab shunt: **(A)** semilunar glandular incision exposing tips of corporal bodies; **(B)** holding sutures are placed in corporal tips to prevent retraction after corporal incision is made; **(C)** removal of distal tunica albugineal exposing cavernosal tissue and allowing easy blood drainage; **(D)** watertight wound closure.

agonists may be administered (intracavernosal or oral) on an interval basis to induce complete detumescence.

If, after repeated first-line interventions over several hours, no resolution of the ischemic priapism can be achieved, advancement to surgical shunts is indicated. In the majority of cases, distal shunts are effective (Fig. 3). Proximal shunts are not more efficacious than distal shunts and have a higher complication rate; thus, proximal shunts should be avoided as first-line surgical intervention.

The most important predictor of maintenance of premorbid erectile function is dependent on the duration of the priapism; thus, rapid intervention is a necessity. Kulmala et al. *(68)* reported that men with less than 24 h of priapism have a 92% probability of returning to premorbid erectile functioning vs only 22% if the priapistic episode extended for more than 7 d.

Nonischemic Priapism Management

The diagnosis of high-flow priapism is usually made by history (perineal trauma is almost always reported by patients) and by physical examination (partial and nonpainful erection). Duplex Doppler ultrasound is a noninvasive modality that allows easy visualization and localization of the arterial-lacunar fistula (Fig. 4A). This form

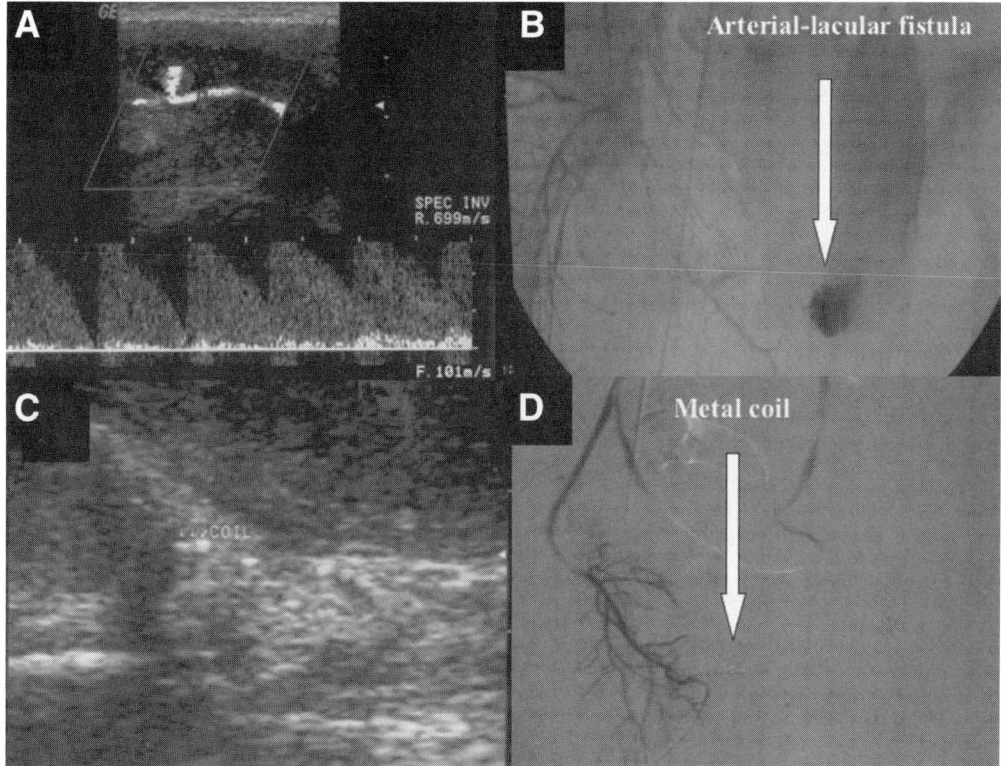

Fig. 4. Arterial priapism: (A) perineal duplex Doppler ultrasound showing arterial lacunar fistula; (B) selective internal pudendal arteriogram documenting arterial lacunar fistula; (C) and (D) selective internal pudendal arteriogram and penile duplex Doppler ultrasound of an impotent man who developed cavernosal artery insufficiency after coil embolization of high-flow priapism.

of priapism is not a compartment syndrome, thus is not a medical emergency. After extensive counseling, selective internal pudendal arteriography and superselective embolization with autologous clot injection will temporarily occlude the lacerated artery allowing the injured vessel to heal. The use of metal coils is associated with permanent and irreversible occlusion of the cavernosal arteries, leading to erectile dysfunction (Fig. 4C,D)

SUMMARY

Ischemic priapism is a pathological pencil erection that persists beyond or is unrelated to sexual stimulation, which requires evaluation and may require emergency management to avoid irreversible corporal fibrosis and permanent erective dysfunction. Arterial, a less common form of priapism, is caused by traumatic unregulated cavernous inflow, thus it is not a compartment syndrome nor a medical emergency. Further research is needed to better understand and manage this potentially devastating condition.

ACKNOWLEDGMENT

This work was supported by grants R01-DK56846 and K01-DK02696 from the National Institute of Diabetes and Digestive and Kidney Diseases.

REFERENCES

1. Papadopoulus I, Kelami A. Priapus and priapism: From mythology to medicine. Urology 1988; 32: 385–386.
2. Callaway T. Unusual case of priapism. London Med Repository 1824; 1: 286.
3. Berger R, Billups K, Brock G, et al. Report of the American Foundation for Urologic Disease (AFUD) Thought Leader Panel for evaluation and treatment of priapism. Int J Impot Res 2001;13(suppl 5): S39–S43.
4. Kulmala RV, Lehtonen TA, Tammela TL. Priapism, its incidence and seasonal distribution in Finland. Scand J Urol Nephrol 1995; 29: 93–96.
5. Eland IA, Van Der Lei J, Stricker BHC, Sturkenboom MJCM. Incidence of priapism in the general population. Urology 2001; 57: 970–972.
6. Adeyoju AB, Olujohungbe AB, Morris J, et al. Priapism in sickle-cell disease; incidence, risk factors and complications—an international multicentre study. BJU Int 2002; 90, 898–902.
7. Banos JE, Bosch F, Farre M. Drug-induced priapism: its etiology, incidence and treatment. Med Toxicol 1989; 4: 46.
8. Junemann KP, Alken P. Pharmacotherapy of erectile dysfunction: a review. Int J Impot Res 1989; 1: 71.
9. Funderburk SJ, Philippart M, Dale G, Cederbaun SD, Vyden JK. Priapism after phenoxybenzamine in a patient with Fabry's disease. N Engl J Med 1984; 290: 60.
10. Law MR, Copland RFP, Armitstead JG, Gabriel R. Labetalol and priapism. Br J Urol 1980; 280: 115.
11. Adams JW, Soucheray JA. Prazosin induced priapism in a diabetic. J Urol 1984; 132: 1208.
12. Bullock N. Prazosin-induced priapism. Br J Urol 1988; 62: 487.
13. Rubin SO. Priapism as a probable sequel to medication. Scand J Urol Nephrol 1968; 2: 81.
14. Duggan ML, Morgan C. Heparin: a cause of priapism? Med J 1970; 63: 1131.
15. Singhal PC, Lynn RI, Scharschmidt LA. Priapism and dialysis. Am J Nephrol 1986; 6: 358.
16. Burke BJ, Scott GL, Smith PJB, Wakerley GR. Heparin-associated priapism. Postgrad Med J 1983; 59: 332.
17. Gralnick H, McKeown LP, Williams SB, Shafer BC, Pierce L. Plasma and platelet von Willebrand's factor defects in uremia. Am J Med 1988; 85: 806.
18. Kem DL, Posey DJ, McDougle CJ. Priapism associated with trazodone in an adolescent with autism. J Am Acad Child Adolesc Psychiatry 2002; 41(7): 758.
19. Lansky MR, Selzer J. Priapism associated with trazodone therapy: case report. J Clin Psychiatry 1984; 45(5): 232–233.
20. Carson CC 3rd, Mino RD. Priapism associated with trazodone therapy. J Urol 1988; 139(2): 369–370.
21. Hanno PM, Lopez R, Wein AJ. Trazodone-induced priapism. Br J Urol 1988; 61(1): 94.
22. Correas Gomez MA, Portillo Martin JA, Martin Garcia B, et al. Trazodone-induced priapism. Actas Urol Esp 2000; 24(10): 840–842.
23. Azadzoi KM, Payton T, Krane RJ, Goldstein I. Effects of intracavernosal trazodone hydrochloride: animal and human studies. J Urol 1980; 144: 1277–1282.
24. Saenz de Tejada I, Ware JC, Blanco R, et al. Pathophysiology of prolonged penile erection associated with trazodone use. J Urol 1991; 145: 60–64.
25. Hyttel J, Larsen JJ, Christensen AV, Arnt J. Receptor-binding profiles of neuroleptics. In: Dyskenesia: Research and Treatment. (Casey DE, Chase TN, Christensen AV, Gerlach J, eds.), Springer-Verlag, New York, NY, 1985, p. 9.
26. Van Rossum JM. The significance of dopamine-receptor blockade for the mechanism of action of neuroleptic drugs. Arch Int Pharmacodyn Ther 1966; 160: 492.
27. Fiorelli RL, Manfrey SJ, Belkoff LH, Finkelstein LH. Priapism associated with intranasal cocaine abuse. J Urol 1990; 143: 581.
28. Rodriguez-Blasquez HM, Cardona PE, Rivera-Herrera JL. Priapism associated with the use of topical cocaine. J Urol 1981; 143: 358.
29. Munarriz R, Hwang J, Goldstein I, Traish AM, Kim NN. Cocaine and ephedrine-induced priapism: case reports and investigation of potential adrenergic mechanisms. Urology. 2003; 62: 187–192.

30. Lakoski JM, Cunningham KA. The interaction of cocaine with central serotonergic neural system: Cellular electrophysiologic approaches. Natl Inst Drug Abuse Res Monogr Ser 1988; 88: 78.
31. Cocores JA, Dackis CA, Gold MS. Sexual dysfunction secondary to cocaine abuse in two patients. J Clin Psychiatry 1986; 47: 384.
32. Hauri D, Spycher M, Bruhlmann W. Erection and priapism: a new physiopathological concept. Urol Int 1983;38:138–145
33. Stackl W, Mee SI Priapism. In: Clinical Urology (Krane RJ, Siroky MB, Fitzpatrick JM, eds.) JB Lippincott, Philadelphia, PA, 1994; pp. 1245–1258.
34. Klein EA, Montague DK, Steiger E. Priapism associated with the use intravenous fat emulsion: case reports and postulated pathogenesis. J Urol 1985; 133: 857.
35. Amris CJ, Brockner J, Larson V. Changes in the coagulability of blood during the infusion of intralipid. Acta Chir Scand 1964; 325(suppl): 70.
36. Brockner J, Amris CJ, Larsen V. Fat infusions and blood coagulation: effect of various fat emulsions on blood coagulability. A comparative study. Acta Chir Scand 1965; 343(suppl): 48.
37. Stiles AD. Priapism following a black widow spider bite. Clin Pediatr 1982; 21: 174.
38. Zelissen PMJ, Stricker BHCh. Severe priapism as a complication of testosterone substitution therapy. Am J Med 1988; 85: 273.
39. Zargooshi J. Priapism as a complication of high dose testosterone therapy in a man with hypogonadism. J Urol 2000; 163(3): 907.
40. Madrid Garcia FJ, Diez Hernandez A, Madronero Cuevas C, Rivas Escudero JA, Delgado Gomez M, Garcia Alonso J. Priapism secondary to testosterone administration in the treatment of delayed puberty. Arch Esp Urol 2001; 54(7): 703–705.
41. Fernando IN, Tobias JS. Priapism in a patient on tamoxifen. Lancet 1989; 1; 436.
42. Hamre MR, Harmon EP, Kirkpatrick DV, Stern MJ, Humbert JR. Priapism as a complication of sickle cell disease. J Urol 1991; 145: 1.
43. Tarry WF, Duckett JW, Snyder HM. Urological complications of sickle cell disease in a pediatric population. J Urol 1987; 138: 592–594.
44. Fowler JEJ, Koshy M, Strub M, Chinn SK. Priapism associated with the sickle cell hemoglobinopathies: prevalence, natural history and sequelae. J Urol 1991; 145: 65–68.
45. Mantadakis E, Cavender JD, Rogers ZR, Ewalt DH, Buchanan GR. Prevalence of priapism in children with sickle cell disease. J Pediatr Hematol/Oncol 1999; 21: 518–522.
46. Jackson N, Franlin IM, Hughes MA. Recurrent priapism following splenectomy for thalassaemia intermedia. Br J Surg 1986; 73: 698.
47. Leifer W, Leifer G. Priapism caused by primary thrombocythemia. J Urol 1979; 121: 254.
48. Winter CC, McDowell G. Experience with 105 patients with priapism: Update review of all aspects. J Urol 1988; 140: 980.
49. Lapan DI, Graham AR, Bangert JL, Boyer JT, Conner WT. Amyloidosis presenting as priapism. Urology 1980; 15(2):167–170.
50. Garcia-Consuegra J, Padron M, Jaureguizar E, Carrascosa C, Ramos J. Priapism and Fabry's disease: a case report. Eur J Pediatr 1990; 149: 500.
51. Bedbrook G. Anonymous. The Care and Management of Spinal Cord Injuries. Springer-Verlag, New York, 1981, p. 155.
52. Baba H, Maezawa Y, Furusawa N, Kawahara N, Tomita K. Lumbar spinal stenosis causing intermittent priapism. Paraplegia 1995; 33: 338–345.
53. Hattori T, Otani T, Ito Y, Takeda H. [A report of two cases of priapism with metastatic penile tumor.] Nippon Hinyokika Gakkai Zasshi [Jap J Urol] 2002; 93(4): 568–572.
54. Casoli E, Di Fiore F, Longobardi S, Intilla O, Pone D. Metastatic penile lesions secondary to transitional cell carcinoma of the bladder: a rare cause of "malignant priapism." Arc Ital Urol Androl 2002; 74(1): 48–49.
55. Morga Egea JP, Ferrero Doria R, Guzman Martinez-Valls PL, et al. Metastasis priapism. Report of four new cases and review of the literature. Arch Esp Urol 2000; 53(5): 447–452.
56. Benson GS. Priapism. AUA Update Series, 1996, Lesson 11, Vol. XV, American Urologic Association, Office of Education, Houston, TX.
57. Pohl J, Pott B, Kleinhans G. Priapism: a three phase concept of management according to aetiology and prognosis. Br J Urol 1986; 58(2): 113–118.

58. Gerstenbluth RE, Kick PS, Srodes AD, Seftel AD. Priapism secondary to hypertriglyceridemia. J Urol 2003; 169(3): 1088.
59. Fernandez Duran AM, Martin Garcia C, Fernandez Gomez J, Jimenez Lopez-Lucendo N, Sampietro Crespo A. Priapism secondary to a bilateral abscess of the corpora cavernosa. Actas Urol Esp 1999; 23(1): 64–66.
60. Bloom DA, Wan J, Key D. Disorders of the male external genitalia and inguinal canal. In Clinical Pediatric Urology, 3rd ed. (Kelalis PI, King LR, Belman AB, eds.), Saunders, Philadelphia, PA, 1992, p. 1023.
61. Saenz de Tejada I, Kim NN, Daley JT, et al. Acidosis impairs rabbit smooth muscle contractility. J Urol 1997; 157(2): 722–726.
62. McAuley I, Munarriz RM, Huang YH, et al. Intracavernosal high dose phenylephrine in the treatment of veno-occlusive priapism: from bench to bedside. Paper presented at AUA meeting, 1999.
63. Goldhaber JI, Weiss JN. Oxygen free radicals and cardiac reperfusion abnormalities. Hypertension 1992; 20: 118–127.
64. Munarriz R, Park K, Huang YH, et al. Reperfusion of ischemic corporal tissue: physiologic and biochemical changes in an animal model of ischemic priapism. Urology 2003; 62: 760–764.
65. Hakim LS, Kulaksizoglu H, Mulligan R, Greenfield A, Goldstein I. Evolving concepts in the diagnosis and treatment of arterial high flow priapism. J Urol 1996; 155(2): 541–548.
66. Witt MA, Goldstein I, Saenz de Tejada I, Greenfield A, Krane RJ. Traumatic laceration of the intracavernosal arteries: the pathophysiology of non-ischemic, high flow, arterial priapism. J Urol 1990; 143: 129.
67. Bodner DR, Lindan R, Leffler E, Kursh E, Resnick MI. The application of intracarvernous injection of vasoactive medications for erection in men with spinal cord injury. J Urol 1987; 138: 138.
68. Kulmala RV, Letonen TA, Tammela TL. Preservation of potency after treatment for priapism. Scand J Urol Nephrol 1916; 30: 313–316.s

# 15 The Acute Scrotum

Gerald C. Mingin, MD
and Hiep T. Nguyen, MD, FAAP

CONTENT

INTRODUCTION
TESTICULAR AND APPENDICAL TORSION
EPIDIDYMITIS/EPIDIDYMO-ORCHITIS
TESTICULAR TRAUMA
SCROTAL AND PERINEAL BURNS
MISCELLANEOUS CAUSES OF ACUTE SCROTUM
SUMMARY
REFERENCES

INTRODUCTION

It is not uncommon for a child, adolescent, or adult to present with scrotal pain, tenderness, or swelling. These patients who present with an acute or subacute scrotum require prompt evaluation. Timely and accurate diagnosis is required to prevent testicular loss. The differential diagnosis is extensive (Table 1), but the diagnosis can be determined based on history, physical examination, and limited laboratory and radiological evaluation.

TESTICULAR AND APPENDICAL TORSION

Torsion of the spermatic cord and testicular/epididymal appendages is one of more common causes of an acute scrotum. Torsion of the former is a true surgical emergency; that of the latter requires no surgical intervention. Although testicular torsion can occur at any age, there is a bimodal distribution in the age of presentation, during the neonatal period and during puberty. Extravaginal torsion is caused by the spermatic cord twisting on itself above the level of the tunica vaginalis and is seen in the neonatal period (Fig. 1). Several explanations, including multiparity, excessive uterine pressure, and a strong cremasteric contraction have been suggested *(1)*.

Intravaginal torsion involves torsion of the spermatic cord within the tunica vaginalis. This so-called bell clapper deformity (Fig. 2) is associated with an abnormal fixation of the testis and epididymis and is most commonly seen in adolescents who present with

From: *Urological Emergencies: A Practical Guide*
Edited by: H. Wessells and J. W. McAninch © Humana Press Inc., Totowa, NJ

Table 1
Differential Diagnosis for Acute/Subacute Scrotum

Testicular torsion
Appendical torsion (testis or epididymis)
Epididymitis/epididymo-orchitis
Inguinal hernia (reducible or incarcerated)
Hydrocele
Trauma (mechanical, burns, or animal/insect bite)
Testicular neoplasms
Spermatocele
Varicocele
Dermatological lesions
Inflammatory vasculitis (Henoch-Schonlein purpura)
Idiopathic scrotal edema
Referred pain

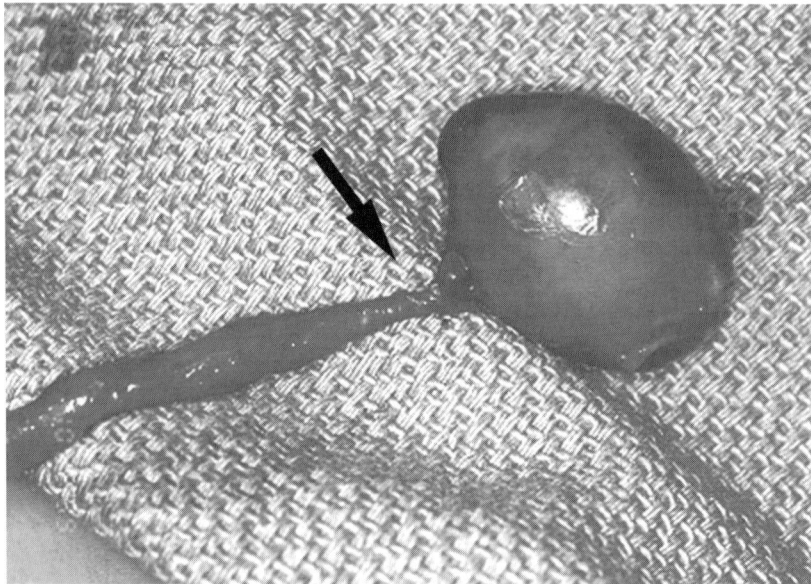

Fig. 1. The left testis of a 3-d-old infant with an extravaginal torsion. Note that the entire cord has twisted above the tunica vaginalis (arrow). The epididymis and testis are enclosed within the tunica; consequently, they are not visualized.

torsion. These patients may also present with intermittent torsion, in which the cord can torse on itself and then spontaneously untwist (Fig. 3).

The appendix testis (Fig. 4A), a müllerian remnant, and the appendix epididymis (Fig. 4B), a Wolffian remnant, are also susceptible to torsion. Torsion of these appendages occurs more commonly during adolescence. It has been suggested that hormonal stimulation during puberty increases their size, making them more susceptible to twisting around their small blood supply.

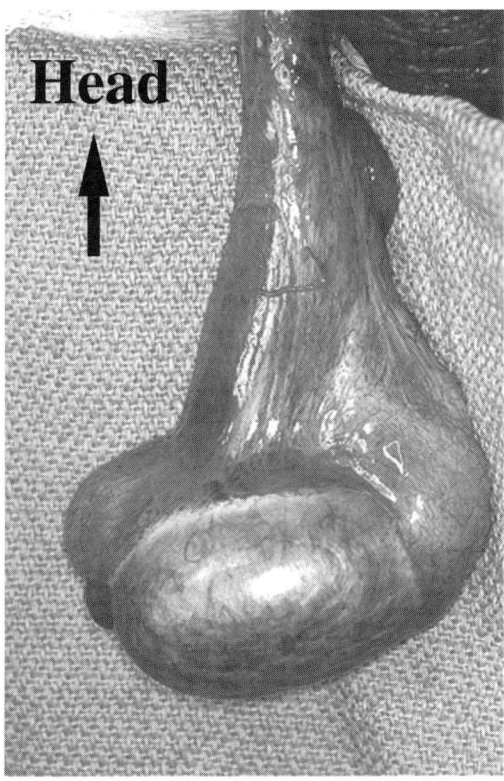

Fig. 2. The right testis of a 14-yr-old boy who presents with intravaginal torsion has the bell clapper deformity, which may predispose to torsion of the spermatic cord.

Clinical Presentation

Typically, patients with intravaginal testicular torsion will present with acute onset of severe scrotal pain, frequently making physical examination difficult. Some patients may only present with pain referred to the ipsilateral lower abdomen. Torsion can occur following trauma or athletic activity; however, in most cases the patient is awakened from sleep. Nausea and vomiting may be associated with testicular torsion; urinary symptoms such as dysuria and urgency are usually absent. Important signs of torsion include a firm testicle riding high in the scrotum, an abnormally transverse orientation of the testis, and the absence of a cremasteric reflex *(2)*. In many cases, acute hydrocele or marked scrotal edema develops when several hours have passed since the onset of the scrotal pain (Fig. 5). Fever and an elevated white blood cell count are not frequently associated with testicular torsion.

In contrast, patients with extravaginal neonatal torsion present with painless swelling and scrotal discoloration. It is often found incidentally on newborn examination, when a firm testis with an associated hydrocele is noted. Interestingly, associated scrotal erythema is not often present, but the overlying skin is discolored by the underlying hemorrhagic necrosis.

Intermittent testicular torsion has a similar presentation to that of intravaginal torsion, except that the episode is self-limited, with resolution of symptoms after the cord spontaneously untwists. Many who present with acute testicular torsion have a history of prior

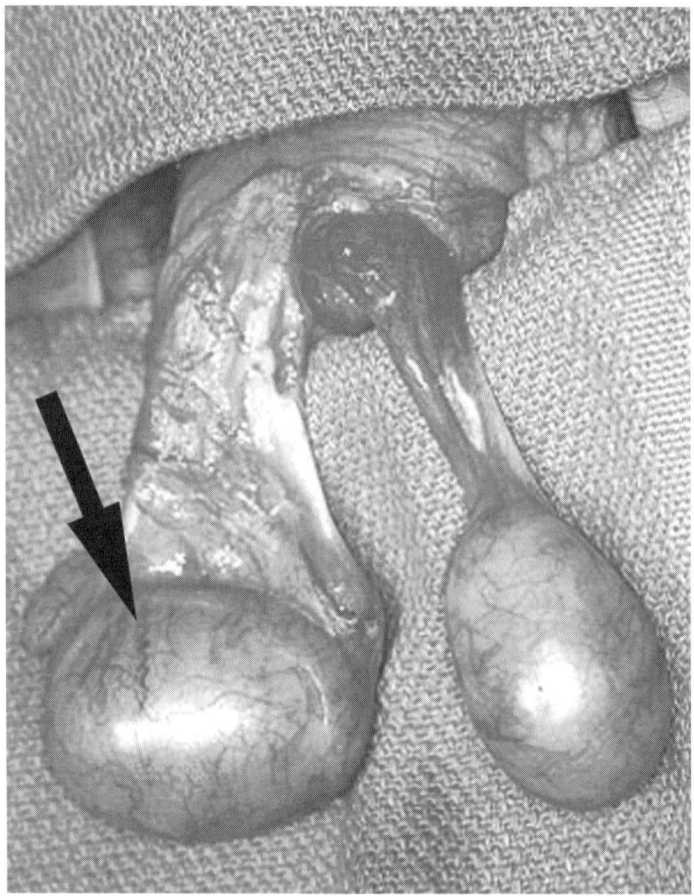

Fig. 3. This patient presented with five previous episodes of acute right testicular pain that spontaneously resolved after 10 to 15 min. On scrotal exploration, a bell clapper deformity was noted on the right side. Note the normal lie of the left testis.

episodes consistent with intermittent testicular torsion. Those with intermittent torsion are likely to have normal physical exam at time of evaluation, when the pain has resolved.

Patients with torsion of the appendix testis or epididymis can also present with pain similar to those with intravaginal testicular torsion. However, the presentation for appendical torsion can be quite variable, from an insidious onset of scrotal discomfort to acute severe scrotal pain. Consequently, it is often difficult to differentiate appendical torsion from other causes of acute scrotum. At the earlier stages, the pain may be localized to the upper pole of the testis or epididymis, and a firm nodule can sometimes be palpated in this region of the scrotum. In some cases, the infarcted appendage can be seen through the scrotal skin as a blue dot, which is considered pathognomic for appendical torsion. In the later stages, scrotal wall edema and erythema can develop, distorting the physical examination. The cremasteric reflex is usually preserved, and the testis should remain mobile.

In those who are suspected of having testicular torsion on a clinical basis, prompt surgical exploration is warranted. Adjunctive radiological tests should only be obtained when their purpose is to confirm the absence of testicular torsion so that surgical explo-

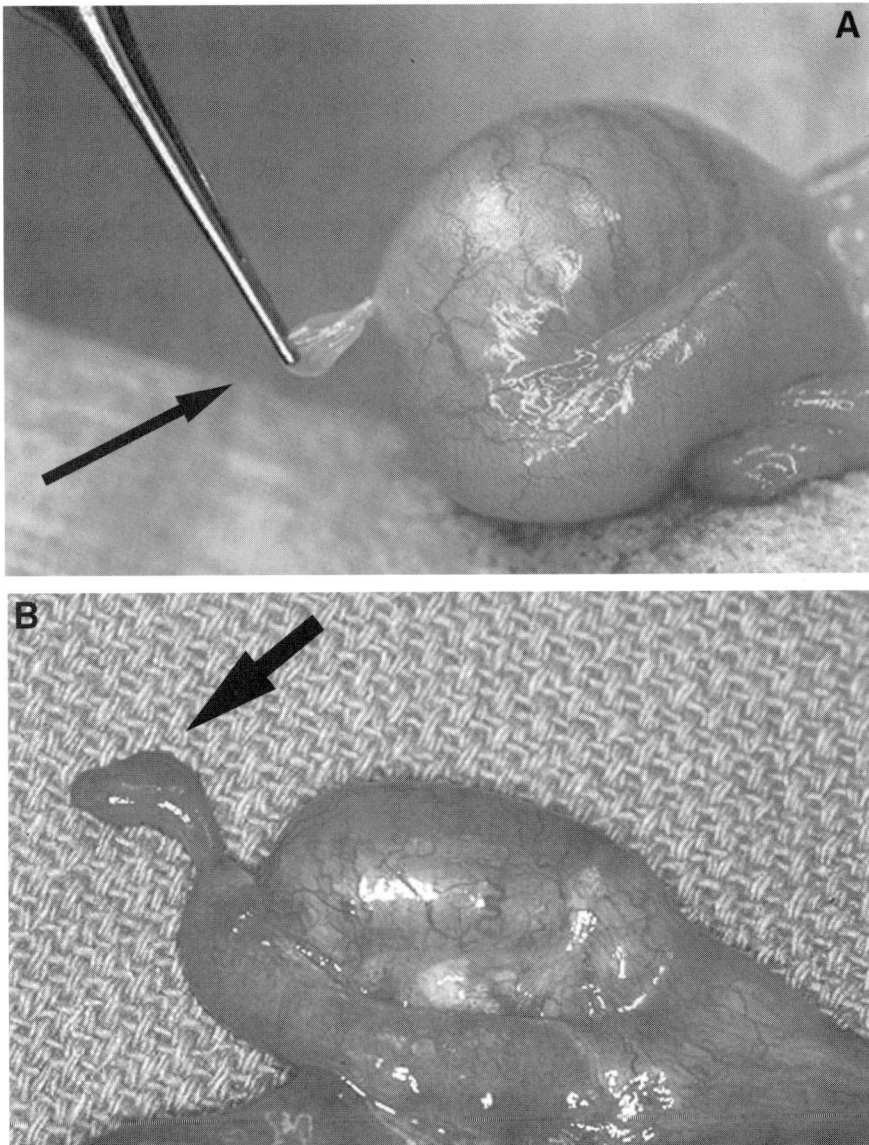

Fig. 4. (A) The appendix testis (arrow). **(B)** The appendix epididymitis (arrow). Both appendages are susceptible to twisting around their small vascular pedicle.

ration can be avoided. In these cases, color or power Doppler ultrasound or scrotal scintigraphy may be obtained. In ruling out testicular torsion, there is no absolute gold standard. False negatives can occur with any of these modalities. The choice of which modality to utilize varies with institution, depending on local experience, availability, and reliability of the tests.

Color Doppler ultrasound studies can assess the anatomy of the scrotum and its content while determining the presence or absence of testicular blood flow (as measured by velocity). The sensitivity of color Doppler ultrasonography is reported to be as high as 90%, with a specificity of 99% *(3)*. Caution must be used in the interpretation of these

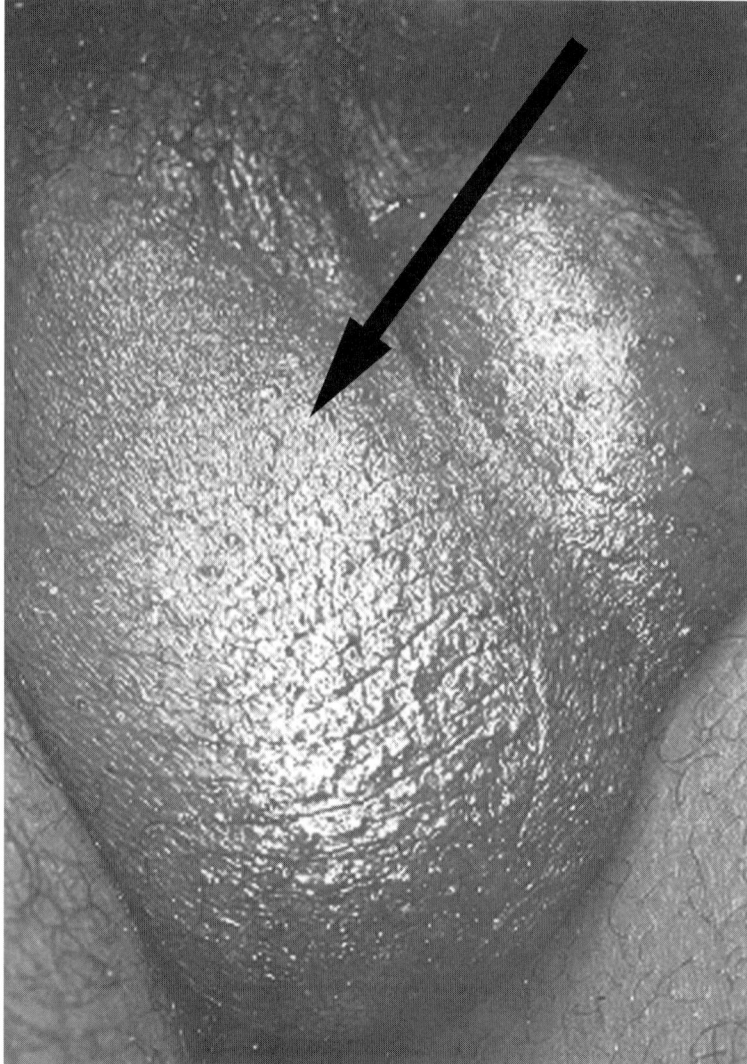

Fig. 5. The scrotum of a 14-yr-old boy who presented with acute right testicular pain. The patient sought medical attention 12 h after the onset of pain. An acute hydrocele (arrow) has resulted, making palpation of the testis more difficult.

studies because almost 40% of patients, especially those younger than 8 yr, may fail to demonstrate flow on the asymptomatic side *(4,5)*. Power Doppler ultrasonography measures blood flow by detecting the number of red blood cells as opposed to the velocity of flow. Although blood flow is more consistently detected in younger children with power Doppler *(4)*, evidence from animal studies suggested that power Doppler and color Doppler are equally efficacious in the detection of torsion *(6)*.

Radionuclide imaging was originally the study of choice for ruling out testicular torsion. However, it only allows for the assessment of blood flow. Its positive predictive value has been reported to be around 75%, with a sensitivity of 90% and a specificity of 89% *(7)*. Hyperemia of the scrotal wall can give false impressions of testicular blood flow. In addition, it is difficult to image children with small scrotal sacs or testis using this study.

Treatment

Faced with a suspected diagnosis of testicular torsion, the patient should be taken to surgery without delay. Manual detorsion may be tried if surgical intervention cannot be done for a period of time. The testis should be turned caudal to cranial and medial to lateral *(8)*. If the first attempt is unsuccessful, the testis should be turned in the opposite direction. If the detorsion is successful, the pain should resolve immediately. However, this process is often very painful, and manual detorsion may not completely correct the obstructed blood flow. Consequently, surgical intervention is still required following manual detorsion.

There are several options for surgical fixation. Traditionally, the testis has been fixed by placing a suture through the tunica albuginea and into the wall of the scrotum. However, recurrent torsion has been reported with this technique. Fixation can be accomplished by securing the testis to the septum or placement into a dartos pouch. For transseptal fixation, the scrotum is opened through an incision in the median raphe; for the pouch fixation, the incision is made transversely, following the skin creases of the scrotum. When using the later method, the dartos pouch is made after the skin is incised. The tunica vaginalis is then entered, and the testis is examined. The spermatic cord should be detorsed to restore blood flow. The affected testis should be placed in a warm sponge and observed for several minutes to determine viability. If it is nonviable, then the necrotic testis should be removed. Exploration of the contralateral testis should also be performed, and in all cases, the contralateral testis must be fixed.

The testicles can be fixed to the median septum with three to four fine, nonreactive, nonabsorbable sutures. These sutures can be brought through the septum, enabling the contralateral side to be fixed concurrently. Alternatively, dartos pouches are created, and fixation relies on scarification of the testis. The tunica vaginalis is everted, and the testicle is placed into the dartos pouch. A nonabsorbable suture is then used to secure the dartos tissue around the cord. This technique is advantageous in that complications such as abscess formation and tubular atrophy are uncommon. In addition, there have been no reported cases of recurrent torsion with this technique. Intermittent torsion is corrected using either of the above techniques on a semiemergent basis.

The treatment of neonatal torsion is controversial. Some suggest that surgical exploration is unnecessary; others advocate immediate surgical exploration and fixation of the contralateral side. It is rare to salvage the affected testis in a patient with unilateral neonatal torsion. In addition, of more than 30 cases of bilateral neonatal torsion reported in the literature, only two testicles have been successfully salvaged *(9)*. The most important reason for exploration in our opinion is to prevent possible unilateral torsion from becoming bilateral anorchia. In the rare case of bilateral neonatal torsion, a more conservative approach can be taken. The newborn's general condition and anesthetic considerations should be evaluated to determine whether to proceed with surgical intervention.

The treatment of twisted testicular appendages is nonsurgical. If the diagnosis is certain, conservative therapy with limitation of activity and administration of nonsteroidal analgesics can be instituted. Most of the symptoms will dissipate once the acute changes of acute necrosis resolve. In rare instances, surgical exploration may be undertaken if conservative management fails. Simple excision of the torsed appendage is curative.

EPIDIDYMITIS/EPIDIDYMO-ORCHITIS

Another common cause of an acute scrotum is inflammation/infection of the epididymis. The infection may also involve the testis (epididymo-orchitis). Although it is an uncommon diagnosis in children *(10)*, it is a more common problem in young adults. Several different etiologies are responsible, including infection, trauma, and anatomical abnormalities.

Bacterial infection is common in patients who are sexually active. However, viral agents such as mumps, coxsackie, echovirus, and adenoviruses have been identified in children with epididymitis *(11,12)*. Traumatic causes include straining or lifting, for which a sudden increase in abdominal pressure causes reflux of sterile urine, leading to epididymal inflammation. Torsion of a testicular appendage can also lead to a reactive epididymitis.

Anatomical abnormalities and dysfunctional voiding are further causes of epididymitis. Insertion of an ectopic ureter into the seminal vesicle as well as bladder outlet obstruction, as in posterior urethral valves, may lead to epididymitis. Detrussor-sphincter dyssynergia, secondary to neurogenic and nonneurogenic bladder dysfunction, will lead to increased bladder pressures, with the possibility of sterile reflux. Finally, epididymitis may be associated with systemic diseases, including sarcoidosis, Kawasaki's disease, and Henoch-Schonlein purpura *(13)*.

Clinical Presentation

The most common presenting symptoms include scrotal swelling, erythema, and pain. Epididymitis is usually an indolent process, but may present in a fashion similar to testicular torsion. Epididymitis is more likely in a patient with a past history of urinary tract infection, urethral catheterization, or urinary tract surgery. Although fever and urinary symptoms such as dysuria, urethral discharge, and hematuria are more common in patients with epididymitis than with testicular torsion, many patients with epididymitis may not have any of these symptoms.

On physical examination, localized epididymal or generalized scrotal tenderness may be found. The cremasteric reflex is usually preserved. Evaluation of the urine often demonstrates pyuria and bacteriuria; however, urine cultures may be sterile in 40% of the cases *(10,13)* because virus can also be an etiological agent.

Scrotal imaging can be used to help distinguish between epididymitis and torsion. In the cases of epididymitis, Doppler ultrasonography or radionuclide imaging demonstrates increased blood flow. On ultrasonography, the testis is often enlarged and has a reactive hydrocele.

Treatment

Epididymitis is treated with a combination of scrotal elevation, nonsteroidal antiinflammatory agents, and antibiotics when appropriate. Patients who are sexually active should be cultured for gonorrhea/chlamydia and treated with an appropriate course of antibiotics. Limitation of activity, scrotal elevation, and application of heat or cold will help alleviate scrotal pain. Urethral instrumentation should be avoided.

In children with suspected epididymitis, a urinalysis and urine culture should be performed. In addition, a voiding cystourethrogram and a renal bladder ultrasound should be obtained to look for anatomical abnormalities such as ectopic ureter if a urinary tract infection is documented. If the above studies are normal, the child should be worked up for unrecognized dysfunctional voiding as a cause for reflux of urine into the epididymis.

TESTICULAR TRAUMA

Testicular trauma is an infrequent occurrence because of the mobility and position of the testicle within the tunica albuginea. The etiology is most often caused by a direct blow that compresses the testicle against the pubic bone *(14)* as a result of a sports injury or motor vehicle accident *(15)*. Blunt trauma accounts for 85% of the cases; the remainder result from penetrating injuries *(16)*. There is a slight preponderance of injuries on the right side, possibly because of the higher riding position of the testicle *(15)*. The majority of patients are between 10 and 30 yr of age.

Types of injuries include testicular contusions with hematoceles and hematoma, testicular rupture, and traumatic dislocation. Hematoceles result from bleeding into the tunica vaginalis; a hematoma develops from intratesticular bleeding. Patients who sustain testicular injury may also present with torsion. Hydroceles and pyoceles may present as delayed sequelae of an acute injury.

Clinical Presentation

In patients with testicular injury, the scrotum may be tense, edematous, ecchymotic, or fail to transilluminate. In these patients, there are often associated findings, such as nausea, emesis, and urinary retention. Because of the nature of the injury and the force required to compress the testicle, other abdominal or pelvic injuries in particular pelvic fractures should be ruled out. This is especially true for testicular dislocation, for which the scrotum will be well developed, but no testicle is palpable within the scrotum. In many cases, the diagnosis is delayed; however, palpation of the inguinal area will reveal a normal testicle.

Urethral injuries are also commonly associated with scrotal trauma. Bleeding at the urethral meatus in association with a pelvic fracture or perineal ecchymosis is an indication for obtaining a retrograde urethrogram. Traumatic torsion will present as a painful high-riding testicle, which may have a transverse lie. Scrotal pain and swelling in the presence of a fever and elevated white blood cell count several days after a traumatic event suggest the presence of a pyocele.

The most useful diagnostic tool in the evaluation of closed testicular trauma is ultrasonography of the scrotum. Intratesticular areas of sonolucency, as well as hyperechoic and hypoechoic regions with poorly defined testicular margins, are suggestive of testicular rupture or hematoma *(14,17,18)*. Absence of testicular blood flow is indicative of traumatic torsion.

Treatment

Patients with penetrating trauma or ultrasound evidence of testicular rupture require immediate surgical exploration. If the diagnosis is uncertain and there is any possibility of an underlying testicular tumor, an inguinal approach is best; otherwise, a transverse scrotal incision is made. In the case of testicular rupture, the devitalized tissue is excised, and the capsule is repaired (Fig. 6A,B). Failure to repair these injuries can lead to persistent pain, abscess formation, and testicular atrophy.

Orchiectomy should be avoided when there is remnant functioning tissue. In the rare occurrence of complete traumatic amputation without scrotal avulsion, prompt

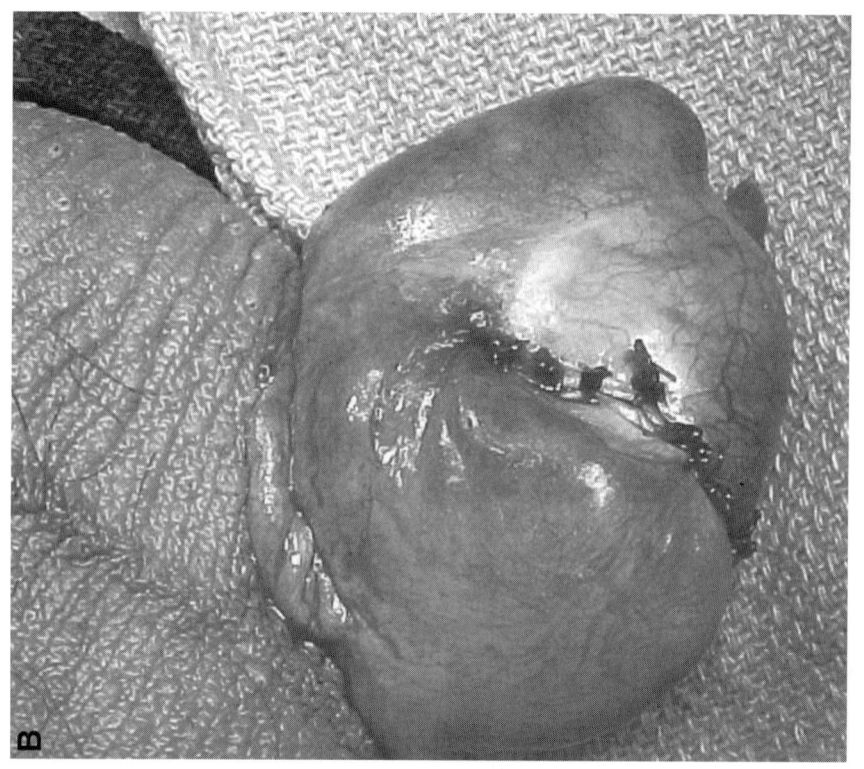
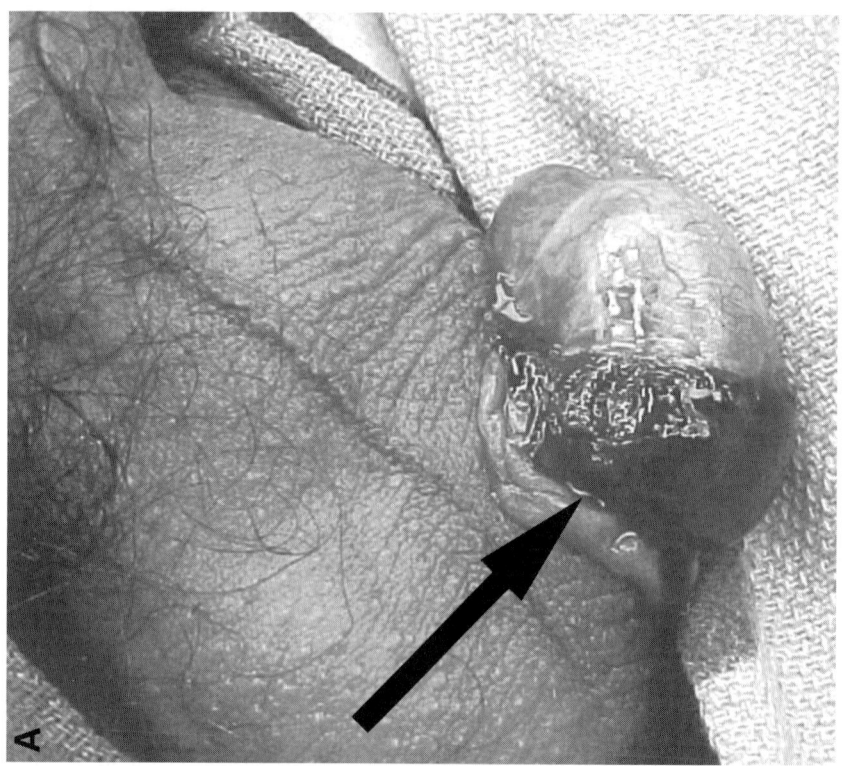

Fig. 6. (**A**) Traumatic rupture of the testicle with devitalized tissue (arrow). (**B**) The devitalized tissue has been excised and the capsule approximated

microsurgical repair of the vessels can be performed. If this is not an option, orchiectomy should be considered. Autotransplantation into a subcutaneous thigh pocket can be attempted; however, the results to date have been disappointing, with atrophy and necrosis more common outcomes *(19)*.

Dog bites to the scrotum are occasionally encountered. These wounds should be debrided, and the patient should be given broad-spectrum antibiotics and tetanus and rabies vaccinations. These wounds should only be closed in the absence of infection *(20)*. Traumatic torsion is corrected by surgical detorsion of the testicle, followed by the placement of the testicle in a dartos pouch. The testicle may be secured in place with a nonabsorbable suture. Testicular dislocation requires immediate surgical reduction. Although closed reduction may be attempted, it is associated with a high failure rate *(21)*. In addition, there is the possibility of torsion or testicular rupture associated with dislocation, which is best managed in an open fashion.

Evacuation of a scrotal or tunical hematoma is controversial. Open evacuation may lead to infection. However, failure to relieve the hematocele can lead to pressure-induced atrophy of the testicle. It is our policy when confronted with a tense subcapsular hematoma to open the tunica albuginea and drain the blood. Patients diagnosed with a mild contusion and no changes in testicular architecture are best managed with bed rest, scrotal elevation, and nonsteroidal anti-inflammatory agents.

SCROTAL AND PERINEAL BURNS

Burns to the scrotum and perineum occur infrequently. Anatomically, the scrotum is protected by the thighs. In combination with the looseness of the scrotal skin and the retraction of the sack by the cremasteric muscles, these features help to protect the testicles. Isolated scrotal burns are uncommon, and most are seen in patients with more extensive burns *(22)*. Scald burns are more common in very young children, whereas flame or electrical burns affect older children.

Treatment depends on the type of burn incurred. Most first-degree and superficial second-degree burns respond to conservative treatment. Michielsen et al. *(23)* reported an 81% success rate in treating these patients with physiological dressings and topical antimicrobials. Of these children, 14% were treated with allografts, for an overall 95% rate of wound healing. Patients with deep second- or third-degree burns will require more surgical procedures; however, those with deep flame or electrical burns suffer a dramatically high incidence of partial penile loss, testicular loss, and groin contractures *(22)*. The outcome of these patients is dictated by the severity of the initial injury.

MISCELLANEOUS CAUSES OF ACUTE SCROTUM

Included in the differential diagnosis for the acute/subacute scrotum are hernias/ hydroceles. In children, a persistent processus vaginalis allows fluid or omentum/bowel to descend into the scrotum, resulting in a communicating hydrocele or hernia, respectively. In adults, hernia results from a weakness in the abdominal wall that allows its content to descend into the scrotum. When pain is present, bowel incarceration in a hernia sac should be considered. Prompt surgical exploration should be undertaken. If the diagnosis is uncertain, Doppler ultrasonography may demonstrate bowel in the inguinal canal or scrotal sac. However, the ultrasonographic findings may be inconclusive. Given the serious, potential complication of ischemic bowel, inguinal exploration should be undertaken when an incarcerated hernia is suspected.

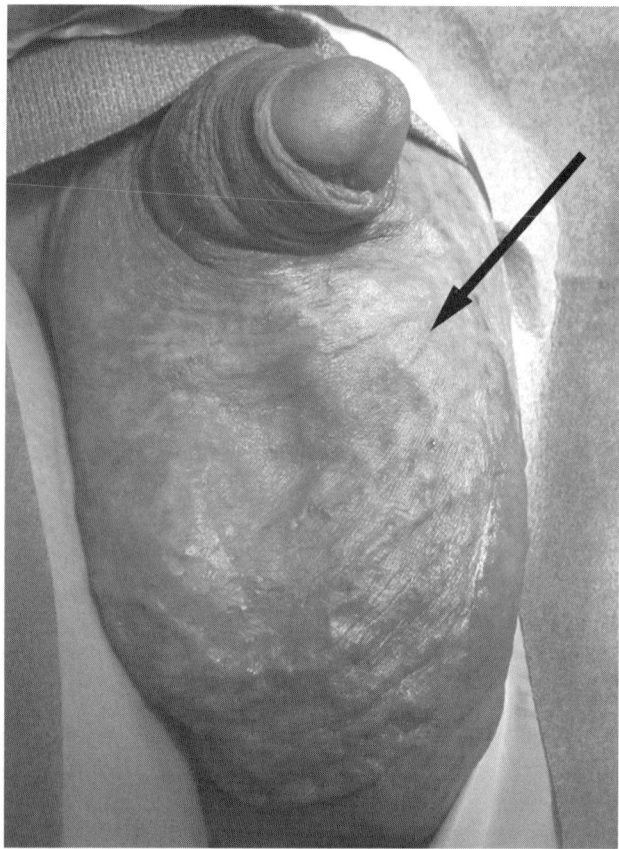

Fig. 7. A varicocele is noted above the left testis (arrow). Note the "wormlike" appearance of the varicocele that often dissipates on recumbence.

Varicocele results from dilation of veins of the pampiniform plexus of the spermatic cord. It is estimated that approx 15% of men have varicocele *(24)*. Its formation is partly caused by increased venous pressure in the left renal vein, collateral venous anastomoses, and incompetent valves of the internal spermatic vein. Occasionally, thrombosis of the varicocele results in inguinal or scrotal pain that is often relieved by assuming the supine position. In most cases, varicocele presents as a painless, compressible mass above or surrounding the testis (Fig. 7).

When symptomatic, treatment of varicocele is indicated. Ligation of the varicocele can be performed using a retroperitoneal, inguinal, or subinguinal approach. Alternatively, angiographic embolization can be performed to occlude the dilated veins. The choice of surgical technique is dependent on the surgeon's familiarity and consideration of potential complications, such as hydrocele formation, varicocele recurrence, and testicular atrophy.

Henonch-Schonlein purpura is a systemic vasculitis that can cause scrotal swelling and pain similar to that of torsion or epididymitis. The cause of the vasculitis is not known, but can involve the testis and/or epididymis *(25)*. Patients with Henonch-Schonlein purpura may have concurrent abdominal or joint pain, nephritis, hematuria, and purpura skin lesions. Scrotal involvement occurs in 35% of patients with Henonch-Schonlein purpura. Typically, the scrotum is diffusely tender with generalized erythema.

Urinalysis often demonstrates hematuria and occasionally proteinuria. Color Doppler ultrasonography or radionuclide scintigraphy shows increased blood flow. Scrotal involvement by Henonch-Schonlein purpura is self-limiting, and observation is usually indicated.

Like Henonch-Schonlein purpura, acute idiopathic scrotal edema is a self-limiting process that results in acute/subacute scrotal swelling *(26)*. Etiological factors include allergic or chemical dermatitis, insect bites, and trauma. Acute idiopathic scrotal edema is usually not associated with erythema, fever, urinary symptoms, hematuria, or pyuria. Pain is likely to be minimal, but pruritus may be significant. The normal testes can be palpated through the thickened scrotal wall. Examination of the perineum should be performed to rule out a contiguous process, such as a perineal abscess, which can also result in scrotal edema. When the diagnosis is unclear, Doppler ultrasonography should be done to evaluate testicular anatomy and blood flow. Acute idiopathic scrotal edema is self-limited and does not require any surgical intervention or antibiotic treatment.

SUMMARY

In summary, any male child who presents with complaints of scrotal pain, tenderness, or swelling should be promptly evaluated. Although the differential diagnosis is extensive, testicular torsion and rupture should be considered based on a through history, physical examination, and appropriate radiological evaluation. However, if testicular torsion is suspected based on history and physical examination, operative management should not be delayed while awaiting radiological confirmation. Testicular salvage is only possible when the diagnosis is considered early in the evaluation of the patient with the acute scrotum.

REFERENCES

1. Barca PR, Dargallo T, Jardon JA, Estevez E, Bautista A, Cives RV. Bilateral testicular torsion in the neonatal period. J Urol 1997; 158: 1957–1959.
2. Rabinowitz R. The importance of the cremasteric reflex in acute scrotal swelling in children. J Urol 1984; 132: 89–90.
3. Baker LA, Sigman D, Mathews RI, Benson J, Docimo SG. An analysis of clinical outcomes using color Doppler testicular ultrasound for testicular torsion. Pediatrics 2000; 105: 604–606.
4. Bader TR, Kammerhuber F, Herneth AM. Testicular blood flow in boys as assessed at color Doppler and power Doppler sonography. Radiology 1997; 202: 559–564.
5. Ingram S, Hollman A. Colour Doppler sonography of the normal pediatric testis. Clin Radiol 1994; 49: 266–267.
6. Lee FT Jr, Winter DB, Madsen FA, et al. Conventional color Doppler velocity sonography vs color Doppler energy sonography for the diagnosis of acute experimental torsion of the spermatic cord. Am J Roentgenol 1996; 167: 785–790.
7. Levy OM, Gittelman MC, Strashun AM, Cohen EL, Fine EJ. Diagnosis of acute testicular torsion using radionuclide scanning. J Urol 1983; 129: 975–977.
8. Kiesling VJ Jr, Schroeder DE, Pauljev P, Hull J. Spermatic cord block and manual reduction: primary treatment for spermatic cord torsion. J Urol 1984; 132: 921–923.
9. Cooper CS, Snyder OB, Hawtrey CE. Bilateral neonatal testicular torsion. Clin Pediatr 1997; 36: 653–656.
10. Siegel A, Snyder H, and Duckett, J.W. Epidymitis in infants and boys: underlying urogenital anomalies and efficacy of imaging modalities. J Urol 1987; 138: 1100–1103.
11. Hermansen MC, Shusid MJ, Sty JR. Bacterial epididymoorchitis in children and adolescents. Clin Pediatr 1980; 19: 812–815.

12. Coran AG, Perlmutter AD. Mumps epididymitis without orchitis. N Engl J Med 1965; 272: 735.
13. Likitnukul S, McCraken GH, Nelson JD. Epididymitis in children and adolescents. A 20-year retrospective study. Am J Dis Child 1987; 141: 41–44.
14. Macdermott JP, Gray BK, Hamilton Stewart PA. Traumatic rupture of the testis. Br J Urol 1988; 62: 179.
15. Schuster G. Traumatic rupture of the testicle and review of the literature. J Urol 1982; 127: 1194–1196.
16. Cass AS. Testicular trauma. J Urol 1983; 129: 299.
17. Lupetin AR. The traumatized scrotum: ultrasound evaluation. Radiology 1983; 148: 203.
18. Friedman SG, Rose JG, Winston MA. Ultrasound and nuclear medicine evaluation in acute testicular trauma. J Urol 1981; 125: 748.
19. Evins SC, Whittle T, Rouse SN. Self emasculation. Review of the literature, report of a case and outline of the objective management. J Urol 1977; 118: 775.
20. Wolf JS, Turzan C, Cattolica EV, Mcaninch JW. Dog bites to the male genitalia: characteristics, management and comparison with human bites. J Urol 1993; 149: 286–289.
21. Lee JY, Cass AS, Streitz JM. Traumatic dislocation of the testes and bladder rupture. Urology 1992; 40: 506–508.
22. Angel C, Shu T, French D, Orihuela E, Lukefahr J, Herndon DN. Genital and perineal burns in children: 10 years of experience at a major burn center. J Pediatr Surg 2002; 37: 99–103.
23. Michielsen D, Van Hee R, Neetens C. Burns to the genitals and the perineum. Br J Urol 1996; 78: 940–941.
24. Steeno O, Knops J, Declerck L, Adimoelja A, van de Voorde H. Prevention of fertility disorders by detection and treatment of varicocele at school and college age. Andrologia 1976; 8: 47–53.
25. Clark WR, Kramer SA. Henoch-Schonlein purpura and the acute scrotum. J Pediatr Surg 1986; 21: 991–992.
26. Qvist O. Swelling of the scrotum in infants and children and non-specific epididymitis: a study of 158 cases. Acta Chir Scand 1956; 110: 417–419.

IV ACUTE URINARY TRACT OBSTRUCTION

16 Renal Colic Resulting From Renal Calculus Disease

Diagnosis and Management

Rajveer S. Purohit, MD, MPH
and Marshall L. Stoller, MD

CONTENTS

    INTRODUCTION
    IMAGING RENAL COLIC
    INTERVENTIONS FOR OBSTRUCTION: SYMPTOMATIC TREATMENTS
    INTERVENTIONS FOR OBSTRUCTION: CURATIVE TREATMENTS
    SPECIAL CONSIDERATIONS
    SUMMARY
    REFERENCES

INTRODUCTION

Colic describes any severe spastic pain originating from distention or obstruction of a hollow organ. In particular, *renal colic* refers to sharp paroxysmal pain originating from spasm in or distention of the renal capsule or ureter or pain resulting from ureteral obstruction. It is perceived as intermittent sharp pain generally originating from the flank and occasionally radiating to the lower abdomen, groin, scrotum, or vulva and has variably been estimated to affect between 1 and 10% of the population at some time in their lives *(1–3)*.

Renal colic can arise from a variety of underlying conditions affecting the urinary tract. Although it has often been associated with pain originating from the passage of calculi through the urinary collecting system, in about 5 to 10% of patients typical renal colic is caused by something other than an obstructing calculus *(4)*. There are four areas of ureteral narrowing where obstruction is most frequent. These include renal calyces, the ureteropelvic junction (UPJ), the pelvic brim as the ureter passes over the iliac vessels, and the ureterovesicular junction.

This chapter reviews the presentation, evaluation, and management of patients who present with renal colic.

From: *Urological Emergencies: A Practical Guide*
Edited by: H. Wessells and J. W. McAninch © Humana Press Inc., Totowa, NJ

History and Physical

The medical history will provide important clues regarding the etiology of patients' pain. Patients with a prior episode of calculi will have between 37 and 50% risk of recurrence during their lifetime. If they had a cystine calculus, the chance of recurrence is significantly higher. In patients with known cardiovascular disease such as atrial fibrillation or atherosclerosis, vascular etiologies of renal colic should be considered.

Other important pertinent medical conditions that may suggest the source of pain include gout, history of trauma, menstrual history, and history of prior retroperitoneal surgeries. In addition, the patients' family history may provide evidence of cystinuria, polycystic kidney disease, or other causes of renal colic. Patients' medications should be reviewed for clues to the source of colic, such as diazides, which may result in triamterene stones.

The physical examination is an important adjunct when evaluating renal colic. Physical examination should include assessment of vital signs. The presence of fever should direct the provider toward infectious etiologies of the pain and increase the urgency of treatment. Examination of distal joints may indicate gout and may suggest the presence of uric acid stones. Location of tenderness or pain on percussion can direct the likely location of the pathology. Renal colic may present with pain in the lower abdomen, but will only rarely present with point tenderness in the lower abdomen or physical signs of peritonitis. If this does exist, the clinician should consider intraperitoneal causes of the acute abdomen. With flank tenderness, the diagnosis of pyelonephritis should be entertained.

Other risk factors for calculi that may become apparent during physical examination include evidence of urinary diversion or pseudohyperparathyroidism. Patients with renal colic often appear restless, continually shifting position, unlike patients who have peritonitis, who rarely move and for whom any movement can be painful.

For patients who present with urosepsis, admission and rapid institution of intravenous antibiotics is mandatory. After drainage of the infected collecting system with either ureteral stent or nephrostomy tube, patients should have vital signs carefully monitored and be given appropriate hydration and pressors as needed. Early blood cultures and urine cultures will help tailor antibiotic therapy more precisely.

Urinalysis

The role of urinalysis (UA) is controversial in the management of renal colic. Prior studies using intravenous urography as the gold standard found an 86 to 100% sensitivity of UA in prediction of calculi in patients with renal colic. If noncontrast computed tomographic (CT) scan is used as the gold standard, with a cutoff of 1 red blood cell (RBC) per high-powered field, the sensitivity of UA is only 81%. Of patients with acute flank pain and hematuria, 40% did not have renal calculi (5). Only 85% of patients presenting with renal colic will have evidence of gross or microhematuria. The absence of blood in the urine does not exclude the diagnosis of urinary stone disease. UA has poor predictive value in determining the etiology of renal colic (6).

However, urinary pH is a significant component of the workup in patients presenting with renal colic. In patients with a known history of calculi, urinary pH may suggest stone composition. Uric acid calculi will form only when urinary pH is consistently less than 5.5, and struvite calculi infected with urease-splitting organisms will only form when urinary pH is greater than 7.2. Microscopic examination of the urine may also demonstrate crystals, suggesting stone composition. Uric acid crystals appear as broken panes of thin glass, thin rectangular crystals suggest calcium phosphate calculi, and "Maltese crosses" suggest calcium oxalate calculi. However, the presence and type of urinary crystals are not definitive in diagnosing either the existence of a stone or its type.

The presence of leukocytes in the urine also may suggest infection or an inflammatory process. In patients with suspected pyelonephritis, urine cultures can be negative if the infection is proximal to an obstructing calculi. Laboratory examination, including complete blood count, electrolytes, and serum creatinine may help determine if infection, hemorrhage, or renal failure may be present. In addition, serum calcium and parathyroid levels may suggest or exclude certain etiologies of urinary stone disease.

Differential Diagnosis

Although renal colic commonly refers to pain from ureteral calculi, its differential is broad (*see* Table 1). By far the most frequent cause of renal colic is distention of the collecting system from obstructing calculi. Onset of pain is frequently acute and severe, and patients will change their position often in the hope of relieving this pain, which is also frequently accompanied by nausea or vomiting.

When calculi are confirmed, localization of pain may suggest stone location. Upper ureteral or renal pelvic dilation is often felt in the flank. With distal stone migration, pain frequently shifts toward the upper quadrant and progressively down the abdomen into the groin and testicle or vulva. Patients with calculi in the right midureter can present with pain at McBurney's point, which may mimic appendicitis; conversely, on the left side, it may mimic diverticulitis. Rarely, renal colic can present with pain on the contralateral side in a phenomenon termed *mirror pain*, which resolves with treatment of the calculus *(7)*.

Stone size often does not correlate with severity of presenting symptoms. Large staghorn calculi can cause minimal discomfort and may present with recurrent infections. Alternatively, a small distal obstructing stone can present with medically uncontrollable colic. Patients with ureterovesicular junction stones can present with urinary urgency or frequency with or without concurrent renal colic.

In evaluating patients with renal colic, vascular etiologies should be expeditiously ruled out. Renal artery aneurysms are increasingly noted incidentally on angiography and, although a rare occurrence, can occasionally rupture *(8)*. Patients may present with a suggestive history and acute onset of usually severe, *continuous* flank pain. Physical examination may reveal flank or abdominal ecchymosis and unstable vital signs responsive to hydration. Diagnosis is confirmed by angiography or CT scan.

In patients with a history of cardiac valve disease or dysrythmias, renal colic should arouse the suspicion of renal infarct from thrombus. Fever and leukocytosis can accompany renal colic, but an elevation in lactate dehydrogenase can help distinguish infarct from pyelonephritis. Presentation can be variable, and accurate diagnosis prior to imaging is difficult.

A retrospective review of 10 patients with 11 cases of acute renal infarct found the mean age to be 67.4 yr, but patients had a broad age range (30–87 yr). In 7 of 10 patients, a predisposing risk of thromboembolic phenomenon was noted, including 6 patients who had chronic atrial fibrillation. Flank pain was found in 10 of the 11 events and nausea and vomiting in 4 cases *(9)*.

On noncontrast CT, patients with renal infarct may have only mild perinephric stranding or renal enlargement *(10)*. Renal hemorrhage secondary to an underlying renal pathology may also present with renal colic. Patients with a bleeding tumor, arterial-venous malformation, or polycystic kidney disease can first present with renal colic.

Table 1
Partial List of Differential Diagnoses of Renal Colic

Retroperitoneal causes
  Renal
    Calculi
    Renal vein thrombosis
    Renal pelvic clot obstruction
    Papillary necrosis
    Transitional cell carcinoma
    Endometriosis
    Fungal bezoar
    Anatomic causes
      Ureteropelvic junction obstruction
      Crossed renal ectopia
      Hematuria loin syndrome
    Renal cell cancer
    Polycystic kidney disease
    Renal hemorrhage
    Trauma
    Pyelonephritis
  Adrenal
    Adrenal tumor
    Adrenal hemorrhage
  Ureteral
    Calculi and causes listed under renal
    Extrinsic compression
      From tumor
      From retroperitoneal fibrosis
      From endometriosis
      Teratoma
    Ureterocele
  Bladder
    Cystitis
    Calculi
    Tumor
  Seminal vesicle
    Ejaculatory duct obstruction
  Prostate
    Prostatitis
    Prostatic abscess
  Vascular etiologies
    Renal artery aneurysm
    Abdominal aortic aneurysm
    Aortic dissection
    Iliac artery aneurysm
  Gynecologic
    Ectopic pregnancy
    Ovarian vein thrombosis
    Endometriosis

(Continued)

Table 1 *(continued)*

    Ruptured ovarian cyst
    Ovarian torsion
Intraperitoneal
    Appendicitis
    Diverticulosis
    Diverticulitis
    Inflammatory bowel disease
    Meckel's diverticula
    Volvulus
    Peptic ulcer disease
    Pancreatitis
    Cholecystitis
    Acute intermittent porphyria
Neuropathic pain
    Referred pain
    Spinal nerve compression
Munchausen's syndrome

Patients may or may not present with any other signs of bleeding depending on the time frame and amount of blood loss. In these patients, definitive diagnosis is made by contrast CT scan; in those with a renal infarct, cardiac evaluation is mandatory.

Intraperitoneal causes of flank pain include diverticulitis, pancreatitis, appendicitis, cholangitis, or small bowel obstruction. Diagnosis can be clarified based on the history, laboratory examination, and imaging tests. In patients who are premenopausal and sexually active, ectopic pregnancy must also be ruled out. This can be ascertained through a careful history of the patients' menstrual cycle and, if needed, pregnancy tests and possibly pelvic ultrasound evaluation.

Clinicians should be conscious of psychogenic causes of renal colic, such as Munchausen's syndrome *(11)*. In two cases reported from the same institution, patients over many years ultimately were given approx 1000 units of blood, and one underwent a nephrectomy after presenting with recurrent flank pain and hematuria. The patients were instilling blood into their bladder and periodically phlebotimizing themselves *(12)*.

Neuropathic pain and referred pain can also mimic renal colic. This pain can be secondary to compression of spinal nerves from a herniated disk or from pain secondary to herpes zoster. Trauma from ingestion of foreign bodies *(13)* or activity that might injure back muscles and cause rhabdomyolysis may also imitate renal colic.

Infectious etiologies unrelated to calculi may present with renal colic. These patients may have leukocytosis, fever, and signs of sepsis on presentation. Acute pyelonephritis may present with lower abdominal or back pain in approx 25% of patients. A retrospective review of 225 patients found that 18.7% presented with nausea and vomiting and 23.1% with ultrasonic evidence of a urinary tract obstruction *(14)*. Perinephric abscesses can present with flank pain in approx 44% of patients and with nausea and vomiting in 64%. In a retrospective review of such problems, Meng et al. found that 24% of patients with perinephric abscesses had renal calculi as a predisposing factor *(15)*.

Calyceal diverticula are another unusual cause of renal colic. Patients are typically asymptomatic, but can become symptomatic if they develop infection or calculi in their diverticula *(16)*. This pain can be chronic *(17)* or acute *(18)*. UPJ obstruction will occasionally present with renal colic. Definitive diagnosis is made by nuclear scintigraphy. Other noncalculus diseases that affect the retroperitoneum can also present as renal colic, including adrenal hemorrhage, papillary necrosis, and for example, acute changes related to hemorrhage from an undiagnosed renal tumor.

IMAGING RENAL COLIC

Prior to institution of pain medications, a definitive diagnosis of calculi should be established because of renal colic's broad differential; consequently, imaging tests play an important role in the diagnosis and management of renal colic.

Plain Films

Plain films of the abdomen (kidney, ureter, bladder [KUB]) are often used as an initial imaging test for those with colic that is suspected of being secondary to calculi (Fig. 1). Plain films not only can help localize stones, but also may help identify the characteristics and shape of calculi. They are often obtained prior to application of contrast for other studies to detect extraosseous calcifications, location, size, and number of stones and assess bowel gas and fecal debris patterns. KUB radiographs frequently do not identify uric acid or indinavir calculi, which are relatively radiolucent.

Plain films alone have a limited sensitivity and specificity when used to evaluate renal colic, although estimates are variable. In patients with intractable renal colic as their only presenting symptom, KUB radiographs had a sensitivity of 95% and specificity of 65%. In a larger cohort of those presenting with flank pain, KUB films have been variously described to have a sensitivity of 44 to 77% and a specificity of 80 to 87% in detecting stones *(19–21)*. The particular radiographic test used to confirm calculi has an impact on the reported efficacy of a KUB radiograph. When noncontrast CT is used as the confirming gold standard, a KUB radiograph has a reported sensitivity of 45% and a specificity of 77% in detecting ureterolithiasis *(22)*.

Data have shown that CT scout radiography is inferior to a dedicated KUB film in detecting the presence of calculi. In a cohort of 60 patients with a single ureteral stone confirmed by CT scan, KUB radiography detected 60% of calculi; the scout CT film detected only 47%. In particular, dedicated KUB radiography was especially superior to CT scout radiography at detecting calculi 3 mm or smaller and those located in the proximal or midureter *(23)*.

KUB films may have some utility as an adjunct to other radiographic tests. The addition of ultrasound to evaluate for ureteral dilation may improve sensitivity to 89% and specificity of detecting calculi to 100% *(24)*. Haddad found similar results in incorporating ultrasound with KUB films, with sensitivities between 94 and 97% and specificities of 90% *(25)*.

Intravenous Pyelography/Excretory Urography

In the past, intravenous pyelography (IVP) was considered the diagnostic imaging modality of choice in patients presenting with renal colic. The scout KUB film may identify calcifications located within the urinary tract, and IVP can help confirm whether these densities lie within the collecting system by noting the presence of a filling defect or proximal ureteral dilatation. IVPs help delineate anatomy and possibly the underlying anomaly of the urinary tract that may contribute to stone growth, such as a UPJ obstruction.

Chapter 16 / Renal Colic 247

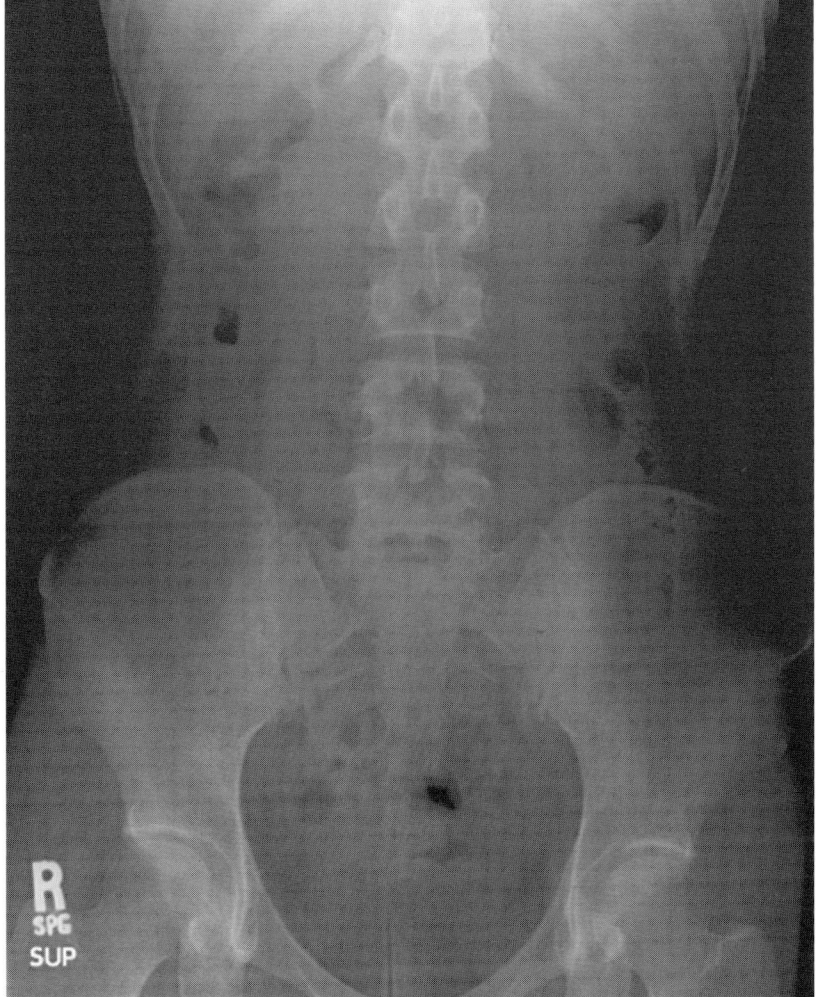

Fig. 1. KUB film of a radioopaque right upper ureteral calculus.

In addition, IVPs can estimate gross and relative renal function by assessing the time and amount of contrast excretion from each kidney. IVP has been reported to have a sensitivity of 75 to 85% and specificity of 90.4 to 91.7% among patients who presented to the emergency room with renal colic secondary to calculi (26).

IVP may help in the evaluation of noncalculus causes of renal colic. Lack of contrast uptake in a kidney, for example, may suggest a renal artery infarct, complete ureteral occlusion, or renal vein thrombosis. The outline of an enlarged polycystic kidney or highly vascular tumors also may be visible on IVP.

Disadvantages of IVP include potential complications resulting from administration of intravenous ionic or nonionic contrast agents, including nephrotoxicity and allergic or anaphylactic reactions. Excessive radiation exposure is a concern because multiple images must be taken, particularly if patients suffer from recurrent stone disease. Accuracy of IVPs is operator dependent because of the judgment required to appropriately time exposures, utilize nephrotomograms and oblique views, or delay films and is impacted by nonoperator-dependent factors, such as suboptimal bowel preparation.

Noncontrast CT

The first report of noncontrast CT scan for the evaluation of renal colic was published in 1995 by Smith et al. *(27)*. They reported on 20 patients who presented with acute flank pain and underwent radiographic testing with noncontrast CT scan and IVP. There were 12 patients who had findings on both tests that were consistent with symptomatic ureteral calculi. In 6 of these patients, both CT and IVP detected calculi; in 5 patients, the CT was positive and the IVP was negative. Subsequent data from the same group but in a larger cohort found that CT had a 97% sensitivity, 96% specificity, 96% positive predictive value, and 97% negative predictive value with confirmation by recovery of spontaneously passed calculi, ureteroscopic stone extraction, successful shock wave lithotripsy (SWL), or utilization of other imaging studies (Fig. 2A) *(28)*. A sensitivity of 94 to 100% and specificity of 94 to 100% have been confirmed in multiple follow-up studies *(20,26,29–32)*. In addition, data suggested that noncontrast CT scan is the study of choice after patients with renal colic are found to have equivocal results by KUB film or ultrasound *(33)*.

Noncontrast CT scans will detect all ureteral calculi except indinivir stones *(34)*. Patients prescribed protease inhibitors with a concurrent history consistent with calculi can be evaluated with secondary signs of obstruction on CT to suggest the diagnosis of indinivir calculi. If the diagnosis is uncertain after noncontrast CT, the addition of intravenous contrast may aid in the diagnosis. In this situation, CT may detect secondary signs of calculi, such as forniceal rupture, as well as provide alternative diagnoses to help explain renal colic, such as a renal infarct, hemorrhage, tumor, or intraperitoneal pathology.

Unlike IVPs, noncontrast CT scans do not directly suggest renal function or degree of obstruction, but indirect signs can provide additional clinical information. One study demonstrated that the severity of periureteral edema was proportional to the amount of obstruction. CT assessment of the extent of perinephric edema was accurate for predicting the extent of obstruction in 94% of patients when compared to excretory urography *(35)*. Interestingly, when results of nuclear scintigraphy were used to corroborate evidence of obstruction on CT, 91% of patients without secondary signs of obstruction by CT indeed had no obstruction on nuclear scan. All patients with severe obstruction had complete obstruction by nuclear scan *(36)*. Other secondary signs of obstruction include unilateral hydronephrosis, perinephric fluid, and asymmetrical perinephric fat stranding (Fig. 2B) *(37)*.

Ureteral calculi can occasionally be difficult to distinguish by CT scan from phleboliths. Attenuation values may vary between urinary calculi and phleboliths: if the mean attenuation value was greater than 311 Hounsfield units, the probability of a calcification being a phlebolith was only 0.03% *(38)*. Stones often demonstrate a soft tissue rim sign not often seen in phleboliths (Fig. 3) *(39)*. However, other data suggested that this sign can be present in up to 8% of phleboliths on CT scan *(40)*.

Ultrasound

Ultrasound alone or in combination with plain films has been utilized for evaluation of renal colic. Calculi may be directly visualized, appearing echogenic with distal acoustic shadowing. Ultrasound can also demonstrate pyeloureteral dilation and the presence of obstruction as well as parenchymal damage from persistent obstruction

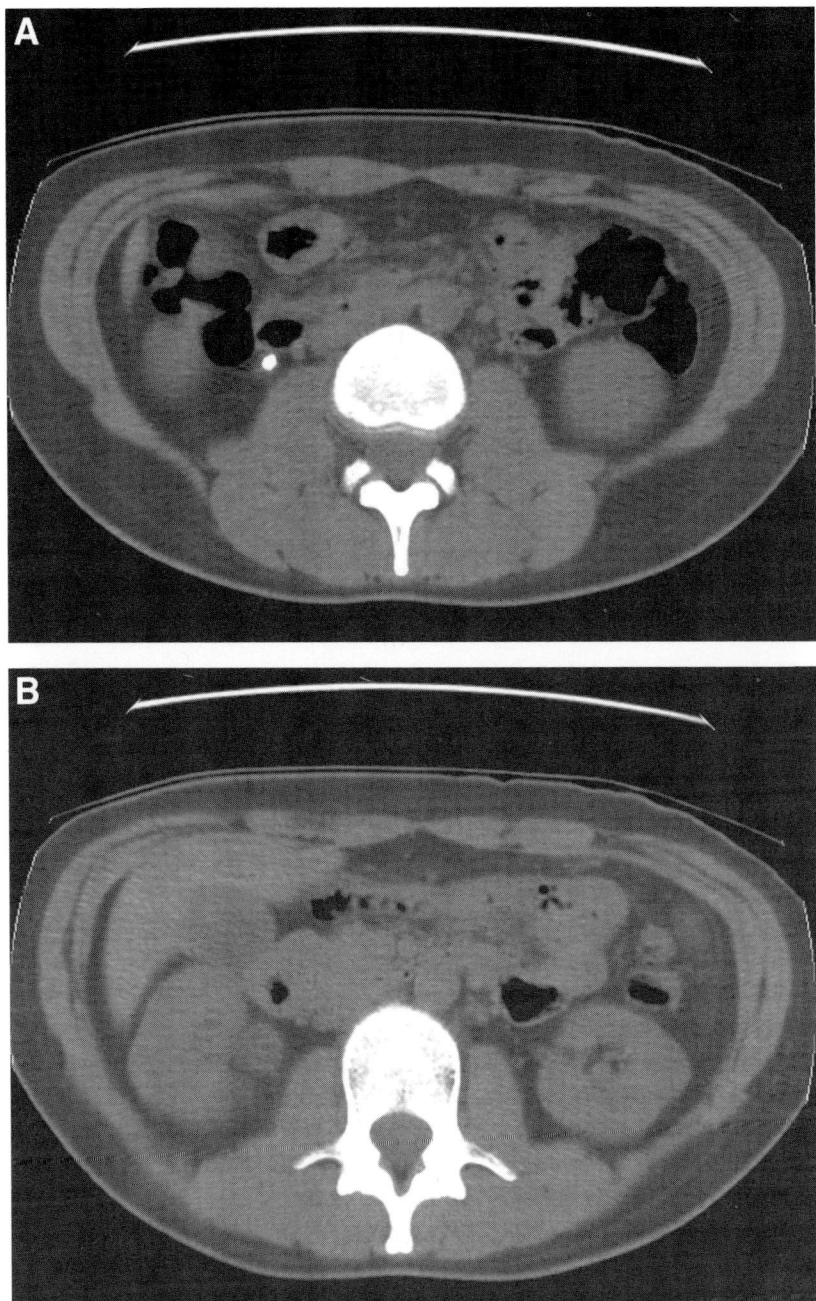

Fig. 2. Computed tomographic noncontrast film: **(A)** right upper ureteral calculus; **(B)** hydronephrosis proximal to stone.

(41). Obstruction can be quantified by evaluating resistive indices, although this is not a reliable technique.

An additional technique that has been utilized to help demonstrate obstruction by ultrasound is noting the absence of the normal urinary jet from the ureteral orifice.

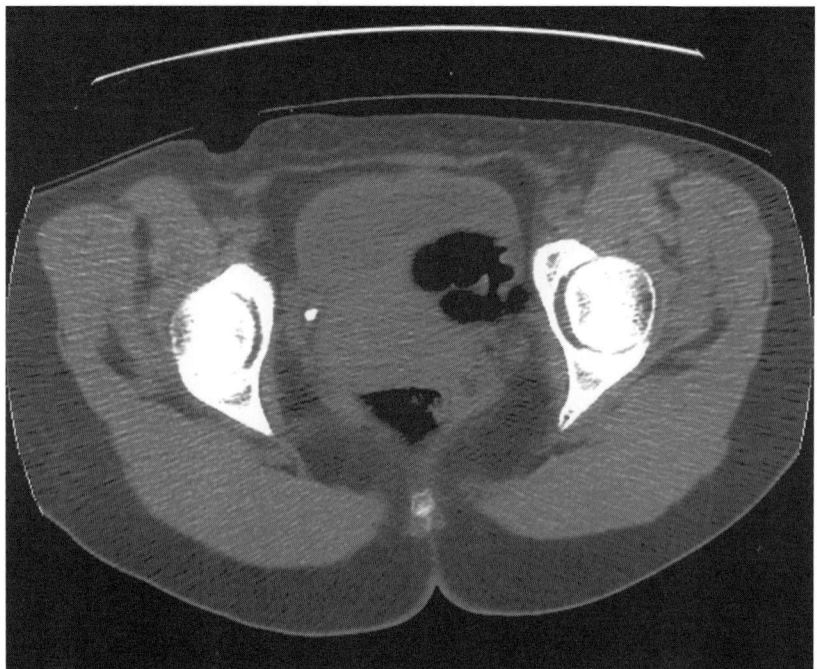

Fig. 3. Computed tomographic noncontrast film demonstrating distal right ureteral calculus.

Magnetic Resonance Imaging

Magnetic resonance imaging is of minimal benefit in the evaluation of renal colic because of difficulty in detecting differential magnetic signal from calculi. However, it may be useful to clarify diagnoses if calculi are not suspected. In patients who do not tolerate intravenous contrast, magnetic resonance imaging can demonstrate areas of infarcted renal tissue, may demonstrate compression of spinal nerves by intravertebral disc disease, and better elucidate underlying pathology after renal hemorrhage.

Renal Scintigraphy

Renal scintigraphy has been suggested as an adjunctive tool to determine the degree of obstruction with the increasing acceptance of noncontrast CT (NCCT) scan for evaluation of renal colic. A study of 49 patients with renal colic who were evaluated with NCCT as well as with aTc-99m DTPA or MAG-3 renogram showed that 34% of patients with secondary signs of obstruction on NCCT had complete obstruction by nuclear scan. Of patients with only moderate hydronephrosis by CT, 18% had complete obstruction by renogram. The authors concluded that nuclear scintigraphic studies can add useful information to the results of CT scan *(36)*. These studies may also play a role in diagnosing UPJ obstruction and renal infarct and can direct treatment in certain circumstances by determining relative renal function. Nuclear scintigraphic studies may have an adjunctive role in special circumstances during evaluation of renal colic.

Nuclear agents utilized for traditional bone scans such as bisphosphonates are typically excreted through the urinary tract. These agents have a high affinity to bind to stones and may occasionally confuse a UPJ obstruction with a large renal pelvic stone. There is evidence that the binding of bisphosphonates to urinary calculi is stone composition dependent.

INTERVENTIONS FOR OBSTRUCTION: SYMPTOMATIC TREATMENTS

Background

The innervation to the kidney is by sympathetic, parasympathetic, and sensory nerve fibers. Sensory afferents travel with sympathetics via thoracic spinal nerves T10–T12. The upper half of the ureter is innervated by the same nerves as the kidney, and the lower half is innervated by the lumbar splanchnic nerves. In addition, the kidneys are innervated by mechanosensitive high-threshold receptors that can be stimulated by distention of the collecting system *(42)*. Pain is often accompanied by accentuated autonomic reflexes, with reflex stimulation of the celiac ganglion, which causes nausea and vomiting.

In models of acute urinary tract obstruction, initially both renal blood flow (RBF) and proximal ureteropelvic pressure increase for 1.5 h. Over the next 4 h, RBF decreases, and pelvic pressure remains high; after this, there is a decline in both RBF and pelvic pressure. These declines nadir at approx 2 wk *(43,44)*. Renal colic is frequently caused by an increase in ureteropelvic pressure from a distal obstruction. This increase causes a prostaglandin-mediated increase in RBF, which in turn increases diuresis, creating a further increase in ureteropelvic pressure. The prostaglandins are believed to act, at least in part, by blocking antidiuretic hormone (ADH) action by interfering with signal transduction mediated by cyclic adenosine monophosphate (cAMP).

Patients treated for renal colic poorly tolerate oral medications because of associated nausea and vomiting. Intravenous formulations of nonsteroidal anti-inflammatory drugs (NSAIDs) are limited, and multiple intravenous opioid options exist. Acetaminophen may provide some pain relief as well as control fevers in patients with infected stones, but may provide inadequate pain relief for severe renal colic.

Nonopioids: NSAIDs

NSAIDs are believed to be useful in the treatment of renal colic by inhibiting the secretion of prostaglandin E_2 (PGE_2). PGE_2 is stimulated by ureteral obstruction and increases the contractility of the ureter. It also dilates the afferent renal artery, thereby increasing urine production and further worsening renal colic. By blocking the effect of PGE_2, NSAIDs should at least theoretically break this cycle in renal colic in addition to decreasing pain. They also reduce RBF and decrease urine production.

The first NSAID studied to treat renal colic was indomethacin *(45,46)*. Early studies showed that naproxen and diclofenac *(47)* also had significant benefit *(48)*. In a meta-analysis of 19 randomized controlled trials published between 1966 and 1992 regarding the use of NSAIDs in renal colic, a statistically significant benefit was found in those who received NSAIDs compared to those receiving a placebo. A relative ratio of 2.34 in providing pain relief was seen in favor of those receiving NSAIDS. In addition, NSAIDs were as effective, if not more so, when compared with other analgesics evaluated *(49)*.

NSAIDs are an attractive alternative to opioids because they do not have addictive potential. In addition, unlike opioids, they do not compound the nausea and vomiting often present in patients with renal colic. Rectal NSAIDs are not effective in relieving renal colic *(50)*.

NSAIDs can have significant adverse effects, including decreased sodium excretion, hyperkalemia, acute renal failure, and papillary necrosis. Under normal circumstances, NSAIDs do not affect RBF or glomerular filtration rate (GFR) *(51)*. If vasoconstrictor tone is increased, prostaglandins are released to vasodilate; in these circumstances,

NSAIDs can substantially decrease RBF and GFR. Concern exists regarding the risk of developing renal failure in those with compromised renal function or severe atherosclerosis; the highest risk of developing renal failure is in patients with cirrhosis, congestive heart failure, hypovolemia, hypotension, nephrotic syndrome, or underlying renal disease. In these patients, RBF is believed to be maintained by prostaglandins, and their inhibition may have an adverse impact on renal function *(52)*.

In addition, NSAIDs, by decreasing RBF, may magnify the delay in return of normal renal function in obstructed kidneys *(53)*. Selective cyclo-oxygenase-2 (COX-2) inhibitors have not been shown to prevent these side effects from occurring *(54)*. Patients given NSAIDs can have an overestimation of ureteral obstruction estimated from ultrasound because of the prolonged renal transit time and increased resistive indices in patients taking these medications *(55,56)*.

KETOROLAC

Ketorolac has become the mainstay of treatment of renal colic partly because of its ready availability as an intravenous formulation *(57)*. In addition to inhibition of PGE_2, ketorolac may act centrally to diminish perception of pain, decrease ureteral wall spasms *(58)*, and potentially decrease ureteral wall edema. Animal studies have shown that it causes an immediate and sustained decrease in RBF and decreases ureteral pressure by 25% *(53)*. An uncontrolled study of 25 patients revealed that intravenous ketorolac was effective in controlling renal colic *(59)*.

Ketorolac has been more effective than meperidine in treating pain from renal colic, and its use promoted earlier discharge from the emergency department *(60)*. In a double-blind, randomized, prospective study of 107 patients, intravenous ketorolac was equivalent to intravenous ketorolac with meperidine and superior to meperidine alone in treating moderate-to-severe renal colic *(61)*. Similar precautions should be maintained when utilizing ketorolac as described for other NSAIDs in the preceding section.

DICLOFENAC

In a randomized, single-blind trial of 41 patients who presented with renal colic to an emergency room in Oslo, Norway, intramuscular diclofenac (75 mg) resulted in a statistically significant reduction in pain compared to those treated with intravenous indomethacin (50 mg; $p < 0.01$). The authors also found a lower incidence of side effects compared to indomethacin. In another double-blind controlled study, diclofenac appeared to be equally effective as high-dose (60 mg) ketorolac in treating renal colic *(62)*. Ketorolac (30 mg) also has provided equivalent pain relief with an equivalent side effect profile compared to intramuscular diclofenac (75 mg) *(63)*.

DIPYRONE

Dipyrone is an NSAID that has not been approved in the United States because of the risk of agranulocytosis. In a meta-analysis of 11 studies on dipyrone, Edwards et al. *(64)* found similar efficacy to other analgesics in treating renal colic. Intramuscular dipyrone was less effective than diclofenac. Side effects reported included dry mouth and somnolence, but no case of agranulocytosis was reported.

PIROXICAM

Intramuscular piroxicam has been as effective as diclofenac with a more rapid onset of action and prolonged effect *(65)*. In a prospective randomized study of 80 patients, fast-acting sublingual piroxicam (40 mg) was as effective as parenteral diclofenac (75 mg) in the treatment of renal colic *(66)*. Both studies reported minimal adverse side effects associated with piroxicam. The sublingual administration is advantageous because it circumvents problems with nausea and vomiting and the need for intravenous access.

SELECTIVE COX-2 INHIBITORS

In vitro, animal and human models have shown that selective COX-2 inhibitors reduce ureteral contractility as well as NSAIDs *(67)*. The risk of renal impairment has not been shown to be lower than NSAIDs *(52)*. Selective COX-2 inhibitors may play an increasing role in treating patients who may otherwise have not been given NSAIDs because of the risk of gastrointestinal complications. More studies are required before this class of drugs can be recommended for routine use in the treatment of renal colic. Evidence has suggested that the use of isosorbide dinitrate with other COX-2 inhibitors may be more efficacious in controlling renal colic than a COX-2 inhibitor alone *(68)*.

Other Nonopioids

DESMOPRESSIN

Increases in intraluminal pressure in patients with obstruction are believed to be caused partly by an ADH-mediated mechanism. An ADH promoter may decrease diuresis and assist in relief of pain associated with renal obstruction *(69)*. Animal models have suggested that desmopressin may decrease intraluminal ureteropelvic pressure and decrease the contractions of circular smooth muscle in the renal pelvis *(70,71)*. Desmopressin may also stimulate central secretion of β-endorphins *(72)*.

A number of trials have evaluated treatment of renal colic with desmopressin. Of patients who presented to the emergency room with renal colic, 61 were entered in a prospective, randomized trial comparing intranasal desmopressin (40 μg) alone with diclofenac (75 mg) alone or with both medications. All groups had equally prompt pain relief as measured by a visual analog scale, but after 30 min, the cohort that received desmopressin alone had slightly higher pain scores *(73)*. Other studies of patients who presented with renal colic found between 44 and 54% *(74)* with complete relief of their symptoms within 30 min of administration of intranasal desmopressin *(75)*.

Evidence suggested that desmopressin may enhance the efficacy of pain relief from NSAIDs *(74)*. These studies found little or no toxicity in those that received desmopressin. Desmopressin may be a useful adjunct to other pain medications because it can be administered rapidly through an intranasal spray, and it works quickly. It could be administered, for example, while patients are waiting for intravenous access.

DROTAVERINE HYDROCHLORIDE

In a multicenter, randomized, double-blind study from Hungary, an antispasmolytic, drotaverine hydrochloride, was effective in controlling pain in renal colic in 79% of patients, compared to 46% who were treated with placebo. Droteravine acts through a cAMP-mediated decrease in cellular calcium uptake and subsequently causes ureteral smooth muscle relaxation. Only minor side effects were reported *(76)*. This medication is not commonly used in the United States, but this study did suggest the potential role of ureteral antispasmolytics in future trials in the treatment of renal colic.

Opioids

Opiates relieve pain through actions on central and spinal opiate receptors. Opiates act quickly, and a variety of parenteral versions are available. In animal studies, opiates do not affect GFR or RBF *(53)*. There is concern that opiates may aggravate nausea and vomiting in patients suffering from renal colic by stimulating the centrally located chemoreceptor trigger zone and delaying gastric emptying. In addition, care should be taken in ensuring adequate urinary drainage in patients who may present with urinary infection because urinary retention can occur. Opiates also are well known to cause sedation, respiratory depression, hypotension, and over time, tolerance and addiction. However, because of presumed efficacy, opiates, particularly meperidine, have commonly been used in the treatment of renal colic *(77)*.

Because of the limited availability of intravenous NSAIDs in the United States, rectal NSAIDs have been compared to opioids, but equivalent efficacy is unclear from the literature *(78,79)*. A significant amount of data suggest that intravenous NSAIDs may have equivalent, if not better, efficacy compared to opioids. In a double-blind, randomized, multicenter clinical trial comparing intravenous ketorolac (60 mg) to intravenous meperidine (50 mg), ketorolac had more rapid and effective pain relief than meperidine alone *(61)*. When intravenous ketorolac (60 mg) was compared to a higher dose of meperidine (100 to 150 mg based on weight) ketorolac, still proved more effective in controlling pain than the opioid *(60)*. Opioids are best utilized as second-tier therapy in the treatment of renal colic after failure of initial treatment with NSAIDs.

Alternative Treatments

TRIGGER POINT

A trigger point related to renal colic is a tender, palpable skeletal muscular "knot" in the ipsilateral back that may induce referred pain to the kidney. In patients with renal colic, the trigger point can be located by placing the patient in a prone position and applying gentle pressure (i.e., from a metal sound) at regular 1-cm intervals between the costal margin, iliac crest, and the vertebral spine. The point of maximum tenderness is believed to be the trigger point. Once it is located, 2 to 3 mL of 1% lidocaine are injected superficially, and 5 to 10 mL can be injected 3 to 5 cm deep.

In a randomized prospective trial, local block of trigger points in patients suffering from renal colic appeared to be more efficacious compared to intravenous butylscopolamine (40 mg) with sulpyrine (500 mg). The trigger point injection group experienced a higher response rate as well as decreased pain after 20 min compared to those without injections *(80)*. The medications used as comparisons in the study are not commonly employed for treatment of colic, and trigger point injection should still be considered experimental.

LOCAL ACTIVE WARMING

Local active warming has been investigated as a nonpharmacological treatment for renal colic that can be utilized before patients arrive in the emergency room. Its advantage lies in the fact that patients can begin it at home, or it can be given in the emergency room before opportunities exist for intravenous medication administration. Local active warming involves the application of an electric heating blanket to portions of the lateral abdomen and lower back. In a prospective randomized study of 100 patients with renal colic, local active warming significantly decreased pain, anxiety, and nausea and compared favorably to passive blanket warming alone *(81)*. Given the low morbidity of this technique, it may prove useful prior to the availability of pain medications.

ACUPUNCTURE

Acupuncture for renal colic involves the placement of needles in the skin at precise points in the body to control pain. Although acupuncture has been used for thousands of years, the scientific mechanism of pain control is unclear. Some data suggest that acupuncture may be useful in the treatment of renal colic. In a prospective randomized study of patients who presented with renal colic and were treated with either acupuncture or Avafortan® (a combination medication containing dipyrone and a spasmolytic), acupuncture was found to have a more rapid onset of action and equal efficacy in providing pain relief. Acupuncture was also noted to have fewer side effects *(82)*. Additional studies are required before acupuncture can be recommended as a routine treatment for renal colic.

INTERVENTIONS FOR OBSTRUCTION: CURATIVE TREATMENTS

Spontaneous Stone Passage

The likelihood of spontaneous stone passage is related to stone size and stone location at time of presentation. Stones 5 mm or smaller and calculi below the sacral-iliac joint are the most likely to pass spontaneously *(83)*. In an analysis of 75 patients diagnosed with unequivocal evidence of ureteral calculi by noncontrast CT and IVP and followed every 2 wk until passage of calculi or intervention occurred, 83% of patients had spontaneous stone passage. This study found that 95% of stones between 2 and 4 mm passed spontaneously, although the time interval to stone passage was highly variable and could take as long as 4 to 5 wk. Authors also confirmed that more distal stones and, interestingly, right-sided stones passed more frequently than proximal stones and left-sided calculi, respectively *(84)*.

Pharmacological Attempts at Stone Passage

If symptomatic calculi are diagnosed as the cause of renal pain, pharmacological treatments may assist in stone passage. Ureteral smooth muscle utilizes an active calcium pump for aid in contractions. Nifedipine, a calcium channel blocker, has been postulated to decrease renal colic by serving as a spasmolytic *(85)*. However, in a prospective double-blind study of patients presenting to the emergency room, nifedipine had no benefit over placebo in providing relief from renal colic *(86)*. However, some data suggested that calcium channel blockers, particularly nifedipine, with the addition of steroids may permit early stone passage.

In a randomized prospective study of 86 patients with ureteral calculi smaller than 15 mm, patients who were given nifedipine (40 mg) and methylprednisolone (16 mg) for up to 45 d had a greater chance ($p = 0.021$) of spontaneous stone passage compared to those who were given methylprednisolone with a placebo *(87)*. A second study evaluated patients with renal colic who presented with unilateral uninfected calculi 2 to 6 (mean

3.9) mm and were randomly assigned either to a control arm of ketorolac, oxycodone/ acetaminophen, and prochloperazine or to a treatment arm of these medications with nifedipine XL (30 mg), prednisone (10 mg), Bactrim DS, and Tylenol. The end point of medical therapy was stone passage. They found that 54% of patients in the control arm and 86% of patients in the treatment arm passed the stone within a mean of 11.15 and 12.60 d, respectively ($p = 0.001$) *(88)*.

Analogously, nitrates have been suggested as capable of relaxing ureteral smooth muscle *(89)*. Nitrates, which have an effect within 2 to 5 min with sublingual administration, may serve as a bridge because of their rapid onset of action before the administration of other pain medications. Care should be taken if infection is suspected behind the obstruction. It has been argued that, in patients with urinary infections, ureteral peristalsis may stop, thereby making passage of stones more difficult *(88)*.

Hydration

Fluid management in patients who present with renal colic is controversial. In patients with obstruction, increased intravascular fluids through intravenous or oral hydration may result in an increase in urine production. This urine production may either cause an increase in renal colic from proximal distention of the collecting system or may permit easier passage of the stone by "flushing" it out of the collecting system. The utility of fluids, although clearly beneficial in providing vascular support in dehydrated or septic patients, has not been demonstrated in clinical trials as useful in treating renal colic or aiding in stone passage. An attempt should be made to make the patient euvolemic, and our belief is that overhydration may exacerbate renal colic.

Surgical Interventions for Calculi

If a stone is determined as the cause of renal colic, then many factors will determine the treatment algorithm, including the size of the calculus and the presence of signs of infection. Intervention for calculi is warranted if conservative treatment fails, if stone appearance suggests that it is unlikely to pass without treatment, if patients develop intractable pain or fever, or if there is evidence of significant renal impairment from the calculus. Special circumstances such as solitary kidney may warrant earlier intervention if the risk of obstruction is high.

URETERAL DECOMPRESSION

In patients with a calculus who develop evidence of infection (i.e., fevers) urinary decompression is mandatory. Options include percutaneous nephrostomy drainage *(90)* or placement of an indwelling ureteral stent and Foley catheter. Although data do not clearly demonstrate the utility of one method of decompression over another, the choice of type of drainage is often institution dependent and contingent on patterns of specialty referrals between urology and interventional radiology.

A prospective randomized study evaluating 42 patients who presented with obstructing ureteral calculi and were treated with either percutaneous nephrostomy or indwelling ureteral stent found that, between the two, differences between time to treatment, time to normalization of fever, and length of stay were not statistically significant. Stent placement was twice as costly as percutaneous nephrostomy drainage *(91)*. If decompression is initiated with a retrograde ureteral stent and is unsuccessful, a nephrostomy tube should be placed.

Stent placement is more successful when used to treat intrinsic obstruction such as ureteral calculi than for obstruction from extrinsic compression *(92)*. In an evaluation of 92 patients who underwent retrograde stent placement, patients with extrinsic obstruction, those with a high degree of obstruction, or patients with a distal obstruction were more likely to fail decompression. Initially, stent placement was successful in 94% of patients with intrinsic obstruction and 73% of patients with extrinsic obstruction. At 3-mo followup, all patients with an initially functioning stent for intrinsic obstruction and only 56% of patients with extrinsic compression had functional ureteral stents *(93)*.

When a decision is made to place a nephrostomy tube, authors have described placement under both ultrasound and fluoroscopic guidance. Stent placement itself may be therapeutic. In a canine model, stents cause dilation of the ureter *(94)*. In a study of 27 patients with ureteral calculi smaller than 10 mm, 83% spontaneously passed their calculi within 2 wk of stent placement *(95)*.

Stents can cause complications, including significant irritative voiding symptoms, hematuria, and flank pain. Indwelling ureteral stents can also cause colicky flank pain similar to renal colic; however, this pain generally occurs with voiding when bladder pressures increase and cause reflux of urine through the stent. Other problems include stent migration, encrustation, and forgotten stents *(16)*.

STONE REMOVAL

Patients with symptomatic ureteral calculi may require stone removal after failed attempts of spontaneous stone passage. However, concern exists about precipitating sepsis by manipulation of the urinary tract in patients harboring infection; therefore, caution is advised prior to extraction of calculi. If gross infection is encountered at the time of stone manipulation, drainage should be established and the procedure terminated. Other options include stone extraction with ureteroscopy, SWL, and laparoscopic or open surgical retrieval. If equipment is available, strong consideration should be made for definitive treatment in afebrile patients.

SPECIAL CONSIDERATIONS

Pregnancy

During pregnancy, mild hydronephrosis is believed to be a normal phenomenon, but can rarely lead to spontaneous rupture of the renal pelvis *(96)*. The incidence of calculi during pregnancy is believed to be equivalent to calculi in nonchildbearing women of the same age *(97)*. Of pregnant women with colic, 80 to 90% present in the third trimester, and 70 to 80% of their calculi pass spontaneously *(98)*. In evaluation of the pregnant patient with suspected renal colic, diagnosis must include other major obstetric complications such as uterine rupture or ectopic pregnancy.

Evaluation and treatment of renal colic in pregnant women must be modified to minimize the risk of radiation to the fetus; consequently, ultrasound has remained the most common first-line test for evaluation of renal calculi in this setting *(99)*. Because of the normal physiological dilation of the ureter during pregnancy (right more than left), hydronephrosis alone has poor sensitivity (34%) and specificity (86%) in the detection of calculi *(100)*. Many urologists have been hesitant to utilize IVP in the evaluation of renal colic in pregnancy not only because of concern about radiation exposure, but also because the fetal skeleton and uterus may obscure visualization of small distal calculi. Various modifications have been proposed, including narrow collimation, low voltages, brief exposure, and prone positioning to minimize the radiation dose delivered to the fetus *(101)*.

Management of pregnant patients with renal colic may become necessary if patients have pain refractory to medications, sepsis, or obstruction in a solitary kidney *(102)*. If intervention is mandatory, multiple options exist, including percutaneous nephrostomy or placement of internal ureteral stents *(103)*. Multiple reports have suggested ureteroscopy is a safe alternative for treatment of ureteral calculi in pregnancy *(104–106)*. SWL is generally believed to be contraindicated in pregnancy because of the potential effects of the shock wave on the fetus, although data on this topic have not been definitive. Prolonged radiation exposure with fluoroscopy and prone patient positioning limit access for percutaneous stone extraction. Techniques to temporize stone pain with a retrograde ureteral stent, percutaneous nephrostomy drainage, or medications should be maximized. After fetal delivery, routine algorithmic approaches can be undertaken.

Renal Transplant

Patients with renal transplants rarely develop or inherit renal calculi. They present in an atypical fashion because of severed nerves that alter their pain perception. Frequently, they will present with signs and symptoms similar to a flulike illness, including tenderness over the graft site, evidence of renal inflammation, or infection that can be mistaken for acute or subacute transplant rejection. In renal transplant recipients in whom calculi are suspected, a NCCT scan is useful in making a definitive diagnosis. Retrograde treatment can be challenging because of the anteriorly located ureteral neocystotomy. SWL may require the patient to be placed in a prone fashion. Percutaneous procedures may best be performed after a CT scan to exclude overlying loops of bowel, and stone size and location will direct treatment strategies.

Pediatric Urolithiasis

Children who present with renal colic will often present with similar signs and symptoms of renal colic as adults. However, because they are often unable to localize their pain or articulate their precise symptoms, renal colic can be confused with other medical or surgical illnesses. Their inability to articulate their complaints may result in a confused diagnosis and may culminate in unhelpful abdominal procedures, such as unnecessary appendectomies. Clinicians should begin with a broad differential and include renal colic in children who present with unexplained pain, discomfort, fevers, hematuria, or a suggestive history.

SUMMARY

Renal colic typically has an acute onset and will affect between 1 and 10% of the population at some time in their lives. It frequently is caused by passage of an ureteral stone. Stone size does not correlate with severity of symptoms. Associated fever, persistent nausea and vomiting, and/or severe pain unresponsive to pharmacological intervention require hospitalization with directed intervention. Urinalysis will reveal microscopic or gross hematuria in 85% of such patients. Lack of blood in the urine does not exclude a urinary stone. The differential diagnosis for acute renal colic is varied. Noncontrast CT is becoming the imaging modality of choice for patients presenting with renal colic. Multiple pharmacological interventions are available to help ease the pain and facilitate stone passage. Initial therapy includes hydration to a euvolemic state and in most instances the stone will pass spontaneously. Those that do not pass on their own can be treated with a variety of techniques.

REFERENCES

1. Holdgate A, Chan T. How accurate are emergency clinicians at interpreting noncontrast computed tomography for suspected renal colic? Acad Emerg Med 2003; 10: 315–319.
2. Shokeir AA. Renal colic: pathophysiology, diagnosis and treatment. Eur Urol 2001; 39: 241–249.
3. Hiatt RA, Dales LG, Friedman GD, et al. Frequency of urolithiasis in a prepaid medical care program. Am J Epidemiol 1982; 115: 255–265.
4. Dalrymple NC, Verga M, Anderson KR, et al. The value of unenhanced helical computerized tomography in the management of acute flank pain. J Urol 1998; 159: 735–740.
5. Bove P, Kaplan D, Dalrymple N, et al. Reexamining the value of hematuria testing in patients with acute flank pain. J Urol 1999; 162: 685–687.
6. Luchs JS, Katz DS, Lane MJ, et al. Utility of hematuria testing in patients with suspected renal colic: correlation with unenhanced helical CT results. Urology 2002; 59: 839–842.
7. Clark AJ, Norman RW. "Mirror pain" as an unusual presentation of renal colic. Urology 1998; 51: 116–118.
8. Power RE, Winter DC, Kelly CJ. A near fatal case of renal colic. J Urol 2001; 165: 1987.
9. Korzets Z, Plotkin E, Bernheim J, et al. The clinical spectrum of acute renal infarction. Isr Med Assoc J 2002; 4: 781–784.
10. Talner L, Vaughan M. Nonobstructive renal causes of flank pain: findings on noncontrast helical CT (CT KUB). Abdom Imaging 2003; 28: 210–216.
11. Gluckman GR, Stoller M. Munchausen's syndrome: manifestation as renal colic. Urology 1993; 42: 347–350.
12. Chew BH, Pace KT, Honey RJ. Munchausen syndrome presenting as gross hematuria in two women. Urology 2002; 59: 601.
13. Li SF, Ender K. Toothpick injury mimicking renal colic: case report and systematic review. J Emerg Med 2002; 23: 35–38.
14. Efstathiou SP, Pefanis AV, Tsioulos DI, et al. Acute pyelonephritis in adults: prediction of mortality and failure of treatment. Arch Intern Med 2003; 163: 1206–1212.
15. Meng MV, Mario LA, McAninch JW. Current treatment and outcomes of perinephric abscesses. J Urol 2002; 168: 1337–1340.
16. Auge BK, Munver R, Kourambas J, et al. Endoscopic management of symptomatic caliceal diverticula: a retrospective comparison of percutaneous nephrolithotripsy and ureteroscopy. J Endourol 2002; 16: 557–563.
17. Wulfsohn MA. Pyelocaliceal diverticula. J Urol 1980; 123: 1–8.
18. Wogan JM. Pyelocalyceal diverticulum: an unusual cause of acute renal colic. J Emerg Med 2002; 23: 19–21.
19. Mutgi A, Williams JW, Nettleman M. Renal colic. Utility of the plain abdominal roentgenogram. Arch Intern Med 1991; 151: 1589–1592.
20. Yilmaz S, Sindel T, Arslan G, et al. Renal colic: comparison of spiral CT, US and IVU in the detection of ureteral calculi. Eur Radiol 1998; 8: 212–217.
21. Roth CS, Bowyer BA, Berquist TH. Utility of the plain abdominal radiograph for diagnosing ureteral calculi. Ann Emerg Med 1985; 14: 311–315.
22. Levine JA, Neitlich J, Verga M, et al. Ureteral calculi in patients with flank pain: correlation of plain radiography with unenhanced helical CT. Radiology 1997; 204: 27–31.
23. Assi Z, Platt JF, Francis IR, et al. Sensitivity of CT scout radiography and abdominal radiography for revealing ureteral calculi on helical CT: implications for radiologic follow-up. AJR Am J Roentgenol 2000; 175: 333–337.
24. Gorelik U, Ulish Y, Yagil Y. The use of standard imaging techniques and their diagnostic value in the workup of renal colic in the setting of intractable flank pain. Urology 1996; 47: 637–642.
25. Haddad MC, Sharif HS, Shahed MS, et al. Renal colic: diagnosis and outcome. Radiology 1992; 184: 83–88.
26. Pfister SA, Deckart A, Laschke S, et al. Unenhanced helical computed tomography vs intravenous urography in patients with acute flank pain: accuracy and economic impact in a randomized prospective trial. Eur Radiol 2003; 13(11): 2513–2520.
27. Smith RC, Rosenfield AT, Choe KA, et al. Acute flank pain: comparison of non-contrast-enhanced CT and intravenous urography. Radiology 1995; 194: 789–794.

28. Smith RC, Verga M, McCarthy S, et al. Diagnosis of acute flank pain: value of unenhanced helical CT. AJR Am J Roentgenol 1996; 166: 97–101.
29. Shokeir AA, Abdulmaaboud M. Prospective comparison of nonenhanced helical computerized tomography and Doppler ultrasonography for the diagnosis of renal colic. J Urol 2001; 165: 1082–1084.
30. Ahmad NA, Ather MH, Rees J. Unenhanced helical computed tomography in the evaluation of acute flank pain. Int J Urol 2003; 10: 287–292.
31. Boulay I, Holtz P, Foley WD, et al. Ureteral calculi: diagnostic efficacy of helical CT and implications for treatment of patients. AJR Am J Roentgenol 1999; 172: 1485–1490.
32. Fielding JR, Fox LA, Heller H, et al. Spiral CT in the evaluation of flank pain: overall accuracy and feature analysis. J Comput Assist Tomogr 1997; 21: 635–638.
33. Kobayashi T, Nishizawa K, Watanabe J, et al. Clinical characteristics of ureteral calculi detected by nonenhanced computerized tomography after unclear results of plain radiography and ultrasonography. J Urol 2003; 170: 799–802.
34. Blake SP, McNicholas MM, Raptopoulos V. Nonopaque crystal deposition causing ureteric obstruction in patients with HIV undergoing indinavir therapy. AJR Am J Roentgenol 1998; 171: 717–720.
35. Boridy IC, Kawashima A, Goldman SM, et al. Acute ureterolithiasis: nonenhanced helical CT findings of perinephric edema for prediction of degree of ureteral obstruction. Radiology 1999; 213: 663–667.
36. German I, Lantsberg S, Crystal P, et al. Non contrast computerized tomography and dynamic renal scintigraphy in the evaluation of patients with renal colic: are both necessary? Eur Urol 2002; 42: 188–191.
37. Dalrymple NC, Casford B, Raiken DP, et al. Pearls and pitfalls in the diagnosis of ureterolithiasis with unenhanced helical CT. Radiographics 2000; 20: 439–447.
38. Bell TV, Fenlon HM, Davison BD, et al. Unenhanced helical CT criteria to differentiate distal ureteral calculi from pelvic phleboliths. Radiology 1998; 207: 363–367.
39. Kawashima A, Sandler CM, Boridy IC, et al. Unenhanced helical CT of ureterolithiasis: value of the tissue rim sign. AJR Am J Roentgenol 1997; 168: 997–1000.
40. Heneghan JP, Dalrymple NC, Verga M, et al. Soft-tissue "rim" sign in the diagnosis of ureteral calculi with use of unenhanced helical CT. Radiology 1997; 202: 709–711.
41. Older RA, Jenkins AD. Stone disease. Urol Clin North Am 2000; 27: 215–229.
42. Al-Chaer ED, Traub RJ. Biological basis of visceral pain: recent developments. Pain 2002; 96: 221–225.
43. Moody TE, Vaughn ED Jr, Gillenwater JY. Relationship between renal blood flow and ureteral pressure during 18 hours of total unilateral urethral occlusion. Implications for changing sites of increased renal resistance. Invest Urol 1975; 13: 246–251.
44. Cadnapaphornchai P, Aisenbrey G, McDonald KM, et al. Prostaglandin-mediated hyperemia and renin-mediated hypertension during acute ureteral obstruction. Prostaglandins 1978; 16: 965–971.
45. Holmlund D, Sjodin JG. Treatment of ureteral colic with intravenous indomethacin. J Urol 1978; 120: 676–677.
46. Holmlund DE, Sjodin JG. Indomethacin in the treatment of ureteral colic. Surg Forum 1978; 29: 639–641.
47. Lundstam S, Sengupta CH, Timbal Y, et al. Diclofenac sodium in renal colic. Practitioner 1984; 228: 704–705.
48. Marsala F, Cavrini P, Bufalino L, et al. Treatment of acute pain of ureteral and biliary colic with naproxen sodium administered by the parenteral route. Int J Clin Pharmacol Res 1986; 6: 495–500.
49. Labrecque M, Dostaler LP, Rousselle R, et al. Efficacy of nonsteroidal anti-inflammatory drugs in the treatment of acute renal colic. A meta-analysis. Arch Intern Med 1994; 154: 1381–1387.
50. Ginifer C, Kelly AM. Administration of rectal indomethacin does not reduce the requirement for intravenous narcotic analgesia in acute renal colic. Eur J Emerg Med 1996; 3: 92–94.
51. Sedor JR, Davidson EW, Dunn MJ. Effects of nonsteroidal anti-inflammatory drugs in healthy subjects. Am J Med 1986; 81: 58–70.
52. Gambaro G, Perazella MA. Adverse renal effects of anti-inflammatory agents: evaluation of selective and nonselective cyclooxygenase inhibitors. J Intern Med 2003; 253: 643–652.

53. Perlmutter A, Miller L, Trimble LA, et al. Toradol, an NSAID used for renal colic, decreases renal perfusion and ureteral pressure in a canine model of unilateral ureteral obstruction. J Urol 1993; 149: 926–930.
54. Brater DC. Effects of nonsteroidal anti-inflammatory drugs on renal function: focus on cyclooxygenase-2-selective inhibition. Am J Med 1999; 107(6A): 65S–70S.
55. Shokeir AA, Abdulmaaboud M, Farage Y, et al. Resistive index in renal colic: the effect of nonsteroidal anti-inflammatory drugs. BJU Int 1999; 84: 249–251.
56. Kinn AC, Larsson SA, Nelson E, et al. Diclofenac treatment prolongs renal transit time in acute ureteral obstruction: a renographic study. Eur Urol 2000; 37: 334–338.
57. Oosterlinck W, Philp NH, Charig C, et al. A double-blind single dose comparison of intramuscular ketorolac tromethamine and pethidine in the treatment of renal colic. J Clin Pharmacol 1990; 30: 336–341.
58. Lennon GM, Bourke J, Ryan PC, et al. Pharmacological options for the treatment of acute ureteric colic. An in vitro experimental study. Br J Urol 1993; 71: 401–407.
59. Larsen LS, Miller A, Allegra JR. The use of intravenous ketorolac for the treatment of renal colic in the emergency department. Am J Emerg Med 1993; 11: 197–199.
60. Larkin GL, Peacock WFT, Pearl SM, et al. Efficacy of ketorolac tromethamine vs meperidine in the ED treatment of acute renal colic. Am J Emerg Med 1999; 17: 6–10.
61. Cordell WH, Wright SW, Wolfson AB, et al. Comparison of intravenous ketorolac, meperidine, and both (balanced analgesia) for renal colic. Ann Emerg Med 1996; 28: 151–158.
62. Stein A, Ben Dov D, Finkel B, et al. Single-dose intramuscular ketorolac vs diclofenac for pain management in renal colic. Am J Emerg Med 1996; 14: 385–387.
63. Cohen E, Hafner R, Rotenberg Z, et al. Comparison of ketorolac and diclofenac in the treatment of renal colic. Eur J Clin Pharmacol 1998; 54: 455–458.
64. Edwards JE, Meseguer F, Faura C, et al. Single dose dipyrone for acute renal colic pain. Cochrane Database Syst Rev 2002; CD003867.
65. Al-Waili NS, Saloom KY. Intramuscular piroxicam vs intramuscular diclofenac sodium in the treatment of acute renal colic: double-blind study. Eur J Med Res 1999; 4: 23–26.
66. Supervia A, Pedro-Botet J, Nogues X, et al. Piroxicam fast-dissolving dosage form vs diclofenac sodium in the treatment of acute renal colic: a double-blind controlled trial. Br J Urol 1998; 81: 27–30.
67. Nakada SY, Jerde TJ, Bjorling DE, et al. Selective cyclooxygenase-2 inhibitors reduce ureteral contraction in vitro: a better alternative for renal colic? J Urol 2000; 163: 607–612.
68. Kekec Z, Yilmaz U, Sozuer E. The effectiveness of tenoxicam vs isosorbide dinitrate plus tenoxicam in the treatment of acute renal colic. BJU Int 2000; 85: 783–785.
69. Grenabo L, Aurell M, Delin K, et al. Antidiuretic hormone levels and the effect of indomethacin on ureteral colic. J Urol 1983; 129: 941–943.
70. Kimoto Y, Constantinou CE. Effects of [1-desamino-8-D-arginine]vasopressin and papaverine on rabbit renal pelvis. Eur J Pharmacol 1990; 175: 359–362.
71. Moro U, De Stefani S, Crisci A, et al. Evaluation of the effects of desmopressin in acute ureteral obstruction. Urol Int 1999; 62: 8–11.
72. Kjaer A. Vasopressin as a neuroendocrine regulator of anterior pituitary hormone secretion. Acta Endocrinol (Copenh) 1993; 129: 489–496.
73. Lopes T, Dias JS, Marcelino J, et al. An assessment of the clinical efficacy of intranasal desmopressin spray in the treatment of renal colic. BJU Int 2001; 87: 322–325.
74. el-Sherif AE, Salem M, Yahia H, et al. Treatment of renal colic by desmopressin intranasal spray and diclofenac sodium. J Urol 1995; 153: 1395–1398.
75. Constantinides C, Kapralos V, Manousakas T, et al. Management of renal colic with intranasal desmopressin spray. Acta Urol Belg 1998; 66: 1–3.
76. Romics I, Molnar DL, Timberg G, et al. The effect of drotaverine hydrochloride in acute colicky pain caused by renal and ureteric stones. BJU Int 2003; 92: 92–96.
77. Eray O, Cete Y, Oktay C, et al. Intravenous single-dose tramadol vs meperidine for pain relief in renal colic. Eur J Anaesthesiol 2002; 19: 368–370.
78. Cordell WH, Larson TA, Lingeman JE, et al. Indomethacin suppositories vs intravenously titrated morphine for the treatment of ureteral colic. Ann Emerg Med 1994; 23: 262–269.

79. Thompson JF, Pike JM, Chumas PD, et al. Rectal diclofenac compared with pethidine injection in acute renal colic. BMJ 1989; 299: 1140–1141.
80. Iguchi M, Katoh Y, Koike H, et al. Randomized trial of trigger point injection for renal colic. Int J Urol 2002; 9: 475–479.
81. Kober A, Dobrovits M, Djavan B, et al. Local active warming: an effective treatment for pain, anxiety and nausea caused by renal colic. J Urol 2003; 170: 741–744.
82. Lee YH, Lee WC, Chen MT, et al. Acupuncture in the treatment of renal colic. J Urol 1992; 147: 16–18.
83. Segura JW, Preminger GM, Assimos DG, et al. Ureteral Stones Clinical Guidelines Panel summary report on the management of ureteral calculi. The American Urological Association. J Urol 1997; 158: 1915–1921.
84. Miller OF, Kane CJ. Time to stone passage for observed ureteral calculi: a guide for patient education. J Urol 1999; 162: 688–690.
85. Bortolotti M, Trisolino G, Barbara L. Nifedipine in biliary and renal colic. JAMA 1987; 258: 3516.
86. Caravati EM, Runge JW, Bossart PJ, et al. Nifedipine for the relief of renal colic: a double-blind, placebo-controlled clinical trial. Ann Emerg Med 1989; 18: 352–354.
87. Borghi L, Meschi T, Amato F, et al. Nifedipine and methylprednisolone in facilitating ureteral stone passage: a randomized, double-blind, placebo-controlled study. J Urol 1994; 152: 1095–1098.
88. Cooper JT, Stack GM, Cooper TP. Intensive medical management of ureteral calculi. Urology 2000; 56: 575–578.
89. Stief CG, Uckert S, Truss MC, et al. A possible role for nitric oxide in the regulation of human ureteral smooth muscle tone in vitro. Urol Res 1996; 24: 333–337.
90. Ng CK, Yip SK, Sim LS, et al. Outcome of percutaneous nephrostomy for the management of pyonephrosis. Asian J Surg 2002; 25: 215–219.
91. Pearle MS, Pierce HL, Miller GL, et al. Optimal method of urgent decompression of the collecting system for obstruction and infection due to ureteral calculi. J Urol 1998; 160: 1260–1264.
92. Docimo SG, Dewolf WC. High failure rate of indwelling ureteral stents in patients with extrinsic obstruction: experience at two institutions. J Urol 1989; 142: 277–279.
93. Yossepowitch O, Lifshitz DA, Dekel Y, et al. Predicting the success of retrograde stenting for managing ureteral obstruction. J Urol 2001; 166: 1746–1749.
94. Lennon GM, Thornhill JA, Grainger R, et al. Double pigtail ureteric stent vs percutaneous nephrostomy: effects on stone transit and ureteric motility. Eur Urol 1997; 31: 24–29.
95. Leventhal EK, Rozanski TA, Crain TW, et al. Indwelling ureteral stents as definitive therapy for distal ureteral calculi. J Urol 1995; 153: 34–36.
96. Satoh S, Okuma A, Fujita Y, et al. Spontaneous rupture of the renal pelvis during pregnancy: a case report and review of the literature. Am J Perinatol 2002; 19: 189–195.
97. Coe FL, Parks JH, Lindheimer MD. Nephrolithiasis during pregnancy. N Engl J Med 1978; 298: 324–326.
98. Horowitz E, Schmidt JD. Renal calculi in pregnancy. Clin Obstet Gynecol 1985; 28: 324–338.
99. Biyani CS, Joyce AD. Urolithiasis in pregnancy. I: pathophysiology, fetal considerations and diagnosis. BJU Int 2002; 89: 811–818.
100. Stothers L, Lee LM. Renal colic in pregnancy. J Urol 1992; 148: 1383–1387.
101. Drago JR, Rohner TJ Jr, Chez RA. Management of urinary calculi in pregnancy. Urology 1982; 20: 578–581.
102. Biyani CS, Joyce AD. Urolithiasis in pregnancy. II: management. BJU Int 2002; 89: 819–823.
103. Meares EM Jr. Urologic surgery during pregnancy. Clin Obstet Gynecol 1978; 21: 907–920.
104. Lifshitz DA, Lingeman JE. Ureteroscopy as a first-line intervention for ureteral calculi in pregnancy. J Endourol 2002; 16: 19–22.
105. Watterson JD, Girvan AR, Beiko DT, et al. Ureteroscopy and holmium:YAG laser lithotripsy: an emerging definitive management strategy for symptomatic ureteral calculi in pregnancy. Urology 2002; 60: 383–387.
106. Shokeir AA, Mutabagani H. Rigid ureteroscopy in pregnant women. Br J Urol 1998; 81: 678–681.

17 Nonurolithic Causes of Upper Urinary Tract Obstruction

Roger K. Low, MD

Contents

INTRODUCTION
URETEROPELVIC JUNCTION OBSTRUCTION
RETROPERITONEAL FIBROSIS
URETEROENTERIC STRICTURES
PAPILLARY NECROSIS
TRANSITIONAL CELL CARCINOMA OF THE URETER
REFERENCES

INTRODUCTION

Renal colic caused by urolithiasis is the most common cause of upper urinary tract obstruction that prompts patients to visit to an acute care facility. Patient care providers must be aware of other less-common urological causes of upper urinary tract obstruction presenting similar to urinary stones. Although few of the clinical entities discussed in this section are true "urological emergencies," a physician's familiarity with all of them will be helpful in the evaluation of any patient thought to have renal colic.

URETEROPELVIC JUNCTION OBSTRUCTION

Ureteropelvic junction obstruction (UPJO) is the most common congenital cause of hydronephrosis. Hydronephrosis results from impaired urinary flow through the ureteropelvic junction (UPJ). Causes for UPJO can be classified as either intrinsic or extrinsic. Intrinsic stenosis is the most common finding. Histological examination of such lesions is characterized by abnormal ureteral musculature or an abnormal ratio of ureteral muscle to collagen (1). Extrinsic lesions compress or kink the UPJ and commonly are caused by either a blood vessel or fibrous band. Crossing blood vessels typically represent an accessory renal artery or lower pole branch supplying the kidney (Fig. 1). It is unclear whether extrinsic lesions are a cause of obstruction or coexist with an intrinsic lesion. It has been theorized that intrinsic stenosis can distort the normal anatomy to give the allusion that extrinsic lesions contribute to obstruction.

From: *Urological Emergencies: A Practical Guide*
Edited by: H. Wessells and J. W. McAninch © Humana Press Inc., Totowa, NJ

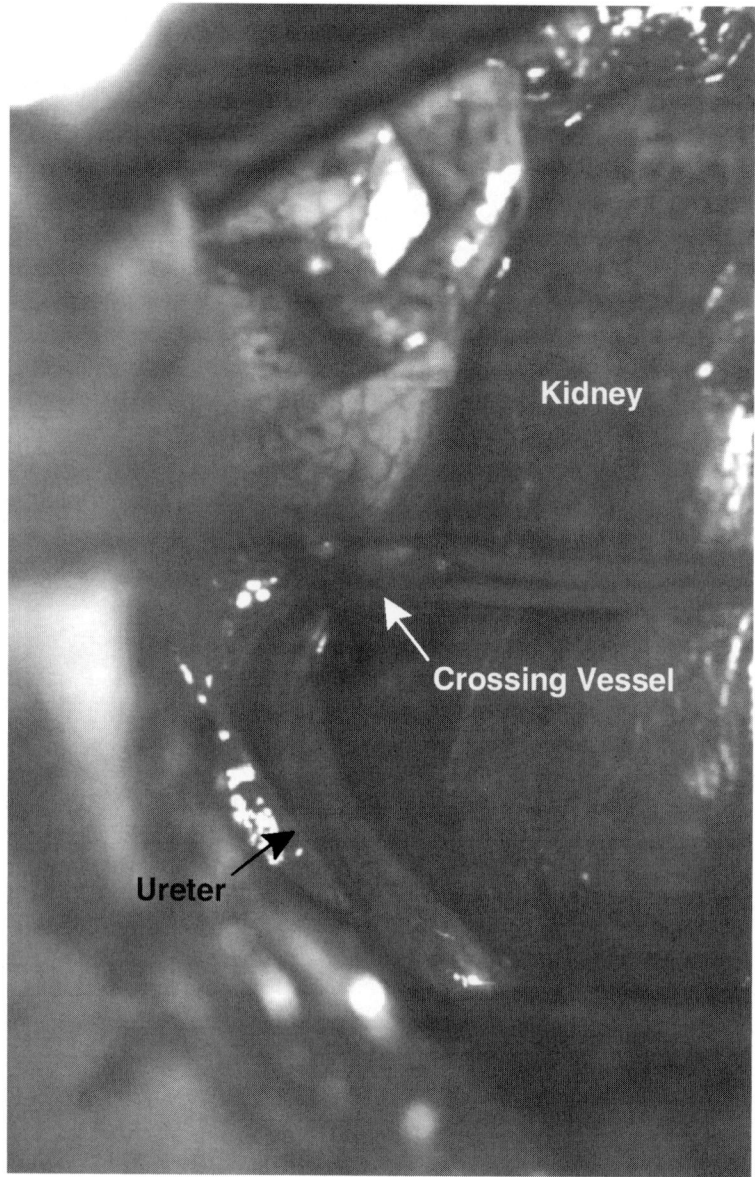

Fig. 1. Operative photo demonstrating anterior crossing vessel at left ureteropelvic junction.

Presentation

The clinical presentation of patients with congenital UPJO has changed related to the development and use of antenatal ultrasonography. Before the widespread use of antenatal ultrasound, patients with congenital UPJO most often presented during childhood. In infants, a palpable abdominal mass was the most common presentation. Infants also present with intestinal colic, failure to thrive, or a febrile illness. Older children typically present with either flank/abdominal pain or symptomatic urinary tract infection. Symptoms often are confused for a gastrointestinal disorder. Hematuria, following only minor trauma, can occur in 15 to 20% of patients.

With the advent of antenatal ultrasonography, most cases of UPJO are now discovered in utero. Hydronephrosis caused by UPJO is the most common abnormality detected on prenatal ultrasound *(2)*. Fetal hydronephrosis is detected in 1% of pregnancies. Congenital UPJ obstruction accounts for 50% of the patients with hydronephrosis; the remainder can be caused by ureterovesicle junction obstruction, vesicoureteral reflux, and ectopic ureter/ureteroceles. Not all fetal hydronephrosis is pathological. Of children demonstrating hydronephrosis on antenatal ultrasonography, 20% have normal imaging after birth *(3)*.

Although less common, some patients with congenital UPJO do not present until adulthood. In adults, UPJO presents with symptoms of flank pain, hematuria, or urinary tract infection. Dietl's crisis refers to severe flank/abdominal pain and nausea/vomiting brought on by drinking fluid. Physiologically, this is explained by a rapid expansion of the kidney that results from diuresis.

Diagnosis

Diagnosis of UPJO is made by eliciting a history of pain brought on by drinking fluids and finding hydronephrosis on imaging studies. Patients typically do not exhibit a fever unless there is an associated infection or renal stone. The choice of initial imaging is ultrasonography in children and noncontrast spiral computed tomography (CT) in adults. Ultrasonography is preferred in children because of its ability to assess patients rapidly for the presence of renal obstruction without exposing them to radiation. In adults, spiral CT has nearly replaced both intravenous pyelography (IVP) and ultrasonography in patients suspected of renal colic. Spiral CT has advantages of being rapid without requiring injection of intravenous contrast (Fig. 2). It is a sensitive test for detecting hydronephrosis and capable of detecting nonurological causes for flank/abdominal pain. Congenital UPJO should be suspected in those patients demonstrating hydronephrosis but without evidence of stone or dilated ureter.

Management

Patients with UPJO rarely present with signs or symptoms necessitating emergent management. Most commonly, patients' symptoms lead to the finding of hydronephrosis by ultrasound or CT, prompting further radiographic imaging. Patients presenting with intractable symptoms of renal colic, signs or symptoms of upper tract infection, or compromised renal function need to be managed emergently.

In most cases, this consists of drainage of the kidney by either internal stenting or external nephrostomy tube. The efficacy of internal stenting vs percutaneous nephrostomy in providing emergent drainage is thought to be similar *(4)*. Most patients prefer to have internal stenting rather than an external nephrostomy for cosmetic and hygienic reasons. Patients with pyonephrosis or an associated large renal stone may benefit from placement of a nephrostomy tube rather than internal stenting. Patients with large renal stones and who contemplate future endoscopic management may prefer to have a nephrostomy placed. If such an approach is considered, a posterior middle or superior calyceal entry is preferred to allow best access for future endopyelotomy.

Symptomatic UPJO is definitively treated after treatment of any associated infection and stabilization of patients' symptoms. Confirmatory imaging with intravenous pyelography or diuretic renography establishes the diagnosis. Patients contemplating endoscopic treatment may benefit from further imaging to establish the presence or absence of a crossing vessel. Magnetic resonance urography may have a role in imaging

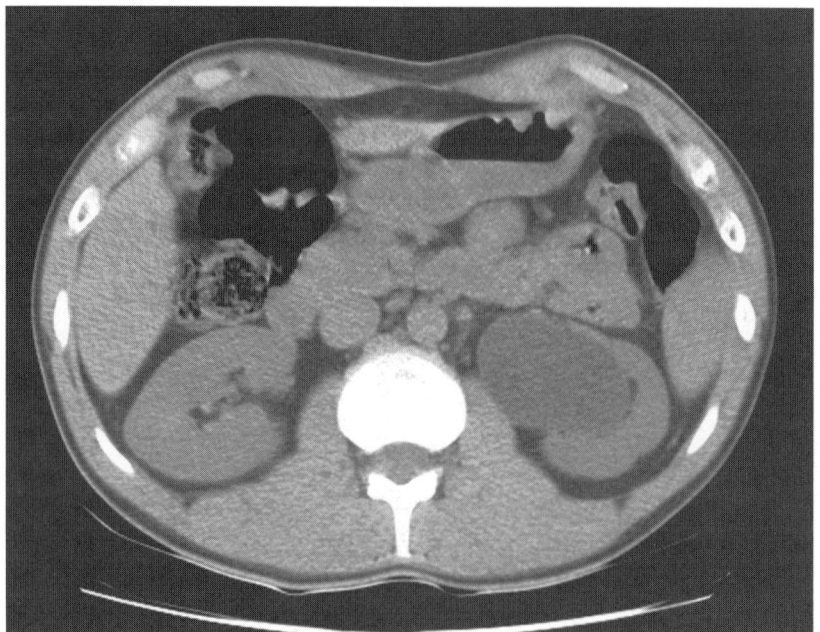

Fig. 2. Noncontrast spiral computed tomography (CT) demonstrating left hydronephrosis caused by ureteropelvic junction obstruction.

patients found to have UPJO. Magnetic resonance urography allows delineation of the UPJO, evaluation for the presence of crossing vessels, and may allow estimation of ipsilateral renal glomerular filtration rate (Fig. 3).

The standard treatment for UPJO is open surgery to excise the stenotic segment or reconstruct the UPJ. There are a variety of open surgical techniques to correct UPJO. The type of repair is dictated by the ureteral insertion and length of stenotic ureter. Adherences to certain surgical principles apply, including creation of a funnel-shaped pelvis with a dependent, tension-free anastomosis. Open surgical techniques are associated with a 90% or better chance of success and represent the gold standard to which all other treatments are compared *(5–7)*.

Many minimally invasive techniques have gained popularity in treating adult UPJO. Minimally invasive techniques include balloon dilation, endoscopic incision, and laparoscopic pyeloplasty. Adverse prognostic factors that affect the success of endoscopic dilation and incision have been established. Prognostic factors that adversely affect success include a long area of stricture, severe hydronephrosis, poor ipsilateral renal function, and the presence of a crossing vessel *(8)*.

The significance of crossing vessels is controversial. Some believe the presence of a crossing vessel precludes treatment with endoscopic incision because of the risk of vessel injury/bleeding and adverse effect on outcome. CT angiography is most useful in detecting the presence of a crossing vessel and delineating the UPJ anatomy. Use of intraureteral ultrasonography also is capable of identifying crossing vessels *(9)*.

The use of balloon dilation to treat primary UPJO has a limited role. Although studies demonstrated 68–80% short-term success rates, long-term follow-up demonstrated inadequate results *(10–12)*. Endoscopic incision of the stenotic segment can be performed in a retrograde ureteroscopic or percutaneous antegrade approach. The retrograde technique evolved paralleling advances in flexible ureteroscopy and instrumentation. The

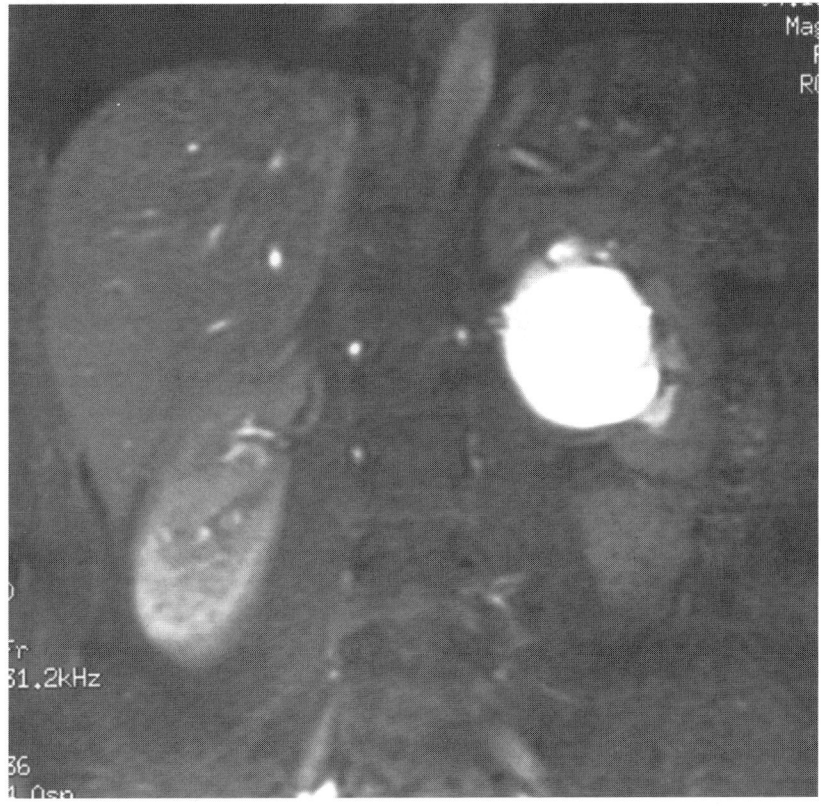

Fig. 3. T-1-weighted magnetic resonance imaging demonstrating left ureteropelvic junction obstruction.

development of small-caliber flexible ureteroscopes (7–10F diameter) and use of the holmium laser for incision offer the ability to treat patients on an outpatient basis or with an overnight hospital stay *(13,14)*.

The Acucise catheter (Applied Medical Technologies, Laguna Hills, CA) is a fluoroscopically positioned device used to incise and dilate the UPJ. The attractiveness of the device is that application requires only standard cystoscopic and fluoroscopic equipment.

Percutaneous endopyelotomy has gained the most acceptance as an alternative therapy to open pyeloplasty for the treatment of UPJO in adults. In comparison to open pyeloplasty, antegrade endopyelotomy is associated with shorter operative times, hospital stay, and convalescence *(15,16)*. Percutaneous endopyelotomy involves gaining percutaneous renal access through a posterior middle calyx and incising the UPJ laterally. A full thickness ureteral incision until retroperitoneal tissue is visualized is required.

Gill and associates described a technique whereby following standard longitudinal endopyelotomy, reapproximation of the incision is performed in a Heineke-Mikulicz fashion using a 5-mm laparoscopic suturing device placed though the nephroscope *(17)*. Closure of the incision in such a fashion reportedly results in a wider caliber UPJ and absence of extravasation, and it requires shorter stenting duration.

A variety of devices can be utilized to incise the ureter, including a cold knife, cutting electrode, or laser. There does not appear to be an appreciable advantage to any particular cutting device. Following incision of the ureter, an indwelling ureteral stent and nephrostomy or universal nephrostomy tube are placed, typically for 4 to 6 wk. A 75 to 90% chance of

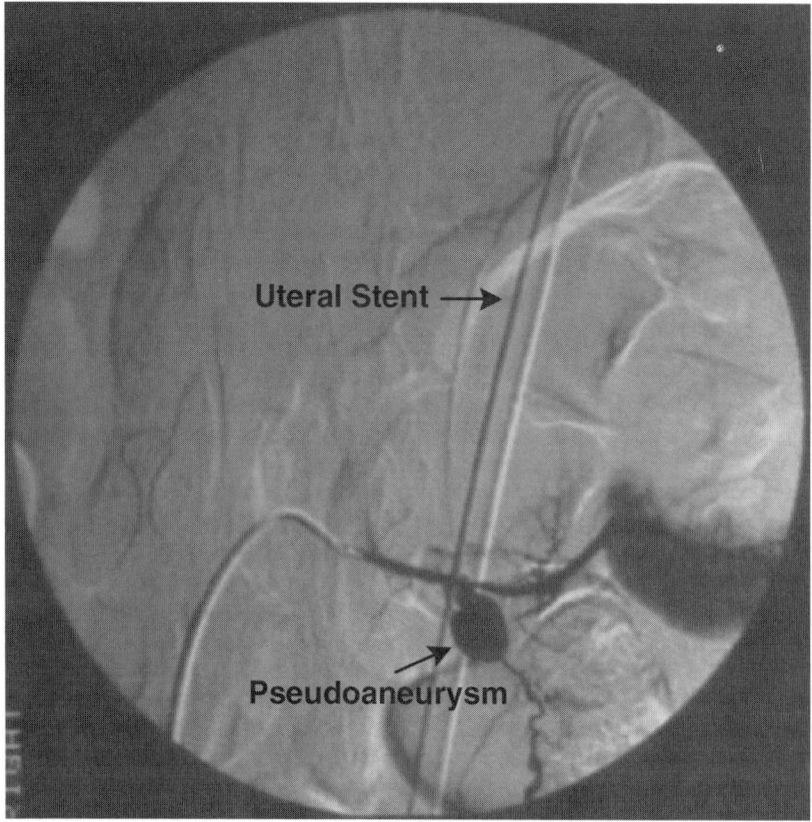

Fig. 4. Pseudoaneurysm of left lower pole renal vessel following endopyelotomy.

success can be expected for treatment of UPJO by endoscopic incision *(18,19)*. Aside from treatment failure, bleeding related to injury of a crossing vessel is the most important risk of endopyelotomy. Figure 4 demonstrates a pseudoaneurysm of a lower pole renal vessel after endoscopic incision of the UPJ. Patients with clinically significant bleeding following endopyelotomy require angiography and embolization of bleeding vessels.

Laparoscopic pyeloplasty was developed in hopes of equaling the success rates offered by open pyeloplasty while maintaining the minimal invasiveness of endopyelotomy. This approach is preferred in patients with poor prognostic variables for endopyelotomy who prefer a minimally invasive approach. Unlike endopyelotomy, open and laparoscopic pyeloplasty allow reduction of redundant renal pelvis and transposition of the UPJ behind any crossing vessels. Currently, the largest review of laparoscopic pyeloplasty patients reveals a 96% radiographic success rate after a mean follow-up of 2.2 yr *(20)*. Their average operative time was 4.2 h, and average hospital stay was 3.3 d.

Use of a robotic system to perform laparoscopic pyeloplasty is under investigation. A preliminary report comparing laparoscopic pyeloplasty with the daVinci Robotic System vs standard laparoscopic pyeloplasty found use of the robotic system feasible and associated with a decrease in operative time compared to standard laparoscopy *(21)*.

Patients with UPJO have a variety of treatment options. Choice of treatment depends on patient priorities and physician experience. Gettman et al. performed a cost analysis of the different treatment modalities for UPJO *(22)*. Primary cost variables included operative time, hospital stay, equipment cost, and success rate. They found ureteroscopic and Acucise endopyelotomy to be the most cost-effective treatment for UPJO.

Prognostic factors affecting success of endopyelotomy should be factored in managing patients with UPJO. Patients with marked hydronephrosis, diminished ipsilateral renal function, and crossing vessels are best served with either laparoscopic or open pyeloplasty. Patients without adverse prognostic factors should be counseled on the 10 to 15% difference in success between endopyelotomy and either laparoscopic or open pyeloplasty. For those choosing endopyelotomy, choice of technique depends primarily on physician preference and equipment availability. For infants and small children, open pyeloplasty remains the treatment of choice. Open pyeloplasty in this population has over a 95% success rate and minimal morbidity.

RETROPERITONEAL FIBROSIS

Retroperitoneal fibrosis (RP) is an uncommon but important cause of upper urinary tract obstruction. It is characterized by the formation of a dense fibrous plaque encasing the aorta and vena cava. Fibrosis typically involves retroperitoneal structures extending from the renal hila to the pelvic brim and the ureters laterally. RP contains a variable cellular inflammatory component consisting of lymphocytes, plasma cells, eosinophils, and polymorphonuclear leukocytes. The hallmark of the disease is entrapment of the ureters, causing hydronephrosis and progressive azotemia.

There are many etiological factors for the formation of RP; however, many cases are idiopathic. RP is associated with use of certain medications, abdominal aortic aneurysm, and retroperitoneal malignancy. Use of the medication methylsergide is most commonly associated with RP. Historically, methylsergide was prescribed for migraine headaches. Approximately 1% of patients taking methylsergide developed RP *(23)*. Methylsergide may act as an allergen stimulating a hypersensitivity or autoimmune response in the retroperitoneum *(24)*. Use of ergot derivatives, certain antihypertensive agents, analgesics, haloperidol, and amphetamines have all been associated with RP *(25)*. RP is also associated with connective tissue diseases such as ankylosing spondylitis, systemic lupus erythmatosis, and polyarteritis nodosa, further suggesting an immune-mediated process for development of RP.

RP is found in up to 23% of patients with abdominal aortic aneurysms *(25)*. It has been theorized that the inflammatory fibrosis results from leakage of aneurysmal lipids into the retroperitoneum *(26,27)*. RP is also associated with certain retroperitoneal tumors. Fibrosis related to malignancy is thought to be caused by a desmoplastic response to tumor cells and is most commonly associated with lymphoma, sarcomas, and carcinoid and metastatic carcinoma from the breast, lung, and gastrointestinal and genitourinary tracts *(28)*. Other than malignancy, radiation, infection, and retroperitoneal trauma have also been associated with RP.

Presentation

The clinical presentation of a patient with RP is typically vague and nonspecific. Most commonly, patients present with noncolicky back or abdominal pain, which is poorly localized *(23)*. Patients also complain of progressive malaise, anorexia and weight loss. Rarely, patients can present with signs of urinary tract infection or anuria. The condition has a reported incidence of 1 in 200,000, with a male predominance of 3:1 *(29)*. Most patients present during their fifth or sixth decade.

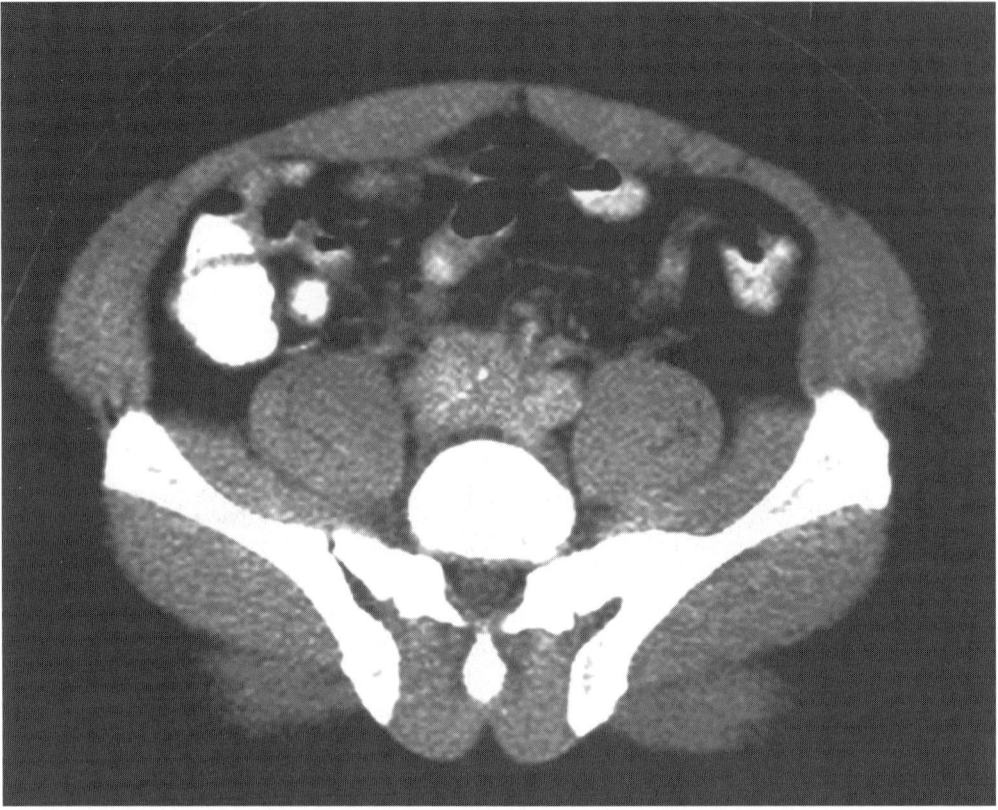

Fig. 5. Computed tomography of pelvis demonstrating retroperitoneal fibrosis surrounding the common iliac vessels.

Clinical signs are related to progressive renal loss and compression of the vena cava. Palpable abdominal mass, lower extremity edema, and hypertension are the most common findings *(23)*. Reports of fibrosis invading gastrointestinal structures resulting in jaundice or intestinal obstruction have been reported *(30,31)*. At presentation, many patients are in poor general health because of prolonged periods of anorexia, weight loss, and progressive renal failure. Laboratory investigation typically demonstrates azotemia and varying degrees of anemia, depending on the severity of renal insufficiency. Elevation of erythrocyte sedimentation rate (ESR) is often found and is an important marker of inflammation. Serial levels of ESR can be utilized to assess the response to medical therapy.

Diagnosis

The diagnosis of RP is best made by CT. RP appears as a soft tissue mass enveloping the aorta and vena cava (Fig. 5). Ureteral involvement and hydronephrosis can be unilateral (20%) or bilateral (68%) *(23)*. Fibrosis typically centers over the sacral promontory, with extension to the renal hila. RP has the same attenuation as muscle and variable enhancement on intravenous contrast administration, depending on the acuity of the disease process.

The differential diagnosis of RP is retroperitoneal hemorrhage, sarcoma, and metastases. Retroperitoneal fibrosis may be difficult to distinguish from retroperitoneal neoplasms. In contrast to RP, which typically causes medial displacement of the

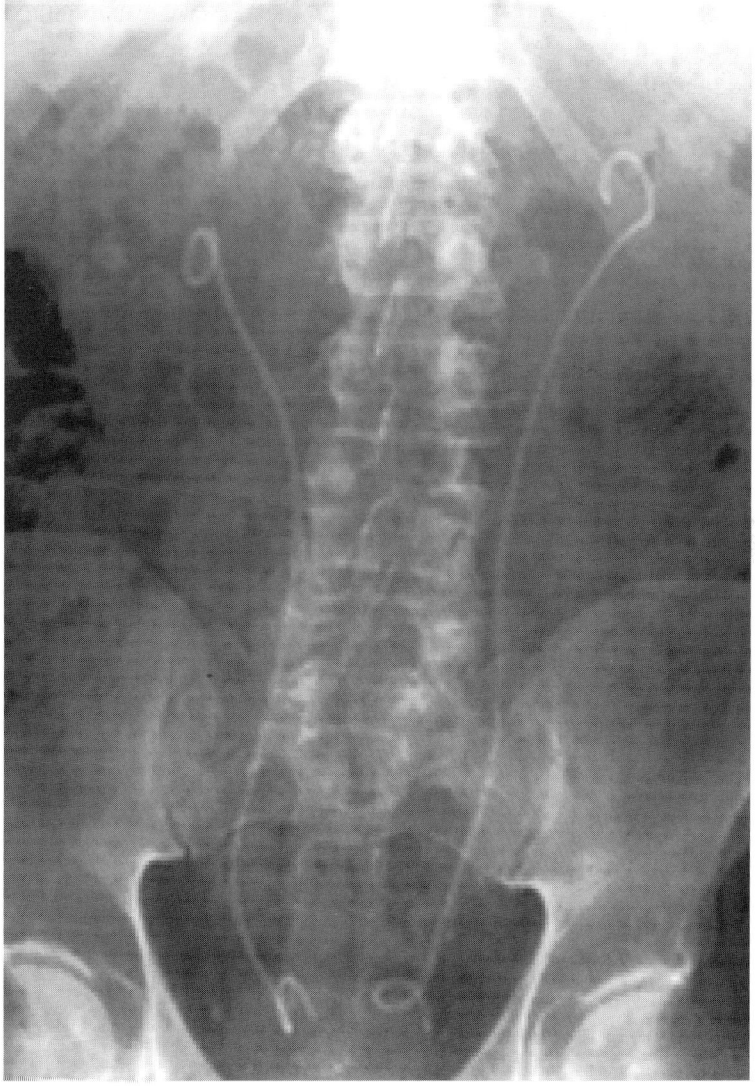

Fig. 6. Abdominal radiograph demonstrating medial deviation of bilateral ureteral stents caused by retroperitoneal fibrosis.

ureters, neoplasms displace the ureters laterally *(32)*. The classic findings of RP on intravenous pyelography are unilateral or bilateral hydronephrosis with delayed contrast excretion and medial deviation and tapering of the ureter(s) at the lumbosacral region *(33)* (Fig. 6). Because most patients have significant renal impairment at the time of presentation, intravenous contrast administration is often not possible. RP by ultrasound appears as a smooth-margined hypoechoic mass centered over the sacral promontory.

Management

The initial management of a patient with RP involves restoration of renal drainage and correction of electrolyte abnormalities. Renal drainage can be achieved by either placement of internal stents or external nephrostomies. Internal stenting is surprisingly easy to perform in most cases of RP.

Once patients have been stabilized, tissue sampling to differentiate RP from cancer is preferred. Tissue samples can be obtained by image-guided, fine-needle aspiration or Tru-cut (Travenol Laboratories, Deerfield, IL) biopsy. Inconclusive tissue sampling is not uncommon because of the acellular nature of RP. Confirmatory diagnosis often requires excisional biopsy at time of laparotomy.

The cornerstone of definitive therapy for RP consists of ureterolysis. The ureters are freed from the surrounding fibrosis for their entire length. Following lysis, ureters are either intraperitonealized or wrapped with omentum to minimize risk of future entrapment. Treatment of both ureters even in the setting of unilateral obstruction is recommended. Relief of ureteral obstruction is successful in approx 90% of cases undergoing surgical ureterolysis *(34)*. Laparoscopic ureterolysis has been reported, but requires longer operating times and expertise in laparoscopy *(35)*.

Ross and Tinckler were the first to report the use of steroids for the treatment of RP in 1958 *(36)*. The use of steroids alone for the treatment of RP is controversial, especially in those without a definitive exclusion of malignancy. Steroids have been useful as an adjunct to ureterolysis and in elderly or debilitated patients who are not ideal surgical candidates. Patients presenting with an elevated ESR, reflecting active inflammation, are most responsive to steroid therapy *(37)*. Other immunosuppressive agents such as tamoxifen and cyclosporin have been used to treat patients with RP *(38,39)*.

URETEROENTERIC STRICTURES

Urinary diversion by creation of ureterosigmoidostomies in a patient with bladder extrophy was first reported in 1852 *(40)*. Bricker later popularized use of an ileal conduit in the 1950s to divert urine following cystectomy *(41)*. Since then, numerous surgical techniques utilizing a variety of bowel segments and configurations are used to provide continent urinary diversions.

Although urinary diversion has vastly improved patient quality of life following cystectomy, the patients are susceptible to a variety of complications, including infection, stone formation, and metabolic derangements. One of the most common complications is development of a ureteroenteric stricture at the anastomosis of the ureter and reconfigured bowel segment. Ureteroenteric strictures occur at a rate of 4 to 8% in patients undergoing urinary diversion *(42,43)*. Most strictures are discovered between 1 and 2 yr following urinary diversion *(44)*. They occur more commonly on the left than the right, believed to be because of ureteral ischemia.

Presentation

The presentation of patients with ureteroenteric strictures is variable. Many patients are asymptomatic and incidental hydronephrosis is found on routine imaging. Others present with flank pain, urinary tract infection, and rarely urosepsis.

Diagnosis

Hydronephrosis can be detected by ultrasonography, intravenous pyelography, or CT. Once detected, further imaging is required to determine the severity, location, and length of stricture. All patients with past continent urinary diversion should be questioned about past difficulties and frequency of catheterizations. Placement of an indwelling catheter should be performed in any patient complaining of abdominal pain or exhibiting bilateral hydronephrosis or signs/symptoms of urinary tract infection.

Management

The initial management of the patient with an anastomotic stricture depends on the condition of the patient and type of past urinary diversion. Patients presenting in urosepsis or renal compromise require immediate establishment of renal drainage prior to definitive management of their stricture. Unlike patients still possessing a bladder, retrograde placement of internal stents is difficult and often impossible in patients with prior urinary diversion. Ureteroenteric anastomoses are often endoscopically inaccessible through an abdominal stoma. As a result, placement of a nephrostomy tube is often necessary to establish renal drainage.

Once renal function has been optimized and any infection cleared, defining the characteristics of the ureteral obstruction is required. Anatomy is best defined with combined antegrade and retrograde contrast studies. Strictures appear as a tapered narrowing of the distal ureter (Fig. 7). They must be distinguished from ureteral filling defects possibly representing recurrent cancer in those with a history of bladder carcinoma. Endoscopic inspection is mandatory in any patient for whom a diagnosis of carcinoma remains uncertain.

Formal reconstruction of the ureter via laparotomy is the traditional treatment for ureteroenteric strictures. Long-term success rates are best with open surgical techniques and range from 76 to 89% *(45,46)*. Minimally invasive techniques have been applied to treat ureteroenteric strictures, but with less success. Balloon dilation is associated with only a 5% long-term patency rate *(46)*. Endoscopic incision has a slightly improved long-term patency rate of 32% *(47)*. Finding poor ipsilateral renal function in patients who were asymptomatic often requires nephrectomy.

PAPILLARY NECROSIS

Papillary necrosis is an uncommon but important etiology to consider in any patient presenting with signs and symptoms of upper urinary tract obstruction. Papillary necrosis is associated most commonly with analgesic abuse, diabetes mellitus, sickle cell disease, and obstructive uropathy *(48–50)*.

The most common cause of papillary necrosis is analgesic abuse. Historically, phenacetin abuse was most commonly implicated; however, recently use of aspirin, acetaminophen, and nonsteroidal anti-inflammatory agents is more common. All of these agents are related to salicylic acid, and their mechanism of action is related to inhibition of prostaglandin biosynthesis. Short-term use of any of these agents can be associated with a spectrum of renal effects, including interstitial nephritis and tubular necrosis *(51)*. There is a dose-dependent correlation between drug consumption and nephropathy *(52)*. Short-term use of these analgesics is associated with transient, self-limited renal changes. Papillary necrosis resulting from destruction of juxtamedullary nephrons predominantly occurs in patients who chronically ingest nonnarcotic analgesics.

Presentation

Patients with papillary necrosis typically present with symptoms of renal colic and urinary tract infection. Upper tract obstruction from papillary necrosis should be considered in any patient with diabetes, sickle cell disease, or chronic analgesic use. A history of arthritis or headache may be elicited from patients with papillary necrosis caused by

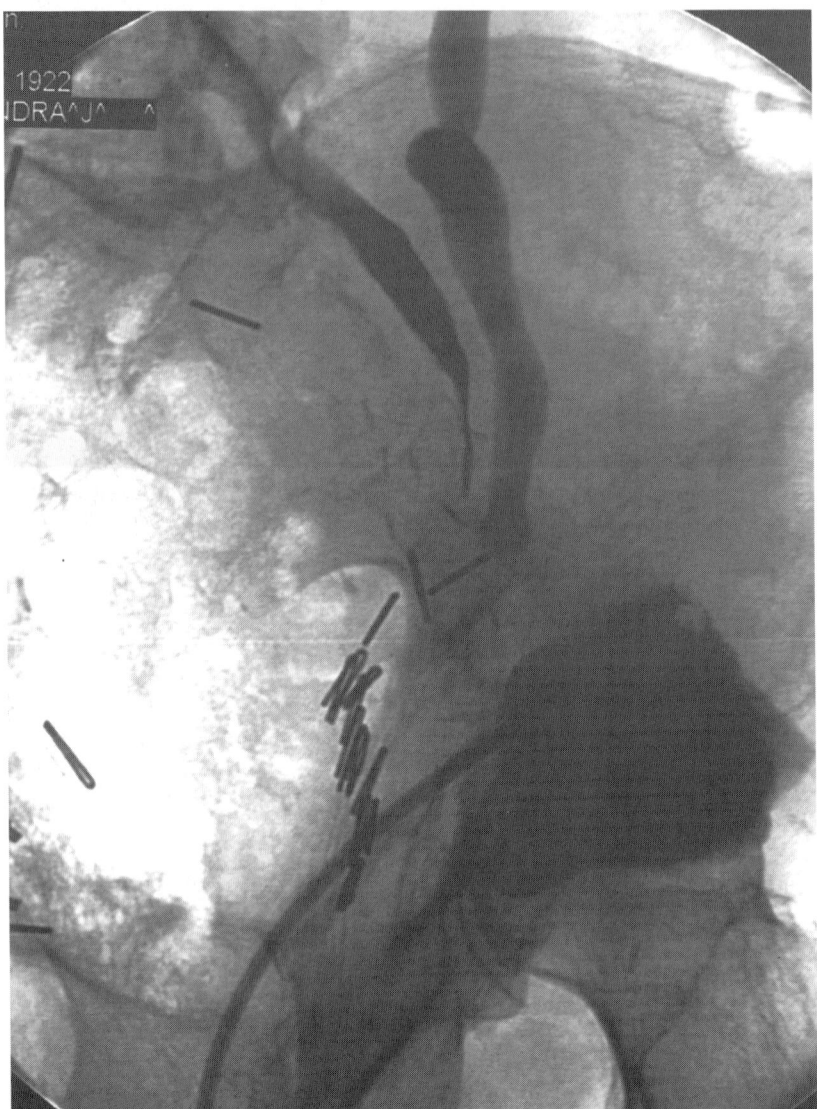

Fig. 7. Bilateral nephrostogram demonstrating bilateral ureteroenteric strictures.

analgesic abuse. Microscopic examination of the urine demonstrates hematuria, pyuria, and often bacteriuria. Occasionally, fragments of papillary renal tissue may be visible on urine microscopy. Patients with associated upper urinary tract infection will manifest fever and leukocytosis. Elevation of the serum creatinine may be caused by preexisting underlying renal compromise, urinary obstruction, or dehydration caused by fever or nausea/vomiting. Papillary necrosis has been associated with renal insufficiency, hyperkalemia, salt wasting, and metabolic acidosis *(51)*.

Diagnosis

Historically, the diagnosis of papillary necrosis has been made by IVP. Renal papillary ulcerations or a radiolucent ureteral filling defect that causes obstruction is the finding on IVP (Fig. 8). Use of noncontrast spiral CT to evaluate patients suspected of renal colic

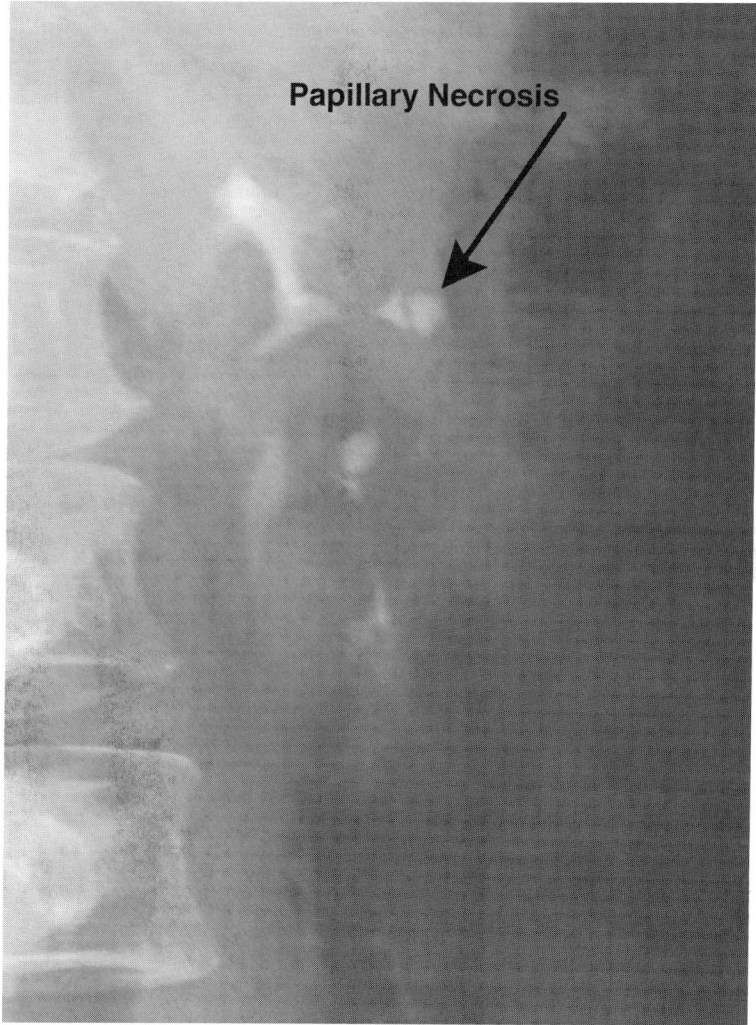

Fig. 8. Intravenous pyelogram demonstrating papillary necrosis.

has increased in popularity. Unlike obstructing ureteral calculi, sloughed papillae do not exhibit high hounsfield units. One must rely on upper tract obstructive changes to make the diagnosis.

Management

The acute management of patients with papillary necrosis is similar to any patient presenting with upper urinary tract obstruction. Patients with intractable symptoms of pain or nausea/vomiting, obstruction contributing to renal compromise, or signs/symptoms of upper urinary tract infection should undergo a procedure to restore renal drainage. Given that many patients with papillary necrosis typically have conditions associated with renal compromise and immunosuppression, decompression is often necessary. Restoration of drainage can be by placement of a nephrostomy or internal stent. Broad-spectrum antibiotics should be given to those suspected of having an infection. Supportive measures, including control of blood sugar in diabetics, is required.

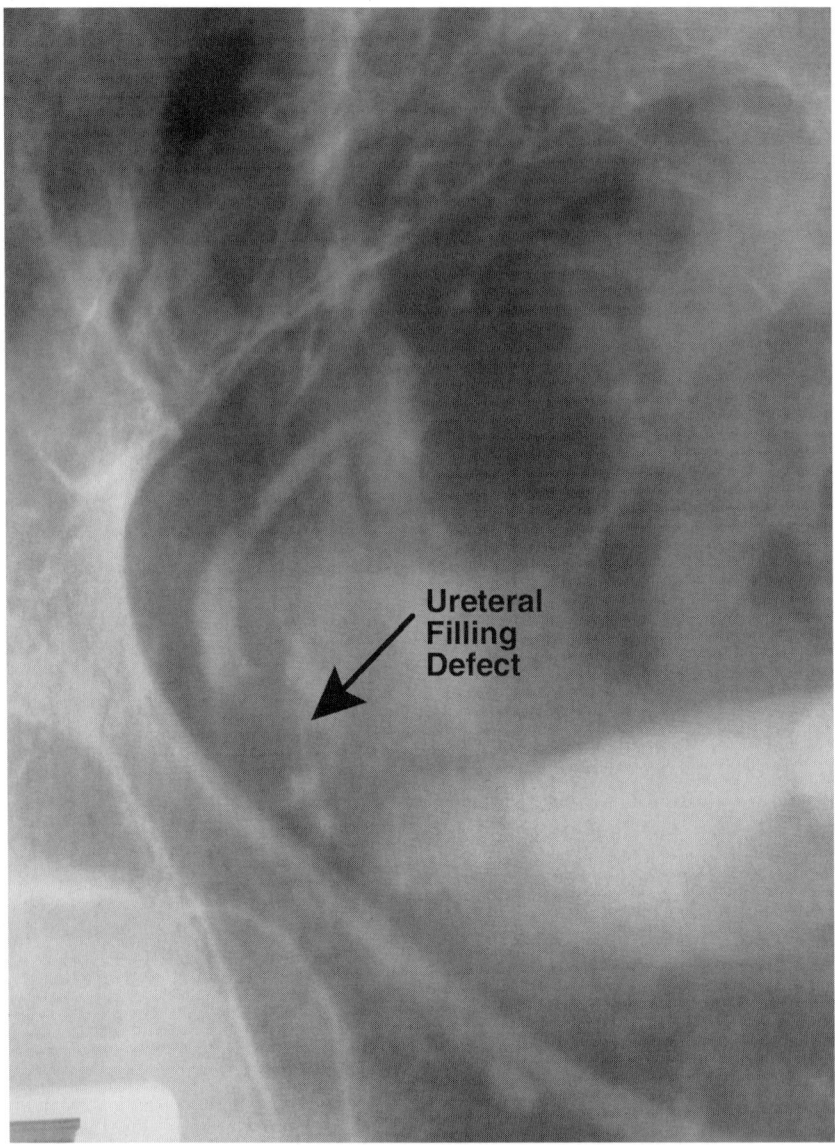

Fig. 9. Filling defect in distal right ureter representing transitional cell carcinoma.

TRANSITIONAL CELL CARCINOMA OF THE URETER

Ureteral obstruction caused by a ureteral tumor is uncommon. Only 5% of urothelial tumors arise in the upper urinary tract, with ureteral tumors accounting for less than 25% *(53,54)*. The majority of ureteral tumors are transitional cell carcinoma (TCC) and occur most frequently in patients with a past history of bladder cancer. Urothelial TCC represents a field-change disease characterized by multiple recurrences over time in different locations. Tobacco use is the most important risk factor for the development of ureteral carcinoma *(55)*. Occupational exposure to chemicals and dyes, analgesic abuse, and cyclophosphamide have also been implicated in the development of upper urinary tract TCC *(56)*.

Presentation

Gross hematuria is the most common presentation of patients with upper urinary tract TCC *(56)*. Unlike patients with bladder cancer, patients may describe passage of vermiform clots suggestive of bleeding originating from the upper urinary tract. Patients may complain of flank pain caused by passage of clots. Not uncommonly, patients are asymptomatic. Anorexia, weight loss, bone pain, and symptoms of advanced disease are uncommon.

Diagnosis

Patients with ureteral tumors rarely present acutely, but more commonly require referral for evaluation of gross hematuria. Traditionally, patients with unexplained hematuria underwent IVP followed by cystoscopy. Increased utilization of ultrasonography and CT in the acute care setting typically reveals hydronephrosis without evidence of an obstructing stone. Ureteral tumors are identified as a radiolucent filling defect on IVP (Fig. 9).

The differential diagnosis of a radiolucent ureteral filling defect includes radiolucent stone, blood clot, sloughed renal papilla, ureteral kink, or vascular impression *(57)*. Uncommon causes include benign fibroepithelial polyp, endometriosis, amyloidosis, fungal ball, or metastases. Further evaluation with ureteroscopic inspection and biopsy is diagnostic. Voided urine cytology alone is not sensitive enough to diagnose most tumors *(58)*.

Management

Nephroureterectomy with excision of a small cuff of bladder is the traditional treatment for patients with upper urinary tract TCC. Laparoscopic nephroureterectomy is feasible and is becoming the standard of care at most academic centers. Endoscopic resection is an option for patients who are a high surgical risk or have compromised renal function, solitary kidneys, or bilateral disease. Prognosis is dependent more on grade and stage of disease than method of treatment *(59,60)*.

REFERENCES

1. Koff SA, Wise HA II. Anomalies of the kidney. In: Adult and Pediatric Urology. (Gllenwater JY, ed.), Mosby, St. Louis, MO, 1996, pp. 2171–2196.
2. Lettgen B, Meyer-Schwickerath M, Bedow W. Prenatal ultrasound diagnosis of the kidneys and efferent urinary tract: possibilities, application and dangers. Monatsschr Kinderheilkunde 1993; 141: 462 467.
3. Dejter SW, Gibbons MD. The fate of infant kidneys with fetal hydronephrosis but initial normal postnatal sonography. J Urol 1989; 142: 661–662.
4. Pearle MS, Pierce HL, Miller GL, et al. Optimal method of urgent decompression of the collecting system for obstruction and infection due to ureteral calculi. J Urol 1998; 160: 1260–1264.
5. Nguyen DH, Aliabadi H, Ercole C, Gonzalez R. Non-intubated Anderson-Hynes repair of ureteropelvic junction obstruction in 60 patients. Urology 1989; 142: 704–706.
6. Notley RG, Beaugie JM. The long-term follow-up of Anderson-Hynes pyeloplasty for hydronephrosis. Br J Urol 1973; 45: 464–467.
7. Persky L, Krause JR, Boltuch RL. Initial complications and late results in dismembered pyeloplasty. J Urol 1977; 118: 162–165.
8. Van Cangh PJ, Nesa S. Endopyelotomy: prognostic factors and patient selection. Urol Clin North Am 1998; 25: 281–288.
9. Bagley DH, Lui JB, Grasso M, Goldberg BB. Endoluminal sonography in the evaluation of the obstructed ureteropelvic junction. J Endourol 1994; 8: 287–292.

10. O'Flynn K, McKelvic G, Steyn J. Endoballoon rupture and stenting for pelvi-ureteric obstruction technique and early results. Br J Urol 1989; 64: 572–574.
11. McClinton S, Steyn JH, Hussey JK. Retrograde balloon dilation for pelviureteric junction obstruction. Br J Urol 1993; 71: 152–155.
12. Osther PJ, Geertsen U, Nielsen HV. Ureteropelvic junction obstruction and ureteral strictures treated by simple high-pressure balloon dilation. J Endourol 1998; 12: 429–431.
13. Hibi H, Yamada Y, Mizumoto H, et al. Retrograde ureteroscopic endopyelotomy using the Holmium:YAG laser. Int J Urol 2002; 9: 77–81.
14. Giddens JL, Grasso M. Retrograde ureteroscopic endopyelotomy using the holmium:YAG laser. J Urol 2000; 164: 1509–1512.
15. Banerjee GK, Ahlawat R, Dalela D, Kumar RV. Endopyelelotomy and pyeloplasty: face to face. Eur Urol 1994; 26: 281–285.
16. Brooks JD, Kavoussi LR, Preminger GM, Scheussler WN, Moore RG. Comparison of open and endourologic approaches to the obstructed ureteropelvic junction. Urology 1995; 46: 791–795.
17. Gill IS, Desai MM, Kaouk JH, Wani K, Desai MR. Percutaneous endopyeloplasty: description of new technique. J Urol 2002; 168: 2097–3102.
18. Clayman RV, Basler JW, Kavoussi L, Picus DD. Ureteronephroscopic endopyletomy. J Urol 1990; 144: 246–251.
19. Thomas R, Monga M, Klein EW. Ureteroscopic retrograde endopyelotomy for management of ureteropelvic junction obstruction. J Endourol 1996; 10: 141–145.
20. Jarrett TW, Chan DY, Charambura TC, Fugita O, Kavoussi LR. Laparoscopic pyeloplasty: the first 100 cases. J Urol 2002; 167: 1253–1256.
21. Gettman MT, Peschel R, Neururer R, Bartsch G. A comparison of laparoscopic pyeloplasty performed with the daVinci Robotic System vs standard laparoscopic techniques: initial clinical results. Eur Urol 2002; 42: 453–458.
22. Gettman MT, Lotan Y, Roerhborn CG, Cadeddu JA, Pearle MS. Cost-effective treatment for ureteropelvic junction obstruction: decision tree analysis. J Urol 2003; 169: 228–232.
23. Koep L, Zuidema GD. The clinical significance of retroperitoneal fibrosis. Surgery 1977; 81: 250–257.
24. Stecker JF Jr, Rawls HP, Devine CJ Jr, Devine PC. Retroperitoneal fibrosis and ergot derivatives. J Urol 1974; 112: 30–32.
25. Buff DD, Bogin MB, Faltz LL. Retroperitoneal fibrosis. A report of selected cases and a review of the literature. N Y State J Med 1989; 89: 511–5161989.
26. Resnick MI, Kursh ED. Extrinsic obstruction the ureter. In: Campbell's Urology. (Walsh PC, Retik AB, Vaugha ED, Wein AJ, eds.), Saunders, Philadelphia, PA, 1998, pp. 387-419.
27. Sakr G, Cynk M, Cowie AG. Retroperitoneal fibrosis. An unusual complication of intra-arterial stents and angioplasty. Br J Urol 1998; 81: 768–769.
28. Thomas MH, Chisolm GD. Retroperitoneal fibrosis associated with malignant disease. Br J Cancer 1973; 28: 453–458.
29. Amis ES Jr. Retroperitoneal fibrosis. AJR Am J Roentgenol 1991; 157: 321–329.
30. Kittredge RD, Nash AD. The many facets of sclerosing fibrosis. Am J Roentgenol Radium Ther Nucl Med 1974; 122: 288–298.
31. Hulnick DH, Chatson GP, Megibow AJ, Bosniak MA, Ruof M. Retroperitoneal fibrosis presenting as colonic dysfunction: CT diagnosis. J Comput Assist Tomogr 1988; 12: 159–161.
32. Persky L, Kursh ED, Feldman S, Resnick MI. Diseases of the retroperitoneum; retroperitoneal fibrosis. In: Campbell's Urology. (Walsh PC, Retik AB, Vaugha ED, Wein AJ, eds.), Saunders, Philadelphia, PA, 1986, pp. 595–601.
33. Webb AJ, Dawson-Edwards P. Malignant retroperitoneal fibrosis. Br J Surg 1967; 54: 508–518.
34. Mikkelsen D, Lepor H. Innovative surgical management of idiopathic fibrosis. J Urol 1989; 141: 1192–1196.
35. Elashry OM, Nakada SY, Wolf JS, Figneshau RS, McDougall EM, Clayma RV. Ureterolysis for external ureteral obstruction: a comparison of laparoscopic and open surgical techniques. J Urol 1996; 156: 1403–1410.
36. Ross JC, Tinckler LF. Renal failure due to periureteric fibrosis. Br J Surg 1958; 46: 58–62.

37. Kardar AH, Kattan S, Lindstedt E, Hanash K. Steroid therapy for idiopathic retroperitoneal fibrosis. J Urol 2002; 168: 550–555.
38. Marzano A, Trapani A, Leone N, Actis GC, Rizzetto M. Treatment of idiopathic retroperitoneal fibrosis using cyclosporin. Ann Rheum Dis 2001; 60: 427–428.
39. Puce R, Porcaro AB, Curti P, et al. Treatment of retroperitoneal fibrosis with tamoxifen: case report and review of literature. Arch Esp Urol 2000; 53: 184–190.
40. Simon J. Ectropia vesical: operation for dissecting the orifices of the ureters into the rectum: temporary success, death, autopsy. Lancet 1852; 2: 568.
41. Bricker EM. Bladder substitution after pelvic evisceration. Surg Clin North Am 1950; 30: 1511.
42. Guiliani L, Gilberti C, Martovana G, et al. Results of radical cystectomy for primary bladder cancer: a retrospective study of more than 2000 cases. Urology 1985; 26: 243.
43. Schmidt JD, Hawtry CE, Flocks RH, Culp DA. Complications, results and problems with ileal diversion. J Urol 1973; 109: 210–216.
44. Malgieri JJ, Perski L. Ileal loop in the treatment for radiation-treated pelvic malignancies: a comparative review. J Urol 1978; 120: 32–34.
45. Kramolowsky EV, Clayman RV, Weyman PJ. Management of ureterointestinal anastomotic strictures: comparison of open surgical and open repair. J Urol 1988; 139: 1195–1198.
46. Dimarco DS, LeRoy AJ, Thieling S, Bergstralh EJ, Segura JW. Long-term results of treatment for ureteroenteric strictures. Urology 2001; 58: 909–913.
47. Wolf JS Jr, Elashry OM, Clayman RV. Long-term results of endoureterotomy for benign and ureteroenteric strictures. J Urol 1997; 158: 759–764.
48. Ellis PS, Pollack HM. The radiologic manifestations of renal papillary necrosis. Semin Nephrol 1984; 4: 77–87.
49. Mujais SK. Renal papillary necrosis in diabetes mellitus. Semin Nephrol 1984; 4: 40–47.
50. Vaamonde CA. Renal papillary necrosis in sickle cell hemoglobinopathies. Semin Nephrol 1984; 4: 48–64.
51. Sabatini S. Analgesic-induced papillary necrosis. Sem Nephrol 1988; 8: 41–54.
52. Buckalew VM Jr, Schey HM. Renal disease from habitual antipyretic analgesic consumption. An assessment of the epidemiologic evidence. Medicine 1986; 65: 291–303.
53. Peterson RO. Renal pelvis. In: Urologic Pathology. (Biello LA, ed.), Lippincott, Philadelphia, PA, 1986, pp. 181–228.
54. Huben RP, Mounzer AM, Murphy GP. Tumor grade and stage as prognostic variables in upper tract urothelial tumors. Cancer 1988; 62: 2016–2020.
55. Jenson OM, Knudsen JB, McLaughlin JK, Sorensen BL. The Copenhagen case-control study of renal pelvis and ureter cancer: role of smoking and occupational exposures. Int J Cancer 1988; 41: 557–561.
56. Hudson MA, Catalona WJ. Urothelial tumors of the bladder, upper tracts, and prostate. In: Adult and Pediatric Urology. (Gillenwater JY, ed.), Mosby, St. Louis, MO, 1996, pp. 1379–1464.
57. Fein AB, McClennan BL. Solitary filling defects of the ureter. Semin Roentgenol 1986; 21: 201–213.
58. Zincke H, Aguilo JJ, Farrow GM, Utz DC, Khan AU. Significance of urinary cytology in the early detection of transitional cell cancer of the upper urinary tract. J Urol 1976; 116: 781–783.
59. Krogh J, Kvist E, Rye B. Transitional cell carcinoma of the upper urinary tract: prognostic variables and post-operative recurrences. Br J Urol 1991; 67: 32–36.
60. Gawley WF, Harney J, Glacken P, Henir M, Rogers A, McKelvie G. Transitional cell carcinoma of the upper urinary tract: some prognostic indicators. Urology 1989; 33: 459–461.

18 Urgent and Emergent Management of Acute Urinary Retention

Ugur Yilmaz, MD and Claire C. Yang, MD

CONTENTS
>INTRODUCTION
>ETIOLOGY
>CLINICAL FINDINGS
>TREATMENT OF ACUTE URINARY RETENTION
>LONG-TERM MANAGEMENT
>SUMMARY
>REFERENCES

INTRODUCTION

Definition

Acute urinary retention (AUR) is the sudden inability to volitionally empty the bladder by urinating (micturition). It is often unexpected and typically painful. A physiological definition of AUR is the inability of the detrusor muscle to produce an intravesical pressure that overcomes urethral closure pressure and to sustain it to empty the bladder. In some cases of AUR, the patient is able to micturate small amounts of urine, but retains large volumes of bladder residual urine. Sustained, untreated urinary retention may lead to urinary infections, hydronephrosis, and acute renal insufficiency or failure.

Prevalence

Among men, the risk of AUR increases with age, and more than 10% of men in the seventh and more than 30% of men in the eighth decade will experience AUR within 5 yr *(1)*. Men with enlarged prostates (an age-related phenomenon) were found to have three times the risk of AUR compared with those without prostatic enlargement *(2)*. Women occasionally present with voiding difficulties and require temporary intermittent catheterization after surgeries related to urinary incontinence *(4)*. In addition, increased residual urinary volume is frequently high in the early postpartum period, whereas the incidence of overt postpartum AUR has been reported as 0.45% *(4,5)*. AUR in children is sometimes difficult to diagnose because many younger children are unable to express the sensation of bladder fullness or inability to void. AUR in children is more

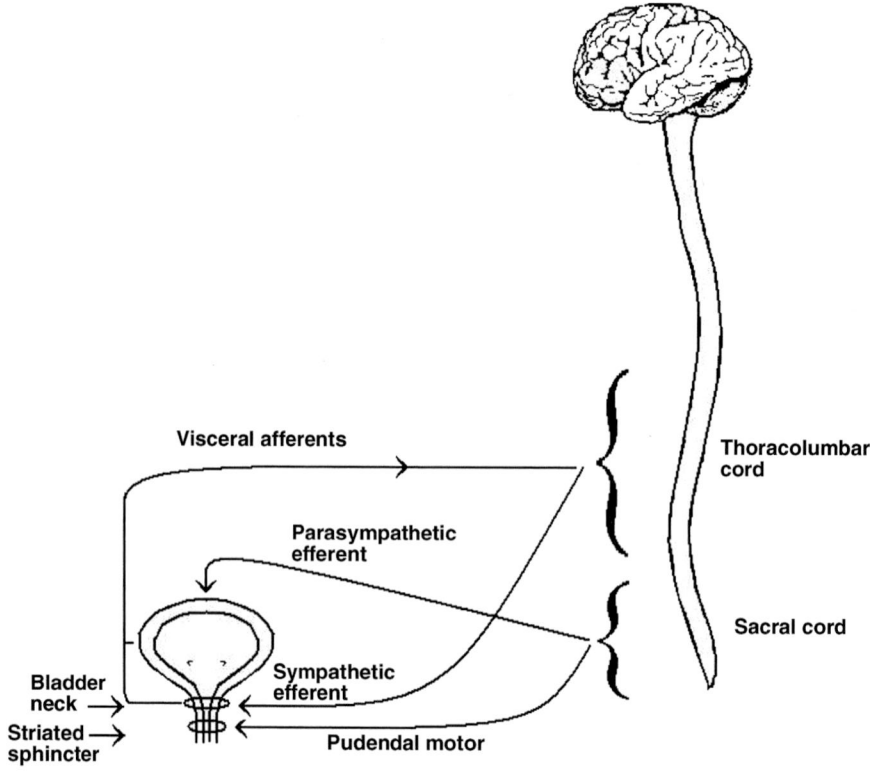

Fig. 1. Dependence of coordinated bladder and sphincter function on intact somatic and autonomic innervation.

frequently because of neurological causes, behavioral voiding dysfunction, and constipation rather than obstruction *(3)*.

Anatomy and Neuroanatomy

The bladder is a smooth muscle viscus that serves as a reservoir for urine. Its function is to store urine until the reservoir is full and to release urine when socially appropriate to do so. Urine storage is achieved through the closure of the bladder neck (also called the internal sphincter) and external striated sphincters, with quiescence of the detrusor muscle, and voiding is achieved with contraction of the detrusor and coordinated opening of the sphincters.

The primary anatomic differences in the lower urinary tract between men and women are the presence of a prostate enveloping the proximal portion of the male urethra and the length of the male urethra. The male adult urethra is typically 16 cm or longer, divided into the prostatic urethra, membranous urethra, bulbar urethra, and penile urethra. The female adult urethra is approx 4 cm.

Coordinated bladder and sphincter function largely depends on intact somatic and autonomic innervation (Fig. 1). Parasympathetic nerves arise at the sacral spinal cord and course through pelvic nerve and pelvic plexus, joining with the thoracolumbar sympathetic efferents that follow a course through the hypogastric plexus. Parasympathetic efferents mediate bladder contraction; sympathetic nerves inhibit the detrusor and

Table 1
Acute Urinary Retention Treatment Algorithm

1. History, physical exam, imaging (if needed)
2. Urethral catheterization or suprapubic cystostomy
3. Labs: urinalysis and Gram stain, urine culture, serum urea nitrogen, creatinine, and electrolytes
4. If serum urea nitrogen and creatinine elevated, observe for postobstructive diuresis
5. If bacteriuria present, begin antibiotics
6. Diagnose underlying cause of AUR, if possible: impaired contractility, bladder outlet obstruction, or both

maintain tone in the bladder neck. Pudendal nerves carry motor innervation from Onuf's nucleus in the sacral spinal cord to innervate the external urethral sphincter. Afferent fibers of these nerves transmit information from the bladder and external urethral sphincter to the lumbosacral spinal cord and central nervous system. Both the somatic and autonomic nerves form reflex loops, also involving central nervous system pathways, to initiate and maintain the bladder storage and voiding functions. Any disruption along the neural pathways results in abnormal bladder function.

AUR may present with varying clinical pictures. A careful diagnostic approach is necessary to manage AUR and to prevent associated complications (Table 1).

ETIOLOGY

The etiological factors of AUR are related to increased bladder outlet resistance, insufficient bladder contractility, or both, with varying frequency of causes among men and women as well as adults and children.

Bladder Outlet Obstruction

Although usually seen in men, bladder outlet obstruction may be encountered in women as well as children (Tables 2 and 3). In both women and men, intravesical foreign bodies such as bladder stones and clot retention following urinary tract bleeding (e.g., bladder tumor, bleeding from kidney) can cause urinary retention. Bladder stones can obstruct the bladder neck or urethra, causing AUR. Antihistamines and α-adrenergic agonists such as ephedrine, pseudoephedrine, phenylephrine, or phenylpropanolamine may increase bladder outlet/urethral resistance and result in AUR.

Lesions of the spinal cord may cause functional obstruction, presenting as bladder neck dyssynergia or detrusor-external sphincter dyssynergia. Dyssynergia, or loss of coordination between the contracting detrusor and opening of the sphincter, can cause AUR as well as result in significant upper urinary tract deterioration in multiple sclerosis, spinal cord injury, and other myelopathic diseases. It can also occur in neurologically intact children and adults, and then is known as dysfunctional voiding. It usually causes chronic urinary retention in children, occurring three times more frequently in males than females *(3)*. In children, congenital lesions of the proximal urethra, such as posterior urethral valves in boys, can cause bladder outlet obstruction.

Prostatic urethral obstruction caused by either benign prostate hyperplasia or prostate cancer occurs frequently in older men. The prostate, which encircles the proximal urethra, grows into the urethral lumen, creating a barrier to efficient urine evacuation. Acute

Table 2
Male Bladder Outlet Obstruction

Bladder neck
   Bladder neck dyssynergia
   Bladder neck contracture
   Clot retention
   Bladder stone
   Drugs that increase bladder neck tone
Prostatic urethra
   Benign prostate hyperplasia
   Prostate cancer
   Acute prostatitis, prostatic abscess
   Posterior urethral valves
Membranous urethra
   Detrusor external sphincter dyssynergia
   Dysfunctional voiding
Penile urethra
   Meatal stenosis
   Paraphimosis
Anywhere in the urethra
   Urethral calculus
   Urethritis
   Stricture
   Urethral tumor or polyp

Table 3
Obstructive Lesions of the Female Lower Urinary Tract

Bladder neck
   Clot retention
   Bladder stone
   Drugs that increase bladder neck tone
Intraurethral lesions
   Tumor
   Meatal stenosis or urethral stricture
   Urethral diverticulum
   Periurethral abscess
   Urethral prolapse
Extrinsic urethral factors
   Pelvic mass/fibroids
   Iatrogenic causes (pubovaginal sling or urethral suspension surgery)
   Pelvic organ prolapse (cystocele, rectocele, uterine prolapse)
Functional causes
   Detrusor external sphincter dyssynergia
   Primary bladder neck dysfunction
   Dysfunctional voiding

bacterial prostatitis is one of the painful causes of AUR, causing retention through urethral edema or possibly through disruption of normal voiding reflexes. Prostatic abscesses frequently cause difficulty urinating, sometimes resulting in AUR. In men, urethral cancer, urethral stricture, and meatal stenosis may also cause AUR.

In women, bladder outlet obstruction is rare (Table 3). Urethral strictures are typically associated with surgical procedures or trauma from catheterization. Intraurethral lesions (malignancy, urethral prolapse) or extrinsic urethral compression by a large uterine myoma or malignant pelvic mass involving the vagina, uterus, or rectum could result in AUR. Pelvic floor relaxation may cause a significant descent of the bladder into the vaginal space, resulting in a cystocele by which part of the bladder lies below the urethral outlet, producing a mechanical obstruction. This obstruction is exacerbated by repeated increases in intraabdominal pressure.

Urethral suspension and sling procedures for stress urinary incontinence are among the frequent causes of postoperative AUR in women. Transient obstruction is usually attributable to urethral edema; however, prolonged obstruction leading to recurrent AUR or chronic urinary retention is seen when excessive tension from the sling or bladder neck suspension procedure compresses the urethra too tightly.

Impaired Detrusor Contractility

Impaired detrusor contractility may result either from neurogenic causes related to disorders of either afferent or efferent neural pathways or from a problem of the bladder muscle itself (myogenic) (Table 4). Acute cerebrovascular accident is one of the transient causes of AUR. The pathophysiology of detrusor areflexia in "cerebral shock" is unclear. Brain tumors located in the posterior fossa and frontal lobe may cause urinary retention.

Acute spinal cord injury causes a flaccid paralysis of the nerves and muscles below the level of the injured segment. During this period, which is called "spinal shock," the detrusor undergoes flaccid paralysis, resulting in AUR. In patients with lesions above the sacral spinal cord, detrusor contractions return after a period of paralysis lasting from a few days up to several months, whereas the retention persists in lesions involving S2 to S4 spinal cord segments.

Urinary retention caused by impaired detrusor contractility also occurs in patients with peripheral polyneuropathies such as diabetic polyneuropathy or chronic alcoholism. In diabetes mellitus, several other factors may also contribute to impaired detrusor contractility, such as polyuria, loss of bladder sensation, functional and structural changes in the detrusor, and chronic overdistension that results in secondary detrusor damage.

Pelvic trauma and abdominopelvic surgery (e.g., pelvic exenteration, abdominoperineal resection, radical hysterectomy) could result in peripheral nerve damage and cause AUR. Herpes zoster infections may cause detrusor muscle paralysis if they involve the pelvic nerves; however, bladder filling sensation is preserved, and the problem resolves as the infection clears.

In children, chronic constipation or fecal impaction impairs detrusor contractility, and treatment of the bowel disorder resolves the associated urinary retention. The pathophysiology may be related to the effects of chronic rectal distension on voiding reflexes.

Chronic infravesical obstruction has also been known to cause impaired bladder contractility resulting in AUR, also called the *decompensated bladder*. Psychogenic urinary retention may be encountered in patients who experience intermittent episodes of acute retention associated with emotional distress.

Table 4
Causes of Impaired Detrusor Contractility

Neurogenic
  Supraspinal level
    Cerebrovascular accident
    Brain tumor
    Parkinsonism
    Multiple sclerosis
  Spinal level
    Spinal shock following spinal injury
    Lesions affecting sacral S2–S4 spinal cord or nerve roots (disc disease, spinal stenosis)
    Sacral spinal cord tumors
    Congenital neurospinal defects (myelomeningocele, lipomeningocele, sacral agenesis)
    Multiple sclerosis, transverse myelitis, other myelopathies
    Guillain-Barré syndrome
    Anogenital herpes
    Shy-Drager syndrome
    Polio
  Infraspinal level
    Peripheral mono- or polyneuropathies
      Diabetes mellitus
      Chronic alcoholism
      Pernicious anemia
      Heavy metal poisoning (lead, mercury)
    Peripheral nerve injury (traumatic or surgical)
Myogenic
  Prolonged, severe obstruction
  Aging
  Tuberculosis
  Radiation cystitis
Other
  Infrequent voiding
  Psychogenic retention
  Postoperative urinary retention
  Constipation
  Chronic pelvic pain syndrome
  Drugs that impair detrusor contractility

CLINICAL FINDINGS

History

When AUR is encountered in an emergency setting, if the patient is aware of a full bladder but is unable to urinate, a brief history should be taken to avoid exacerbating conditions such as urethral trauma or stricture with overzealous urethral catheterization. The detailed history can be deferred until after the emergency procedure.

Past medical history may reveal a systemic neurological disease, diabetes mellitus, end-stage genitourinary or pelvic malignancy, or recent genitourinary, abdominal, or pelvic surgical procedures.

The duration of urinary retention, other relevant urinary symptoms, and identification of precipitating factors such as recent fluid overload and alcohol intake should be noted. A previous history of urinary retention should prompt an analysis of precipitating factors. Older patients should be carefully evaluated for the history of benign prostatic hyperplasia and prostate cancer in men and endometrial disease and cervical cancer in women. Gonorrhea is often associated with urethral stricture disease.

Many medications, including sympathomimetics, anticholinergics, antihistamines, antidepressant drugs, narcotics, antipsychotics, and sedatives, may precipitate AUR. Acute retention is also commonly encountered after general or regional anesthesia.

Symptoms

The clinical presentation of AUR is usually easily recognized in patients with intact bladder sensation. A recent history of urinary symptoms such as increased urinary frequency, dysuria, decreased force and caliber of urinary stream, terminal dribbling, and hesitancy should warn the clinician about urinary retention. Hematuria may be a manifestation of clot retention within the bladder. Absence of voiding for an extended time, flank or abdominal pain, and a sense of fullness in the pelvic region may be the only symptoms in patients with AUR but without normal bladder sensation.

Physical Examination

Inspection may reveal a lower abdominal mass or fullness, particularly if the patient is thin. Percussion of a distended bladder produces a high-pitched, dull sound. If the bladder is either palpable or percussable in the adult, it indicates at least 400 cc of urine in the bladder. The urethral meatus should be carefully examined for the presence of meatal stenosis in both sexes and urethral caruncles in females. Phimosis may be found in boys or men, but is not usually the primary cause of retention. Urethral stricture may be palpable along the urethra. Inspection may also reveal genital herpetic lesions.

Rectal digital examination is important for diagnosing an enlarged or indurated prostate in older men. Anal sphincter tone and a bulbocavernosus reflex should be checked to assess the neurological integrity of the sacral spinal nerves. In females, a bimanual examination is important to detect uterine, cervical, or other gynecologic mass. Rarely, genital or pelvic masses may only be detected after emptying the bladder; thus, it might be necessary to perform a rectal or bimanual examination following catheterization. The urine volume obtained with catheterization must be measured and documented, and the catheter is usually left in place.

Frequently, the patient may be unaware of AUR or unable to clearly communicate symptoms; therefore, retention should be considered in any patient with a known or suspected pelvic trauma, spinal cord injury, stroke, or other acute neurological diseases likely to alter pelvic sensations or the ability to communicate symptoms.

Imaging

If the history and physical examination are inconclusive, pelvic ultrasonography is the easiest and quickest imaging method for detecting a distended bladder. It can also detect the presence of a foreign body, calculus, clot retention, or an enlarged prostate. Gynecologic masses such as uterine myoma are easily detected by ultrasound. Renal ultrasonography may reveal complications of AUR, such as hydronephrosis, renal calculus disease, or the presence of pyonephrosis. A kidney, ureter, bladder (KUB) film will detect approx 80% of stone disease and spinal anomalies such as spina bifida. Urinary retention can manifest as a faintly opaque bladder shadow in the pelvis. Computed tomography is important for the follow-up of mass lesions; however, it is not necessary or cost-effective for the diagnosis of AUR.

Laboratory Evaluation

Laboratory tests are not useful for the diagnosis of AUR, but labs drawn at the time of the initial evaluation or after urinary drainage is achieved will be helpful for further patient management. Urinalysis may be useful for diagnosing the primary causes of AUR, such as an infection. Complete blood count will be necessary to rule out infectious complications such as pyelonephritis. The levels of serum urea nitrogen and creatinine are necessary to assess the impact on renal function. In addition, they may predict the development of postobstructive diuresis (*see* "Immediate Postdrainage Management").

TREATMENT OF ACUTE URINARY RETENTION

The treatment objectives of AUR are to establish urinary drainage, learn as much as possible about the cause of AUR for future management, and minimize harm to the urethra.

Urethral Catheterization

Typically, the first maneuver to treat AUR is Foley catheter placement. Compared to suprapubic drainage, urethral drainage is generally more expeditious and less morbid.

With children, it is crucial to do no harm. If a few simple attempts to catheterize a child's urethra are unsuccessful, then extensive instrumentation should be avoided, and one should proceed to suprapubic cystostomy.

In women, urethral instrumentation is seldom a significant problem. The only situation is the case of female hypospadias, for which the urethral meatus is within the vaginal canal and not easily visualized. The adult female urethra is approx 4 cm long and is in the midline. Thus, the hypospadiac meatus has to be located along the anterior vaginal wall, within 4 cm of its usual position. Placing a gloved fingertip of the nondominant hand deep on the anterior vaginal wall while sliding a 14 or 16F coude tip catheter (with the tip up) along the finger should cannulate the meatus. In women with significant uterine prolapse, visualizing the urethral orifice may be difficult if the uterus is not reduced.

Urethral catheterization in men can be problematic; in situations other than a routine urethral catheterization, intravenous or intramuscular antibiotics prior to instrumentation should be considered. Generous urethral lubrication can greatly facilitate urethral catheterization. ("Float it in on a river of lube," attributed to Dr. William H. Boyce, Bowman Gray School of Medicine, Winston-Salem, NC.) Sterile, water-soluble lubricant can be loaded into a 10-cc syringe and injected directly into the urethra. When necessary, 2% lidocaine jelly can be used, and 15 to 20 min are needed for the full effect of the anesthetic on the urethral tissues.

The first attempts at urethral catheterization can be with a 16 or 18F Foley catheter. Smaller caliber catheters (e.g., 8F pediatric feeding tubes) may be able to negotiate narrow strictures, but sometimes they are not stiff enough to pass through a resistant, scarred passage.

In passing any instrument or catheter into the male urethra, grasp the penile shaft and gently stretch it upward, perpendicular to the body. Insert the catheter slowly. When the catheter reaches the bulbar urethra (usually signaled by a little resistance), bend the penis down toward the scrotum to lever the catheter tip through the membranous urethra. If Foley catheter passage is not successful, use of a similar size coude tip catheter can be the next step. The coude tip catheter has a curved tip that points anteriorly to facilitate passage through the male bulbous urethra. The raised bleb on the connector end points in the same direction as the curved tip to help the operator keep the catheter oriented properly.

If neither of these is successful, there are other techniques to negotiate the problematic male urethra. Only trained practitioners should perform all of these techniques because the risks of urethral perforation and other sequelae (e.g., transurethral perforation of the rectum) are high in inexperienced hands. These techniques are as follows:

1. Urethral strictive dilation with van Buren or Goodwin sounds. The urethra should be dilated to two or three sizes larger than the caliber of the stricture. As with all instrumentation, the tip of the sounds should hug the anterior wall of the urethra to avoid perforation in the posterior wall of the bulbar urethra.
2. Place a guide wire through the urethra into the bladder and pass a Councill catheter over it. A Councill catheter is identical to a Foley catheter except that it has a small hole in the tip.
3. For stylet-guided catheter placement, a stylet (also called a Mandarin guide) must have a gentle curve at the end, mimicking the curve of the bulbar urethra.
4. Filiforms and followers can be used. Filiforms are long, slender nylon rods used to "snake" through urethral obstructions into the bladder. Once the filiform is passed into the bladder, a series of graduated followers, which are hollow tubes threaded onto the shank of the filiform, are used to dilate the obstruction.
5. Flexible or rigid cystoscopy, if easily available in the clinic, is invaluable in negotiating the difficult urethra. A guide wire can be passed into the bladder under direct vision, and then Goodwin sounds or a Councill catheter can be passed over it.

Suprapubic Cystostomy

PUNCH CYSTOSTOMY

If all reasonable attempts to establish urethral drainage have failed and the patient's condition requires immediate urinary drainage, a "punch" cystostomy tube can be placed. This procedure is generally reserved for those patients who have not had lower abdominal or pelvic surgery via an abdominal incision (owing to significant risk of intestinal adhesion to the lower abdominal wall, through which the cystostomy tube is placed), are not anticoagulated, and do not have known bladder tumors. A punch cystostomy should be performed by an experienced practitioner.

OPEN SUPRAPUBIC TUBE

In massive pelvic trauma or if the patient is not a candidate for punch cystostomy, a formal suprapubic tube can be placed in the operating room, often in conjunction with other operative procedures. The bladder should be inspected for complete integrity, and perforations can be repaired simultaneously. In some situations, a suprapubic tube placed next to hardware stabilizing the pelvic ring may not be desirable. In this case, a large Foley catheter with a closed-system pelvic suction drain may be the best option.

Immediate Postdrainage Management

Once urinary drainage is achieved, a urine specimen should be sent for urinalysis and culture. In the presence of infected urine, antibiotics should be started, particularly if the catheterization was traumatic. The patient should be monitored for postobstructive diuresis if azotemic. The most common form of diuresis occurs because of the urea load accumulated during the period of urinary retention. After relief of the obstruction, the release of excess urea and water is typically self-limiting (24–48 h) until normovolemia is attained.

An uncommon but potentially life-threatening form of postobstructive diuresis occurs when there is a massive, salt-wasting diuresis, persisting even after normovolemia has been achieved. Serum electrolytes and fluid replacement must be carefully monitored after relief of the urinary retention if the patient has urine output greater than 200 mL per hour.

If the bladder has been massively distended for a long period, bladder hemorrhage may occur following decompression. Keeping the bladder free of clots to maintain catheter patency may be a challenge.

In select cases when the patient is an outpatient, reasonably healthy, and reliable, clean intermittent catheterization can be initiated instead of Foley catheterization to avoid complications of indwelling catheterization.

LONG-TERM MANAGEMENT

AUR is frequently transient, and once the inciting event is resolved (removal of medication, treatment of infection, resection of obstructing prostate), spontaneous voiding is possible. A voiding trial can be performed using the "fill-and-pull" method, by which the bladder is filled with sterile saline via the indwelling catheter to the patient's capacity ($\leq$450 cc), and then the catheter is removed. The patient is then asked to void, and the amount voided is measured. If there is more than 200 cc postvoid residual, then the patient may be at risk for recurrent urinary retention.

If the cause of the AUR is not reversible, long-term management of urinary retention can be via indwelling urethral or suprapubic catheter or with clean intermittent catheterization. The patient's overall health, physical and cognitive capacity, and social support will determine which type of management is most appropriate.

SUMMARY

AUR is a true urologic emergency. The etiologies are related to bladder outlet obstruction, impaired detrusor contractility, or both. Bladder drainage is necessary to relieve pain, and avoid complications of infection, uremia, and irreversible renal damage. The diagnosis of AUR is typically straightforward. Treatment by urethral catheterization is the first-line treatment. Placement in males and children may be complicated, and require suprapubic cystotomy. Immediate postdrainage sequelae include postobstructive diuresis and hematuria.

REFERENCES

1. Emberton M, Anson K. Acute urinary retention in men: an age old problem. BMJ 1999; 318 (7188): 921–925.

2. Jacobsen SJ, Jacobson DJ, Girman CJ, et al. Natural history of prostatism: risk factors for acute urinary retention. J Urol 1997; 158(2): 481–487.
3. Gatti JM, Perez-Brayfield M, Kirsch AJ, et al. Acute urinary retention in children. J Urol 2001; 165: 918–921.
4. Austin P, Spyropoulos E, Lotenfoe R, Helal M, Hoffman M, Lockhart JL. Urethral obstruction after anti-incontinence surgery in women: evaluation, methodology, and surgical results. Urology 1996; 47(6): 890–894.
5. Carley ME, Carley JM, Vasdev G, et al. Factors that are associated with clinically overt postpartum urinary retention after vaginal delivery. Am J Obstet Gynecol 2002; 187(2): 430–483.
6. Porter JR, Takayama TK, Defalco AJ. Traumatic posterior urethral injury and early realignment using magnetic urethral catheters. J Urol 1997; 158: 425–430.

V   Iatrogenic Complications

19 Vesicovaginal Fistula and Ureteral Injury During Pelvic Surgery

Craig V. Comiter, MD and Christina Escobar, MD

CONTENTS

INTRODUCTION
VESICOVAGINAL FISTULA
URETEROVAGINAL FISTULA
SUMMARY
REFERENCES

INTRODUCTION

Because of the proximity of the bladder and ureters to the uterus, iatrogenic injuries are a well-described complication of gynecologic surgery. If unrecognized, complications such as vesicovaginal fistula (VVF) and ureterovaginal fistula (UVF) may occur. VVF ranks as the second most common genitourinary tract injury, with the second highest cause of malpractice claims *(1,2)*. Given the morbidity suffered by the patient and the medicolegal implications realized by the surgeon *(3)*, the avoidance, recognition, and subsequent treatment of these complications is an important issue. This chapter focuses on iatrogenic causes of VVF and ureteral injuries, strategies to prevent and recognize them, and management of postoperative complications.

VESICOVAGINAL FISTULA

Definition and Etiology

A VVF is an anomalous communication between the bladder and the vagina. In developing countries, the most common cause is obstructed labor *(4–7)*, which causes pressure necrosis of the bladder base and urethra, resulting in significant tissue loss *(8)*. In West Africa, prolonged labor results in VVF at a rate of 1 to 3 per 1000 deliveries *(4)*. In more developed countries in which women have better access to more modern obstetric care, obstetric fistulas are much less common. In such areas, fistula formation most commonly results from iatrogenic injury during pelvic surgery *(9–12)*.

In fact, 90% of VVFs in North America result from gynecologic surgery *(13)*. Abdominal and vaginal hysterectomies are the most common causative factors, accounting for 75%

From: *Urological Emergencies*
Edited by: H. Wessells and J. W. McAninch © Humana Press Inc., Totowa, NJ

of all VVFs *(12,14,15)*. The risk of fistula formation following hysterectomy is approx 0.1% *(9–12)*. Other iatrogenic causes include injury during laparoscopic pelvic surgery, antiincontinence procedures, gastrointestinal pelvic surgery, and pelvic radiation *(16,17)*. Noniatrogenic fistulas may result from locally advanced pelvic malignancy *(15,18)*, tuberculous infection *(19)*, and foreign bodies *(20–22)*.

Pathogenesis

The foremost mechanisms of VVF formation following vaginal or abdominal hysterectomy are (1) unrecognized cystotomy or insufficiently repaired cystotomy, resulting in urinoma formation with subsequent fistulization to the vaginal cuff *(23)*, and (2) vaginal cuff sutures that inadvertently incorporate the posterior bladder, resulting in necrosis and fistula formation *(24)*. The mechanism of postradiation VVF is progressive obliterative endarteritis *(8)*.

Prevention

The most common factors that increase the risk of posthysterectomy VVF include previous pelvic radiation, prior uterine surgery, and a history of endometriosis. In addition, previous cervical conization *(8)*, distorted anatomy secondary to fibroids or adnexal mass *(25)*, and steroid use *(26)* have been affiliated with increased risk of VVF. Therefore, elective hysterectomy in a high-risk patient should be performed by an experienced surgeon with the availability of urological assistance if necessary *(27)*.

The bladder's proximity to the cervix and anterior vaginal wall render it susceptible to injury during hysterectomy. Prevention of inadvertent bladder injury is best accomplished by adherence to basic principals of surgery, namely, a thorough knowledge of surgical anatomy, as well as adequate surgical exposure and hemostasis. During hysterectomy, the bladder is most likely to be injured supratrigonally, at the level of the vaginal cuff. Sharp dissection, rather than the use of cautery or swabs, should be used to dissect the bladder off the uterus *(12,28)*. Moreover, the bladder should be continuously decompressed during pelvic surgery with an indwelling catheter. If bleeding occurs, specific ligation of the bleeding site is preferred to excessive cautery. Prior to ligation of the uterosacral ligaments, adequate mobilization of the inferior and lateral aspects of the bladder is essential, and the ligaments should be taken close to the uterus to avoid injury to the bladder *(29)*. When extensive pelvic and perivesical fibrosis are encountered, *intentional* anterior cystotomy may be performed to prevent *accidental injury* to the bladder base *(30)*.

If injury is suspected, the bladder should be filled with fluid to localize any leakage site. Repair of the injury should not be attempted until tissues are adequately mobilized *(31)*. Urological consultation is recommended, and the cystotomy should be closed with self-absorbing suture (SAS) in multiple layers. If the closure is tenuous, interposition of adjacent well-vascularized tissue between the cystotomy repair and the vagina is recommended. The bladder should be drained via indwelling catheter for 2–3 wk postoperatively, with catheter removal only after cystographic confirmation of complete healing.

Presentation

Bladder injuries not recognized during surgery may present immediately postoperatively or up to 3 wk later. Radiation-induced fistulas may present up to 20 yr postradiation *(8,36)*. Patients typically present with continuous daytime and nighttime leakage per

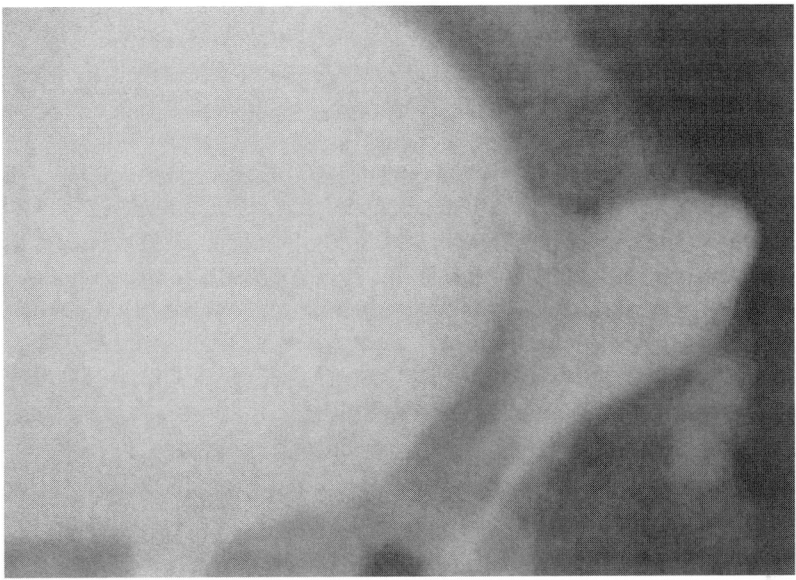

Fig. 1. Lateral cystogram demonstrating vesicovaginal fistula.

vagina *(32)*. Depending on the size of the fistula, varying amounts of urine may be voided vs leaked per vagina. Patients may initially present with postoperative abdominal/pelvic pain and ileus secondary to urinoma formation *(23)* prior to frank fistulization of the urinoma to the vagina.

Diagnosis

The differential diagnosis of clear fluid per vagina includes urine, lymph, peritoneal fluid, fallopian tube exudates, and vaginal discharge *(33)*. A high creatinine level confirms the diagnosis of urinary fistula. Identifying the origin of leakage—ureter, bladder, or proximal urethra—is the most important first step *(13)*.

Vaginal examination with a speculum is mandatory for identifying the fistulous site, most commonly at the apex of the vaginal vault. With a large fistula, a bladder catheter may be visible or palpable per vagina. If the exam is unrevealing and suspicion remains high, methylene blue or indigo carmine can be instilled into the bladder via urethral catheter, and leakage may be observed per vagina.

Alternatively, the diagnosis may be confirmed by cystography (Fig. 1). Cystoscopy is indicated to identify the relation of the fistulous opening to the ureteral orifices, to document free urinary outflow from each ureter, and to assess bladder capacity and rule out concomitant foreign body. With a patient who has a history of genitourinary carcinoma, biopsy is necessary to rule out recurrent malignancy *(32)*.

Concomitant UVF must be excluded because the incidence of UVF exceeds 10% in patients with a VVF *(3,14,30)*. Intravenous urography and retrograde ureteropyelography are useful for identifying hydronephrosis, ureteral obstruction, and fistula formation. If the diagnosis remains uncertain, the bladder may be catheterized and filled with blue dye while the patient is given oral pyridium. The vagina can be packed with gauze, and the patient asked to ambulate with a plugged urethral catheter. Blue staining confirms VVF; orange staining confirms UVF *(34)*.

Concomitant Stress Incontinence

Any woman with a prior history of urinary incontinence must be adequately evaluated prior to fistula repair, with multichannel videourodynamics if indicated. Because of the continuous leakage per vagina, the patient may not notice stress incontinence. However, an investigation suggested that stress incontinence perceived as new onset following VVF repair may have been present before the repair was undertaken (35). Repair of anatomic abnormalities contributing to stress incontinence may be performed concomitantly with fistula surgery (via abdominal or vaginal route) and may avoid the need for a further surgical procedure. Most important, incontinence surgery has not been demonstrated to increase fistula recurrence (36).

Management

Although most cases of VVF will ultimately require surgery for definitive cure, conservative management should be offered for small fistulas uncomplicated by ischemia, radiation, or malignancy. Continuous urethral catheter drainage plus oral antimuscarinics and antibiotics have been associated with a 2 to 10% closure rate (3,12,26,37,38). However, once the fistulous tract becomes epithelialized (usually 4–6 wk), catheter drainage is unlikely to aid fistula closure (3). A trial of deepithelialization has been advocated for mature small fistulas (1–3 mm) using silver nitrate, mechanical curettage (39), or electrocautery (40). In addition, the use of fibrin glue (41–43) and Nd-YAG laser welding (44) has been anecdotally successful for sealing small fistulas.

For large VVFs and for the majority of smaller ones that fail conservative management, surgery is required for definitive repair. The routine use of preoperative urethral catheterization is controversial. Although bladder drainage may reduce skin excoriation and patient discomfort, catheterization exacerbates bladder sensitivity, intravesical inflammation, and the risk of urinary infection. The author therefore recommended that any indwelling catheter be removed at least 1 wk prior to surgery, and that the urine should be sterilized with broad-spectrum antibiotics at least 24 h prior to surgery. Preoperative estrogen replacement (oral or vaginal) is recommended in postmenopausal women (45), and any vaginal yeast infection should be treated with an oral or vaginal antifungal agent.

Timing of Surgery

If a bladder injury or ureteral injury is recognized during pelvic surgery, urological consultation is recommended at this critical time, and immediate repair is warranted. The immediate repair of such bladder and ureteral injuries is covered in other chapters of this volume.

Although surgery had traditionally been deferred for 3 to 6 mo following the injury to allow maximum resolution of the inflammation and edema, it is now commonplace to proceed to earlier and even immediate repair of iatrogenic VVF. A waiting period is still recommended for a fistula related to obstetrical trauma to allow the ischemic tissue to declare itself fully. Similarly, with radiation-induced VVF, the surgeon should wait until the size of the fistula has stabilized, as verified by serial vaginal and cystoscopic examination. For these fistulas associated with obliterative endarteritis, a waiting period of at least 12 mo is recommended (8).

As many series document excellent success rates with early fistula repair (9,24,46–50), early surgical intervention for uncomplicated VVF caused by iatrogenic injury is

Table 1
Principles of Surgical Repair for Vesicovaginal Fistula

Preoperative
  Timing of repair
  Vaginal vs abdominal approach
  Health of tissues
    Estrogenization
    Steroid use
    Radiation
  Planning of concomitant procedures
    Stress incontinence surgery
    Prolapse surgery
    Augmentation cystoplasty
    Ureteral surgery
Intraoperative
  Good exposure of fistulous site
  Wide mobilization of tissues
  Tension-free approximation of tissue
  Watertight closure
  Multilayer repair with nonoverlapping suture lines
  Interposition flaps
Postoperative
  Avoidance of infection
  Maximal and continuous bladder drainage
  Adequate estrogenization
  Prevention of bladder spasms

now recommended. In addition, early repair avoids the discomfort associated with urinary leakage (odor, skin excoriation, urinary tract infection) as well as the adverse psychological and medicolegal impact of prolonged urinary leakage (25).

SURGICAL TECHNIQUE

The principles of surgical repair are as follows: The fistula tract must be adequately exposed, and the fistula repair should be tension-free, watertight, multilayered with nonoverlapping suture lines and should remain uninfected (Table 1). Whether the approach is vaginal, abdominal, or a combination of both routes, the initial attempt at repair has the highest success rate (4,8). The best approach should depend on the patient's anatomy, location of the fistula, and reconstructive considerations; these decisions must be individualized for each case. Compared to abdominal surgery, the transvaginal approach is associated with significantly decreased morbidity and length of hospitalization (51).

ABDOMINAL APPROACH

All VVFs can be approached transabdominally. Abdominal repair is recommended, however, when the fistulous opening cannot be adequately exposed vaginally; simultaneous bladder augmentation is planned; or simultaneous ureteral surgery/ureteroneocystotomy is planned.

The patient is placed in the supine position with the legs slightly abducted to allow access to the vagina. Through a Pfannenstiel or lower abdominal midline incision, an intraperitoneal or extraperitoneal approach to the bladder may be utilized. Packing the vagina is often helpful to temporarily seal the fistula so that the bladder can be filled through a urethral catheter.

Extraperitoneal Approach

The bladder dome is elevated, and dissection is carried posterior to the bladder and anterior to the vagina, down toward the fistulous tract. After the fistula is identified, a small opening is made sharply in the tract, and the bladder wall can be dissected off the tract. The vaginal opening and the bladder opening are each closed in two layers using 2-0 SAS *(31)*. Perivesical or extraperitoneal fibrofatty tissue may be interposed between the two layers. Alternatively, a peritonotomy may be used to harvest an omental flap, or the peritoneal reflection itself may be interposed between the bladder and vaginal closures. A transvesical extraperitoneal approach has also been described in which the fistulous tract is excised transvesically *(52,53)*.

Intraperitoneal Approach

The bladder is approached transperitoneally, and the bladder is bisected down to the fistula. The bladder and vagina are widely mobilized from each other, and the fistula is excised. The bladder and vagina are each closed in two layers using 2-0 SAS *(54,55)*. When operating transperitoneally, harvesting an omental graft is more straightforward. If omentum does not easily reach the site of repair, a rotational flap based on the right gastroepiploic artery may be mobilized and secured between the bladder and vaginal closure with 3-0 SAS *(56)*. A suprapubic tube is placed in addition to the urethral catheter to allow maximal bladder drainage. A Penrose drain should be placed and brought out through a separate stab wound.

Vaginal Approach

Most VVFs are amenable to transvaginal repair. A vaginal operation is far less burdensome for patients than is an abdominal approach *(15,31,57,58)*. Contraindications to the vaginal approach include severe vaginal stenosis and an inability to tolerate the dorsal lithotomy position (e.g., because of muscular contraction/spasticity). If the fistula encroaches on the ureteral orifices, transurethral placement of ureteral stents is indicated. For access to the vagina, the patient is positioned in dorsal lithotomy. Urethral and suprapubic catheters are placed, and the fistulous tract should be dilated with lacrimal duct probes and pediatric urethral sounds until an 8F Foley catheter, which may be used for traction, can be inserted into the bladder. The vaginal wall surrounding the fistula is instilled with saline to aid with subsequent dissection. The fistula is circumscribed sharply, and the incision is extended as an inverted J, with the long arm of the J ending at the vaginal apex (Fig. 2).

Vaginal wall flaps (2–4 cm wide) are created anteriorly, posteriorly, and laterally. The perivesical fascia is exposed, and the circumscribed fistulous tract is left intact. Excision of the tract may unnecessarily enlarge the fistula and might increase the risk of bleeding. Furthermore, the fibrous ring of the fistula can help improve the strength of the repair by providing a strong anchor for suture placement *(32)*. The intrafistula catheter is removed, and the tract is closed transversely with interrupted 2-0 SAS (Fig. 3).

A second closure layer is placed perpendicular to the first layer in an imbricating fashion, incorporating the perivesical fascia and detrusor muscle 5 mm from the previous closure. Integrity of the closure is tested by filling the bladder via the urethral catheter. The distal vaginal flap is excised, and the proximal flap is advanced anteriorly at least

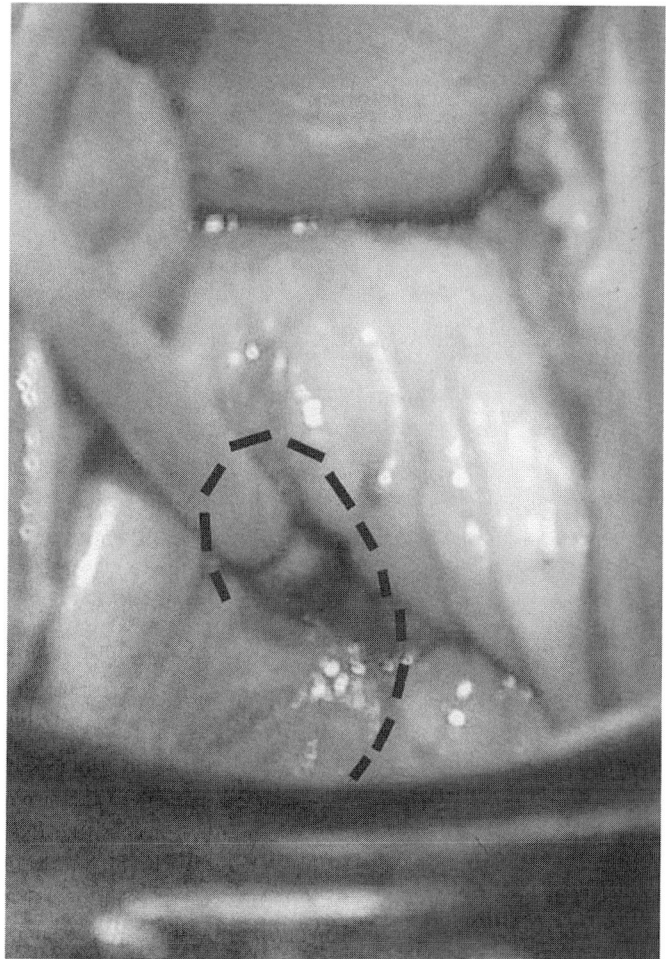

Fig. 2. Fistulous tract is dilated, and 8F Foley catheter is inserted. Inverted J incision aids with raising vaginal wall flaps anteriorly, posteriorly, and laterally.

2 to 3 cm beyond the fistula repair. This third layer is closed with a running 2-0 SAS, covering the site of repair with healthy vaginal tissue, while avoiding overlapping suture lines (Fig. 4).

Interposition Grafts

In cases of recurrent fistulas, radiation or ischemic (obstetric) fistulas, and when the fistula is high in the vaginal vault or associated with poor tissue quality, the interposition of another source of healthy tissue is recommended (Table 2) *(59)*. In addition to the same basic principles of achieving a watertight, tension-free, uninfected repair, realizing a reliable closure often involves the need for interposing a well-vascularized tissue flap. When operating transabdominally, omental fat interposition is usually straightforward, and if increased mobility is necessary, the flap should be based on the right gastroepiploic artery *(56,60)*. Alternatively, the peritoneal reflection of the cul-de-sac may be interposed between the bladder and vagina to help prevent refistulization *(51)*. Other choices of vascularized tissue include the appendix epiploica of the colon *(26)*, a

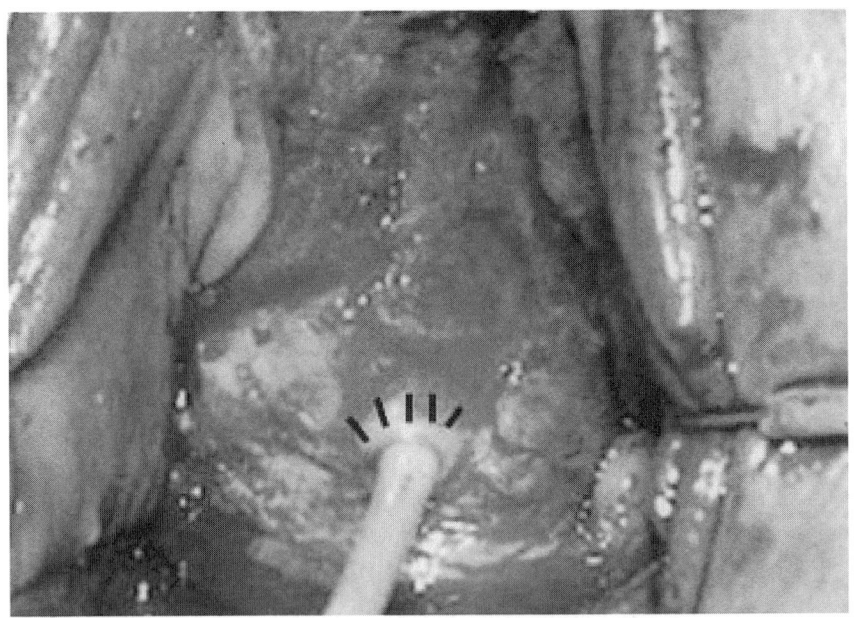

Fig. 3. Catheter is removed, and fistula is closed with 3-0 self-absorbing suture.

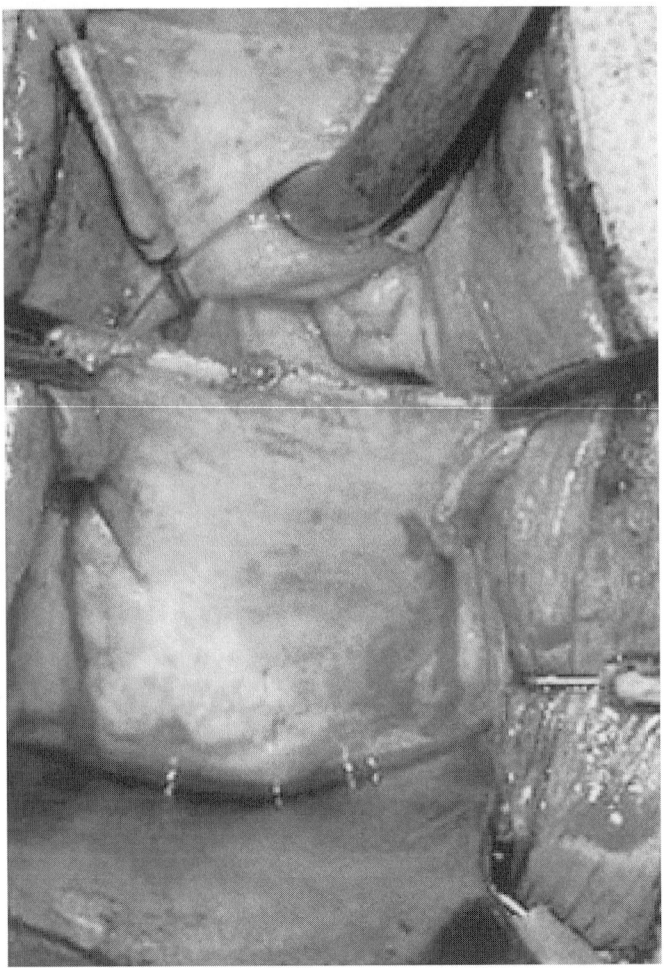

Fig. 4. Vaginal wall flap is advanced anteriorly 3 cm beyond the fistula repair.

Table 2
Tissue Interposition During Vesicovaginal Fistula Repair

Abdominal approach
    Greater omentum
    Peritoneal reflection
    Appendix epiploica of colon
    Myofacial rectus flap
    Posterior bladder wall advancement flap
Vaginal approach
    Labial fat graft (Martius flap)
    Peritoneum
    Sartorius
    Gluteus
    Gracilis

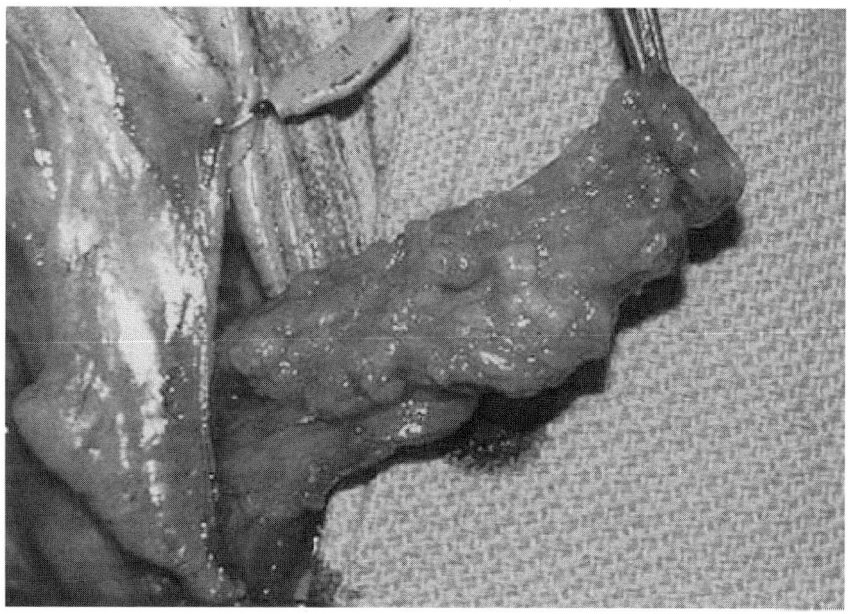

Fig. 5. Vascularized labial fat pad with blood supply based inferiorly on the inferior labial artery.

myofascial rectus flap *(61)*, or an advancement flap derived from the posterosuperior bladder wall *(62)*.

When approaching the recurrent fistula transvaginally, the most popular flap derives from the labial fat pad, which can be tunneled under the labia minora to the site of repair (Fig. 5) *(63,64)*. We prefer to use a peritoneal flap, which obviates the need for extravaginal harvesting. This technique was first described by Raz et al. *(51)* and involves dissecting the posterior vaginal wall flap posteriorly toward the cul-de-sac. The preperitoneal fat and peritoneum are sharply mobilized caudally. The peritoneal flap can then be advanced over the repair with interrupted 3-0 SAS (Fig. 6).

Other reconstructive techniques have been described using sartorius, gluteus, rectus, and gracilis muscle *(65–70)*. These muscular and myocutaneous flaps are recommended for large radiation or ischemic fistulas *(8,65)*.

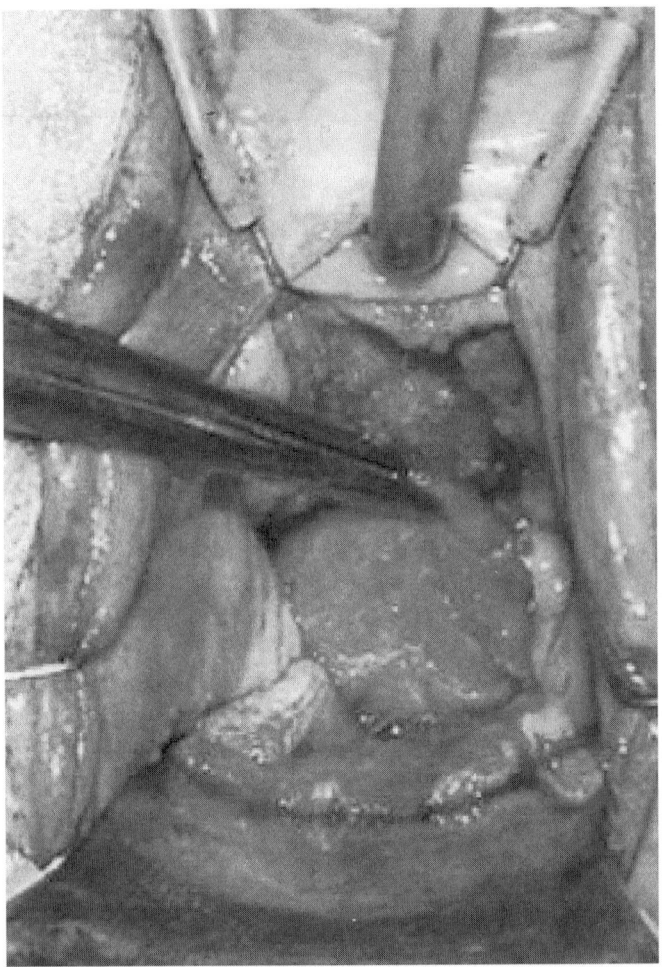

Fig. 6. Preperitoneal fat and peritoneum are mobilized in a caudal direction and sutured into position over the initial two-layer repair.

Postoperative Care

The vagina should be packed with an antibiotic-impregnated gauze for several hours to reduce the likelihood of vaginal wall hematoma formation. Maximal bladder drainage is recommended, and urethral and suprapubic catheters should remain on gravity drainage until the urine is clear of any blood. The urethral catheter may be removed after the urine clears only if it poses a threat of mucosal irritation at the site of repair (bladder neck or trigonal fistula). Oral antibiotics are recommended while urinary catheters are in place to minimize the risk of infection (8). Bladder spasms should be treated with oral or rectal antimuscarinics because bladder overactivity has been postulated to compromise healing of the repair (71). Oral or topical estrogen has been demonstrated to promote healing (57,72).

Cystography should be performed at 2 to 3 wk postoperatively to document complete healing of the fistula, with discontinuation of antimuscarinics at least 24 h prior to voiding trial. If the fistula is healed and the patient voids to completion following removal of the urethral catheter, the suprapubic tube should be removed. If persistent fistula is noted during cystography, catheter drainage is recommended for an additional 6 wk. Persistent leakage at 6 wk requires repeat operative repair. Following successful repair, patients should avoid douching and vaginal intercourse for 3 mo.

Success Rates

Although success rates vary in the literature, approx 85 to 90% of VVFs caused by gynecologic iatrogenic surgical injury are repaired successfully at the first attempt *(9,11,14,46,48,55,73–76)*. At the our institution, success rates in excess of 80% have been achieved in repair of recurrent VVF. Other centers of excellence report similar results *(31,51)*. Success rates for radiation-induced fistulas are lower, ranging from 50 to 80% *(49,60,65)*.

Complications

Early complications include vaginal bleeding, bladder spasms, and urinary or vaginal infection *(32)*. Intraoperative bleeding should be controlled with suture ligation, minimizing electrocautery. Postoperative bleeding is usually controlled by vaginal packing and bed rest. Bladder spasms can be treated with cholinolytics, and vaginal or urinary infections may be managed with appropriate oral antibiotics.

Late complications include unrecognized ureteral injury, vaginal stenosis and foreshortening, and fistula recurrence *(32)*. Vaginal shortening or stenosis usually results from excessive resection of vaginal tissue during posterior flap advancement. Delayed recognition of a ureteral injury is best managed initially by percutaneous nephrostomy, followed by definitive surgical repair after the inflammation has subsided. Cystoscopic approaches are contraindicated because distention of the bladder may lead to VVF recurrence. Recurrent fistula mandates reoperation, which is typically delayed for several months to allow the inflammation to subside. Interposition of vascularized tissue is always recommended for repair of recurrent VVF.

URETEROVAGINAL FISTULA

Definition and Etiology

A UVF may be defined as an abnormal communication involving the ureter and the vagina. This condition arises from an ectopic ureteral insertion into the vagina. It is rarely congenital, and more commonly is acquired, usually from a transmural injury to the ureter during pelvic surgery. An obstruction of the distal ureter leads to continued extravasation of urine and failure of the ureteral defect to heal. The most common cause of UVF is gynecologic surgery, most commonly after total abdominal hysterectomy for either benign or malignant disease *(77)*. Fistulas may also occur after prolonged or difficult delivery secondary to the pressure effect of the fetus on the distal ureter, resulting in necrosis *(78)*.

The ureter is vulnerable during pelvic surgery because it lies close to the rectum and female reproductive organs within the pelvis. With laparoscopic pelvic surgery becoming more common, inadvertent electrocautery of the distal ureter, especially in laparoscopic hysterectomy, during ligation of the uterine artery is reported *(79)*. Others argue that the ureter is most vulnerable during laparoscopic surgery when the cardinal ligament is dissected and divided below the uterine vessels *(80)*. Ureteral injury reportedly occurs in 0.5 to 1% of all pelvic surgeries *(81)* and in 1.4 to 2% of patients undergoing radical hysterectomy *(82,83)*.

UVFs occur when a ureteral leak persists, and the urine makes its way to the vaginal cuff. This adverse outcome of ureteral injury with its associated incontinence negatively affects the quality of life for the patient and causes anxiety on the part of the surgeon *(84,85)*. Any unexplained abdominal or flank pain or costovertebral angle tenderness, especially if fever is present, should alert the surgeon to the possibility of a ureteral injury. Often, there are no symptoms of ureteral injury or obstruction before urinary incontinence occurs. The usual UVF presentation is one of a sudden onset of urinary leakage from the vagina 1 to 4 wk postoperatively *(84,85)*. In addition to the constant incontinence, the patient voids normally because the contralateral ureter provides normal filling of the bladder.

Assessment and Investigation

Several studies may provide a diagnosis. In a female with vaginal leakage after pelvic surgery, a double dye test may differentiate between VVF and UVF *(86)*. To perform this test, the vagina is packed, and methylene blue is given intravenously; red carmine is instilled intravesically. The vaginal pack will stain red if a VVF is present and blue if a UVF is present. An intravenous urogram will demonstrate varying degrees of hydronephrosis (Fig. 7) and may demonstrate an occasional silent kidney *(87)*. If intravenous urogram fails to reveal the fistula, a retrograde ureteropyelography will usually demonstrate the location and magnitude of the fistula.

Management

The objectives in management of a UVF are to preserve renal function, prevent or treat urinary sepsis, and cure the incontinence. Treatment options include observation, internal drainage via ureteral stent, external drainage via percutaneous nephrostomy, open surgical repair, and nephrectomy. However, controversy surrounds the role, if any, of protective nephrostomy drainage and the timing of surgical intervention. Some surgeons advocate immediate surgical repair of the damaged ureter once the diagnosis is certain; although others advocate early drainage of the upper tract followed by delayed ureteral repair *(14,88–93)*. There are reports of spontaneous healing of UVFs *(14,84,94)*.

When the diagnosis of UVF is made, the surgeon must define the degree of ureteral obstruction distal to the fistula site. If distal ureteral obstruction remains, spontaneous healing of the fistula is extremely unlikely. The recommendation for both diagnostic and therapeutic reasons is to perform ureteral catheterization in addition to retrograde ureteropyelography. If a ureteral catheter is unable to be passed, the diagnosis of a distal obstruction is confirmed. If a stent can be placed to bypass the fistula, spontaneous healing is likely without further intervention *(94–96)*. The best-suited patients for nonsurgical management are those with unilateral ureteral injury, documented ureteral continuity, mild-to-moderate obstruction, and minimal extravasation. It is advantageous to attempt ureteral stenting to ensure decompression of the renal unit while simultaneously increasing the chance of healing. Conservative management has been successful when the radiographic criteria were met, even when ureteral stenting failed *(94)*. In a patient who is nonoperatively managed, upper tract improvement and resolution of ureteral extravasation need to be documented on follow-up evaluation.

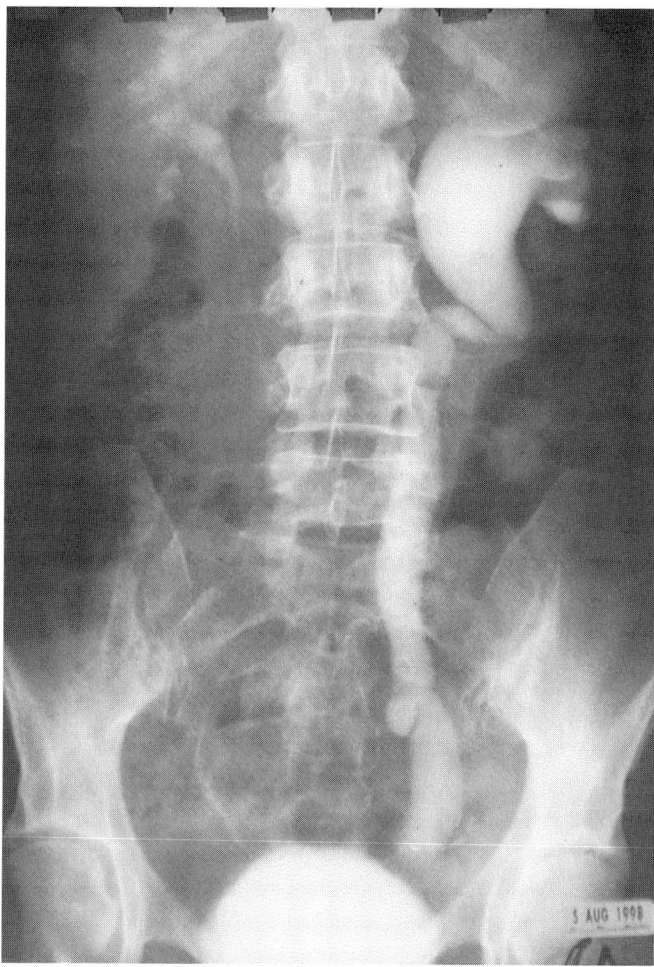

Fig. 7. An intravenous urogram will demonstrate varying degrees of hydronephrosis.

ENDOSCOPIC TECHNIQUES

Successful ureteral stenting may be achieved through several recently described endourological techniques. One option is the use of rigid ureteroscopy with low-flow irrigation to pass a 0.89-mm Glide wire retrograde across the ureteral injury (96,97). The advantage of ureteroscopy is direct visualization of the wire and improvement of the fulcrum at the level of the ureteral orifice, which increases the likelihood of achieving stenting.

If retrograde ureteral stenting is unsuccessful, antegrade percutaneous nephrostomy drainage may be attempted under local anesthesia. By placing the nephrostomy, the obstruction is relieved, and access for antegrade ureteral intubation is made available. Percutaneous nephrostomy is the first choice for a patient with infection or one who is too ill for general anesthesia or retrograde manipulation. A period of observation after percutaneous nephrostomy to allow for spontaneous healing of the damaged ureter was advocated by some (98,99). The spontaneous healing rate in highly selected individuals is reported as greater than 50% following nephrostomy (98,99).

In the majority of patients, a prolonged course of external drainage is less than desirable and antegrade stenting on an elective basis is recommended. In the event that antegrade stenting fails, a combination of antegrade-retrograde stenting technique may succeed. After passing one to two antegrade wires, cystoscopic removal of the bladder wire is performed. When tension is applied to both ends of the working wire, a retrograde ureteral stent is often able to pass across the fistula. Once a stent is placed, there is a 50 to 70% chance that the UVF will heal without the need for open surgical intervention *(96,98–100)*. In a study by Selzman et al. *(100)*, eight women with UVFs underwent stent placement. All except one had the stent left in place for 4 to 8 wk. All seven patients had resolution of the fistula when the stent was left in for this amount of time and the ureter was given the chance to heal. The only complication was one stricture, which developed after stent removal and was repaired endoscopically. Because of the chance of ureteral stricturing, close follow-up is needed *(94)*.

Surgical Repair

If neither antegrade nor retrograde ureteral access is achievable or even an option, open surgical repair is indicated. Controversy regarding the timing of the fistula repair is present because it is a reoperative procedure. Some surgeons recommend a cooling down period to allow the inflammation to resolve. In this instance, a percutaneous nephrostomy is performed to allow for drainage of infection and to protect the kidney *(93,101)*. Some advocate nephrostomy only in the face of azotemia and urosepsis *(84)*. Drainage of the upper tract will not necessarily solve the incontinence because some urine will proceed down the ureter and out the vagina through the fistula.

During a laparoscopic case, the chance of thermal injury to the ureter is a possibility, which may turn a less-invasive case into a debilitating one. In these circumstances, bipolar electrocautery is safer than unipolar because it reduces thermal spread *(80)*. To take this a step further, bipolar scissors are recommended over 5-mm forceps because it is thought they allow energy to be applied more accurately *(79)*.

Should a burned ureter occur and there is no urine extruding from one ureteral orifice on cystoscopy, a double-J stent should be placed for 6 wk. This course of action is based on the belief that a burned ureter develops immediate mucosal edema that prevents urine passage. The double-J stent prevents fistula formation by diverting the urine while the ureter has a chance to heal. If cystoscopy reveals that a stent should be placed, even if the ureter is not really damaged, no harm is done. However, if a burned ureter is not stented, a fistula with its related morbidity may form *(80)*.

A movement toward early repair of the UVF is made because it is such a distressing complication and involves a great deal of distress for the patient and anxiety for the surgeon. Early surgical repair may be undertaken if there is no significant urosepsis and renal function is relatively well preserved *(86–88,102)*. Goodwin and Scardino were the first to demonstrate that early repair is achievable with excellent results *(14)*.

Operative repair of the UVF is governed by several principles. All abnormal ureter should be removed, little attempt should be made to confine the surgery extraperitoneally, continuity between a normal ureter and bladder should be reestablished, and adequate drainage should be maintained *(87)*. On occasion, end-to-end ureteroureterostomy may be performed *(84,85,89)*, but only in the case of limited inflammation and ureteral loss, so that as much of a tension-free anastomosis may be created as possible. Frequently, ureteroneocystostomy is the favored repair. Ureteroneocystostomy involves a bypass of the site of ureteral injury, eliminating the need for direct localization of the injured ureter by a difficult dissection *(90)*.

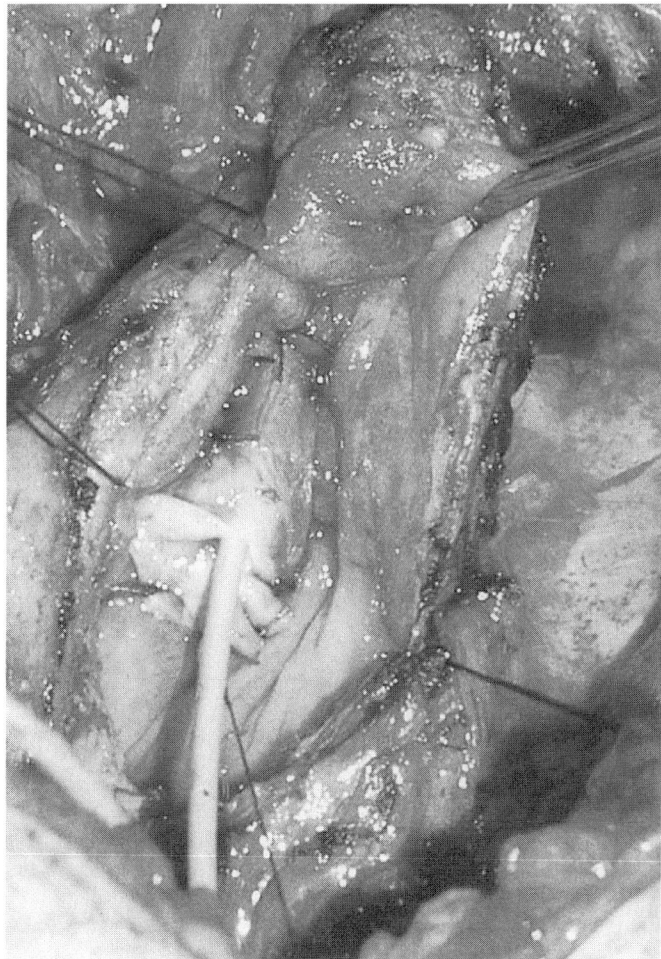

Fig. 8. A psoas bladder hitch.

The length of the ureteral segment needed to bypass, which depends on the location of the injury and obstruction, and the degree of ureteral and bladder mobility will dictate the method of implantation. In the majority of cases, a direct ureteroneocystostomy can be performed, often aided by a psoas bladder hitch (Fig. 8) to relieve any tension of the anastomosis *(82,84,91,103)*. The majority of reports revealed that, by using sound surgical principles, almost 100% success can be achieved with ureteral reimplantation *(82,84,88,91,100,104)*. Goodwin and Scardino *(14)* recommended using an antireflux submucosal tunnel in each patient; others did not feel this measure is necessary *(77,82)*. We believe that ureteroneocystostomy without the use of an antirefluxing anastomosis lowers the risk of postoperative ureteral obstruction.

If the injury to the ureter is distal, a psoas hitch is usually sufficient to render the anastomosis free of tension. A Boari flap replacement of the distal ureter may be employed when the obstructive segment lies proximally or when there are multiple sites of obstruction. A Boari flap is also used in the face of a pelvic abscess cavity, which allows the surgeon to perform the anastomosis of the ureter to the bladder away from any foci of infection *(84)*. A report by Falandry of 14 cases of UVF repair with a cuffed reimplantation with a tubular bladder plasty demonstrated no anastomotic stenosis or leak *(104)*. In the instance of high or long ureteral strictures, a more complex reconstruction such as transureteroureterostomy, renal decensus, renal autotransplantation, or ileouretero-cystoplasty may be necessary.

A nephrectomy or percutaneous ureteral occlusion should only be undertaken as a last resort *(105,106)*. Goodwin and Scardino *(14)* established that treatments other than nephrectomy can successfully treat UVF. In a series performed before 1958 by Lee and Symmonds, 48% of their patients required a nephrectomy *(107)*, whereas a 25-yr series by Goodwin and Scardino culminating in 1980 reported only a 5% nephrectomy rate.

Conclusion

UVF is a rare complication of pelvic surgery, most often following total abdominal hysterectomy and radical hysterectomy. Some degree of distal obstruction with concomitant transmural injury results in constant urinary extravasation, with fistulization to the vaginal cuff. Urinary incontinence usually follows 1 to 4 wk postoperatively without previous symptoms. Intravenous urogram and ureteropyelography are adequate studies to demonstrate the location of the injury and the degree of distal obstruction and to provide information necessary to formulate an appropriate plan of treatment. The goals of treatment center on renal preservation, treatment of urosepsis, relief of any obstruction, and alleviation of incontinence.

Advances in endourological procedures have made retrograde or antegrade ureteral stenting prudent in patients with unilateral injury, only mild-to-moderate obstruction, minimal extravasation, and some demonstrable ureteral continuity. Percutaneous nephrostomy is indicated in patients with complete ureteral obstruction or obstruction with simultaneous infection. Patients who are not candidates for ureteral stenting and who fail conservative management need definitive surgical repair. The procedure of choice is reimplantation of the healthy ureter into a mobilized bladder. In the event of a proximal ureteral injury, a psoas hitch, Boari flap, or even transureteroureterostomy or ileal ureteral replacement may be required. Percutaneous ureteral occlusion or nephrectomy should only be used as a last resort.

SUMMARY

Iatrogenic injuries are a well-described complication of gynecological surgery. The proximity of the ureters and the bladder to the cervix and anterior vaginal wall render them susceptible to injury during gynecological and pelvic operations. Iatrogenic injury, if unrecognized and untreated, can result in vesicovaginal fistula or ureterovaginal fistula—an anomalous communication between the bladder or ureter and the vagina. The avoidance, recognition, and subsequent treatment of these complications are important issues, given the morbidity suffered by the patient and the medicolegal implications realized by the surgeon.

REFERENCES

1. Medical Defense Union. Risk management in obstetrics and gynaecology. J Med Def Union 1991; 2: 36–39.
2. Ward CJ. Analysis of 500 obstetric gynecologic malpractice claims. Causes and prevention. Am J Obstet Gynecol 1991; 165: 298–304.
3. Gerber GS, Schoenberg HW. Female urinary tract fistulas. J Urol 1993; 142: 229–236.

4. Elkins TE. Surgery for the obstetric vesico-vaginal fistula. A review of 100 operations in 82 patients. Am J Obstet Gynecol 1994; 170: 1108–1118.
5. Kelly J. Vesico-vaginal and recto-vaginal fistulae. J R Soc Med 1992; 85: 257–258.
6. Hilton P, Ward A. Epidemiological and surgical aspects of urogenital fistulae: a review of 25 years' experience in Nigeria. Pelvic Floor Dysfunct 1998; 9: 189–194.
7. Danso KA, Martey JO, Wall LL, Elkins TE. The epidemiology of genito-urinary fistulae in Kumasi, Ghana. Int Urogynaecol J 1996; 7: 117–120.
8. Dmochowski R. Surgery for vesicovaginal fistula, urethrovaginal fistula, and urethral diverticulum. In: Campbell's Urology, 8th ed. (Walsh PC, Retik AB, Vaughan ED, Wein AJ, eds.), Saunders, Philadelphia, PA, pp. 1195–1217.
9. Blandy JP, Badenoch DF, Fowler CG, Jenkins BJ, Thomas NWM. Early repair of iatrogenic injury to the ureter or bladder after gynaecological surgery. J Urol 1991; 146: 761–765.
10. O'Conor V. Review of experience with vesico-vaginal fistula repair. J Urol 1980; 123: 367–369.
11. Tancer ML. The post-total hysterectomy (vault) vesicovaginal fistula. J Urol 1980; 123: 839–840.
12. Tancer ML. Observations on prevention and management of vesicovaginal fistula after total hysterectomy. Surg Gynecol Obstet 1992; 175: 501–506.
13. Romics I, Kelemen Z, Fazakas Z. The diagnosis and management of vesicovaginal fistulae. BJU Int 2002; 89: 764–766.
14. Goodwin WE, Scardino PT. Vesicovaginal and uretherovaginal fistulas: a summary of 25 years of experience. J Urol 1980; 123: 370–374.
15. Lee RA, Symmonds RE, Williams TJ. Current status of genitourinary fistula. Obstet Gynecol 1988; 72: 313–319.
16. Hedlund H, Lindstedt E. Urovaginal fistulas: 20 years experience with 45 cases. J Urol 1987; 137: 926–928.
17. Kadar N, Lemminerling L. Urinary tract injuries during laparoscopic assisted hysterectomy: causes and prevention. Am J Obstet Gynecol 1994; 170: 47–48.
18. Janeschek G, Mack D, Hetzel H. Urinary diversion in gynecologic malignancies. Eur Urol 1988; 14: 371–376.
19. Ba-Thike K, Thane A, Nan O. Tuberculous vesicovaginal fistula. Int J Gynecol Obstet 1996; 37:127–130.
20. Szabl P. Bladder stone formation on a swallowed knife blade and spontaneous passage through a vesicovaginal fistula. Br J Urol 1995; 76:659–660.
21. Goldstein I, Wise GJ, Tancer ML. A vesicovaginal fistula and intravesical foreign body: a rare case of the neglected pessary. Am J Obstet Gynecol 1990; 163: 589–591.
22. Binstock MA, Semrad N, Dubow L, Watring W. Combined vesicovaginal-ureterovaginal fistulas associated with a vaginal foreign body. Obstet Gynecol 1980; 76: 918–921.
23. Kursch ED, Morse RM, Resnik MI, Persky L. Prevention and development of a vesicovaginal fistula. Surg Gynecol Obstet 1988; 166: 409–412.
24. Zimmern PE, Ganabathi K, Leach GE. Vesicovaginal fistula repair. Urol Clin North Am 1994; 2: 87–97.
25. Smith GL, Williams G. Vesicovaginal fistula. BJU Int 1999; 83: 564–569.
26. Rackley RR, Appell RA. Vesicovaginal Fistula: Current Approach. AUA Update Series. Lesson 21, Volume 17, Lippincott Williams & Wilkins, Philadelphia, PA, 1998.
27. Neale G. Clinical analysis of 100 medico-legal cases. Br Med J 1993; 307: 1483–1487.
28. Schleicher DJ, Ojengbede OHA, Elkins TE. Urologic evaluation after closure of vesico-vaginal fistulae. Urogynaecol J 1993; 4: 262–264.
29. Chassar-Moir J. Vesico-vaginal fistulae as seen in Britain. J Obstet Gynaecol Br Com 1983; 80: 598–601.
30. Symmonds RE. Incontinence: vesical and urethral fistulas. Clin Obstet Gynecol 1984; 27: 499–514.
31. Stothers L, Chopra A, Raz S. Vesicovaginal fistula. In: *Female Urology*, 2nd ed. (Raz S, ed.), Saunders, Philadelphia, PA, 1996, pp. 492–506.
32. Comiter CV, Vasavada S, Raz S. Vesico-vaginal fistula. In: Atlas of the Urologic Clinics of North America—Vaginal Surgery. (Raz S, ed.), Williams and Wilkins, Baltimore, MD, 2000, pp. 133–140.
33. Muntz HG, Goff BA, Thor AD, Tarraza HM. Post-hysterectomy carcinoma of the fallopian tube mimicking a vesicovaginal fistula. Obstet Gynecol 1992; 79: 853–856.

34. O'Brien WM, Lynch JH. Simplification of double-dye test to diagnose various types of vaginal fistulas. Urology 1990; 36: 456.
35. Hilton P. Urodynamic findings in patients with urogenital fistulae. Br J Urol 1998; 81: 539–542.
36. Arrowsmith SD. Genitourinary reconstruction in obstetric fistulas. J Urol 1994; 152: 403–406.
37. O'Conor VJ. Nonsurgical closure of vesicovaginal fistulae. Trans Am Assoc Genito Urin Surg 1938; 31: 255–258.
38. Davits RJAM, Miranda SI. Conservative treatment of vesicovaginal fistulas by bladder drainage alone. Br J Urol 1991; 68: 155–156.
39. Aycinea JF. Small vesicovaginal fistula. Urology 1977; 9: 543–545.
40. Stovsky MD, Ignatoff JM, Blum MD, et al. Use of eletrocoagulation in the treatment of vesicovaginal fistulas. J Urol 1994; 152: 1443–1444.
41. Hedelin H, Nilson AE, Teger-Nilsson AC, Thorsen G. Fibrin occlusion of fistulas postoperatively. Surg Gynecol Obstet 1982; 154: 366–368.
42. Petersson S, Hedelin H, Jansson I, Teger-Nilsson AC. Fibrin occlusion of a vesicovaginal fistula. Lancet 1979; 1: 933–934.
43. Kanaoka Y, Hirai K, Ishiko O, Ogita S. Vesicovaginal fistula treated with fibrin glue. Int J Gyneacol Obstet 2001; 73: 147–149.
44. Dogra PN, Nabi G. Laser welding of vesicovaginal fistula. Int Urogynecol J Pelvic Floor Dysfunct 2001; 12:69–70.
45. Thacker HL Current issues in menopausal hormone replacement therapy. Cleve Clin J Med 1996; 63: 344–353.
46. Wang Y Hadley HR. Nondelayed transvaginal repair of high lying vesicovaginal fistula. J Urol 1990; 144: 34–36.
47. Robertson JR. Vesicovaginal fistulas. In: Disorders of the Female Urethra and Urinary Incontinence. (Slate WG, ed.), Williams and Wilkins, Baltimore, MD, 1982, pp. 242–249.
48. Persky L, Herman G, Guerrier K. Non delay in vesicovaginal fistula repair. Urology 1979; 13: 273–275.
49. Raz S, Little NA, Juma S. Female urology. In: Campbell's Urology, 6th ed. (Walsh PC, Retik AB, Stamey TA, eds.), Saunders, Philadelphia, PA, 1992, pp. 2782–2828.
50. Eliber KS, Kaveler E, Rodriguez LV, Rosenblum N, Raz S. Ten-year experience with transvaginal vesicovaginal fistula repair with tissue interposition. J Urol 2003; 169: 1033–1036.
51. Raz S, Bregg KJ, Nitti VW, Sussman E. Transvaginal repair of vesicovaginal fistula using a peritoneal flap. J Urol 1993; 150: 56–59.
52. Cetin S, Tazicioglu A, Ozgur S, Ilker Y, Dalva I. Vesicovaginal fistula repair: a simple suprapubic transvesical approach. Int Urol Nephrol 1988; 20: 265–268.
53. Gelabert A, Arango OJ, Borau A, Coronado J. Rectangular vesical flap. Exptraperitoneal suprapubic approach to close vesicovaginal fistulae. Acta Urol Belg 1988; 56: 64–67.
54. O'Conor VJ, Sokol JK. Vesicovaginal fistula from the standpoint of the urologists. J Urol 1951; 66: 579–585.
55. O'Conor VJ, Sokol JK, Bulkley GJ, Nanninga JB. Suprapubic closure of vesicovaginal fistula. J Urol 1973; 109: 51–54.
56. Wein AJ, Malloy TR, Greenberg SH, Carpiniello VL, Murphy JJ. Omental transposition as an aid in genitourinary reconstructive procedures. J Trauma 1980; 20: 473–477.
57. Barnes R, Hadley H, Johnston O. Transvaginal repair of vesicovaginal fistulas. Urology 1977; 10: 258–260.
58. Little NA, Juma S, Raz S. Vesicovaginal fistulae. Semin Urol 1989; 7: 78–85.
59. Hedlund H, Lindstedt E. Urovaginal fistulas: 20 years of experience with 45 cases. J Urol 1987; 137: 926–928.
60. Bissada SA, Bissada NK. Repair of active radiation-induced vesicovaginal fistula using combined gastric and omental segments based on the gastroepiploic vessels. J Urol 1992; 147: 1368–1370.
61. Salup RR, Julian TB, Linag MD, et al. Closure of large postradiation vesicovaginal fistulas with rectus abdominis myofascial flap. Urology 1994; 44: 130–131.
62. Gil-Vernet JM, Gil-Vernet A, Campos JA. New surgical approach for treatment of complex vesicovaginal fistula. J Urol 1989; 141: 513–516.

63. Martius H. Die operative wiedeherstellung der volkommen fehlenden harnorohre und des schiessmuskels derselben. Zentralbl Gynakol 1928; 52: 480–486.
64. Margolis T, Elkins TE, Seffah J, et al. Full-thickness Martius grafts to preserve vaginal depth as an adjunct in the repair of large obstetric fistulas. Obstet Gynecol 1994; 84: 148–152.
65. Obrink A, Bunne G. Gracilis interposition in fistulas following radiotherapy for cervical cancer: a retrospective study. Urol Int 1978; 33: 370–376.
66. Byron RL Jr, Ostergard DR. Sartorius muscle interposition for the treatment of the radiation-induced vaginal fistula. Am J Obstet Gynecol 1969; 104: 104–107.
67. Stirnemann H. Treatment of recurrent recto-vaginal fistula by interposition of a gluteus maximus muscle flap. Am J Proctol 1969; 20: 52–54.
68. Menchaca A, Akhyat M, Gleicher N, Gottlieb L, Bernstein J. The rectus abdominis muscle flap in a combined abdominovaginal repair of difficult vesicovaginal fistulae. A report of three cases. J Reprod Med 1990; 35: 565–568.
69. Tancer ML. A report of 34 instances of urethrovaginal and bladder neck fistulas. Surg Gynecol Obstet 1993; 177: 77–80.
70. Patil U, Waterhouse K, Laungani G. Management of 18 difficult vesicovaginal and urethrovaginal fistulas with modified Ingelman-Sundberg and Martius operations. J Urol 1980; 123: 653–656.
71. Carr LK, Webster G. Abdominal repair of vesicovaginal fistula. Urology 1996; 48: 10–11.
72. Jonas U, Petro E. Genito-urinary fistulas. In: Clinical Gynecologic Urology. (Stanton SL, ed.), Mosby, St. Louis, MO, 1984, pp. 238–255.
73. Nesrallah LJ, Srougi M, Gittes RF. The O'Conor technique: the gold standard for supratrigonal vesicovaginal fistula repair. J Urol 1999; 161: 566–568.
74. Kristensen JK, Lose G. Vesicovaginal fistulas: the transperitoneal repair revisited. Scand J Urol Nephrol 1994; 157(suppl):101–105.
75. Akman RY, Sargin S, Ozdemir G, Yazicioglu A, Cetin S. Vesicovaginal and ureterovaginal fistulas: a review of 39 cases. Int Urol Nephrol 1999; 31: 321–326.
76. Blaivas JG, Heritz DM, Romanzi LI. Early vs late repair of vesicovaginal fistulas: vaginal and abdominal approaches. J Urol 1995; 153: 1110–1112.
77. Symmonds RE. Ureteral injuries associated with gynecologic surgery: prevention and management. Clin Obstet Gynecol 1976; 19: 623–644.
78. Hosseini SY, Roshan YM, Safarinejad MR. Ureterovaginal fistula repair after vaginal delivery. J Urol 1998; 160: 829.
79. Nouira Y, Oueslati H, Reziga H, Horchani A. Ureterovaginal fistulas complicating laparoscopic hysterectomy: a report of two cases. Eur J Obstet Gynecol Reprod Biol 2001; 96: 132–134.
80. Tamussino K, Lang P, Breinl E. Ureteral complications with operative gynecologic laparoscopy. Am J Obstet Gynecol 1998; 178: 967–970.
81. Mattingly RF, Borkowf HI. Acute operative injury to the lower urinary tract. Clin Obstet Gynaecol 1978; 5: 123–149.
82. Brown RB. Surgical and external ureteric trauma. Aust N Z J Surg 1977; 47: 741–746.
83. Baltzer J, Kaufmann C, Ober KG, Zander J. Complications in 1,092 radical abdominal hysterectomies with pelvic lymphadenectomies. Geburtshilfe Frauenkeild 1980; 40: 1–5.
84. Mandal AK, Sharma SK, Vaidyanathan S, Goswami AK. Ureterovaginal fistula: summary of 18 years experience. Br J Urol 1990; 65: 453–456.
85. Murphy DM, Grace PA, O'Flynn JD. Ureterovaginal fistula: a report of 12 cases and review of the literature. J Urol 1982; 128: 924–925.
86. Raghavaiah NV. Double-dye test to diagnose various types of vaginal fistulas. J Urol 1975; 112: 811.
87. Benchekroun A, Lachkar A, Soumana A, et al. Ureterovaginal fistulas. 45 cases. Ann Urol (Paris) 1988; 32: 295–299.
88. El Ouakdi J, Jlif H, Boujnah B, Ayed M, Zmerli S. Uretero-vaginal fistula. Apropos of 30 cases. J Gynecol Obstet Biol Reprod (Paris) 1989; 18: 891–894.
89. Badenoch DF, Tiftaft RC, Thakar DR, Fowler CG, Blandy JP. Early repair of accidental injury to the ureter or bladder following gynaecological surgery. Br J Urol 1987; 59(6): 516–518.
90. Beland G. Early treatment of ureteral injuries found after gynecological surgery. J Urol 1977; 118: 25–27.

91. Witeska A, Kossakowski J, Sadowski A. Early and delayed repair of gynecological ureteral injuries. Wiad Lek 1989; 42: 305–308.
92. Meirow D, Moriel EZ, Zilberman M, Farkas A. Evaluation and treatment of iatrogenic ureteral injuries during obstetric and gynecologic operations for non-malignant conditions. J Am Coll Surg 1994; 178: 144–148.
93. Onoura VC, al-Mohalhal S, Youssef AM, Patil M. Iatrogenic urogenital fistulae. Br J Urol 1993; 71: 176–178.
94. Peterson DD, Lucey DT, Fried FA. Nonsurgical management of ureterovaginal fistula. Urology 1974; 4: 677–680.
95. Kihl B, Nilson AE, Pettersson S. Ureteroneocystotomy in the treatment of postoperative ureterovaginal fistula. Acta Obstet Gynecol Scand 1982; 61: 341–346.
96. Patel A, Werthman PE, Fuchs GJ, Barbaric AL. Endoscopic and percutaneous management of ureteral injuries, fistulas, obstruction, and strictures. In: Female Urology, 2nd ed. (Raz S, ed.), Saunders, Philadelphia, PA, 1996, pp. 521–538.
97. Lingeman JE, Wong MY, Newmark JR. Endoscopic management of total ureteral occlusion and ureterovaginal fistula. J Endourol 1995; 9: 391–396.
98. Lask D, Abarbanel J, Luttwak Z, Manes A, Mukamel E. Changing trends in the management of iatrogenic ureteral injuries. J Urol 1995; 154: 1693–1695.
99. Dowling RA, Corriere JN, Sandler CM. Iatrogenic ureteral injury. J Urol 1986; 135: 912–915.
100. Selzman A, Spirnak J, Kursh ED. The changing management of ureterovaginal fistulas. J Urol 1995; 153: 626–628.
101. Godunov BN, Loran OB, Gazimaomedov GA, Kaprin AD. The diagnosis and treatment of ureterovaginal fistulae. Urol Nefrol (Mosk) 1997; 6: 44–47.
102. Bennani S, Joual A, El Mrini M, Benjelloun S. Ureterovaginal fistulas. A report of 17 cases. J Gynecol Obstet Biol Reprod (Paris) 1996; 25: 56–59.
103. Server G, Alonso M, Ruiz JL, Osca Garcia JM, Jimenez Cruz JF. Surgical treatment of ureterovaginal fistulae caused by gynecologic surgery. Actas Urol Esp 1992; 16: 1–4.
104. Falandry L. Uretero-vaginal fistulas: diagnosis and operative tactics. Apropos of 19 personal cases. J Chir (Paris) 1992; 129: 309–316.
105. Reddy PK, Moore L, Hunter D, Amplatz K. Percutaneous ureteral fulguration: a nonsurgical technique for ureteral occlusion. J Urol 1987; 138: 724–726.
106. Papanicolaou N, Pfister RC, Yoder IC. Percutaneous occlusion of ureteral leaks and fistulae using nondetachable balloons. Urol Radiol, 1985; 7: 28–31.
107. Lee RA, Symmonds RE. Ureterovaginal fistula. Am J Obstet Gynecol 1971; 109: 1032–1035.

20 Endoscopic Perforation and Complications of BCG Therapy

Nathan F. E. Ullrich, MD,
Sanjay Ramakumar, MD, *and Bruce L. Dalkin,* MD

CONTENTS

    INTRODUCTION
    PERFORATION DURING BLADDER BIOPSY AND TRANSURETHRAL
        RESECTION OF BLADDER TUMOR
    UPPER TRACT INJURY DURING URETEROSCOPY
    COMPLICATIONS OF PERCUTANEOUS NEPHROLITHOTOMY
    COMPLICATIONS OF BACILLUS CALMETTE-GUÉRIN THERAPY
    SUMMARY
    REFERENCES

INTRODUCTION

Minimally invasive and organ-sparing treatments for benign and malignant conditions have improved therapeutic outcomes and quality of life, but unique adverse events are associated with these interventions. The endoscopic treatment of bladder cancer may cause morbidity as a result of disease progression, intraoperative complications, and side effects of therapy. Acute bleeding and ureteral obstruction owing to tumor progression or therapy are reviewed elsewhere in this book (Chapters 13 and 18). Bladder perforation during transurethral resection can lead to tumor dissemination, abdominal distension, and permanent bladder fibrosis. During percutaneous upper urinary tract surgery, injury to the colon, duodenum, lung and great vessels can lead to life-threatening infection, pulmonary compromise, and exsanguination. Systemic infection with bacillus calmette geurin (BCG) during the course of immunotherapy for bladder or upper tract urotehlial cancer, although rare, may lead to fatal sepsis if not promptly recognized and aggressively treated.

PERFORATION DURING BLADDER BIOPSY AND TRANSURETHRAL RESECTION OF BLADDER TUMOR

Incidence

Bladder perforation is the most common complication of transurethral bladder surgery, with large series reporting 1.3 to 12% perforation rates *(1–3)*. These reported rates include perforations noted by the surgeon during the operation and those that became clinically apparent postoperatively. The actual incidence of perforation is probably higher, however. In a prospective study in which patients were evaluated by cystogram before and after random bladder biopsies were performed, 9 of 25 patients had extravasation of contrast postoperatively *(4)*. As with traumatic bladder rupture, iatrogenic injuries can be classified as intraperitoneal or extraperitoneal; the majority (83–88%) of perforations are extraperitoneal *(5,6)* and occur most commonly while resecting tumors on the lateral and posterior wall of the bladder *(1)*.

Perforation is reported as more common in female patients, thought to be caused by a thinner bladder wall *(2)*. It is also more common in patients who require more than one session to resect their tumor completely *(3)*; this may be caused by larger tumor size or problems with vision during resection.

Sequelae

Bladder perforation during endoscopy usually does not add significant morbidity, but has correlated with an increased rate of other complications. Dick et al. observed that patients with endoscopic perforation had a twofold risk of infection and hemorrhage requiring transfusion and a threefold risk of sepsis *(1)*. Rarely, urinoma can result from endoscopic perforation. Extravesical tumor seeding following perforation while resecting transitional cell carcinoma has been reported, but is rare *(7,8)*. Another rare complication of perforation during transurethral bladder surgery that has been reported is transurethral resection (TUR) syndrome from excessive absorption of irrigating solution *(9)*.

Prevention

Measures to prevent perforation during transurethral surgery involve application of basic endourological principles. Avoiding overdistention during resection or biopsy is crucial. With overdistention, the bladder wall is stretched and thinned, reducing the margin for error. When resecting large tumors, a systematic approach is safest. Resection should proceed from superficial to deep. Maintaining hemostasis during resection also increases safety by decreasing vision problems caused by excessive bleeding in the operative site.

Another intraoperative risk factor for perforation is adductor muscle contraction while resecting lateral tumors (often called the obturator reflex). General anesthesia and paralysis will prevent this problem; however, anesthesia practice considerations often direct patients toward short-acting general anesthesia agents or regional anesthetic. Although no specific measures can be taken to avoid stimulating the adductor muscles, if this problem is encountered during resection, extra caution and judicious use of electrocautery with short, controlled strokes of the resecting loop can reduce the risk of perforation. In addition, preoperative antibiotics and sterilization of the urine are important to reduce infective consequences of perforation should it occur.

Treatment

Significant perforations should be apparent to the surgeon at the time of the operation, and delayed presentation of unrecognized perforation is very rare *(1)*. A perforation can be recognized by extravesical fat protrusion from the resection site or a visible hole in the case of a large intraperitoneal perforation. A high index of suspicion is warranted when resecting a large tumor with distorted anatomy. An intraoperative cystogram can be performed if there is any doubt, but this is rarely necessary.

Conservative management is preferred, with urethral catheter drainage for at least 7 d postoperatively and broad-spectrum antibiotic coverage while the catheter is in place. As with traumatic bladder rupture, which is discussed in Chapter 3, almost all extraperitoneal perforations can be managed this way. Although operative repair is mandatory in traumatic intraperitoneal rupture, iatrogenic intraperitoneal perforation can often be managed conservatively as well in select cases. If significant intraperitoneal extravasation of urine and irrigant is noted or expected, a peritoneal drain can be placed percutaneously using radiological guidance. A cystogram may be performed prior to catheter removal to confirm bladder healing. A urinoma can be drained by computed tomography (CT)- or ultrasound (US)-guided percutaneous drain *(10)*.

Operative management is recommended for intraperitoneal perforations that are very large or in a bladder or patient at high risk of healing compromise (i.e., from radiation or formalin changes, immunosuppression, diabetes, etc.). Surgical repair should be undertaken through a midline or Pfannenstiel incision and open cystotomy with multiple-layer closure using absorbable suture and closed suction drain. The bladder has an extensive blood supply, and debridement of devitalized tissue is rarely necessary. A urethral catheter or suprapubic tube should be left in place, and a cystogram demonstrating no extravasation should be performed prior to catheter removal. The patient should be maintained on antibiotics for 5 to 7 d after repair and for 3 to 5 d at the time of catheter removal.

UPPER TRACT INJURY DURING URETEROSCOPY

Incidence

Injury to the ureter is the most common reported complication during ureteroscopy, but serious injuries have become less frequent with the advent of new equipment and with increased experience. Reported rates of perforation range from 0.3 to 17%. Reviewing 10 large series, including 5400 patients, we found the combined perforation rate was 2.8%, with 11% of these injuries requiring an open operation for acute repair *(11–20)*. Reporting of minor ureteral injuries is inconsistent among series in the literature, but these injuries have occurred with a certain frequency regardless of experience and equipment and rarely have clinical significance *(21)*. Newer semirigid or flexible ureteroscopes and increased surgeon experience appear to reduce the risk of serious ureteral perforation *(13,22)*.

Relevant Anatomy

The ureter is supplied by three to nine arteries, with an average of five *(21)*. The arterial supply runs longitudinally between the adventitia and the muscularis medially above the pelvic brim and laterally below, and most segments do not have a dual supply; this is important to remember during repair and in assessing injury severity.

The layers of the ureter are composed of a mucosa of transitional epithelium, a lamina propria that caries the mucosal blood supply, and a muscularis with longitudinal and circular fibers. The muscularis has fewer circular fibers in the proximal segment and in the intramural ureter, which may predispose to perforation in these areas *(23)*.

The three areas of narrowing in the ureter include the ureterovesical junction, the pelvic brim where the iliac vessels cross, and the ureteropelvic junction. In addition, two regions that may be vulnerable to perforation are the curve in the pelvic ureter where its orientation transitions from posterolateral to anteromedial and the curve over the psoas muscle.

Types of Injury

Ureteral injuries range in severity and clinical consequences. Mucosal injury is quite common, with reported rates as high as 24.5% *(15)* and is rarely reported by authors. More extensive mucosal lesions can involve stripping of the mucosa or creation of a false passage by the tip of the beak or by an accessory such as a lithotripsy device, laser fiber, basket, or alligator grasper.

Perforation is a full-thickness injury. There can be significant fluid and urine extravasation with perforation, and an untreated or inadequately drained perforation can result in urinoma or abscess.

Rarely, ureteroscopy can result in avulsion of the ureter. Avulsion can be complete or partial, and in severe cases, ureteral blood supply can be compromised with extensive devitalization.

The final category of ureteral injury is thermal injury from accessories used for intracorporeal lithotripsy or fulguration of ureteral lesions. Electrohydraulic or ultrasonic lithotriptors appear to have the most potential for ureteral injury, with an increased safety margin using a laser device, although a retrospective review by Teichman et al. found no difference in complication rate between electrohydraulic lithotripsy and holmium laser lithotripsy *(24)*.

Prevention

Routine ureteroscopy is a safe procedure, but does carry inherent risks even in the most skilled hands. Careful planning and execution can increase safety and chances of success. A brief review of measures that may reduce complication rates follows.

PATIENT SELECTION

A number of patient factors can contribute to the incidence of and increase morbidity from ureteral perforation. A history of retroperitoneal surgery, radiation therapy, or previous extensive ureteral manipulation has been shown to increase the perforation rate *(25)*, likely caused by relative immobility of the ureter in the retroperitoneum and impaired vascular supply. Impacted stones or a large intrarenal stone burden may increase the perforation rate, but this is dependent on the skill of the operator. Patients should be free of urinary tract infection prior to ureteroscopy, both because intrarenal reflux occurs with irrigation and because extravasation of infected urine can lead to retroperitoneal abscess.

PATIENT PREPARATION

Patients should be given preoperative antibiotics, and sterile preparation and technique should be used for ureteroscopy. Choice of anesthesia technique is changing with the use of smaller flexible or semirigid scopes and outpatient ureteroscopy. In the era of rigid ureteroscopy, general or regional anesthesia was mandatory to prevent patient movement. Monitored sedation has been shown to be safe for ureteroscopy with newer equipment and techniques *(26)*, but when long procedures are anticipated, an immobilizing technique may be advisable. Preoperative imaging with intravenous urogram may be helpful in planning complex ureteroscopic procedures, but is not mandatory.

INTRAOPERATIVE TECHNIQUE

Use of a guide wire can facilitate introduction of the ureteroscope and allows insertion of a stent at any time during the procedure. Good vision is imperative for ureteroscopy both during introduction and while manipulating a stone or lesion. Care should be taken to flush all equipment to prevent air bubbles. Irrigation improves vision, but periodic drainage is necessary to prevent excessive intrarenal pressure. If vision becomes poor at any time, the procedure should be aborted.

Liberal use of intraoperative imaging also increases safety and allows for early identification of injury. A retrograde ureterogram should be performed at the start of any ureteroscopy and can be repeated to confirm an injury. Fluoroscopic guidance should be used while advancing guide wires and may be helpful in difficult ureteroscope advancement.

Many ureteric injuries occur when excessive force is applied to extract large calculi. When attempting ureteroscopic stone extraction, a method of intraluminal lithotripsy, such as electrohydraulic, ultrasonic, or laser lithotripter, should be available, and stones should be fragmented to a size that passes easily. If a stone becomes impacted during extraction with a basket and the basket cannot be disengaged, the basket handle should be removed and the ureteroscope advanced alongside the basket sheath for fragmentation of the stone.

Diagnosis and Management

DIAGNOSIS

Most ureteral perforations are detected by vision intraoperatively. A perforation may not be noticed until the end of the procedure, however, and the entire course of the ureter should always be visualized at the completion of the procedure while withdrawing the scope. If an injury is suspected, it may be visualized by extravasation on a retrograde pyelogram, but this does not need to be a routine step.

An unrecognized injury may not be easily identified because signs and symptoms are nonspecific. A patient may complain of flank pain, but pain is usually absent in a large perforation. There may be a slight increase in serum creatinine or serum urea nitrogen if there is significant urine extravasation. An unrecognized perforation may present late as a urinoma, which can be identified by US or CT.

MANAGEMENT

Most ureteral perforations can be managed conservatively. Routine ureteral stenting after ureteroscopy is currently controversial, but possibly unnecessary *(26,27)*. A stent should be placed whenever significant ureteral trauma results from ureteroscopy even without perforation to avoid postoperative obstruction. If perforation does occur, all attempts should be made to place a ureteral stent, although patients have been successfully managed without *(27,28)*. If a stent cannot be placed retrograde, a percutaneous nephrostomy should be placed, and placement of an antegrade internal stent should be attempted *(29)*.

Recommendations and practice patterns vary regarding the duration of stenting after ureteral perforation, with most authors reporting 2–6 wk of stenting. Experimental data on an animal model showed no benefit from ureteral catheters beyond 3 wk *(30)*.

Contrast imaging showing no extravasation should be performed prior to stent removal. A urethral catheter should be left in place for several days to prevent reflux and extravasation of urine while voiding and may be left in place longer for high-risk injuries.

Extensive perforations and avulsions may require surgical reconstruction. In our review, 11% of ureteral injuries were repaired operatively *(12–21)*. Immediate repair is preferable. If the repair is undertaken after 10 d from the time of injury, maximum inflammation, edema, and distortion of anatomy are encountered, making the operation difficult, and decrease chances of successful outcome. If delayed repair is necessary, it should be undertaken after 3 to 6 mo, with interval urinary diversion using percutaneous nephrostomy.

Type of repair depends on the extent and location of the injury. A detailed discussion of operative ureteral reconstruction is found in Chapter 2. Distal perforations can be repaired by ureteral neocystostomy with or without Boari flap or psoas hitch. Mid- and proximal ureteral perforations without extensive devitalization can be repaired by ureteroureterostomy or transureteral-ureterostomy. However, transureteral-ureterostomy should be avoided in patients with a history of stone disease or upper tract urothelial carcinoma, and most patients undergoing ureteroscopy have one of these conditions. An avulsion or extensively devitalized ureter may require complex reconstruction with ileal substitution, autotransplant, or nephrectomy.

Rarely, an unrecognized or inadequately diverted ureteral injury results in urinoma from extravasation. This complication can be difficult to diagnose, but can be seen using US or CT. Percutaneous drainage with or without closed-suction drainage is the treatment of choice, and antibiotic coverage should be provided *(31)*.

COMPLICATIONS OF PERCUTANEOUS NEPHROLITHOTOMY

Classification of Injury

Perforation injuries during percutaneous nephrolithotomy (PNL) can occur during access to create the nephrostomy tract or during endoscopic manipulation. Access complications can include thoracic, liver, spleen, bowel, or vascular injury, as well as injury to the renal collecting system. Injuries incurred during endoscopic manipulation usually involve the collecting system and can result in urinary fistula or urinoma.

Injury During Access

Technique

Many urologists perform PNL through existing nephrostomy tracts established preoperatively by an interventional radiologist, but it can be advantageous to create the nephrostomy tract at the time of PNL for placement that allows the most direct approach to the stone. Initial collecting system access is gained using a 22- or 18-gage needle through which a wire is threaded (Seldinger technique). Position is confirmed using fluoroscopy. The nephrostomy tract is then dilated over the wire using flexible fascial dilators or by balloon dilation. A working wire and a safety wire are then maintained during the procedure.

Once the tract is created, a nephroscope can be introduced through an access sheath or over the working wire. Fluoroscopy with the aid of contrast administration can define collecting system anatomy and can alert the urologist to potential injury prior to dilation or manipulation, which may reduce morbidity from a perforation injury.

THORACIC INJURY

When accessing the upper pole, there is always potential for transversing the pleural space, particularly if a supracostal approach is used. Entering the pleural space can result in pneumothorax or hydrothorax. Incidence of thoracic injury is reported as 0.1 to 3.2% *(32–35)*. Most pleural injuries incurred during access for PNL are minor and can be managed conservatively *(33)*. Urine extravasation into the chest is rare and should always be drained to reduce morbidity. Careful examination of pleural anatomy using fluoroscopy before introducing a needle for access is crucial for avoiding thoracic injury. Postoperative chest radiography or fluoroscopic examination should be performed after upper pole access procedures or if any suspicion for thoracic injury exists *(33)*.

SOLID ORGAN INJURY

Injury to the liver or spleen is an uncommon complication of percutaneous renal access. A significant injury manifests as bleeding, which is proportional to the magnitude of the tissue damage *(36)*. Treatment should follow principles of penetrating liver or spleen trauma and can be conservative, involving bed rest, serial blood count, and interval imaging using CT. Failure of blood count to stabilize or hemodynamic instability mandate intervention with surgical exploration or angiography and embolization.

BOWEL INJURY

Bowel injury is rare during percutaneous renal surgery and often results from patients with anatomic variations or prior abdominal surgery. Reported incidence is 0.2 to 0.8 % *(37–39)*. An excessively lateral approach or a mobile kidney can also increase the risk of colonic injury *(38)*. Extraperitoneal colon injury can be managed conservatively with internal urinary system stenting and drainage. Using the percutaneous tube as a colostomy tube has been described *(37)*. When the connection between the urinary system and colon is sealed, the tube and stent can be removed and the resulting colocutaneous fistula managed conservatively until it closes. Intraperitoneal colon injury requires immediate abdominal exploration and repair *(38)*.

Duodenal injury during PNL has also been successfully managed conservatively *(40)*.

Perforation During Endoscopic Manipulation

Once a nephrostomy tract is created and a nephroscope is introduced, perforation can occur as a result of endoscopic manipulation or stone fragmentation using ultrasonic, laser, or electrohydraulic lithotriptors or during extraction of stone fragments using a basket or grasper. Extravasation during PNL is relatively common, but rarely results in morbidity. After PNL, an antegrade ureteral catheter and nephrostomy tube should be left in place. Routine postoperative nephrostogram should be performed 24 to 48 h after PNL to detect extravasation prior to removal of nephrostomy or ureteral catheter.

Unrecognized extravasation can lead to serious morbidity and can be life threatening *(41,42)*. If extravasation is encountered, antegrade ureteral stent placement should be performed, and nephrostomy and urethral catheter should be left in place. If nephrostomy output remains high, retained obstructing stone fragments should be suspected.

Once extravasation has resolved on follow-up nephrostogram, tubes and stents can be removed. Prolonged urinary extravasation can lead to infection, urinoma, or urinary fistula. Acutely, extravasation during PNL procedures can lead to excessive fluid absorption. Fluid absorption should be treated with diuresis and electrolyte monitoring and management.

Prevention

As with all procedures, careful planning and vigilance for complications are required to reduce morbidity during PNL. Use of preoperative imaging for high-risk patients and intraoperative fluoroscopy of all patients reduces the chance of injury. Urinary tract infection should be detected by routine preoperative culture and treated prior to PNL. All patients should be given preoperative antibiotics. Intraoperatively, careful technique should be employed to avoid collecting system injury, and a safety wire and working wire should always be used. If vision is impaired by bleeding, the procedure should be abandoned with an interval procedure to complete stone removal. Postoperative imaging should be utilized to identify unrecognized injuries.

COMPLICATIONS OF BACILLUS CALMETTE-GUÉRIN THERAPY

Background

Bacillus Calmette-Guérin (BCG) is used as an intravesical agent for treating superficial bladder cancer. Indications include carcinoma *in situ* and superficial tumors at high risk for recurrence, including T1 lesions of any grade, and T0 tumors that are high grade, multifocal, or frequently recurrent. BCG therapy regimens usually consist of an induction phase of six weekly instillations, followed by a maintenance program of periodic instillations continued indefinitely. Adverse effects of BCG therapy include local and systemic reactions, which may be immune mediated or infectious and can be classified as true complications or side effects. Adverse side effects are quite common with BCG therapy, but major complications are infrequent.

Mechanism of Action

BCG is a live, attenuated mycobacterium and is believed to act on superficial bladder cancer by inducing a local inflammatory reaction *(43)*. The mycobacterium is ingested into the urothelium and induces the local release of cytokines, some of which initiate the recruitment of cytotoxic and helper lymphocytes *(44,45)*. The primary cytokines released are interferon-γ and interleukin-2, and these cytokines are believed to produce the majority of systemic side effects *(46)*.

Local Side Effects

Local side effects occur in 27 to 90% of patients receiving BCG therapy *(47,48)*. The most common are dysuria, hematuria, urgency, and frequency. These side effects are symptoms of the local inflammatory reaction from BCG instillation. Local side effects can usually be treated symptomatically using nonsteroidal anti-inflammatory agents and pyridium or anticholinergics. Urine and blood cultures should be obtained. It may be necessary to withhold treatment briefly, but these reactions do not preclude further treatment.

Immune-Mediated Systemic Symptoms

Fever, myalgias, and malaise may accompany local side effects or may occur alone. These systemic reactions are reported in 1 to 17% of patients on BCG programs *(47,48)*. Systemic symptoms are similar to those seen with systemic administration of cytokines and are likely caused by cytokine release in response to BCG. Symptomatic therapy with antipyretics or nonsteroidal anti-inflammatory agents can be used to treat systemic effects, and urine and blood cultures should be obtained. As with local side effects, BCG therapy may need to be withheld temporarily, but may be resumed after resolution of symptoms. Prophylactic antipyretic and anti-inflammatory treatment with or without prophylactic isoniazid and pyridoxine may prevent or minimize such reactions in subsequent instillations.

Infectious Complications

Systemic Infection and Sepsis

Systemic mycobacterial infection is a rare, but serious complication of intravesical BCG therapy. Incidence of systemic infection is reported as 0.4 to 0.7% in contemporary series *(48)*. It is characterized by much higher fevers than seen in cytokine-mediated reactions, with temperatures greater than 103°F and shaking chills. The clinical picture is similar to that for bacterial sepsis, with progression to hemodynamic instability, respiratory distress, multisystem organ failure, and disseminated intravascular coagulation. It has been proposed that BCG sepsis may have a component of delayed-type hypersensitivity *(49)*.

Treatment consists of supportive therapy, with hospital admission for aggressive hydration, and may require invasive monitoring and mechanical ventilation. A full septic workup with blood, urine, and sputum cultures as well as chest X-ray to exclude bacterial causes is required. After obtaining cultures, antimicrobial therapy should be initiated, with parenteral broad-spectrum antibiotics and antimycobacterial therapy.

The optimal antimicrobial regimen for systemic BCG infection is not completely agreed on, but isoniazid, rifampin, and prednisone or prednisolone are included in most recommendations *(49,50)*. Adding prednisolone has been shown to increase survival in an animal model of BCG sepsis *(51)*, and 80% survival for BCG sepsis in humans has been reported with 300 mg isoniazid, 600 mg rifampin, and 40 mg prednisone daily *(49)*. The rationale for steroid use comes from the theory of delayed-type hypersensitivity reaction in BCG sepsis. For patients not initially responding to isoniazid, rifampin, and steroids, 1200 mg ethambutol may be added.

Cycloserine use in BCG sepsis is controversial. Some authors recommended cycloserine for the first 5 d of BCG sepsis treatment because of its rapid onset of action *(49)* and because of a survival advantage in mice *(51)*. However, currently used strains of BCG are resistant to cycloserine *(52)*.

Patients who have had septic complications should not be given further BCG therapy.

Granulomatous Disease

Granulomatous BCG infection is infrequently encountered in patients on intravesical programs. The prostate is the most common site of granulomatous disease, with rates as high as 27% reported *(49)*. Many patients are asymptomatic, are only discovered on digital rectal examination, and do not require treatment. Symptomatic granulomatous prostatitis should be treated with 3 to 6 mo of 300 mg isoniazid and 600 mg rifampin.

Epididymo-orchitis can also occur with BCG therapy and may require epididymectomy if refractory to 3 to 6 mo of isoniazid, rifampin, and pyridoxine. Hepatitis and pneumonitis are rare granulomatous complications of BCG treatment. They may be diagnosed by characteristic lesions on chest X-ray or CT, and liver biopsy may be necessary. Fever, malaise, and respiratory compromise are typical, as are elevated liver enzymes. Most patients with hepatitis and pneumonitis require hospitalization acutely and should be treated with isoniazid and rifampin for 6 mo. Ethambutol or steroids may be added during the acute phase of this complication. Granulomatous disease rarely can occur in the bladder and bone marrow as well. Pyridoxine replacement should be given with isoniazid treatment to prevent seizures. All patients with granulomatous disease should have appropriate cultures to rule out bacterial causes of their illness. BCG therapy can be resumed with caution after granulomatous complications have resolved, and patients should be pretreated with 300 mg isoniazid and pyridoxine starting the day prior to instillation and continuing for a total of 3 d.

Prevention

Infectious complications of BCG therapy are thought to result from systemic absorption, most commonly through disrupted mucosal surfaces. To avoid systemic absorption, BCG instillation should be delayed in the setting of gross hematuria, a traumatic catheterization, active stricture disease, ulcerated tumors, and urinary tract infection. An interval of 2 to 3 wk after bladder tumor resection is required before initiating BCG therapy. Patients should be periodically cultured while on therapy programs, and BCG should be instilled by gravity only. Contraindications to BCG therapy include active tuberculosis infection, immunosuppression, pregnancy or lactation, and acute urinary tract infection. Intravesical therapy is safe in the setting of vesiculoureteral reflux *(53)*.

SUMMARY

Bladder perforation during transurethral surgery is a relatively common complication. It can usually be managed conservatively with catheter drainage and antibiotics. Careful endoscopic technique and recognition of perforation intraoperatively are the keys to preventing morbidity because of this complication.

Upper tract perforation is the most common complication of ureteroscopy. Conservative therapy with stenting is the preferred treatment, but surgical reconstruction is required in severe cases. Newer endoscopes and increased experience may reduce the incidence of perforation, but careful technique, including gentle manipulation, use of intraoperative fluoroscopy, always maintaining good vision, and working with a safety wire, are mandatory for reducing morbidity from this complication.

Mild local and systemic side effects of BCG intravesical therapy for superficial bladder cancer are common and are probably directly related to the immunological mechanism of action against bladder cancer. Symptomatic treatment is sufficient for such adverse effects. Severe systemic and granulomatous infectious complications can occur, but are infrequent. Antimycobacterial therapy is required for BCG infection, and severe cases can be life threatening. Avoiding BCG instillation in the setting of compromised mucosal barriers is essential for preventing systemic absorption.

REFERENCES

1. Dick A, Barnes R, Hadley H, Bergman RT, Ninan CA. Complications of transurethral resection of bladder tumors: prevention, recognition and treatment. J Urol 1980; 124(6): 810–811.
2. Mitchell JP. Transurethral resection for neoplasm of the bladder. In: Endoscopic Operative Urology. (Wright PSG, ed.), Bristol, UK, 1981, pp. 341–363.
3. Collado A, Chechile GE, Salvador J, Vicente J. Early complications of endoscopic treatment for superficial bladder tumors. J Urol 2000; 164: 1529–1532.

4. Siegler LJ, Addonidio JC, Fernandez R, Shutte H. Incidence and treatment of bladder perforation following bladder biopsy. Urol 1985; 26(1):10–11.
5. Richardson JR Jr, Leadbetter GW Jr. Non-operative treatment of the ruptured bladder. J Urol 1975; 114: 213–216.
6. Mulkey AP Jr, Witherington R. Conservative management of vesical rupture. Urology 1974; 5: 426–430.
7. Mydlo JH, Weinstein R, Shah S, et al. Long-term consequences from bladder perforation and/or violation in the presence of transitional cell carcinoma: results of a small series and a review of the literature. J Urol 1999; 161(4): 1128–1132.
8. Ohguchi N, Sakaida N, Okamura A, et al. Extravesical tumor implantation caused by perforation during transurethral resection of a bladder tumor: a case report. Int J Urol 1997; 4(5): 516–518.
9. Ekengren J, Conner P, Lindholm M, Hahn RG. Fluid absorption during transurethral bladder surgery. Scand J Urol Nephrol 1995; 29(4): 519–520.
10. Vansonnenberg E, Mueller PR, Ferrucci JT Jr. Percutaneous drainage of 250 abdominal abscesses and fluid collections. Radiology 1984; 151: 337–341.
11. Shuster TG, Hollenbeck BK, Faerber GJ, Wolf JS Jr. Complications of ureteroscopy: analysis of predictive factors. J Urol 2001; 166(2): 538–540.
12. Hollenbeck BK, Shuster TG, Faerber GJ, Wolf JS Jr. Comparison of outcomes of ureteroscopy for ureteral calculi above and below the pelvic brim. Urol 2001; 58(3): 351–356.
13. Jeromin L, Sosnowski M. Ureteroscopy in the treatment of ureteral stones: over 10 years experience. Eur Urol 1998; 34(4): 344–349.
14. Harmon WJ, Serson PD, Blute ML, Patterson DE, Segura JW. Ureteroscopy: current practice and long term complications. J Urol 1997; 157(1): 28–32.
15. Francesca F, Scattoni V, Nava L, et al. Failures and complications of transurethral ureteroscopy in 297 cases: conventional rigid instruments vs small caliber semirigid ureteroscopes. Eur Urol 1995; 28: 112–115.
16. Kranolowsky EV. Ureteral perforation during ureterorenoscopy: treatment and management. J Urol 1987; 138: 36–38.
17. Peh OH, Lim PH, Ng FC, et al: Holmium laser lithotripsy in the management of ureteric calculi. Ann Acad Med Singapore 2001; 30(6): 563–567.
18. Assimos DG, Patterson LC, Taylor CL. Changing incidence and etiology of iatrogenic ureteral injuries. J Urol 1994; 152(6): 2240–2246.
19. Andersen JR, Ostri P, Jansen JE, Kristensen JK. A retrospective evaluation of 691 ureteroscopies: indications, procedures, success rate and complications. Urol Int 1993; 51(4): 191–197.
20. Kostakopoulos A, Sofras F, Karayiannis A, Kranidis A, Dimopoulos C. Ureterolithotripsy: report of 1000 cases. Br J Urol 1989; 63(3): 243–244.
21. Houffman JL. Ureteroscopic injuries to the upper urinary tract. Urol Clin North Am 1989; 16(2): 249–254.
22. Weinberg JJ, Ansong K, Smith AD. Complications of ureteroscopy in relation to experience: a reported survey and author experience. J Urol 1987; 137: 384.
23. Stoller ML, Wolf JS Jr, Hofman R, et al. Ureteroscopy without balloon dilation: an outcome assessment. J Urol 1992; 147: 1238.
24. Teichman JM, Rao RD, Rogenes VJ, Harris JM. Ureteroscopic management of ureteral calculi: electrohydraulic vs holmium:YAG lithotripsy. J Urol 1997; 158(4): 1357–1361.
25. Stackl W, Marberger M. Late sequelae of the management of ureteral calculi with the ureterorenoscope. J Urol 1986; 136: 386.
26. Cheung MC, Lee F, Leung YL, et al. Outpatient ureteroscopy: predictive factors for postoperative events. Urology 2001; 58(6): 914–918.
27. Chen YT, Chen J, Wong WY, et al. Is ureteral stenting necessary after uncomplicated ureteroscopic lithotripsy? A prospective, randomized controlled trial. J Urol 2002; 167(5): 1977–1980.
28. Benjamin JC, Donaldson PJ, Hill JT. Ureteric perforation after ureteroscopy. Conservative management. Urology 1987; 29(6): 623–624.
29. Lang EK. Antegrade ureteral stenting for dehiscence, stricture and fistulae. AJR Am J Roentgenol 1984; 143: 795–801.

30. McDonald JH, Falons JA. Experimental ureteral stricture: ureteral regrowth following ureterotomy with and without intubation. J Urol 1960; 84: 52.
31. Vansonnenberg E, Mueller PR, Ferrucci JT Jr. Percutaneous drainage of 250 abdominal abscesses and fluid collections. Radiology 1984; 151: 337–341.
32. Segura JW, Patterson DE, LeRoy AJ, Williams HJ, et al. Percutaneous removal of kidney stones: review of 1000 cases. J Urol 1985; 134: 1077.
33. O'Donnell A, Schoenberger C, Weiner J, Tsou E. Pulmonary complications of percutaneous nephrostomy and kidney stone extraction. South Med J 1988; 81: 1002.
34. Fernstrom I, Johannson B. Percutaneous pyelithotomy. A new extraction technique. Scand J Urol Nephrol 1976; 10: 257.
35. Lee WJ, Smith AD, Cubelli V, Badlani GH, et al. Complications of percutaneous nephrolithotomy. AJR Am J Roentgenol 1987; 148(1): 177–180.
36. Kondas J, Szentgyorgyi E, Vaczi L, Kiss A. Splenic injury: a rare complication of percutaneous nephrolithotomy. Int Urol Nephrol 1994; 26: 399.
37. Leroy AJ, Williams HJ, Bender CE, Segura JW, et al. Colon perforation following percutaneous nephrostomy and renal calculus removal. Radiology 1985; 155: 83.
38. Vallancien G, Capdeville R, Veillon B, Charton M, Brisset JM. Colonic perforation during percutaneous nephrolithotomy. J Urol 1985; 134: 1185.
39. Rodrigues Netto N Jr, Lemos GC, Fiuza JL. Colon perforation following percutaneous nephrolithotomy. Urology 1988; 32(3): 223–224.
40. Ahmed M, Reeve R. Iatrogenic duodeno-cutaneous fistula at percutaneous nephrolithotomy managed conservatively. Br J Urol 1995; 75: 416.
41. Carson CC, Nesbitt JA. Peritoneal extravasation during percutaneous lithotripsy. J Urol 1985; 134: 725.
42. Dimberg M, Norlen H, Hoglund N, Allgen LG. Absorption of irrigating fluid during percutaneous transrenal lithotripsy. Scand J Urol Nephrol 1993; 27: 463.
43. Ratliff TL. The role of the immune response in bacillus Calmette-Guérin for bladder cancer. Eur Urol 1992; 21: 17–21.
44. Ratliff TL, McCarthy R, Telle WB, et al. Purification of a mycobacterial adhesion for fibronectin. Infect Immunol 1993; 61: 1889–1894.
45. Kurota K, Brown EJ, Telle WB, et al. Characterization of bacillus Calmette-Guérin by human bladder tumor cells. J Clin Invest 1993; 91: 69–76.
46. Pattard JJ, Saint F, Velotti F, et al. Immune response following intravesical bacillus Calmette-Guérin instillations in superficial bladder cancer: a review. Urol Res 1998; 26: 155–159.
47. Lamm DL, Stogdill VD, Stogdill BJ, et al. Complications of bacillus Calmette-Guérin immunotherapy in 1278 patients with bladder cancer. J Urol 1986; 135: 272–274.
48. Lamm DL. Complications of bacillus Calmette-Guérin immunotherapy. Urol Clin North Am 1992; 19: 565–572.
49. Lamm DL, van der Meijden PM, Morales A, et al. Incidence and treatment of complications of bacillus Calmette-Guérin intravesical therapy in superficial bladder cancer. J Urol 1992; 147: 596–600.
50. Durek C, Rusch-Gerdes S, Jocham D, et al. Interference of modern antibacterials with bacillus Calmette-Guérin viability. J Urol 1999; 162: 1959–1962.
51. DeHaven JI, Traynellis C, Riggs DR, et al. Antibiotic and steroid therapy of massive systemic bacillus Calmette-Guérin toxicity. J Urol 1992; 147: 738–742.
52. Durek C, Rusch-Gerdes S, Jocham D, et al. Sensitivity of BCG to modern antibiotics. Eur Urol 1999; 37: 21–25.
53. Heney NM, Koontz WW, Barton B, et al. Intravesical thiotepa vs mitomycin C in patients with Ta, T1, and TIS transitional cell carcinoma of the bladder: a phase III prospective randomized study. J Urol 1988; 140: 1390–1393.

VI Newborn Urological Emergencies

21 The Exstrophy–Epispadias Complex

Richard W. Grady, MD

CONTENTS

INTRODUCTION
ANATOMIC FEATURES
INCIDENCE
ANTENATAL DIAGNOSIS
PREOPERATIVE CARE
OPERATIVE INTERVENTION: METHODS AND TIMING
POSTOPERATIVE CONSIDERATIONS
SUMMARY
REFERENCES

INTRODUCTION

Children born with congenital anomalies in the exstrophy–epispadias complex include children with epispadias, classic bladder exstrophy, cloacal exstrophy, and exstrophy variants. These congenital defects are considered pediatric urological emergencies because early repair (at less than 48–72 h of age) can be done more easily. Furthermore, newborn repair is associated with improved success rates compared to exstrophy repair later in life. Because the bladder exstrophy–epispadias complex is not a lethal condition, children with bladder exstrophy or epispadias can survive untreated. Before the modern era of surgery and anesthesia, some patients with bladder exstrophy survived untreated into adulthood. However, the morbidity bladder exstrophy patients experienced was often severe because of bladder and kidney infection, skin breakdown, and tumor formation in the bladder plate. Reports exist of such patients with classic bladder exstrophy living into their eighth decade *(1)*. In contrast, until recently, patients born with cloacal exstrophy almost universally died shortly after birth from electrolyte abnormalities and malnutrition.

ANATOMIC FEATURES

The primary features of exstrophy involve an absence of the anterior bladder wall and dorsal urethra with an associated absence of the anterior abdominal wall overlying it (Fig. 1). The urothelium of the bladder and urethra is thus exposed to the environment. With cloacal exstrophy, the cecal plate is also exposed to the environment and rests

From: *Urological Emergencies: A Practical Guide*
Edited by: H. Wessells and J. W. McAninch © Humana Press Inc., Totowa, NJ

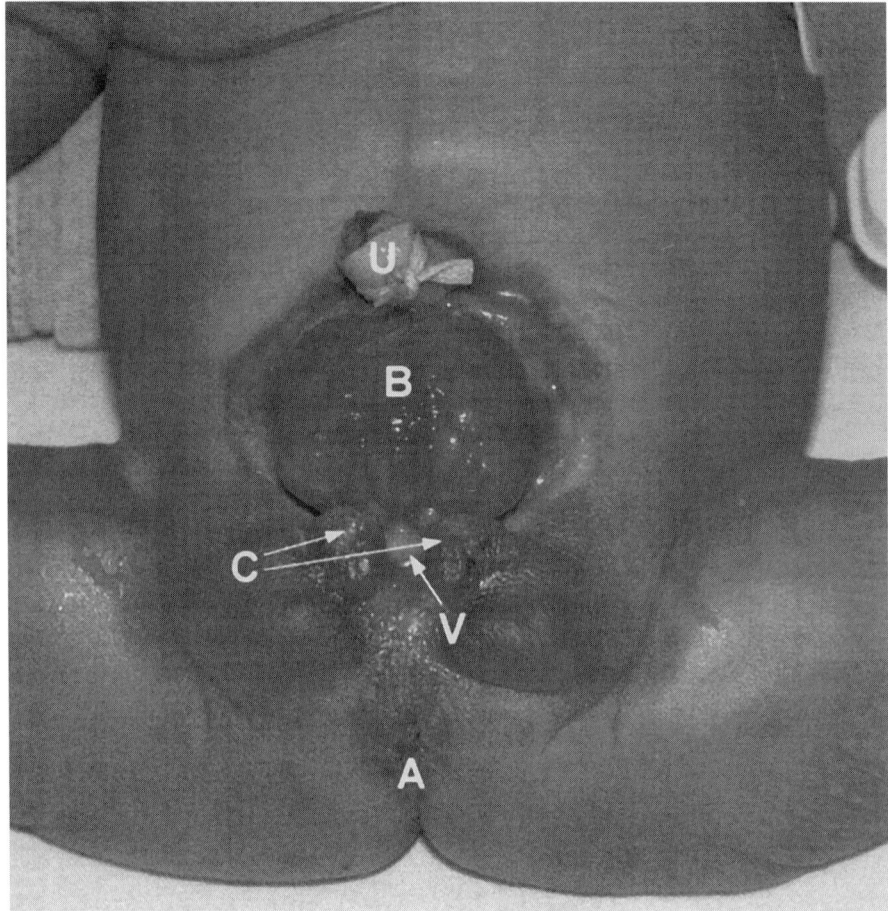

Fig. 1. Female neonate with bladder exstrophy. **B,** exstrophic bladder; **C,** clitoral bodies; **V,** vagina; **U,** umbilical cord; **A,** anus.

between two bladder halves (Fig. 2). Considerable variation exists in the size and compliance of the bladder plate at birth; some bladders are quite small and inelastic, whereas others appear large and compliant.

At birth, the urothelium is usually normal in appearance. However, ectopic bowel mucosa or polypoid lesions consistent with cystitis cystica or glandularis may be present. If left untreated and without meticulous protection after birth, the exposed urothelium will undergo squamous metaplasia in response to acute and chronic inflammation. Other inflammatory changes such as cystitis cystica and/or glandularis will also be seen. When left chronically exposed to the environment, the areas of squamous metaplasia often undergo malignant degeneration to adenocarcinoma or squamous cell carcinoma *(1,2)*.

Classic exstrophy and epispadias share a low incidence of anomalies affecting organ systems other than the genitourinary tract and bony pelvis. In contrast, patients with cloacal exstrophy have associated anomalies more often than not *(3,4)*. These anomalies can affect the upper urinary tract, intestines, skeletal system, and neurological system. A possible reason for this is that the cloacal exstrophy defect occurs much earlier in development, affecting subsequent development of related structures, including the spine, kidneys, and hindgut (Table 1).

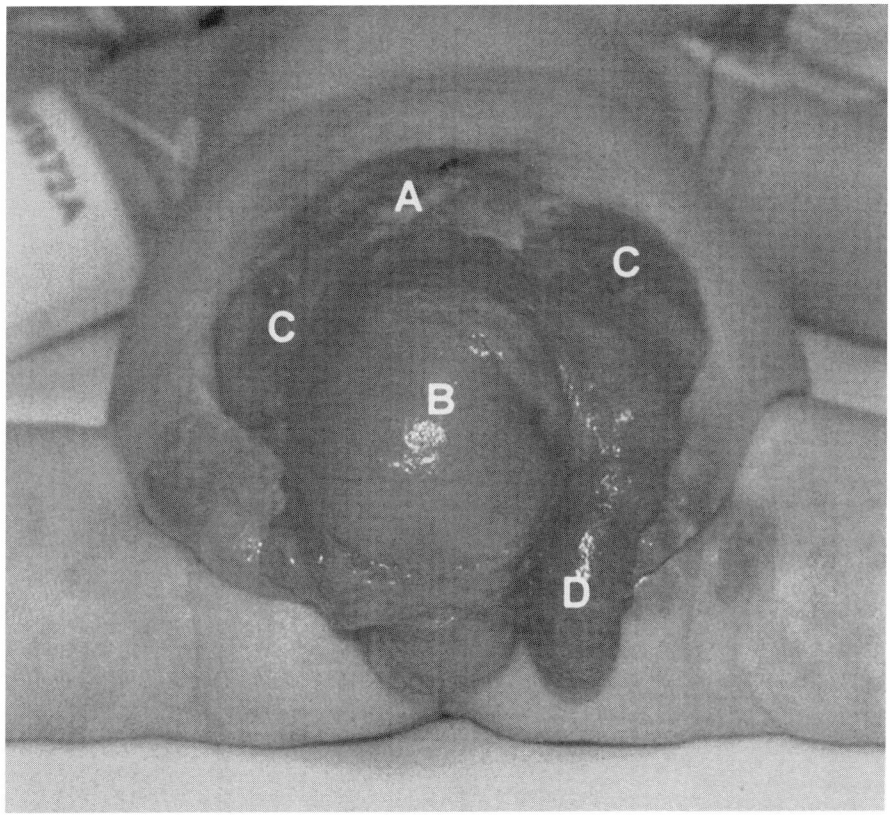

Fig. 2. Male neonate with cloacal exstrophy. (**A**) Small omphalocele status post treatment with silvadene; (**B**) hindgut plate; (**C**) exstrophic bladder halves; (**D**) intussuscepted ileum.

INCIDENCE

Bladder exstrophy occurs at a rate of 1 per 10,000 live births to 1 per 50,000 live births *(5,6)*. This anomaly has long been recognized to occur more commonly in males than females, with a ratio of 2.3–4:1 reported in the literature *(7,8)*. Cloacal exstrophy occurs even more rarely, with an incidence of 1:200,000 to 400,000 live births *(9)*.

Genetic factors involved in exstrophy remain incompletely defined. To date, 18 familial cases of bladder exstrophy have been reported, the most recent of which describes a mother and son with bladder exstrophy *(10)*. In 1984, a survey of pediatric urologists and surgeons reported 9 cases related to 2500 index cases of bladder exstrophy; this same series also reported on cases of twins and noted discordance in both fraternal as well as identical twinships *(11)*. Furthermore, in a study population of greater than 6 million births with 208 reported cases of exstrophy, no case had a family history for this anomaly *(12)*.

Current recommendations on counseling about risk of recurrence in a sibling of a patient with exstrophy cite an estimate of about 1% and a 1:70 chance of transmission to the progeny of an affected parent *(10)*. Based on these findings, bladder exstrophy appears likely to be multifactorial rather than genetically based; environmental factors may play a significant role in the cause of the exstrophy–epispadias complex.

Table 1
Affected Organ Systems in the Exstrophy–Epispadias Anomalies

Deformation	Cloacal exstrophy	Cloacal exstrophy variant	Classic exstrophy	Epispadias
Exstropic bladder	+	+	+	(−)
Open bladder neck	+	±	+	±
Reflux	+	±	+	±
Genitalia				
Epispadias	+ serve	±	+	+ (can be minor)
Failure of Müllerian duct function	++	+	(−)	(−)
Pelvis				
Lack of pelvic floor support	++	+>++	+	(−)
Pubis symphysis diastasis	++	+>++	+	+
Renal				
Ectopia	++	+	(−)	(−)
Dysplasia	+	+	(−)	(−)
Spine				
Vertebral	++	+	(−)	(−)
Lipomeningocele	+	+	(−)	(−)
Meningomyelocele	rare	rare	rare	(−)
Abdominal wall				
Omphalocele	++	++	(−)	(−)
Intestine				
Short bowel absent large bowel	++	±	(−)	(−)
Imperforate anus	++	++	(−)	(−)
Neurology				
Paraplegia	±	±	(−)	(−)
Limb deformity	±	±	(−)	(−)

ANTENATAL DIAGNOSIS

Prenatal identification of exstrophy is possible, although many cases remain undiagnosed until birth. The bladder may be visualized at 11 to 12 wk of gestation and the kidneys at 14 to 15 wk; both become more obvious with advanced gestational age, so ultrasonography can reliably detect exstrophy before the 20th wk of gestation (13–15). Absence of the bladder is a hallmark of exstrophy, but several findings also suggest the diagnosis. These include the presence of normal kidneys in association with a low-set umbilical cord. Sonographic examination may also reveal a semisolid mass protruding from the abdominal wall in addition to the above findings (16,17). Gearhart and coworkers reviewed the antenatal ultrasonographic studies of 25 women who delivered live infants with exstrophy. They noted the following:

- An absent bladder in 71% of the studies
- A lower abdominal protrusion in 47% of the studies
- An anteriorly displaced scrotum with a small phallus in 57% of the male fetuses
- A low-set umbilical cord in 29% of the studies
- An abnormal iliac crest widening in 18% (15).

Because urine production is normal for these fetuses, amniotic fluid levels should be normal. Prenatal diagnosis allows optimal perinatal management of these infants, including delivery near a pediatric center equipped to treat babies with this unusual anomaly. Any affected fetuses are still not detected antenatally *(18)*. In Gearhart's review of 29 antenatal studies of 17 children born with exstrophy, only 3 children were identified before delivery despite the presence of findings to suggest the diagnosis *(15)*.

Subtle findings such as low umbilical cord insertion and the location of the genitalia will only be seen if the fetus is examined in a sagittal alignment with the spine. Because of the abnormal genitalia findings, the diagnosis is easier to make in males than females. Iliac crest widening can also be seen during the routine prenatal evaluation of the lumbosacral spine that is performed to evaluate for myelomeningocele. The iliac angle will be about 110° rather than the 90° normally seen *(19)*.

Antenatal diagnosis of cloacal exstrophy is also possible. Austin et al. *(20)* reported the typical findings associated with cloacal exstrophy in utero, including

- Nonvisualization of the bladder
- A large midline infraumbilical anterior wall defect
- Omphalocele
- Myelomeningocele
- Widened pubic arches
- Lower extremity defects
- Renal anomalies

In a review of 22 patients with cloacal exstrophy, all or some of these findings could be identified antenatally for 19 patients.

Antenatal diagnosis has many benefits. It allows the expectant parents the opportunity to anticipate and plan for a child who will have significant anomalies at birth. The early counseling should include the expertise of a pediatric urologist experienced in the treatment of bladder exstrophy because the overall prognosis of these children is excellent if initially treated at medical centers with physicians experienced in the treatment of this disorder. So, antenatal identification also permits parents to have these children delivered at a tertiary medical center equipped to provide multidisciplinary consultation and services.

Because these congenital anomalies are rare, health care providers who lack insight and knowledge of them often counsel prospective parents of these patients. The resultant counseling of these families by health care providers who are unaware of the true potential of patients with these birth defects can result in overly pessimistic assessments. This is unfortunate in view of the very satisfactory long-term outcome and life expectancy with appropriate management. Discussions regarding treatment options, including therapeutic abortion, should include pediatric surgeons and urologists familiar with the care of these children.

PREOPERATIVE CARE

To prevent trauma to the exposed bladder plate after delivery, the umbilical cord should be ligated with silk suture rather than a plastic or metal clamp. The exstrophic bladder should be protected against the elements by whatever means available. We prefer a hydrated gel dressing such as Vigilon (C. R. Bard Inc, Covington, GA). This type of dressing protects the bladder plate and stays in place to allow handling of the infant with minimal risk of trauma to the bladder. We have used this dressing for over 2 mo for infants who could not undergo immediate repair because of severe prematurity; we noted minimal inflammation of the bladder at the time of total primary repair. The exposed bladder may be covered with plastic wrap as an acceptable alternative. Either dressing should be replaced daily. The bladder should be irrigated with normal saline with each diaper change. Other authors have advocated the use of a humidified air incubator with no dressing at all to minimize bladder trauma *(21)*.

Routine use of intravenous antibiotic therapy in the pre- and postoperative periods decreases the chance for infection. These children should also undergo ultrasonography to assess the kidneys preoperatively and to establish a baseline examination for later ultrasonographic studies. A spinal sonographic examination should also be obtained if sacral dimpling or other signs of spina bifida occulta are noted on physical examination.

Preoperative care of children with cloacal exstrophy is more involved. Because the care of patients with cloacal exstrophy involves multiple organ systems, these patients are optimally cared for at a tertiary medical center. As a result of the advances in neonatal care and intravenous nutrition, the survival of neonates with cloacal exstrophy is quite high. Mortality in this time period is usually caused by concomitant anomalies that affect the cardiovascular or pulmonary systems in these patients rather than directly as a result of the cloacal exstrophy.

In the past, mortality was high for these patients because of poor nutritional and fluid support. With hyperalimentation and surgical sparing of the hindgut to preserve salt and water, the cloacal exstrophy patient has a good prognosis. The initial hospitalization may be significant, however. Preoperative studies include ultrasonography and karyotyping. Sonographic examination allows the evaluation of the upper urinary tracts, internal genital structures, and spinal cord. Magnetic resonance imaging may also evaluate spinal abnormalities. Magnetic resonance imaging of the pelvis is also useful to characterize the anatomy in the pelvis *(22)*.

Because the genital anomalies associated with cloacal exstrophy may cause confusion in accurately identifying the sex of the baby, karyotyping is indicated to define the chromosomal sex. The decision to gender reassign is usually based on the assessment of reconstruction potential. This should only be done by a team very experienced in the care of the patient with cloacal exstrophy patient. Antenatal imprinting may result in behavioral patterns that follow the genetic sex. This has resulted in sex conversion to the genetic sex in later years for some of these children who previously had been gender reassigned.

OPERATIVE INTERVENTION: METHODS AND TIMING

Bladder Exstrophy

Despite the innumerable operations that have been applied to the treatment of exstrophy, operations for bladder exstrophy currently fall largely into two strategies. The first includes operations designed to remove the exstrophic bladder and replace it with a form of urinary diversion. The second includes reconstructive procedures designed to reconstruct the bladder either in multiple stages or in a single stage. Surgeon preference, patient anatomy, previous surgical procedures, availability of tertiary care facilities, and access to medical care all play a role in which operative procedures are chosen.

No standard of care exists for this patient population. However, because of the complexity of exstrophy, specialists with an interest in the exstrophy–epispadias complex best manage these patients by tailoring their care to each patient's situation.

As currently described, the staged approach to bladder exstrophy reconstruction includes the following steps:

1. Initial bladder closure, ideally in the newborn period
2. Epispadias repair, usually performed at 12 to 18 mo of age, but may be combined with initial bladder closure, especially if initial bladder closure is delayed beyond 6 mo of age
3. Bladder neck reconstruction, usually performed at 4 to 5 yr of age or when age is appropriate for toilet training and bladder is capacity adequate

Mitchell, Kelley, and others have repopularized a single-stage approach to the functional reconstruction of exstrophy *(22a)*. The goals of this approach include bladder closure, optimization of urinary continence, and correction of epispadias in a single operative procedure. Single-stage reconstruction of the exstrophied bladder is best done in the newborn period for several reasons. The procedure is technically easier in the newborn period than when done in an older child. It also offers theoretical advantages as it may maximize the opportunity for normal bladder development and the potential for urinary continence.

The delayed use of the total disassembly technique with primary reconstruction (Mitchell technique or complete primary repair of exstrophy technique) in older children with untreated exstrophy has been shown to be less successful than when used in the newborn period *(23)*. The bony pelvis also remains pliable in the newborn period so that osteotomies may be avoided in some cases, usually if closure can be performed within the first 72 h of life.

In the newborn period, we perform primary exstrophy closure using general inhalation anesthesia. We advise against the use of nitrous oxide during primary closure because it may cause bowel distension, which decreases surgical exposure during the operation and increases the risk of wound dehiscence. Some authors advocate the use of nasogastric tube drainage to decrease abdominal distension in the postoperative period *(24)*. We do not use nasogastric suction in most patients, but routinely use a one-time caudal block to reduce the inhaled anesthetic requirement during the procedure.

For patients older than 3 d or newborns with a wide pubic diastasis, pelvic osteotomy will facilitate closure and strengthen the anterior pelvic support, which may potentiate later urinary continence *(25,26)*.

Children with epispadias can be managed operatively in a similar fashion to that described for bladder exstrophy.

Cloacal Exstrophy

Management of the genitourinary system for patients with cloacal exstrophy remains challenging. Many factors have an impact on the surgical approach to these patients, including the severity of the underlying anatomic anomalies, availability of tertiary care facilities, surgeon experience with cloacal exstrophy, and the effects of previous surgical procedures. A specific standard of care does not exist for this patient population. Because of the complexity of exstrophy, specialists with an interest in the exstrophy–epispadias complex should manage these patients so that their care may be optimized.

As with the management of classic bladder exstrophy, physicians caring for these patients approach the surgical management of the lower urinary tract of these patients with a strategy of functional reconstruction or urinary diversion. Urinary diversion involves excision of the exstrophic bladder plates and creation of a urinary reservoir from the gastrointestinal system. Functional reconstruction of the urinary tract may proceed in a staged or single-stage approach, depending on the physician team responsible for care and patient anatomy.

POSTOPERATIVE CONSIDERATIONS

After a primary reconstructive procedure for exstrophy, the patient must be immobilized to decrease lateral stresses on the closure. A spica cast for 3 wk to prevent external hip rotation and optimize pubic apposition can facilitate early discharge and home care. Modified Buck's traction has been used by many groups for a period of 3 to 4 wk. A posterior lightweight splint can be used in newborns when the child is out of traction to facilitate home care and early removal of traction. Over the years, we have tended not to use Buck's traction to facilitate earlier discharge and ease of care. External fixation devices have also been advocated by several centers. Fixator pins for these devices should be cleaned several times a day to reduce the chance for infection. Internal fixation may be necessary in older patients.

Because of the high incidence of vesicoureteral reflux, we prescribe low-dose suppressive antibiotic therapy for all newborns after bladder closure. This is continued until vesicoureteral reflux is corrected or is proven to resolve spontaneously. Postoperative factors that appear to have a direct impact on the success of initial closure include

- Postoperative immobilization
- Use of postoperative antibiotics
- Ureteral stenting catheters
- Adequate postoperative pain management
- Avoidance of abdominal distension
- Adequate nutritional support
- Secure fixation of urinary drainage catheters *(27,28)*.

SUMMARY

Children born with the exstrophy–epispadias complex are routinely treated early in life. Early treatment appears to increase the success of surgical intervention and to reduce the morbidity associated with treatment. Surgical techniques continue to advance in the treatment of this urological congenital anomaly.

REFERENCES

1. O'Kane HO, Megaw JM. Carcinoma in the exstrophic bladder. Br J Surg 1968; 55(8): 631–635.
2. Gupta S, Gupta IM. Ectopia vesicae complicated by squamous cell carcinoma. Br J Urol 1976; 48(4): 244.
3. Beckwith JB. The congenitally malformed. VII. Exstrophy of the bladder and cloacal exstrophy. Northwest Med 1966; 65(5): 407–410.
4. Diamond DA, Jeffs RD. Cloacal exstrophy: a 22-year experience. J Urol 1985; 133(5): 779–782.
5. Engel RM. Exstrophy of the bladder and associated anomalies. Birth Defects Orig Artic Ser 1974; 10(4): 146–149.
6. Lattimer JK, Smith MJ. Exstrophy closure: a follow-up on 70 cases. J Urol 1966; 95(3): 356–359.
7. Ives E, Coffey R, Carter CO. A family study of bladder exstrophy. J Med Genet 1980; 17(2): 139–141.
8. Epidemiology of bladder exstrophy and epispadias: a communication from the International Clearinghouse for Birth Defects Monitoring Systems. Teratology 1987; 36(2): 221–227.
9. Ziegler M, Duckett JW, Howell JG. Cloacal exstrophy. In: Pediatric Surgery. (Welch J, ed.). Year Book Medical Publishers, Chicago, IL, 1986, pp. 567–583.
10. Messelink EJ, Aronson DC, Knuist M, Heij HA, Vos A. Four cases of bladder exstrophy in two families. J Med Genet 1994; 31(6): 490–492.
11. Shapiro E, Lepor H, Jeffs RD. The inheritance of the exstrophy-epispadias complex. J Urol 1984; 132(2): 308–310.

12. Jeffs RD. Exstrophy, epispadias, and cloacal and urogenital sinus abnormalities. Pediatr Clin North Am 1987; 34(5): 1233–1257.
13. Paidas MJ, Crombleholme TM, Robertson FM. Prenatal diagnosis and management of the fetus with an abdominal wall defect. Semin Perinatol 1994; 18(3): 196–214.
14. Pinette MG, Pan YQ, Pinette SG, Stubblefield PG, Blackstone J. Prenatal diagnosis of fetal bladder and cloacal exstrophy by ultrasound. A report of three cases. J Reprod Med 1996; 41(2): 132–134.
15. Gearhart JP, Ben-Chaim J, Jeffs RD, Saunders RC. Criteria for the prenatal diagnosis of classic bladder exstrophy. Obstet Gynecol 1995; 85(6): 961–964.
16. Jaffe R, Schoenfeld A, Ovadia J. Sonographic findings in the prenatal diagnosis of bladder exstrophy. Am J Obstet Gynecol 1990; 162(3): 675–678.
17. Barth RA, Filly RA, Sondheimer FK. Prenatal sonographic findings in bladder exstrophy. J Ultrasound Med 1990; 9(6): 359–361.
18. Skari H, Bjornland K, Bornstad-Ostensen A, Hauger G, Emblem R. Consequences of prenatal ultrasound diagnosis: a preliminary report on neonates with congenital malformations. Acta Obstet Gynecol Scand 1998; 77(6): 635–642.
19. Sanders R. Prenatal diagnosis of bladder and cloacal exstrophy and related conditions. In: The Exstrophy-Epispadias Complex: Research Concepts and Clinical Applications. (Gearhart JP Hatthou R, ed.), Kluwer Academic/Plenum, New York, NY, 1999, pp. 5–8.
20. Austin PF, et al. The prenatal diagnosis of cloacal exstrophy. J Urol 1998; 160(3 Pt 2): 1179–1181.
21. Churchill B, Merguerian PA, Khoury AE, Husmann DA, McLorie GA. Bladder exstrophy and epispadias. In: Pediatric Urology. (O'Donnell B, Koff S, eds.), Reed Elsevier, Oxford, UK, 1997, pp. 495–508.
22. Meglin AJ, Balotin RJ, Telinck JS, Fishman EK, Jeffs RD, Ghaed V. Cloacal exstrophy: radiologic findings in 13 patients. AJR Am J Roentgenol 1990; 155(6): 1267–1272.
22a. Grady R, Mitchell M. Surgical technique for one stage reconstruction of the exstrophy–epispadias complex. In: Campbell's Urology, 8th ed. (Walsh P, Retik A, Vaughan D Jr., et al., eds.), Saunders, Philadelphia, 2002, pp. 2192–2205.
23. Hafez AT, Elsherbiny MT, Ghoneim MA. Complete repair of bladder exstrophy: preliminary experience with neonates and children with failed initial closure. J Urol 2001; 165(6 Pt 2): 2428–2430.
24. Gearhart JP, Jeffs JD. State-of-the-art reconstructive surgery for bladder exstrophy at the Johns Hopkins Hospital. Am J Dis Child 1989; 143(12): 1475–1478.
25. Aadalen RJ, et al. Exstrophy of the bladder: long-term results of bilateral posterior iliac osteotomies and two-stage anatomic repair. Clin Orthop 1980 Sep; (151): 193–200.
26. Ben Chaim J, Laufer M, Matzkin M. [Current management of bladder exstrophy]. Harefuah 2000; 138(6): 505–509.
27. Lowe FC, Jeffs RD. Wound dehiscence in bladder exstrophy: an examination of the etiologies and factors for initial failure and subsequent success. J Urol 1983; 130(2): 312–315.
28. Husmann DA, McLorie GA, Churchill BM. Closure of the exstrophic bladder: an evaluation of the factors leading to its success and its importance on urinary continence. J Urol 1989; 142(2 Pt 2): 522–524; discussion 542–543.

22 Intersex Conditions

Richard W. Grady, MD

CONTENTS
INTRODUCTION
EVALUATION
DIAGNOSIS
MANAGEMENT
SUMMARY
REFERENCES

INTRODUCTION

The term *ambiguous genitalia* or *intersex* includes many different developmental abnormalities of the external sexual structures. Any infant in whom there is discordance between the appearance of the external genitalia and the karyotype may be considered to have ambiguous genitalia or an intersex condition. Reported incidence of these conditions varies widely depending on how broadly the term is defined. However, conservative estimates would place the incidence from 1:1500 to 15,000 live births *(7)*.

Intersex conditions may be the result of a variety of underlying causes (Table 1). For instance, genotypic females may be highly androgenized and may appear to have androgenized genitalia (Fig. 1); an XY infant may exhibit an external appearance of female genitalia.

EVALUATION

For both medical and social reasons, intersex conditions are considered urgent urological conditions to evaluate and treat. Particular care must be made to identify those patients with endocrinological abnormalities that can be rapidly life threatening, such as certain forms of congenital adrenal hyperplasia (CAH) that are salt wasting. Evaluation of serum chemistries should be performed if there is a suspicion of such abnormalities. Many states have also instituted screening programs that include the assessment of 17-hydroxyprogesterone, a serum steroid precursor used in the evaluation of 21-hydroxylase deficiency, the most common form of CAH.

From: *Urological Emergencies*
Edited by: H. Wessells and J. W. McAninch © Humana Press Inc., Totowa, NJ

Table 1
Categories and Characteristics of Disorders With Ambiguous Genitalia

Diagnosis	Defect	External appearance	Karyotype, internal status
Female pseudohermaphroditism	Fetal exposure to virilizing substances:	Virilization depends on extent of androgen exposure *in utero*; mild clitoromegaly to fully male-appearing phallus	46,XX Ovarian tissue only Mullerian structures present
Congenital adrenal hyperplasia Progestin induced Maternal androgen induced Indeterminate	Appearing within the fetus Coming from the mother	No palpable gonads	
Male pseudohermaphroditism Androgen insensitivity Androgen receptor defect (5α-reductase) Vanishing testis syndrome	Several possible defects, including: Defective androgen synthesis Target tissue insensitivity to androgen Failure of mullerian regression	Variable presentations, including Near-normal male Inguinal hernias Cryptorchidism	46,XY Testicular tissue only Wolffian structures present Mullerian structures may be present
Persistent mullerian duct syndrome Indeterminate	Other uncertain causes Hypospadias	Small phallus Intermediate genitalia Near-normal or normal female	
Mixed gonadal dysgenesis	Developmental defect	Usually incompletely virilized male: Small phallus Cryptorchidism Hypospadias	Most 46,XY/45,XO Testis, streak gonad present Mullerian structures may be present on the side of the streak gonad

Pure gonadal dysgenesis	Developmental defect	Often initially normal; infertility, lack of sexual development noted later	46,XX; 46,XY; 45,XO Bilateral streak gonads Underdeveloped mullerian structures
True hermaphroditism	Developmental defect	Female with clitoromegaly Variable presentations: Male with hypospadias, undescended testes	46,XX (~70%); remainder 46,XY or mosaic Testicular and ovarian tissues are both present (separate or as ovotestis) Wolffian and mullerian structures may both be present
Others:		External male genitalia severely compromised	46,XY Testes present
Cloacal exstrophy Aphallia Microphallus	Developmental defect	Cloacal exstrophy: bifid phallus and scrotum	Wolffian structures present

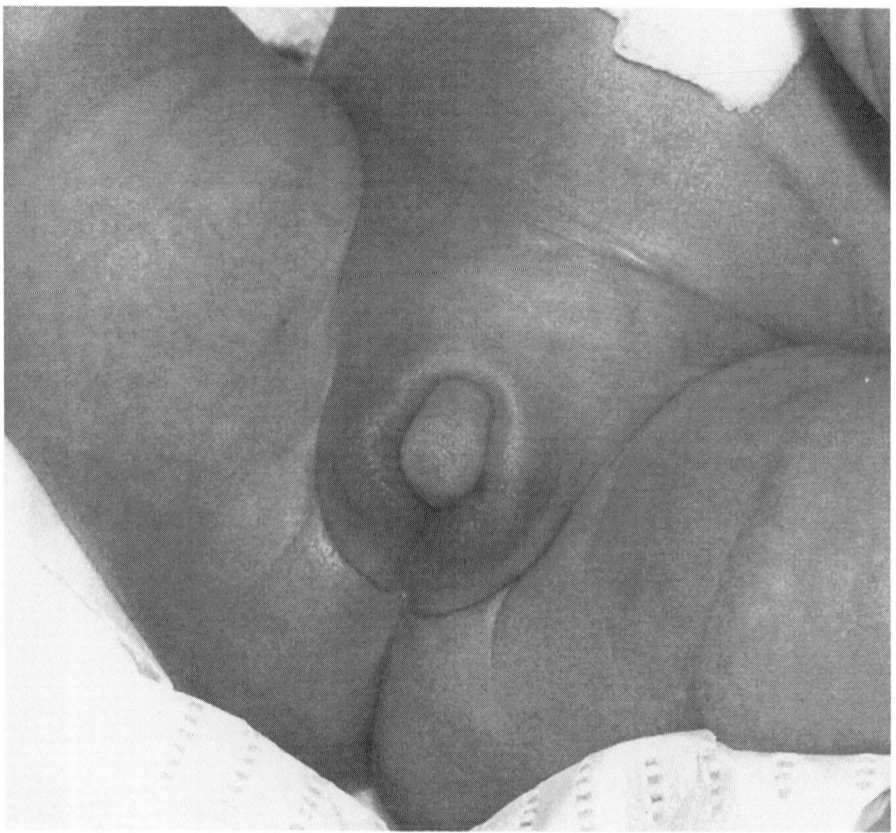

Fig. 1. Androgenized genitalia in karyotypic (XX) baby girl with congenital adrenal hyperplasia.

Evaluation and management of ambiguous genitalia is challenging both medically and socially. It is important for health care providers to be sensitive to the medical and social challenges in these situations, when the baby's gender may not be obvious. It remains a truism that one of the first questions a family is asked after a child's birth relates to determining the sex of the child. As a consequence, health care providers should discuss this issue thoughtfully with parents when their child is born with genital ambiguity. Typically, parents are told that their child has a birth defect that has interfered with the usual way of determining the sex of their infant. Medical terminology may be confusing for many parents, and the situation may feel overwhelming for them.

The initial medical evaluation and treatment are focused on an evaluation of the underlying condition and a determination of the most appropriate gender of rearing for the infant. In some medical centers, a gender assessment team exists that includes medical geneticists; pediatric surgeons, urologists, and endocrinologists; cytogeneticists; psychiatrists; and reproductive endocrinologists. These teams meet on a regular basis to discuss the evaluation and management of new and ongoing cases. At the Children's Hospital and Regional Medical Center in Seattle, Washington, a gender assessment team has been in existence for more than 20 yr. Determination of the underlying cause of the intersex condition may take longer than gender assignment and in some cases is never completely determined. When possible, identification of the underlying cause will permit more effective therapeutic interventions and counseling regarding the underlying inheritance patterns.

Initial discussions with the families of infants with intersex conditions often set the tone for future interactions. Health care providers should be sensitive to the family's need to have information repeated. Often, a discussion of genital development and embryology is helpful to parents to understand how the precursor structures in a fetus may become phenotypically male or female depending on genetic and hormonal influences. To increase parental understanding, line drawings and diagrams are often useful, as are a review of the baby's physical examination findings. Ideally, family members should become familiar and comfortable enough with the underlying condition that they can actively participate in the decision-making process regarding gender of rearing. Some experts suggest that the families with an intersexed child consider delaying naming the baby, announcing the birth, or registering the birth until more information is known *(2)*.

DIAGNOSIS

History

A careful history may offer clues to the underlying diagnosis. Infertile aunts or partially virilized uncles may suggest a familial X-linked disorder such as some forms of androgen insensitivity. A family history of unexplained neonatal death suggests CAH. Maternal exposure to exogenous or endogenous androgens or estrogens should also be investigated.

Physical Examination

A detailed physical examination of the newborn genitalia is essential. Key components of the exam include the following:

- Symmetry of the external genitalia
- Presence and location of palpable gonads
- Extent of virilization
- Presence of additional anomalies

The most important part of the examination is palpation for the presence or absence of gonads in the labioscrotal compartment. A gonad that has descended into this compartment is typically a testis, and the patient is a karyotypic male, although there are exceptions (e.g., SRY+ XX male and uterine hernia inguinalae). In the absence of palpable gonads in an otherwise phenotypic male, no definitive gender assignment should be made until further evaluations are performed, including hormonal studies and radiographic imaging studies.

Additional findings to be noted on physical exam include phallus size, location of urethral opening, appearance and pigmentation of labiosacral folds, and other associated anomalies. Observing the baby urinate may also be necessary to locate the position of the urethral meatus. The extent of external virilization may be documented using the Prader classification system (Table 2). Other physical findings to note include phallic configuration and diameter, including the glans, and the extent of fusion of the labioscrotal folds.

Imaging Studies

Ultrasonography can be a useful imaging modality to identify internal gonads, although pelvic ultrasonography is not generally considered sensitive enough to

Table 2
Prader Classification

Prader classification	Features
I	Hypertrophic clitoris with otherwise normal external female genitalia
II	Hypertrophic clitoris with urogenital sinus
III	Hypertrophic clitoris, narrow and deep urogenital sinus, high urethrovaginal confluence
IV	Phallus with small urogenital opening
V	Normal external male genitalia

confirm their absence if gonads are not visualized. Pelvic ultrasonography can also document the presence of uterine structures in an externally virilized female. It is most helpful to perform this study immediately after birth when the maternal estrogen effect increases the thickness of the endometrial lining of the infant uterus. After the maternal estrogen effect decreases, the uterus becomes significantly more difficult to visualize.

Magnetic resonance imaging with intravenous gadolinium or laparoscopic exploration of the pelvis are the most accurate methods to evaluate pelvic anatomy in this population and should be used when indicated. Improved magnetic resonance imaging technology makes this an increasingly attractive imaging modality to evaluate these children, although some children require deep sedation or general anesthesia to obtain an adequate study if they cannot hold still.

Before reconstructive surgery, retrograde fluoroscopic studies of the introitus can be particularly helpful to assess the extent of urethrovaginal fusion and the length of the urogenital sinus (Fig. 2). Retrograde studies may also provide more anatomic information by outlining the vagina, cervical impression, and uterus.

Karyotyping

Genetic evaluation by karyotype should also be performed as soon as possible even if prenatal chromosome testing was previously performed. Usually, peripheral blood karyotypes are adequate unless the patient has a mosaic karyotype with another cell line restricted to gonadal tissue *(3)*. In this case, a gonadal biopsy may be necessary to confirm the karyotype.

Laboratory Studies

Babies born with ambiguous genitalia should undergo a metabolic evaluation, including serum electrolytes (both after birth and several days later if CAH is a possibility). Laboratory studies of serum testosterone, dihydrotestosterone, follicular stimulating hormone, luteinizing hormone, and estrogen will help determine gonadal function and the integrity of the hypothalamic–pituitary–gonadal axis. Other possible laboratory studies include serum 17-hydroxyprogesterone. Levels of this hormone are elevated in the serum of infants with the most common form of CAH, 21-hydroxylase deficiency. Mullerian inhibiting substance may also be useful in select cases if karyotyping shows an XY pattern, but the infant is agonadal *(4)*.

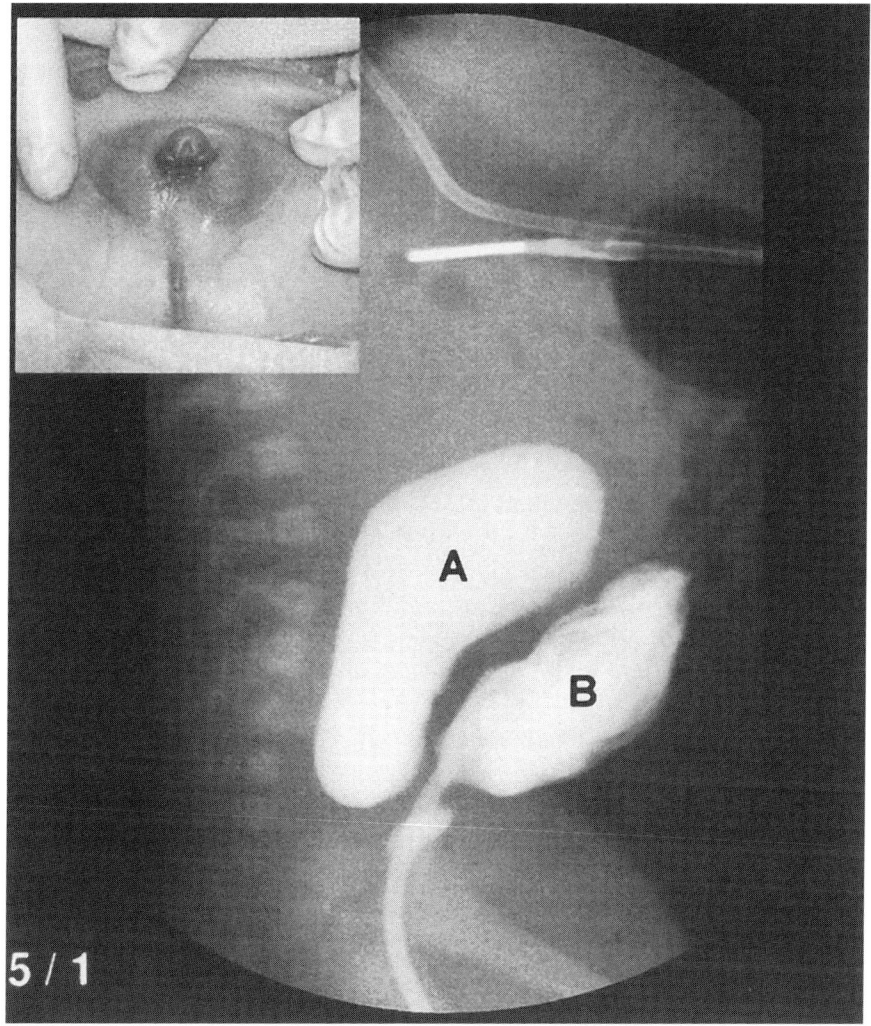

Fig. 2. Female neonate born with a cloacal anomaly. Retrograde fluoroscopic study demonstrating the (**A**) vagina and (**B**) bladder. Inset photo demonstrates single perineal opening.

To adequately assess the potential for testosterone production for some of these children, human chorionic gonadotropin (hCG) may be administered and the subsequent hormonal response measured. Several different protocols have been described. They involve daily or weekly hCG injection for several weeks *(5)*. hCG injections are useful to assess not only the potential for testosterone production, but also to target tissue response to testosterone if it is made *(5)*.

Molecular genotype analysis has also become commercially available that may be valuable in the evaluation of some intersex conditions. GeneDX (www.genedx.com) offers molecular genotyping for X-linked androgen receptor involved in some androgen insensitivity conditions. Enzyme assays from cultured genital skin fibroblasts to assess ligand binding to the androgen receptor and 5-α-reductase binding activity may also be helpful in the diagnosis of some androgen insensitivity cases *(2)*.

MANAGEMENT

Careful communication with the family is essential in cases of ambiguous genitalia. It is vitally important to avoid definitive gender assignment until data are collected and interpreted and discussions are held between the medical team and the family. Gender-specific pronouns are typically avoided when speaking to the family about the infant until a decision is made by the family and the medical team regarding the gender of rearing. A focused effort to obtain these studies and engage in these discussions in a timely fashion is important not only to assist the family in coping with the social stress of having a child with gender ambiguity, but also to ensure that potentially life-threatening conditions, such as CAH, are recognized early.

The primary decision in the management of these patients focuses on the gender of rearing. This decision is based on several factors, including the specific pathophysiology, the chance for spontaneous pubertal development, the anticipated capacity for satisfactory sexual intercourse and orgasm, fertility potential, and risk for gonadal tumors, such as gonadoblastoma when Y chromosomal material is present in a dysgenetic testis (6). For instance, patients with complete androgen insensitivity often are felt to be served best by a female gender assignment because the prospects of additional virilization and anticipated capacity for sexual intercourse and fertility are felt to be poor with a male gender assignment. Hormonal stimulation with hCG or testosterone may be helpful to assess the potential for virilization in some intersex cases.

Each child must be considered individually when making gender assessment decisions. Few long-term studies exist regarding the function and quality of life of patients born with intersex conditions. However, renewed interest in open, honest communication with the families and children born with these conditions may help provide answers to some of these questions in the future (7). Consultation with specialists to plan for the appropriate medical and surgical management ideally involves pediatric endocrinologists, pediatric surgeons or urologists, and psychiatry or psychology services along with a medical genetics and cytogenetics team.

In specific conditions, specific medical therapy is required. Patients diagnosed with CAH require glucocorticoid therapy to suppress excessive adrenal androgen secretion. They may also require mineralocorticoids if they have a salt-losing form of CAH. Typically, oral cortisol is used for glucocorticoid replacement, and oral fludrocortisone is used for mineralocorticoid replacement. Long-term hormonal management may be indicated for some patients. This is particularly important for those infants with CAH who will require replacement for glucocorticoid and mineralocorticoid deficiency.

Timing and extent of surgical correction for ambiguous genitalia remain controversial (1). It is important to inform families fully about the complex psychosocial issues related to surgical correction in addition to the medical risks and benefits. Labioscrotal reduction may be beneficial for some virilized female patients. Phallic reconstructive surgery may also be important to create a cosmetically acceptable end function for those patients with intersex conditions who are undervirilized and have been assigned a male gender status. Issues of timing of surgery currently focus on the benefits of achieving true informed consent by waiting until patients are old enough to decide for themselves vs the disadvantage of longer recovery times and potentially poorer surgical outcomes compared to when these operations are done in early childhood.

The ultimate success for an infant with ambiguous genitalia may depend as much on the quality and extent of psychosocial support as on sophisticated medical and surgical management. In recognition of this, many gender assessment teams are fully integrating psychiatric services from infancy into the management of these patients and their families.

Complex family dynamics will also have a profound impact on children born with ambiguous genitalia. Honest and informed communication between the family and the health care provider is important to create trust and understanding with this emotionally charged issue.

Follow-Up

The generalist must play a central role during follow-up care for the infant with ambiguous genitalia because a large number of consulting services are typically involved, including medical genetics, endocrinology, urology, and psychiatry. Long-term psychosocial support for the family and the child should be provided. Patient-based support groups are an excellent resource for both the children and families. For those patients requiring ongoing medical management for hormonal replacement, a primary care physician will also need to be an active participant.

SUMMARY

The evaluation and management of children with ambiguous genitalia remains challenging medically and socially. Despite technological advances, and improved medical understanding of the causes of intersex conditions, no absolute answers exist in the care of these patients and their families. It is important for health care provides to be sensitive to the medical and social challenges in these situations and remain up to date on the current body of knowledge in this field.

REFERENCES

1. Dreger AD. "Ambiguous sex" or ambivalent medicine? Hastings Center Rep 1998; 28(3): 24–35.
2. Lee PA. Ambiguous genitalia. In: Pediatric Endocrinology. (Sperling MA, ed.), Saunders, Philadelphia, 2002.
3. Kocova M, Siegel SF, Wenger SL, et al. Detection of Y chromosome sequences in a 45X/46XXq- patient by Southern blot analysis of PCR-amplified DNA and fluorescent *in situ* hybridization (FISH). Am J Med Genet 1995; 55: 483–488.
4. Rey R, Belville C, Nihoul-Fekete C, et al. Evaluation of gonadal function in 107 intersex patients by means of serum anti-mullerian hormone measurement. J Clin Endocrin Metab 1999; 84: 627–633.
5. Almaglier M, Saenger P, Linder BL. Phallic growth after hCG: a clinical index of androgen responsiveness. Clin Pediatr 1993; 32: 329–336.
6. Lerman S, McAleer IM, Kaplan GW. Sex assignment in cases of ambiguous genitalia and it s outcome. Urology 2000; 55: 8–12.
7. Glassberg K. Gender assignment and the pediatric urologist. J Urol 1999; 161: 1308–1310.

23 Posterior Urethral Valves

Hiep T. Nguyen, MD, FAAP

CONTENT

INTRODUCTION
ANATOMY AND PATHOPHYSIOLOGY
CLINICAL PRESENTATION
EVALUATION
TREATMENT
FOLLOW-UP MANAGEMENT
SUMMARY
REFERENCES

INTRODUCTION

Posterior urethral valves (PUVs) are membranes that act as one-way valves impairing the antegrade flow from the bladder and upper urinary tract. They are the most common forms of congenital urethral obstruction, with an incidence of 1 in 8,000 to 25,000 live male births *(1)*. Children with PUVs present with a wide spectrum of symptoms, from minor voiding dysfunction to end-stage renal disease (ESRD) and death. Proper initial treatment and long-term management are essential to maintain good bladder and renal function.

ANATOMY AND PATHOPHYSIOLOGY

In 1919, Young et al. first published a description of PUVs based on their observations in a small number of cases, which includes those who have been previously instrumented *(2)*. According to Young's classification, type I valves are those that originate from the urethral crest of the distal verumontanum and fan across the urethra lumen to fuse anteriorly. Type II valves originate at the verumontanum and pass along the posterior urethral wall toward the bladder neck. It was subsequently recognized that these are not obstructive, but are hypertrophied muscle fibers of the superficial trigone. The type III valve is a membrane that originates distal to the verumontanum near the bulbomembranous junction and spans transversely across the urethra.

It has been suggested that the Young's classification of PUVs may be incorrect. Modern endoscopic studies *(3)* suggest that all patients with valves have the same diaphragmatic configuration, which is iatrogenically altered by urethral instrumentation.

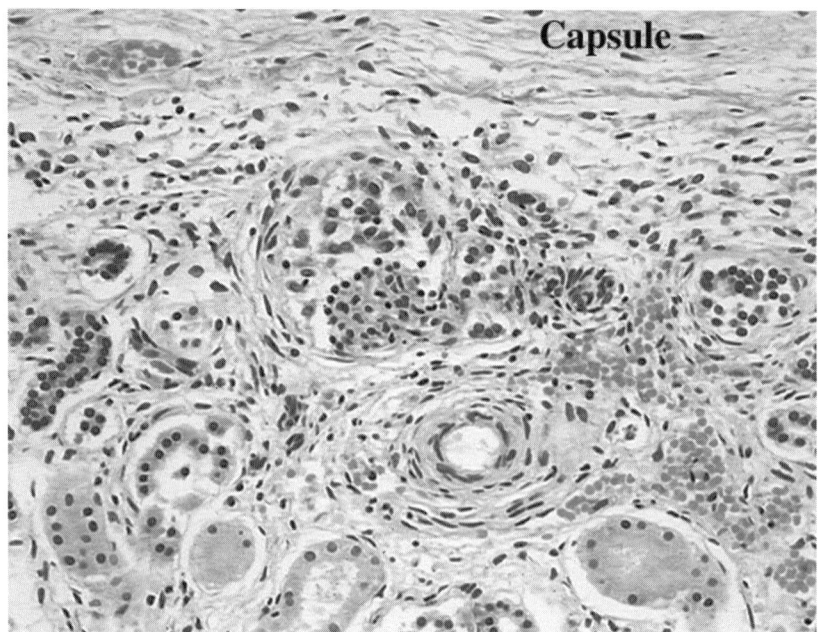

Fig. 1. Evidence of dysplasia from the kidney of a fetus at 24 wk gestation with posterior urethral valves and severe oligohydramnios. Note the lack of nephrogenesis at the periphery and normal tubules.

The etiology of PUVs remains unknown. By the eighth week of gestation, the prostatic urethra develops from the urogenital sinus. The distal segments of the mesonephric and paramesonephric ducts are absorbed into this region, forming the ejaculatory ducts and the prostatic utricle, respectively. As a result of the expanding ejaculatory ducts and prostatic utricle, the verumontanum forms on the floor of the prostatic urethra. During this process, the mesonephric ducts move from an anterolateral position to a posterior one. It is hypothesized that aberrant movement of the mesonephric ducts into the urethral wall results in PUVs *(4)*. It is observed that PUVs have occurred in siblings, twins, and successive generations, suggesting a polygenetic pattern of inheritance *(5)*.

PUVs have a wide range of effects on the urinary tract depending on the severity of urethral obstruction. The nature of injury appears to be caused by high-pressure storage and emptying of urine, producing characteristic changes to the urinary tract. In response to the high voiding pressures, the prostatic urethra dilates, in some cases to a volume equivalent to that of the bladder. Histological studies of fetal valve bladder demonstrated hypertrophy and hyperplasia of detrusor smooth muscle and increased connective tissue *(6)*. Similarly, the bladder neck is hypertrophied and rigid. Despite these changes, the bladder neck does not cause further obstruction, and these changes usually resolve with ablation of the valves *(7)*.

High bladder filling and voiding pressure lead to poor drainage of urine from the upper tract and the development of vesicoureteral reflux, which in turn result in dilation of the ureters. Ureterectasis compromises peristalsis and further impairs drainage of urine from the upper tract. Variation in competency of the vesicoureteral junctions may direct the high pressure generated by the bladder to one renal unit, sparing the other from the damaging effects of obstruction *(8)*.

The renal damage induced by PUVs is caused by renal dysplasia and obstructive uropathy. In almost all patients with PUVs, there is some degree of renal dysplasia, characterized by disorganization of renal parenchyma and the presence of embryonic tubules, cartilage, cysts, and mesenchymal connective tissue (Fig. 1). Some studies suggested that the renal dysplasia is caused by interference of high pressures with the normal differentiation of metanephric mesenchyme *(9,10)*. Other studies proposed that renal dysplasia is caused by an abnormal position of the ureteral bud along the mesonephric duct *(11)*.

Regardless of the mechanisms, the renal dysplasia observed in patients with PUVs appears to be irreversible. In addition to renal dysplasia, almost all patients with PUVs have some component of obstructive uropathy. This form of renal damage is characterized by glomerular and tubular dysfunction and to some degree is potentially reversible. It is observed that up to 60% of the valve patients have tubular impairment of concentration and acidification *(12)*. This leads to a pathological high urine output and electrolyte imbalances *(13)*. Finally, the high urine output can cause further dilation of the urinary tract, worsening the degree of hydronephrosis and bladder dysfunction *(14)*.

Besides the urinary system, the effects of PUVs can be observed in the pulmonary system. The amniotic fluid volume is primarily dependent on urine production after the first trimester of gestation. Oligohydramnios resulting from inadequate fetal urine production interferes with the normal development of the lungs. The proposed mechanism for pulmonary hypoplasia includes physical restriction of fetal breathing movements, resulting in a small chest cavity and reduced chest wall motion *(15,16)*; and restriction of amniotic fluid to the lung buds, resulting in decreased branching of the bronchial tree and alveoli formation *(17–19)*. The degree of pulmonary hypoplasia varies depending on the severity of the PUVs.

CLINICAL PRESENTATION

Patients with PUVs may present with a wide range of symptoms, from minor voiding dysfunction to death *(20)*. With the advent of routine maternal ultrasonography, 45–55% of patients with PUVs are detected antenatally *(21–23)*. Characteristic findings on antenatal ultrasonography include a dilated/thickened bladder with a keyhole sign and hydroureteronephrosis (Fig. 2); however, these findings have only a 40% positive predictive value *(24,25)*.

Abnormal renal architecture observed on prenatal ultrasound (US) might further suggest the presence of clinically significant obstruction. Increased echogenicity compared to the liver denotes underlying renal pathology, such as interstitial, tubular, or vascular renal diseases (Fig. 3) *(26)*.

As defined by a fetal renal cortex less than 2 mm thick, the finding of cortical atrophy is observed in some patients with PUVs *(27)*. In addition, the presence of cortical cysts is highly suggestive of renal dysplasia. Furthermore, it is observed on multivariate analysis that the presence of oligohydramnios on prenatal US is predictive of the presence of obstruction *(28)*. Finally, in addition to the above ultrasonographic findings, signs of fetal distress and intrauterine growth failure may be present in a fetus with PUVs.

Despite screening with prenatal US, a significant number of patients with PUVs are missed, especially when the maternal US is performed early in pregnancy. Newborns may present with an abdominal mass caused by dilated bladder, hydroureteronephrosis, or urinary ascites *(29)*. Older infants may present with urinary tract infection (UTI)/

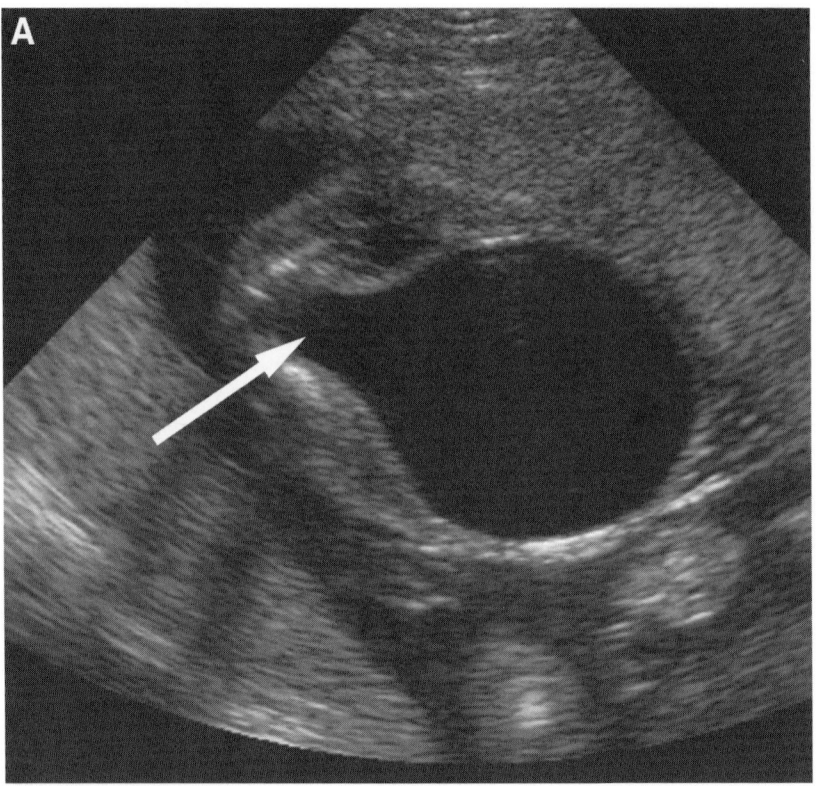

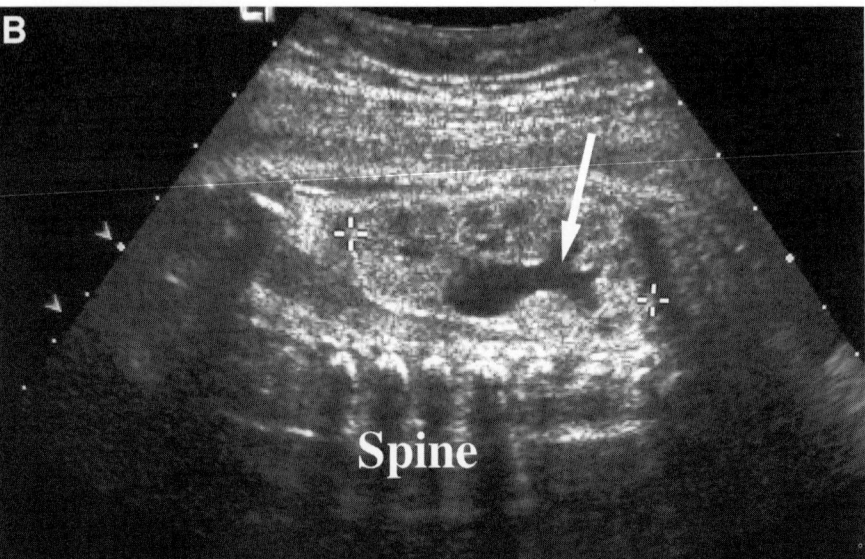

Fig. 2. Ultrasound of a fetus at 30 wk gestation with posterior urethral valves. **(A)** Note the dilated bladder and posterior urethra (arrow). There is associated **(B)** hydronephrosis (arrow) and **(C)** oligohydramnios (arrow).

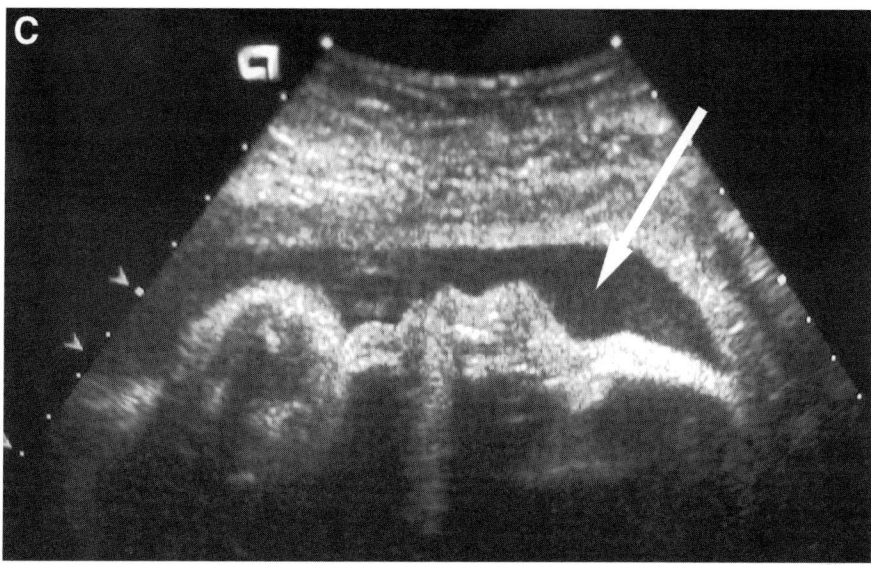

Fig. 2. *(Continued)*

sepsis or renal insufficiency *(30)*. Some children with PUVs do not present until much later, with UTI, renal colic, or voiding complaints such as urinary frequency, dribbling, or urinary incontinence *(31)*. The majority have good renal function, and it would be uncommon for these older patients to present with renal insufficiency.

EVALUATION

All male infants with significant prenatal hydronephrosis should be evaluated to rule out PUVs. In addition to PUVs, the differential diagnosis for these patients includes prune belly syndrome, bilateral ureteropelvic junction obstruction, bilateral vesicoureteral reflux, bilateral ureterovesical junction obstruction, congenital urethral atresia, and anterior urethral valves. A thorough radiological evaluation is necessary to make an accurate diagnosis.

A postnatal US should first be performed. Because dehydration is common during the first 48 h of life, US studies performed before this time may underestimate the degree of hydronephrosis *(32)*. In addition, a voiding cystourethrogram (VCUG) should be performed regardless of whether the patient is voiding normally. This should be performed using a 5F feeding tube rather than a balloon catheter because the latter may obscure bladder anatomy.

When performing a VCUG, cyclical filling and voiding should be done to distend the bladder and urethra. Inadequate distension or poor voiding may miss vesicoureteral reflux or dilation of the prostatic urethra (Fig. 4) *(33)*. Vesicoureteral reflux is seen in approx 50% of the patients with PUVs *(34,35)*. An oblique view of the urethra is essential to demonstrate an elongated and dilated urethra with an elevated bladder neck seen in patients with PUVs (Fig. 5).

Finally, a myelin-associated glycoprotein 3 radionuclide renal scan may be useful in evaluation patients with PUVs. The renal scan provides information concerning renal perfusion and function, although assessment of urinary drainage may not be accurate because of the relative immaturity of the newborn kidney *(36)*.

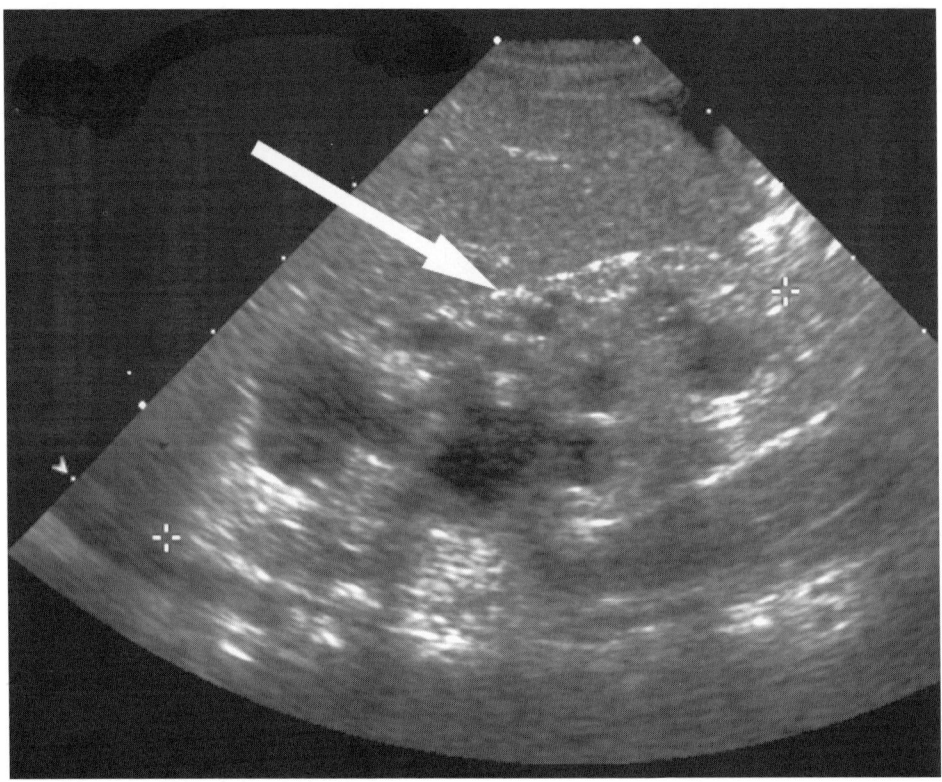

Fig. 3. Ultrasound of the right kidney in a 4-d-old infant with posterior urethral valves. Note the increased echogenicity compared to the liver and cysts in the periphery suggestive of renal dysplasia.

Once the diagnosis of PUVs is made, laboratory evaluation of renal function and electrolytes should be obtained. Because of the functioning of the placenta, serum creatinine values obtained during the first 48 h of life do not reflect the renal function of newborns with PUVs. After 48 h, an elevation in serum creatinine and serum urea nitrogen and a decrease in serum bicarbonate levels is seen in most patients. In those with severe renal function, hyperkalemia may be present and requires prompt treatment. Because patients with PUVs have tubular dysfunction and subsequent high urine output, serum electrolytes should be monitored.

TREATMENT

Once the diagnosis of PUVs is made, prompt relief of obstruction is needed. In newborns with PUVs, a 5 or 6F catheter without a balloon should be placed. Foley catheters may be used; however, they can be associated with poor upper tract drainage caused by either bladder volume displacement or irritation of the bladder by the balloon *(37)*. Because of the dilated posterior urethra and elevated bladder neck, it may be difficult to navigate the catheter into the bladder. A coude tip catheter or catheter with a malleable guide may be used to avoid misplacement.

After catheter placement, US studies should be performed to confirm that the catheter is not coiled in the posterior urethra. Serial creatinine measurements after 7 to 10 d of

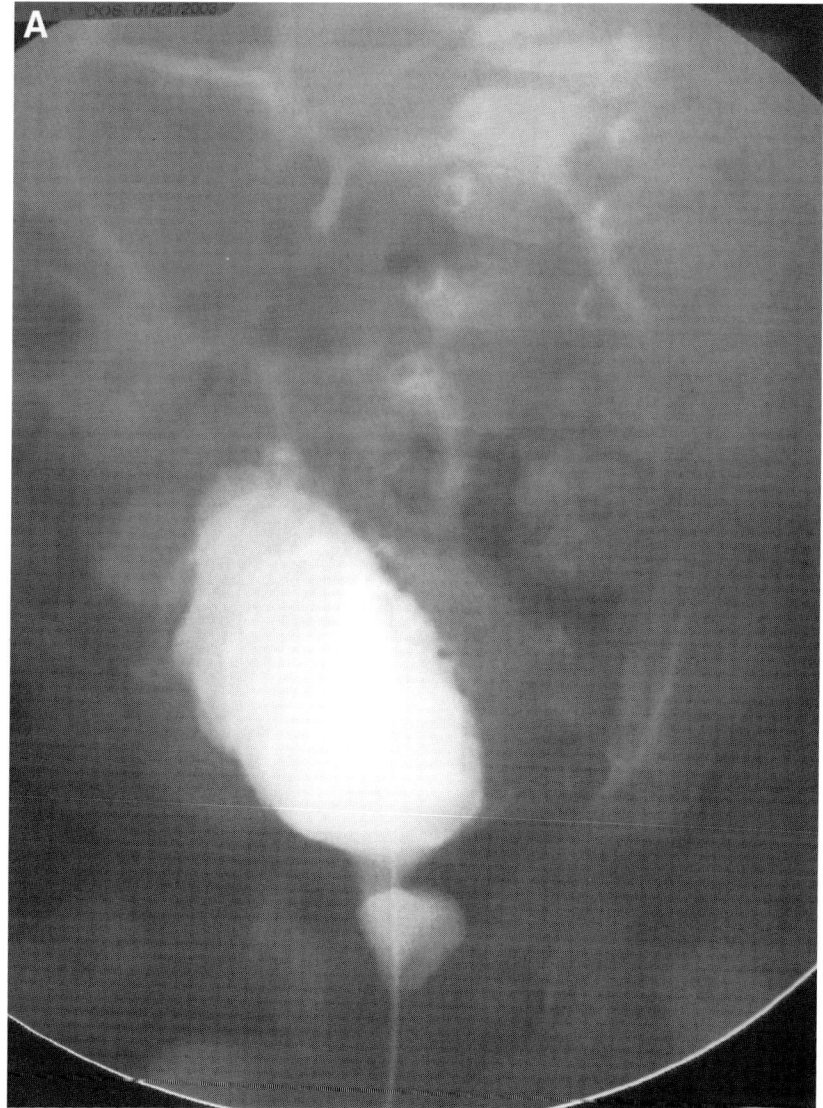

Fig. 4. (A) Voiding cystourethrogram (VCUG) performed with one filling cycle did not demonstrate any vesicoureteral reflux. **(B)** Cyclic VCUG demonstrated grade V reflux into the right kidney.

catheter drainage will establish the patient's nadir value. Newborns with PUVs should be started on prophylactic antibiotics to prevent UTI.

After stabilization with catheter drainage, most infants can undergo endoscopic valve ablation. Historically, PUVs were ablated with open procedures, or suprapubic catheters were left in place *(38)*. However, these procedures had a high risk of damaging the bladder and urethra. With the development of pediatric endoscopic equipment, most infants with PUVs can safely undergo endoscopic valve ablation.

Using a 5F cystourethroscope or an 8.5F resectoscope, incision of the valves is made with a Bugbee electrode, hook, laser, or cold knife at the 4 and 8 o'clock positions. Incision at the 12 o'clock position may be necessary to open the urethral lumen (Fig. 6).

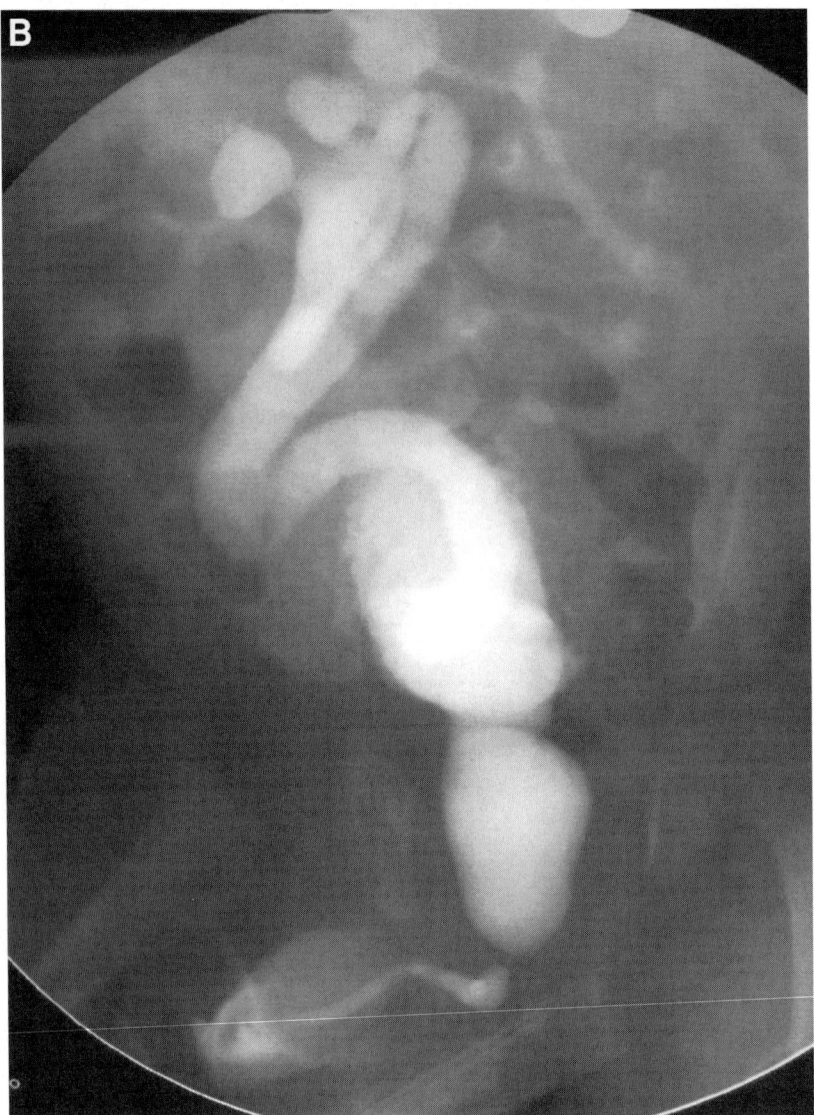

Fig. 4. *(Continued)*

Careful understanding of the infant's urethral anatomy is needed to prevent damage to the urethral sphincter and the formation of the urethral stricture. Some authors have recommended not using electrocautery to prevent these complications. If the procedure is difficult or if there is a lot of bleeding, a catheter should be left in place for 24 h. Otherwise, a catheter is usually not needed after valve ablation.

Alternatives for initial treatment of infants with PUVs include vesicostomy and upper urinary tract diversion. For very small or premature infants, a cutaneous vesicostomy may be performed, allowing valve ablation to be delayed until the child is older. It appears to be safe with comparable long-term results to endoscopic treatment *(39)*. Vesicostomy may also be a good option in some valve patients with severe reflux, allowing improvement in the dilation of the upper urinary tract *(40)*. However, this procedure is also associated with a higher complication rate (up to 40%), the most common is severe UTI *(41)*.

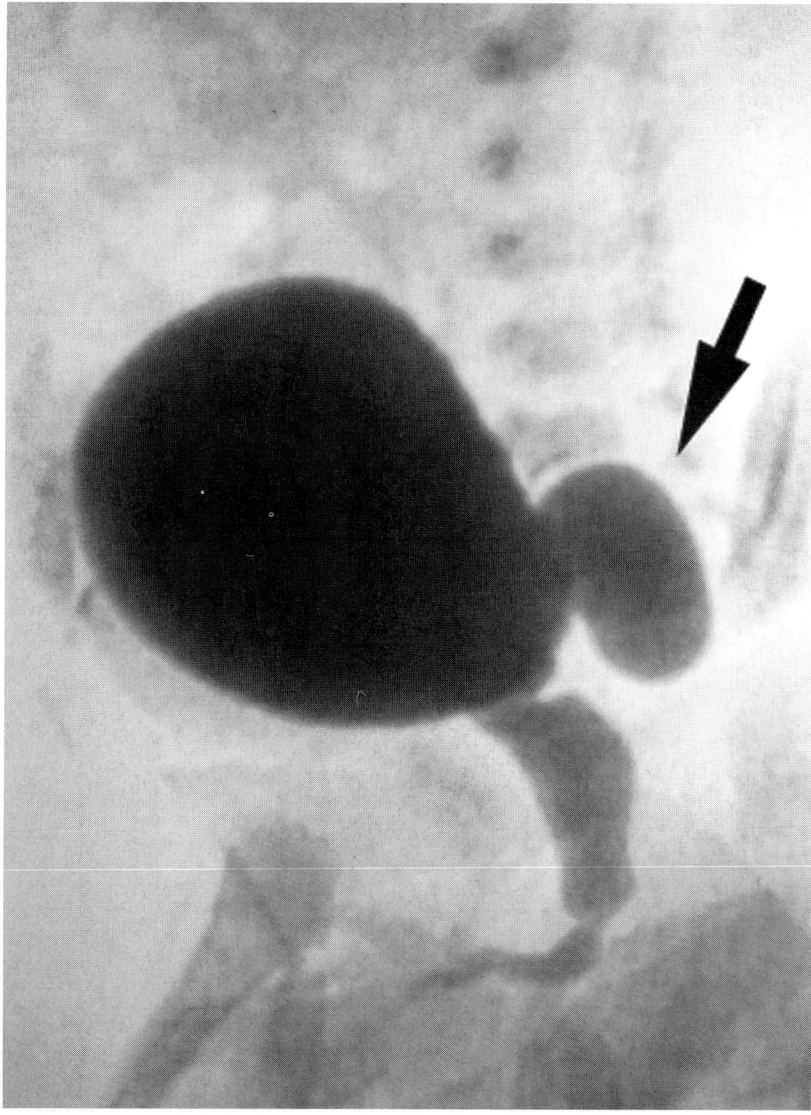

Fig. 5. Dilated posterior urethra with an elevated bladder neck can be seen in this oblique view of a voiding cystourethrogram. Note the presence of a bladder diverticulum (arrow), which can serve as a pressure pop-off mechanism.

Another option for treatment of PUVs is diversion above the level of the bladder with a cutaneous ureterostomy or pyelostomy. Although it is safe *(42,43)*, it remains to be demonstrated that upper tract drainage is superior to endoscopic treatment or vesicostomy. In addition, the patients with upper urinary tract diversion will be required to undergo additional reconstructive surgeries.

Currently, most pediatric urologists recommend treating PUVs initially with endoscopic ablation and observing for improvement in hydronephrosis and renal function. For those with decreasing hydronephrosis and creatinine levels, no additional surgical procedure is needed. A vesicostomy should be considered in those who cannot undergo valve surgery for technical reasons (significantly premature or small urethra) or have a

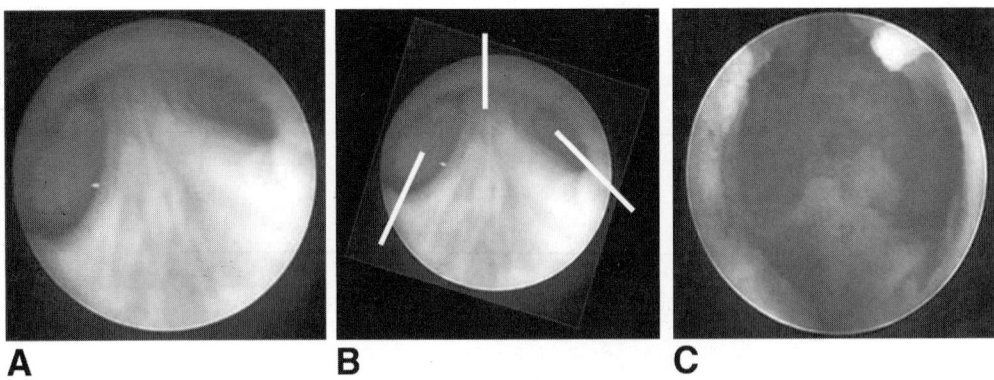

Fig. 6. Endoscopic view of posterior urethra (**A**) before and (**C**) after valve ablation. (**B**) Incisions are made in 4 and 8 o'clock positions; if needed, an incision can also be made at the 12 o'clock position.

bladder that does not drain efficiently despite valve ablation. If the patient's creatinine levels remain greater than 2.0 mg/dL with persistent severe hydronephrosis and it has been demonstrated that there is good bladder emptying, upper tract diversion may be considered to preserve renal function. It is uncommon for most patients with PUVs to require upper tract diversion.

FOLLOW-UP MANAGEMENT

After diagnosis and initial treatment, close follow-up is essential to preserve bladder and renal function. Following valve ablation, a VCUG and urodynamic study should be obtained to confirm complete valve ablation and that the resting bladder pressures are within safe levels (<30 cm H_2O). It is not uncommon for patients with PUVs to have persistent hydroureteronephrosis following valve ablation. Chronic dilation of the ureter and pelvis will not resolve immediately and does not likely represent continued obstruction from the ureterovesical junction *(44)*.

In most patients with PUVs, progressive renal insufficiency following newborn creatinine level stabilization is primarily caused by underlying renal dysplasia rather than continued obstruction *(44)*. A Tc-99m dimercaptosuccinic acid (DMSA) or myelin-associated glycoprotein 3 renal scan should be obtained after 4 wk of life to determine baseline differential renal function and identify nonfunctioning units. Because acidosis and salt-wasting nephropathy are commonly observed in patients with PUVs, frequent electrolyte evaluation should be performed to help tailor medical management.

Vesicoureteral reflux occurs in 50 to 75% of patients diagnosed with PUVs *(45–47)*. Most studies indicated that, in the majority of patients, the reflux resolves following valve ablation, but resolution may occur up to 3 yr later *(45)*. Reflux into nonfunctioning renal units is not likely to resolve *(35)*. However, a nonfunctioning reflux unit should be retained until adequate bladder function is achieved because it may be used for a ureteral augmentation if bladder capacity/compliance is inadequate *(48)*.

If the reflux into functioning units persists or there is a breakthrough infection on prophylactic antibiotic, a urodynamic study should be performed to evaluate bladder function. If it is abnormal, treatment with anticholinergic therapy should be considered prior to thinking about surgical reimplantation. Surgical correction of reflux in valve patients should be reserved for those who fail medical management or have significant reflux that interferes with normal voiding. Ureteral reimplantation performed in a valve bladder that has not been properly managed medically has a high complication rate *(49)*.

In patients with PUVs, long-term outcome is dependent on maximizing good bladder function. Long-term follow-up of patients with PUVs demonstrates discrete patterns of abnormal bladder function *(50)*. In infants and young children, urodynamic evaluation often demonstrates poor compliance; in older children, instability with uninhibited detrusor contractions predominates. In contrast, postpubertal patients with PUVs develop myogenic failure with large bladder volumes and weak, unsustained voiding contractions *(51–53)*.

It is suggested that the progressive bladder failure is partly caused by polyuria resulting from the urine concentrating defect seen in patients with PUVs *(14)*. Urine production in these patients can range up to 3 to 6 L/d. In addition, many of these patients lack normal bladder sensation, allowing them to hold large urine volumes at high intravesical pressures without pain. Over time, the chronic distention at high pressures may lead to change in bladder compliance and contractility. To alter the natural history of the valve bladder, early identification of bladder dysfunction allows medical management such as anticholinergic therapy, double voiding, intermittent catheterization, or nighttime bladder drainage, depending on urodynamic findings.

Despite appropriate medical and surgical management, some patients with PUVs will progress to renal insufficiency/failure in follow-up. Adequate renal function is necessary not only for fluid homeostasis and clearance of metabolic waste, but also for providing an adequate metabolic environment for somatic growth. Renal function must increase as the child grows to keep up with the increased metabolic demands needed for growth.

ESRD occurs in 25 to 50% of patients with PUVs *(54,55)*. One-third of these patients progress to ESRD within the first few months of life, and two-thirds progress during adolescence *(54)*. In one study in which patients with PUVs were followed for at least 10 yr, 32% had poor renal function, 6% had chronic renal insufficiency, 15% had ESRD, and 10% died of renal failure *(56)*.

Renal insufficiency/failure in patients with PUVs is likely caused by several factors, including bladder function, infection, residual obstruction, and hyperfiltration *(57,58)*. Several studies suggested that initial treatments, whether primary valve ablation, vesicostomy, or upper tract diversion, are equally effective in preserving renal function and allowing for somatic growth *(42,59)*.

The most important factor in determining eventual renal function appears to be the degree of renal dysplasia *(44)*. It not only affects renal function early in life, but also limits the potential for the kidneys to grow and meet the metabolic needs of somatic growth. Although bladder dysfunction, infection, and obstruction can be diagnosed and managed, dysplasia and hyperfiltration are not presently correctable. Consequently, some patients with PUVs will progress to renal insufficiency/failure and thus require close follow-up.

Finally, patients with PUVs may develop problems with sexual function *(60)*. Erection and libido appear to be normal in patients without renal failure and impaired in patients with ESRD. Woodhouse et al. observed that 48% of their adult patients with PUVs had slow or dry ejaculation; in the majority, this was because of failure of posterior urethra to generate contractile forces; very few had retrograde ejaculation. Of their patients who underwent semen analysis, 40% had poor motility or oligospermia, and 60% had viscous semen with a pH above 8.0, suggestive of prostatic and seminal vesicle dysfunction. Very few patients actually fathered children.

SUMMARY

In summary, posterior urethral valves is a common cause of congenital bladder outlet obstruction. In the past, children with posterior urethral valves were diagnosed after presenting with urinary tract infection, hematuria, urinary incontinence, or renal dysfunction. Today, the majority is diagnosed *in utero*. Appropriate radiological evaluation includes a renal/bladder ultrasound, a voiding cystourethrogram, and functional assessment of the kidneys such as nuclear renal scan. Treatment includes endoscopic ablation of the valves, vesicostomy, and rarely, upper tract drainage. However, long-term follow-up is necessary because the complications of posterior urethral valves may not be evident until several years.

REFERENCES

1. Casale AJ. Early ureteral surgery for posterior urethral valves. Urol Clin North Am 1990; 17: 361–372.
2. Young HH, Frontz RH, Baldwin TC. Congenital obstruction of the posterior urethra. J Urol 1919; 3: 289.
3. Dewan PA, Zappala SM, Ransley PG, Duffy PG. Endoscopic reappraisal of the morphology of congenital obstruction of the posterior urethra. Br J Urol 1992; 70: 439–444.
4. Stephens FD, Smith ED, Hutson JM. Congenital anomalies of the urinary and genital tracts. In: Isis Medical Media, Oxford, UK, 1996.
5. Livne PM, Delaune J, Gonzales ET Jr. Genetic etiology of posterior urethral valves. J Urol 1983; 130: 781–784.
6. Workman SJ, Kogan BA. Fetal bladder histology in posterior urethral valves and the prune belly syndrome. J Urol 1990; 144: 337–339.
7. Bauer SB, Dieppa RA, Labib KK, Retik AB. The bladder in boys with posterior urethral valves: a urodynamic assessment. J Urol 1979; 121: 769–773.
8. Kaefer M, Keating MA, Adams MC, Rink RC. Posterior urethral valves, pressure pop-offs and bladder function. J Urol 1995; 154: 708–711.
9. Glick PL, Harrison MR, Noall RA, Villa RL. Correction of congenital hydronephrosis in utero III. Early mid-trimester ureteral obstruction produces renal dysplasia. J Pediatr Surg 1983; 18: 681–687.
10. Maizels M, Simpson SB Jr. Primitive ducts of renal dysplasia induced by culturing ureteral buds denuded of condensed renal mesenchyme. Science 219: 509–510.
11. Henneberry MO, Stephens FD. Renal hypoplasia and dysplasia in infants with posterior urethral valves. J Urol 1980; 123: 912–915.
12. Dinneen MD, Duffy PG, Barratt TM, Ransley PG. Persistent polyuria after posterior urethral valves. Br J Urol 1995; 75: 236–240.
13. Gonzales ET Jr. Posterior urethral valves and bladder neck obstruction. Urol Clin North Am 1978; 5: 57–73.
14. Koff SA, Mutabagani KH, Jayanthi VR. The valve bladder syndrome: pathophysiology and treatment with nocturnal bladder emptying. J Urol 2002; 167: 291–297.
15. Harding R. Fetal pulmonary development: the role of respiratory movements. Equine Vet J 1997; Suppl, 32–39.
16. Thurlbeck WM. Prematurity and the developing lung. Clin Perinatol 1992; 19: 497–519.
17. Kitterman JA, Chapin CJ, Vanderbilt JN, et al. Effects of oligohydramnios on lung growth and maturation in the fetal rat. Am J Physiol Lung Cell Mol Physiol 2002; 282: L431–439.
18. Kitagawa H, Pringle KC, Zucollo J, et al. Early fetal obstructive uropathy produces Potter's syndrome in the lamb. J Pediatr Surg 2000; 35: 1549–1553.
19. Nakamura Y, Harada K, Yamamoto I, et al. Human pulmonary hypoplasia. Statistical, morphological, morphometric, and biochemical study. Arch Pathol Lab Med 1992; 116: 635–642.

20. Hendren WH. Posterior urethral valves in boys. A broad clinical spectrum. J Urol 1971; 106: 298–307.
21. Hutton KA. Posterior urethral valves. Br J Urol 1994; 74: 134.
22. Jee LD, Rickwood AM, Turnock RR. Posterior urethral valves. Does prenatal diagnosis influence prognosis? Br J Urol 1993; 72: 830–833.
23. Dinneen MD, Dhillon HK, Ward HC, Duffy PG, Ransley PG. Antenatal diagnosis of posterior urethral valves. Br J Urol 1993; 72: 364–369.
24. Montemarano H, Bulas DI, Rushton HG, Selby D. Bladder distention and pyelectasis in the male fetus: causes, comparisons, and contrasts. J Ultrasound Med 1998; 17: 743–749.
25. Abbott JF, Levine D, Wapner R. Posterior urethral valves: inaccuracy of prenatal diagnosis. Fetal Diagn Ther 1998; 13: 179–183.
26. Brenbridge AN, Chevalier RL, Kaiser DL. Increased renal cortical echogenicity in pediatric renal disease: histopathologic correlations. J Clin Ultrasound 1986; 14: 595–600.
27. Grignon A, Filion R, Filiatrault D, et al. Urinary tract dilatation in utero: classification and clinical applications. Radiology 1986; 160: 645–647.
28. Oliveira EA, Diniz JS, Cabral AC, et al. Prognostic factors in fetal hydronephrosis: a multivariate analysis. Pediatr Nephrol 1999; 13: 859–864.
29. Adzick NS, Harrison MR, Flake AW, deLorimier AA. Urinary extravasation in the fetus with obstructive uropathy. J Pediatr Surg 1985; 20: 608–615.
30. Dinneen MD, Duffy PG. Posterior urethral valves. Br J Urol 1996; 78: 275–281.
31. Nguyen HT, Peters CA. The long-term complications of posterior urethral valves. BJU Int 1999; 83: 23–28.
32. Wiener JS, O'Hara SM. Optimal timing of initial postnatal ultrasonography in newborns with prenatal hydronephrosis. J Urol 2002; 168: 1826–1829.
33. Papadopoulou F, Efremidis SC, Oiconomou A, et al. Cyclic voiding cystourethrography: is vesicoureteral reflux missed with standard voiding cystourethrography? Eur Radiol 2002; 12: 666–670.
34. Churchill BM, McLorie GA, Khoury AE, Merguerian PA, Houle AM. Emergency treatment and long-term follow-up of posterior urethral valves. Urol Clin North Am 1990; 17: 343–360.
35. Hoover DL, Duckett JW Jr. Posterior urethral valves, unilateral reflux and renal dysplasia: a syndrome. J Urol 1982; 128: 994–997.
36. Lythgoe MF, Gordon I, Anderson PJ. Effect of renal maturation on the clearance of technetium-99m mercaptoacetyltriglycine. Eur J Nucl Med 1994; 21: 1333–1337.
37. Jordan GH, Hoover DL. Inadequate decompression of the upper tracts using a Foley catheter in the valve bladder. J Urol 1985; 134: 137–138.
38. Gonzales ET Jr. Alternatives in the management of posterior urethral valves. Urol Clin North Am 1990; 17: 335–342.
39. Walker RD, Padron M. The management of posterior urethral valves by initial vesicostomy and delayed valve ablation. J Urol 1990; 144: 1212–1214.
40. Krahn CG, Johnson HW. Cutaneous vesicostomy in the young child: indications and results. Urology 1993; 41: 558–563.
41. Noe HN, Jerkins GR. Cutaneous vesicostomy experience in infants and children. J Urol 1985; 134: 301–303.
42. Reinberg Y, de Castano I, Gonzalez R. Prognosis for patients with prenatally diagnosed posterior urethral valves. J Urol 1992; 148: 125–126.
43. Hendren WH. Complications of ureterostomy. J Urol 1978; 120: 269–281.
44. Tietjen DN, Gloor JM, Husmann DA. Proximal urinary diversion in the management of posterior urethral valves: is it necessary? J Urol 1997; 158: 1008–1010.
45. Close CE, Carr MC, Burns MW, Mitchell ME. Lower urinary tract changes after early valve ablation in neonates and infants: is early diversion warranted? J Urol 1997; 157: 984–988.
46. Scott JE. Management of congenital posterior urethral valves. Br J Urol 1985; 57: 71–77.
47. Johnston JH. Vesicoureteric reflux with urethral valves. Br J Urol 1979; 51: 100–104.
48. Bellinger MF. Ureterocystoplasty: a unique method for vesical augmentation in children. J Urol 1993; 149: 811–813.

49. Warshaw BL, Hymes LC, Trulock TS, Woodard JR. Prognostic features in infants with obstructive uropathy due to posterior urethral valves. J Urol 1985; 133: 240–243.
50. Peters CA, Bolkier M, Bauer SB, et al. The urodynamic consequences of posterior urethral valves. J Urol 1990; 144: 122.
51. Holmdahl G, Hanson E, Hanson M, Hellstrom AL, Sillen U, Solsnes E. Four-hour voiding observation in young boys with posterior urethral valves. J Urol 1998; 160: 1477–1481.
52. Holmdahl G, Sillen U, Hanson E, Hermansson G, Hjalmas K. Bladder dysfunction in boys with posterior urethral valves before and after puberty. J Urol 1996; 155: 694–698.
53. Holmdahl G, Sillen U, Bachelard M, Hansson E, Hermansson G, Hjalmas K. The changing urodynamic pattern in valve bladders during infancy. J Urol 1995; 153: 463–633.
54. Smith GH, Canning DA, Schulman SL, Snyder HM 3rd, Duckett JW. The long-term outcome of posterior urethral valves treated with primary valve ablation and observation. J Urol 1996; 155: 1730.
55. Sheldon CA, Churchill BM, McLorie GA, Arbus GS. Evaluation of factors contributing to mortality in pediatric renal transplant recipients. J Pediatr Surg 1992; 27: 629.
56. Parkhouse HF, Barratt TM, Dillon MJ, et al. Long-term outcome of boys with posterior urethral valves. Br J Urol 1988; 62: 59.
57. McGuire EJ, Woodside JR, Borden TA, Weiss RM. Prognostic value of urodynamic testing in myelodysplastic patients. J Urol 1981; 126: 205.
58. Brenner BM, Meyer TW, Hostetter TH. Dietary protein intake and the progressive nature of kidney disease: the role of hemodynamically mediated glomerular injury in the pathogenesis of progressive glomerular sclerosis in aging, renal ablation, and intrinsic renal disease. N Engl J Med 1982; 307: 652–659.
59. Krueger RP, Hardy BE, Churchill BM. Growth in boys and posterior urethral valves. Primary valve resection vs upper tract diversion. Urol Clin North Am 1980; 7: 265.
60. Woodhouse CR, Reilly JM, Bahadur G. Sexual function and fertility in patients treated for posterior urethral valves. J Urol 1989; 142: 586–588.

24 Spina Bifida

Hiep T. Nguyen, MD, FAAP

CONTENTS

INTRODUCTION
PATHOGENESIS
DIAGNOSIS AND INITIAL MANAGEMENT
URODYNAMIC FINDINGS AND TREATMENT
FOLLOW-UP AND MANAGEMENT
COMPLICATIONS OF AUGMENTATION CYSTOPLASTY
SUMMARY
REFERENCES

INTRODUCTION

Abnormal development of the spinal canal and cord is the most common cause of neurogenic bladder dysfunction in children. Spina bifida, also known as myelodysplasia, is a general term that describes various abnormal conditions affecting spinal cord function. Meningocele occurs when the meninges without neural elements extend beyond the vertebral canal. When the meninges are accompanied by neural elements, a myelomeningocele results. Lipomyelomeningocele occurs when fatty tissue has developed within the cord structures, and all elements evaginate beyond the vertebral canal.

In the United States, the incidence of myelodysplasia is approx 1 of 1000 births *(1)*. However, this rate decreased over the last 20 yr because of improved prenatal care and pregnancy termination following fetal detection of the problem.

Myelodysplasia produces a wide spectrum of effects on bladder function and consequently on renal function. In addition, it is a dynamic problem that changes as the child grows. Consequently, accurate assessment and regular follow-up are needed to prevent complications such as infection, urinary incontinence, and loss of renal function.

PATHOGENESIS

Around the day 18 of gestation, the neural groove, derived from neural ectoderm, deepens and fuses to form the neural tube. This process begins in the center and proceeds both cranially and caudally. Around the fourth week of gestation, formation of the neural tube is completed, and vertebral development begins. The vertebral arches fuse poste-

From: *Urological Emergencies: A Practical Guide*
Edited by: H. Wessells and J. W. McAninch © Humana Press Inc., Totowa, NJ

riorly to produce the spinous processes *(2)*. Myelodysplasia develops when the caudal end of the neural tube and vertebral arches do not fuse normally. Causative factors include maternal exposure to teratogens or medications, excessive heat *(2)*, and deficiency of folic acid *(3)*. Maternal ingestion of 400 µg of folate per day in women of childbearing age reduces the incidence of spina bifida by 50%. In addition, there appears to be a genetic component, with an increased incidence (2–5%) of a second child in the family developing myelodysplasia *(4)*.

Myelomeningocele accounts for approx 90% of the cases of spinal dysraphism *(5)*. The most common level of spinal cord affected is the lumbosacral region (47%); lesions in the lumbar (26%), sacral (20%), thoracic (5%), and cervical (2%) regions occur less commonly *(6)*. Most spinal defect sacs protrude posteriorly, but on occasion can be anterior, presenting as a pelvic mass. The meningocele is usually covered with a thin layer of tissue that could be easily disrupted, allowing cerebrospinal fluid to leak. The neurological lesion produced by spinal dysraphism is variable, depending on the neural elements present in the meningocele. In addition, it is often difficult to predict the type of neurological lesion in a child with spina bifida.

The level of bony vertebral defect does not correlate with the type of neurological lesion present; the height of bony level defect may differ from the level of spinal cord lesion by 1 to 3 vertebrae in either direction *(6)*. In addition, one side of the body may be more affected than the other. In children with high-level lesions, the spine is often reconstituted in the sacral region, allowing for the preservation of sacral reflex function *(7)*.

Besides the spinal cord abnormalities, 85% of children with spina bifida have associated Arnold-Chiari malformation, a condition in which the cerebellar tonsils herniate down through the foramen magnum, obstructing the fourth ventricle and preventing the cerebrospinal fluid from entering the subarachnoid space surrounding the brain and spinal cord. This malformation leads to development of hydrocephalus. In addition, children with spina bifida may have associated gastrointestinal, genitourinary, and cardiac anomalies. Of interest, there is a higher incidence of renal fusion anomalies and cryptorchidism *(8)*.

DIAGNOSIS AND INITIAL MANAGEMENT

Early diagnosis of spina bifida may be made by sampling maternal serum α-fetoprotein. Obtained within 24 wk of gestation, an elevated value greater than three times the standard deviation indicates a 70% risk of myelodysplasia *(9)*. Fetal ultrasonography alone is not accurate in diagnosing spinal dysraphism, but when combined with an elevated α-fetoprotein has an 80% sensitivity and 99% specificity.

Because the mode of delivery can affect the severity of the neurological outcome *(8,10)*, early diagnosis is essential for prenatal counseling and planning of delivery. Fetal intervention has been performed between 25 and 29 wk of gestation *(11)*. Although the incidence of abnormal bladder function does not seem to be significantly affected *(12)*, the incidence of hydrocephalus has drastically decreased. Currently, fetal intervention is only available in selected medical centers.

It is usually recommended that children with spina bifida undergo cesarean section to reduce the incidence of paralysis *(10)*. Sterile precautions should be taken after delivery to minimize the chance of infecting the central nervous system. Proper support staff, including neurosurgery, pediatric urology, orthopedics, neonatology, specialized nursing, and social service, should be assembled to provide comprehensive care for the affected child and his or her family. Radiographic evaluation with ultrasonography or computed tomography should be performed to assess for associated anomalies such as Arnold-Chiari malformation.

Initial management consists of closure of spinal defect within 24 to 48 h. Fewer than 5% of children who underwent spinal closure had a change in neurological status as a result of surgery *(13)*. Consequently, urodynamic evaluation can be delayed until it is safe for the patient to be on his or her back or side for the test. Prior to urodynamic evaluation, clean intermittent catheterization (CIC) should be instituted if the patient cannot void spontaneously. Serum creatinine, urine analysis/culture, and measurement of postvoid residual should also be performed to assess the baseline status of bladder function. The normal bladder capacity for a newborn is 10 to 15 mL with an acceptable postvoid residual of less than 5 mL. Renal ultrasonography should also be performed during the newborn period; approx 15% of newborns with spina bifida will have abnormalities detected by radiologic evaluation *(14)*.

URODYNAMIC FINDINGS AND TREATMENT

Urodynamic evaluation is needed to help counsel parents regarding their child's future bladder and sexual function *(15,16)*. It is estimated that 95% of children with spina bifida have abnormal lower urinary tract function *(17)* (Fig. 1). At birth, 10 to 30% of newborns with myelodysplasia will have impairment of upper urinary tract function *(18)*. Without appropriate diagnosis and treatment, 50% will have upper tract deterioration by 5 yr of age *(19)*. Appropriate medical management has reduced the incidence of upper tract deterioration and the need for future lower urinary tract reconstruction *(20)*.

Urodynamic studies performed during the newborn period indicated that 57% of children with spina bifida have detrusor contraction; 43% have an areflexic bladder *(7)*. As assessed by electromyography, intact sacral reflux is present in 40% of the affected newborns; partial denervation is seen in 24% and complete denervation in 36% *(16)*.

Detrusor sphincter dyssynergy (DSD) develops when the external sphincter fails to decrease its activity during a detrusor contraction. DSD is present in 49%; the external sphincter is synergic only in 19% *(21)*. The finding of DSD is an important prognostic factor. Within the first 3 yr of life, 71% of the children with DSD develop urinary tract deterioration, compared to 17% with synergy and 23% with complete denervation *(22)*. Importantly, those with synergy who had upper tract deterioration only did so when they developed DSD, and those with complete denervation developed increased urethral resistance because of fibrosis.

Children with myelodysplasia who are at high risk for urinary tract deterioration should be aggressively treated with CIC with or without anticholinergic therapy. The integrity of the upper urinary tract depends on storage and emptying of urine at low pressure. Compliance is a measurement of the bladder's storage capacity, defined as a change in volume per change in pressure. Bladders with less than 20 mL/cm H_2O have decreased compliance.

Another measurement of the bladder's storage characteristic is detrusor leak point pressure (DLLP), the bladder pressure during filling when urinary leakage occurs. DLLP greater than 40 cm H_2O is associated with a higher risk of renal damage *(23)*. Normal voiding pressure varies from 55 to 80 cm H_2O in boys and 30 to 65 cm H_2O in girls *(24)*.

Treatment for decreased bladder compliance, elevated DLLP, or voiding pressure with CIC and/or anticholinergic therapy reduces the incidence of upper tract deteriora-

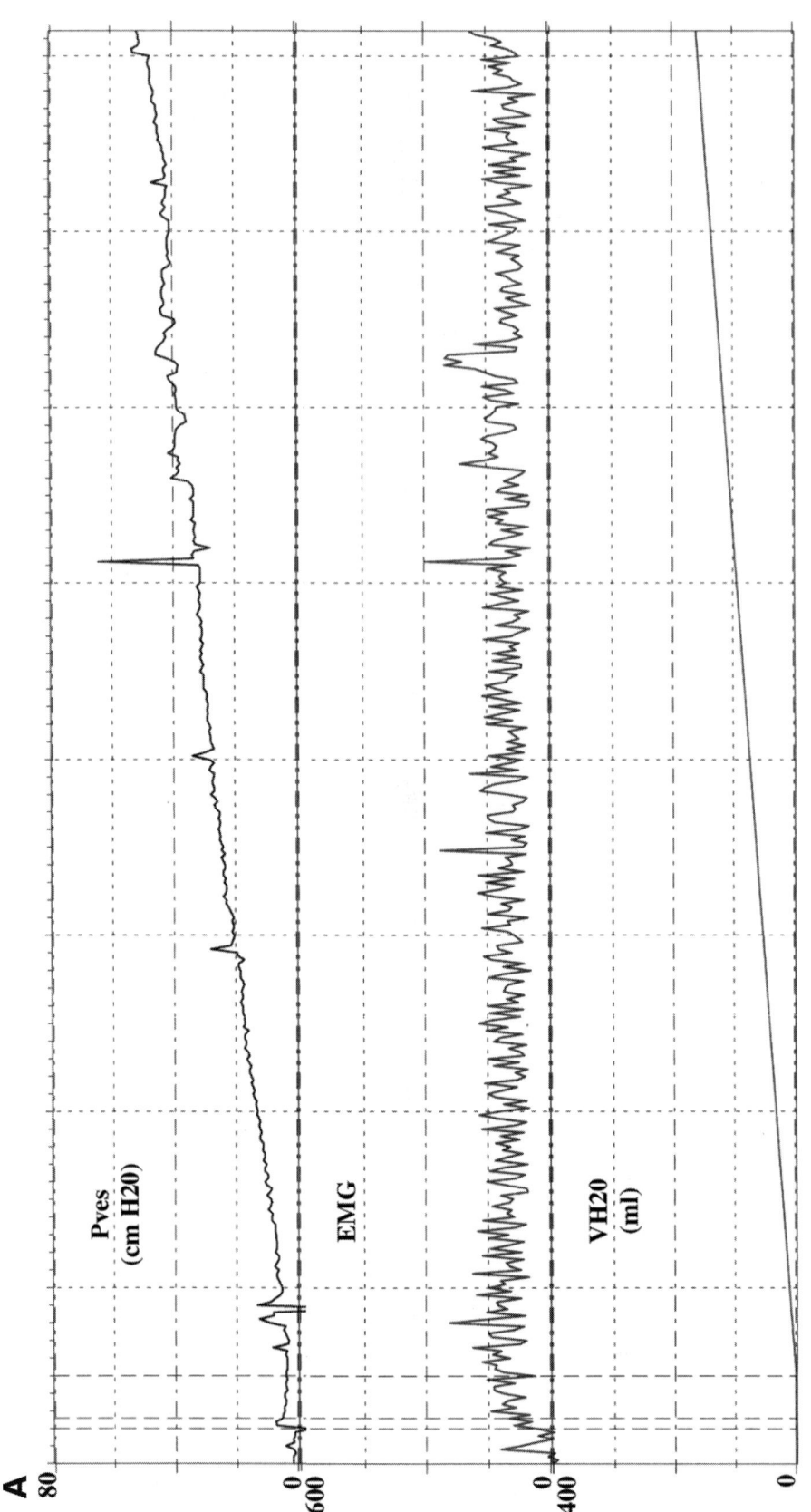

Fig. 1. (*Continued*)

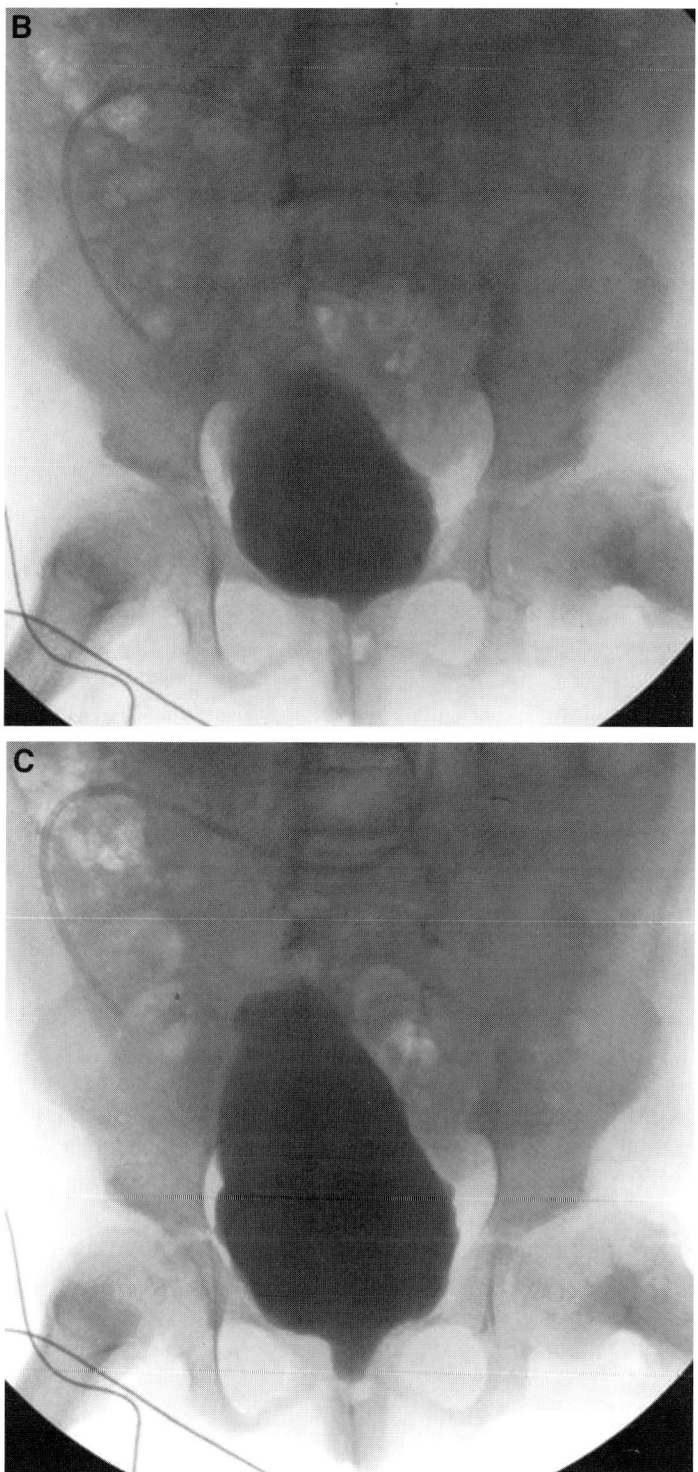

Fig. 1. (A) Urodynamic evaluation of a 6-yr-old girl with lumbosacral myelomeningocele. Note the poor compliance (high Dp/Dv) and decreased bladder capacity (estimated normal capacity at 240 mL). **(B)** Simultaneous fluoroscopic image of the bladder at 60 mL demonstrates trabeculation of the bladder without vesicoureteral reflux. **(C)** Simultaneous fluoroscopic image of the bladder at 160 mL demonstrates an open bladder neck, but no leakage to an active urinary sphincter. EMG, electromºyogram.

tion to 8 to 10% *(25,26)*. In the rare cases that do not respond to medical management, a vesicostomy may be performed *(27)*.

CIC performed in the neonate is safe with very few complications *(17)*. Although 42% of children on CIC had chronic bacteriuria, only 5% developed febrile urinary tract infection. CIC initiated in the neonatal period is easier for the parents to learn and for the children to accept as they grow older *(17,28)*. Similarly, anticholinergics such as oxybutynin have been shown to help improve bladder function with minimal side effects. Currently, there is evidence that starting anticholinergic therapy early may alter bladder growth and development and improve eventual bladder function *(29)*.

FOLLOW-UP AND MANAGEMENT

The neurological lesion in children with spina bifida changes over time, especially in early infancy *(30)* and during puberty *(31)*. The changes may be caused by tethering of the spinal cord, development of syrinx or hydromyelia of the cord, shunt malfunction, or partial herniation of brain stem or cerebellum. Magnetic resonance imaging is useful in identifying anatomic details of the spinal cord and central nervous system. However, it is not a functional study and cannot provide precise information regarding neurological changes.

Changes in bladder function may often be the first sign of problems in the spinal cord or central nervous system. Consequently, it is recommended that children with myelodysplasia be followed with renal ultrasonography and urodynamics study at least once a year *(16)*. New onset of urinary tract infection, hydronephrosis, or urinary incontinence should prompt more urgent evaluation.

Vesicoureteral reflux is present in 3 to 5% of newborns with spina bifida *(32)*. Reflux is usually found in bladders with poor compliance or DSD *(26,26)*. If bladder dysfunction is not managed, 30 to 40% will develop reflux. Although antibiotic prophylaxis prevents recurrent infection, treatment with CIC and anticholinergics allows resolution of reflux in 30 to 55% of patients *(32)*. Antireflux surgery should be reserved for patients who have recurrent urinary tract infection or persistent reflux despite maximal medical management or are undergoing surgery to increase bladder outlet resistance. Antireflux surgery is effective as long as complete bladder emptying can be attained *(33)*.

As the child grows, urinary continence becomes an important consideration for both the child and parents. For the majority of the patients, acceptable urinary continence can be obtained with CIC and anticholinergic therapy. Urodynamic findings can help guide treatment, allowing for the addition of other medications, such as α-sympathomimetic agents to increase urethral resistance. When medical therapy fails to achieve urinary continence, augmentation cystoplasty with ileum, colon, or stomach can be performed to increase bladder capacity and improve compliance. When urethral resistance is inadequate, bladder neck reconstruction, fascial sling, collagen injection, or artificial sphincter can be used to increase the continence mechanisms. Potential complications of surgery for increasing bladder outlet resistance include difficulty with catheterization, creation of false passage, and recurrent incontinence. On rare occasions, complete urinary diversion may be required to achieve urinary continence.

Sexual function becomes an important concern for most adults with spina bifida. Lack of understanding of sexual issues is in part caused by lack of education, mental handicaps, poor manual dexterity, and overprotective parents *(34)*. Boys with spina bifida reach puberty at the same age as their normal counterparts. In contrast, breast development and menarche occurs, on the average, 2 yr earlier in girls with spina bifida *(35)*.

It was observed that approx 70% of the male patients with spina bifida had erections, 65% could ejaculate, and 30% fathered children *(36,37)*. Reproductive function is usually preserved in men with neurological lesions at or below S1; only 50% of patients with higher lesions have adequate sexual function *(38)*. Of the female patients, 70% are able to become pregnant. Most have an uneventful pregnancy, although problems with urinary incontinence and the need for cesarean section more commonly occur *(39)*.

COMPLICATIONS OF AUGMENTATION CYSTOPLASTY

Although augmentation cystoplasty has helped to preserve renal function and urinary incontinence in children with spina bifida, it is not without potentially serious complications, such as metabolic derangement, infection, stone formation, and bladder perforation. When intestinal segments are placed in continuity with the urinary tract, hyperchloremic metabolic acidosis can develop. The segments absorb ammonia and chloride from the urine, creating a large chronic acid load and overwhelming the body's acid-base control mechanisms *(40)*. Clinical signs and symptoms of severe metabolic acidosis include lethargy, weakness, fatigue, anorexia and polydipsia.

In contrast, when gastric segments are augmented to the bladder, hypochloremic, hypokalemic metabolic alkalosis can develop *(41)*. The gastric mucosa prevents the absorption of chloride and acid, but secrets hydrogen chloride. The alkalosis is more pronounced following a gastrointestinal illness when the patient is also losing acid through vomiting *(42)*.

Bacteriuria is a common problem following bowel augmentation cystoplasty. The majority of patients with ileal augmentation cystoplasty and on CIC have chronic colonization with bacteria *(43)*. However, fewer than 15% develop febrile urinary tract infection *(44,45)*. Interestingly, patients with gastric augmentation have fewer symptomatic lower urinary tract infection than those augmented with ileum or colon, but the incidence of pyelonephritis is the same in both groups *(46)*.

Treatment of asymptomatic bacteriuria is usually not recommended; however, antibiotic treatment should be considered for fever, new-onset incontinence, suprapubic pain, hematuria, malodorous urine, or increased mucus production *(45)*. Often, increasing the frequency of catheterization will reduce the number of bacteria in the bladder and resolve the infection. Periodic bladder irrigation is also helpful in preventing the accumulation of mucus, which can interfere with complete bladder drainage and serve as a nidus for infection.

Bladder calculi occur in 8 to 52% of patients with augmented bladder *(47,48)*. Most stones are struvite in composition (Fig. 2). Likely etiological factors include chronic bacteriuria with urea-splitting organisms, incomplete emptying, mucus accumulation, and foreign bodies such as staples or nonabsorbable sutures *(49)*. Like urinary infection, bladder stones are less common in patients who have gastric augmentation cystoplasty *(50)*. Bladder calculi can be treated through an endoscopic or percutaneous approach *(51)*. After rendering the patient stone free, aggressive irrigation and catheterization should be performed to reduce the chance of recurrence.

The most serious complication of bowel augmentation cystoplasty is delayed bladder perforation in 2 to 15% of patients with augmented bladder. These perforations commonly occur within the bowel segment rather than at the bladder–bowel anastomosis. Contribution factors include bladder overdistention, blunt abdominal trauma, trauma

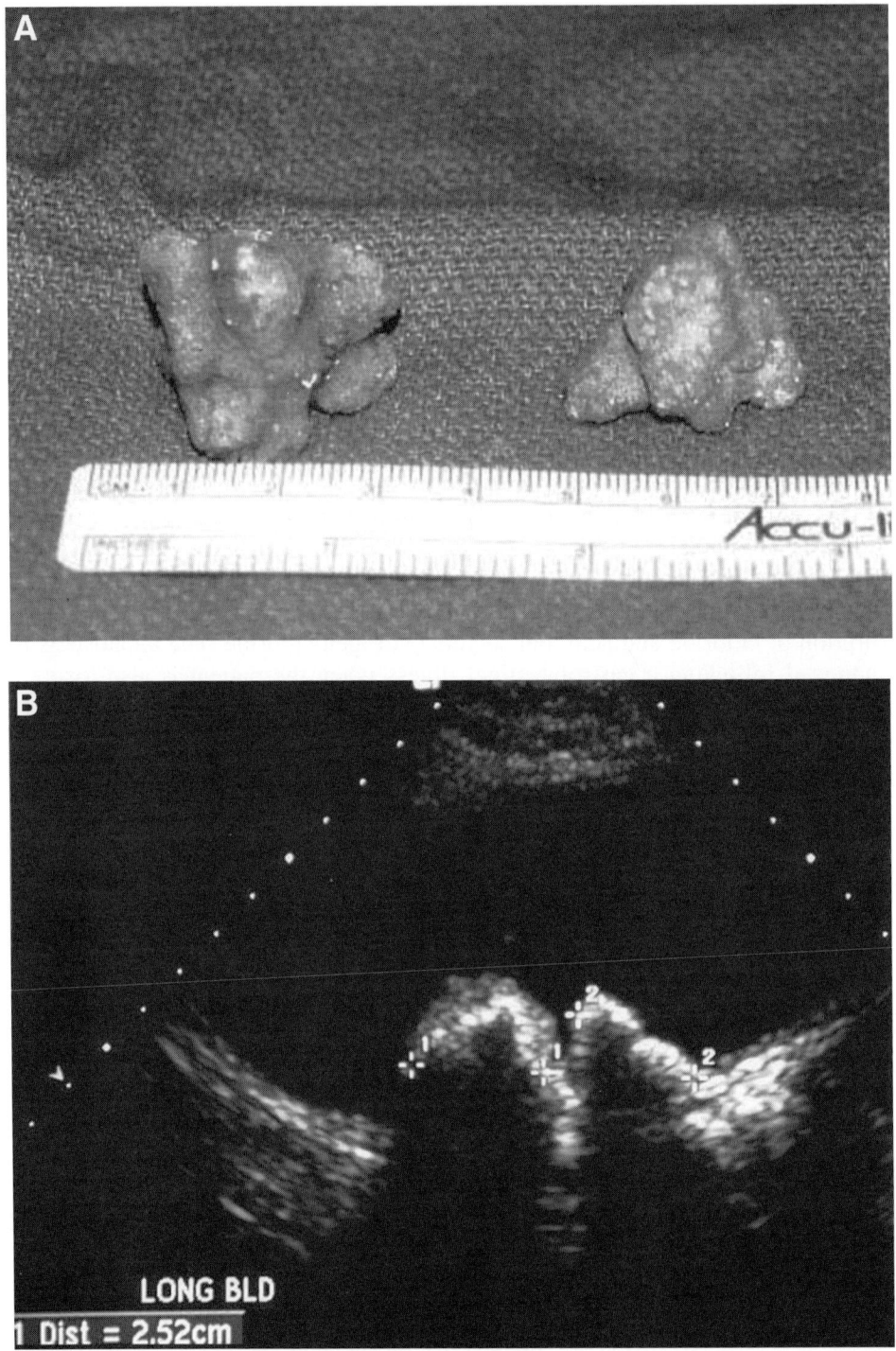

Fig. 2. (A) Ultrasonography demonstrating two large stones in the augmented bladder of a 10-yr-old child with spina bifida. **(B)** Stone analysis demonstrated struvite composition, and the child had chronic proteus bacteriuria.

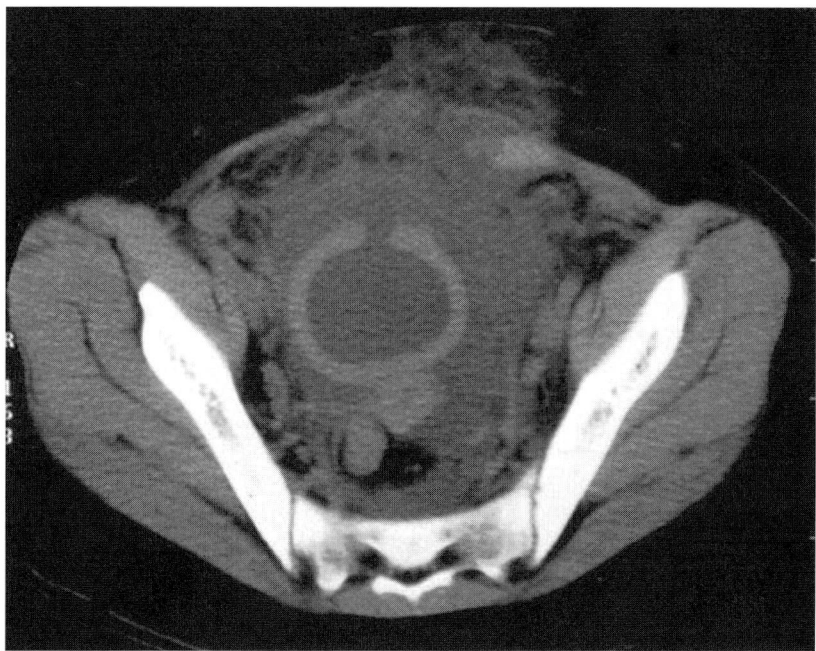

Fig. 3. Computed tomography demonstrated a bladder perforation in a 16-yr-old girl with an ileal augmentation cystoplasty.

from CIC, chronic urinary tract infection, local bowel wall ischemia, and adhesions that cause shearing during bladder filling and emptying. In some studies, there appears to be a slightly higher risk of bladder perforation in bladder augmented with sigmoid colon *(52)*; others demonstrate a higher risk in ileal augmented bladder *(53)*.

Presenting signs and symptoms may include abdominal pain, distention, fever, or septic shock *(54)*. Because of impaired sensation, patients with spina bifida and augmented bladder may present late during the course of the illness.

Any patients with augmented bladder and abdominal pain should be evaluated for bladder perforation. Contrast cystography or computed tomography can be used to diagnose bladder perforation *(55,56)* (Fig. 3).

Patients who are severely ill should undergo immediate surgical exploration and drainage. In patients in more stable condition, percutaneous/catheter drainage and antibiotics can be tried initially. However, if clinical improvement does not occur rapidly, surgical intervention is then recommended.

SUMMARY

In summary, neurogenic bladder and sphincteric dysfunction commonly occur in children with abnormal development of the spinal canal and cord. Urodynamic evaluation is essential in order to identity the specific type of bladder and sphincteric dysfunction. Those children with unfavorable urodynamic parameters should be aggressively treated with intermittent catheterization and anticholinergic therapy. Some children with spina bifida may eventually require urological reconstructive surgery. These patients will require close follow-up in order to be monitored for potentially morbid surgical and metabolic complications.

REFERENCES

1. Stein SC, Feldman JG, Friedlander M, Klein RJ. Is myelomeningocele a disappearing disease? Pediatrics 1982; 69: 511–514.
2. Sutherland RS, Mevorach RA, Baskin LS, Kogan BA. Spinal dysraphism in children: an overview and an approach to prevent complications. Urology 1995; 46: 294–304.
3. Czeizel AE, Dudas I. Prevention of the first occurrence of neural-tube defects by periconceptional vitamin supplementation. N Engl J Med 1992; 327: 1832–1835.
4. Scarff TB, Fronczak S. Myelomeningocele: a review and update. Rehabil Lit 1981; 42: 143–146, 192.
5. Stark GD. Spina Bifida: Problems and Management. Blackwell Scientific, Oxford, UK, 1977.
6. Bauer SB, Labib KB, Dieppa RA, Retik AB. Urodynamic evaluation of boy with myelodysplasia and incontinence. Urology, 1977; 10: 354–362.
7. Pontari MA, Keating M, Kelly M, Dyro F, Bauer SB. Retained sacral function in children with high level myelodysplasia. J Urol 1995; 154: 775–777.
8. Selzman AA, Elder JS, Mapstone TB. Urologic consequences of myelodysplasia and other congenital abnormalities of the spinal cord. Urol Clin North Am 1993; 20: 485–504.
9. Kraus SR, Boone TB. Pediatric neurogenic bladder: etiology and diagnostic evaluation. In: Pediatric Urology Practice. (Gonzales ET, Bauer SB, eds.), Lippincott, Williams, and Wilkins, Philadelphia, PA, 1999, pp. 365–381.
10. Luthy DA, Wardinsky T, Shurtleff DB, et al. Cesarean section before the onset of labor and subsequent motor function in infants with meningomyelocele diagnosed antenatally. N Engl J Med 1991; 324: 662–666.
11. Adzick NS, Sutton LN, Crombleholme TM, Flake AW. Successful fetal surgery for spina bifida. Lancet 1993; 352: 1675–1676.
12. Holmes NM, Nguyen HT, Harrison MR, Farmer DL, Baskin LS. Fetal intervention for myelomeningocele: effect on postnatal bladder function. J Urol 2001; 166: 2383–2386.
13. Kroovand RL, Bell W, Hart LJ, Benfield KY. The effect of back closure on detrusor function in neonates with myelomeningocele. J Urol 1990; 144: 423–424.
14. Bauer SB. The management of spina bifida from birth onwards. In: Paediatric Urology. (Whitaker RH, Woodard JR, eds.), Butterworths, London, UK, 1985, pp. 87–112.
15. McGuire EJ, Woodside JR, Borden TA, Weiss RM. Prognostic value of urodynamic testing in myelodysplastic patients. 1981. J Urol 2002; 167: 1049–1053.
16. Lais A, Kasabian NG, Dyro FM, Scott RM, Kelly MD, Bauer SB. The neurosurgical implications of continuous neurourological surveillance of children with myelodysplasia. J Urol 1993; 150: 1879–1883.
17. Joseph DB, Bauer SB, Colodny AH, Mandell J, Retik AB. Clean, intermittent catheterization of infants with neurogenic bladder. Pediatrics 1989; 84: 78–82.
18. Chiaramonte RM, Horowitz EM, Kaplan GW, Brock WA. Implications of hydronephrosis in the newborn with myelodysplasia. J Urol 1986; 136: 427–429.
19. Bauer SB, Hallett M, Khoshbin S, et al. Predictive value of urodynamic evaluation in newborns with myelodysplasia. JAMA 1984; 252: 650–652.
20. Wu HY, Baskin LS, Kogan BA. Neurogenic bladder dysfunction due to myelomeningocele: neonatal vs childhood treatment. J Urol 1997; 157: 2295–2297.
21. Sidi AA, Aliabadi H, Gonzalez R. Enterocystoplasty in the management and reconstruction of the pediatric neurogenic bladder. J Pediatr Surg 1987; 22: 153–157.
22. Bauer SB, Koff SA, Jayanthi VR. Voiding dysfunction in children: neurogenic and non-neurogenic. In: Campbell's Urology. (Walsh P, Retik AB, Wein A, eds.), Saunders, Philadelphia, PA, 2002, pp. 2231–2260.
23. McGuire EJ, Woodside JR, Borden TA, Weiss RM. Prognostic value of urodynamic testing in myelodysplastic patients. J Urol 1981; 126: 205–209.
24. Blaivas JG, Labib KL, Bauer SB, Retik AB. Changing concepts in the urodynamic evaluation of children. J Urol 1977; 117: 778–781.
25. Geraniotis E, Koff SA, Enrile B. The prophylactic use of clean intermittent catheterization in the treatment of infants and young children with myelomeningocele and neurogenic bladder dysfunction. J Urol 1988; 139: 85–86.

26. Edelstein RA, Bauer SB, Kelly MD, et al. The long-term urological response of neonates with myelodysplasia treated proactively with intermittent catheterization and anticholinergic therapy. J Urol 1995; 154: 1500–1504.
27. Mandell J, Bauer SB, Colodny AH, Retik AB. Cutaneous vesicostomy in infancy. J Urol 1981; 126: 92–93.
28. Lindehall B, Moller A, Hjalmas K, Jodal U. Long-term intermittent catheterization: the experience of teenagers and young adults with myelomeningocele. J Urol 1994; 152: 187–189.
29. Park JM, Bauer SB, Freeman MR, Peters CA. Oxybutynin chloride inhibits proliferation and suppresses gene expression in bladder smooth muscle cells. J Urol 1999; 162: 1110–1114.
30. Spindel MR, Bauer SB, Dyro FM, et al. The changing neurourologic lesion in myelodysplasia. JAMA 1987; 258: 1630–1633.
31. Begeer JH, Meihuizen de Regt MJ, HogenEsch I, Ter Weeme CA, Mooij JJ, Vencken LM. Progressive neurological deficit in children with spina bifida aperta. Z Kinderchir 1986; 41: 13–15.
32. Flood HD, Ritchey ML, Bloom DA, Huang C, McGuire EJ. Outcome of reflux in children with myelodysplasia managed by bladder pressure monitoring. J Urol 1994; 152: 1574–1577.
33. Jeffs RD, Jonas P, Schillinger JF. Surgical correction of vesicoureteral reflux in children with neurogenic bladder. J Urol 1976; 115: 449–151.
34. Joyner BD, McLorie GA, Khoury AE. Sexuality and reproductive issues in children with myelomeningocele. Eur J Pediatr Surg 1998; 8: 29–34.
35. Coakley RM, Holmbeck GN, Friedman D, Greenley RN, Thill AW. A longitudinal study of pubertal timing, parent-child conflict, and cohesion in families of young adolescents with spina bifida. J Pediatr Psychol 2002; 27: 461–473.
36. Decter RM, Furness PD 3rd, Nguyen TA, McGowan M, Laudermilch C, Telenko A. Reproductive understanding, sexual functioning and testosterone levels in men with spina bifida. J Urol 1997; 157: 1466–1468.
37. Sandler AD, Worley G, Leroy EC, Stanley SD, Kalman S. Sexual function and erection capability among young men with spina bifida. Dev Med Child Neurol 1996; 38: 823–829.
38. Woodhouse CR. The sexual and reproductive consequences of congenital genitourinary anomalies. J Urol 1994; 152: 645–651.
39. Bomalaski MD, Teague JL, Brooks B. The long-term impact of urological management on the quality of life of children with spina bifida. J Urol 1995; 154: 778–781.
40. Koch MO, McDougal WS. The pathophysiology of hyperchloremic metabolic acidosis after urinary diversion through intestinal segments. Surgery 1985; 98: 561–570.
41. Gosalbez R Jr, Woodard JR, Broecker BH, Warshaw B. Metabolic complications of the use of stomach for urinary reconstruction. J Urol 1993; 150: 710–712.
42. Adams MC, Bihrle R, Rink RC. The use of stomach in urologic reconstruction. Am Urol Assoc Update Series 1995; 122.
43. Schlager TA, Dilks S, Trudell J, Whittam TS, Hendley JO. Bacteriuria in children with neurogenic bladder treated with intermittent catheterization: natural history. J Pediatr 1995; 126: 490–496.
44. Bakke A, Digranes A, Hoisaeter PA. Physical predictors of infection in patients treated with clean intermittent catheterization: a prospective 7-year study. Br J Urol 1997; 79: 85–90.
45. Zhanel GG, Harding GK, Guay DR. Asymptomatic bacteriuria. Which patients should be treated? Arch Intern Med 1990; 150: 1389–1396.
46. Kaefer M, Tobin MS, Hendren WH, et al. Continent urinary diversion: the Children's Hospital experience. J Urol 1997; 157: 1394–1399.
47. Barroso U, Jednak R, Fleming P, Barthold JS, Gonzalez R. Bladder calculi in children who perform clean intermittent catheterization. BJU Int 2000, 85: 879–884.
48. Palmer LS, Franco I, Kogan SJ, Reda E, Gill B, Levitt SB. Urolithiasis in children following augmentation cystoplasty. J Urol 1993; 150: 726–729.
49. Kronner KM, Casale AJ, Cain MP, Zerin MJ, Keating MA, Rink RC. Bladder calculi in the pediatric augmented bladder. J Urol 1998; 160: 1096–1098.
50. Kaefer M, Hendren WH, Bauer SB, et al. Reservoir calculi: a comparison of reservoirs constructed from stomach and other enteric segments. J Urol 1998; 160: 2187.
51. Cain MP, Casale AJ, Kaefer M, Yerkes E, Rink RC. Percutaneous cystolithotomy in the pediatric augmented bladder. J Urol 2002; 168: 1881–1882.

52. Pope JCI, Rink RC. Surgical options in the management of the neurogenic bladder. In: Pediatric Urology Practice. (Gonzales ET, Bauer SB, eds.), Lippincott, Williams, and Wilkins, Philadelphia, PA, 1999, pp. 401–419.
53. Bauer SB, Hendren WH, Kozakewich H, et al. Perforation of the augmented bladder. J Urol 1992; 148: 699–703.
54. Worley G, Wiener JS, George TM, et al. Acute abdominal symptoms and signs in children and young adults with spina bifida: 10 years' experience. J Pediatr Surg 2001; 36: 1381–1386.
55. Braverman RM, Lebowitz RL. Perforation of the augmented urinary bladder in nine children and adolescents: importance of cystography. AJR Am J Roentgenol 1991; 157: 1059–1063.
56. Rushton HG, Woodard JR, Parrott TS, Jeffs RD, Gearhart JP. Delayed bladder rupture after augmentation enterocystoplasty. J Urol 1988; 140: 344–346.

Index

A

Abdominal distention, 42
Abdominal pain, 41, 51, 52, 117, 125, 189, 197, 264, 265, 269, 273, 287, 371
   bladder trauma, 41, 51
   in acute urinary retention, 287
   in endoscopic perforation, 316
   in retroperitoneal and upper tract hemorrhage, 189
   in upper urinary tract infection, 117, 125
   in upper urinary tract obstruction, 275
Abscess, 50, 53, 54, 60, 87, 102, 104, 110, 115, 121–132, 135–138, 141, 143, 144, 151, 158, 161, 178, 183, 184, 194, 216, 224, 231, 233, 237, 244, 245, 284, 309, 318, 325
   epididymal, 74
   in pelvic trauma, 285, 287
   in penile trauma, 96
   in priapism, 216
   in retroperitoneal and upper tract hemorrhage, 183–185
   in urethral trauma, 53, 54, 60
   perinephric, 115, 122–134, 197, 245, 259
   prostatic, 135–138, 145, 244, 284, 285
   renal, 10, 20, 115, 121–136, 141, 178, 189, 194, 216, 244, 245, 259, 326
   retroperitoneal, 10, 189, 197, 244, 318
   surgical drainage, 123–126, 129, 132
Acrolein, 203, 205
Acute pyelonephritis, 116–123, 127, 128, 132, 133, 245, 259
Adrenal hyperplasia, 340
   congenital, 339
Adrenocorticotropic hormone, 183, 186
Al-Ghorab procedure, *see* shunts
Ambiguous genitalia, 339, 340, 344–347
Amoxicillin, 86, 92, 118, 119, 133
Ampicillin, 118–121, 133, 136

Aneurysm, 172, 182, 187–192, 195–200, 243, 244, 269
Angiography, 50
   renal, 172, 191, 192, 196, 243, 266, 268, 321
   in renal trauma and vascular injury, 8, 21, 199
Antibiotics, 48, 73, 82, 107, 118, 120, 149, 150, 153, 155, 159, 162, 167, 232, 235, 242, 275, 283, 288, 290, 298, 304, 305, 316, 317, 322–324, 336, 355, 371
   in acute protatitis, 323
   in abscess, 53, 54, 60, 87, 129, 143, 144, 151, 161
   renal, 115, 121–128, 136, 326
   retroperitoneal, 318
Anuria,
   renal, 180, 269
   in renal trauma, 180
Arterioureteral fistula, 198
Arteriovenous fistula, 21, 101, 188, 198–200
Arteriovenous malformation, 184, 188, 190, 193, 196, 199
Artificial urinary sphincter, 54
Aspiration, 137, 174, 179, 180, 218, 272
   of renal abscess, 124
Autotransplantation, renal, 195

B

Bacteria, 48, 50, 54, 86, 115–118, 121, 125, 128, 132–134, 148–150, 153–157, 161–164, 167, 204, 324, 326, 369
   in epididymitis, 135, 136, 141–145, 158, 232, 237
   in prostatitis, 135–137, 141, 145, 285, 323
   in urethritis, 135–137, 141–145
Bacille Calmette-Guerin, 315–326
BCG; *see* Bacille Calmette-Guerin
Benign prostatic hyperplasia, 139, 287
Biopsy, 186–190, 194–200, 205, 272, 277, 297, 316, 323, 325, 344

Bladder, 6, 30–35, 39–55, 58, 59, 64, 65, 67, 100, 115, 116, 118, 123, 125, 136, 139, 149, 202–206, 208, 210, 216, 232, 244–246, 257, 272, 273, 276, 277, 281–290, 295–301, 303–306, 308–310, 315–317, 322, 324, 329, 345, 349–355, 357–360, 363–371, 204
   overdistention, 52, 53, 316, 369
   perforation of, 40, 53, 56, 205, 289, 316, 317, 326, 369, 371, 374
   during transurethral resection of the prostate, 315, 325
   tumor resection, 324
   posterior urethral valves, 232, 283, 284, 349–362
   rupture of, 37–40, 43–48, 52–58, 65, 100, 125, 238, 245, 257, 316, 317, 325, 374
   trauma to, 6, 31–48, 51–59, 64–69, 216, 232, 238, 244, 245, 285–290, 298, 312, 313, 316, 317, 324, 333, 334, 369
Bladder augmentation, 299
Bladder neck, 43, 51, 69, 282, 284, 304, 332, 335, 349, 353, 354, 357, 360, 367, 368
   injury, 40, 48–55, 65, 67, 283, 285, 313, 350
Bleeding, 13, 20, 26, 29, 77, 79, 82, 158, 192–196, 266, 268
   bladder, 6, 50, 202–208, 211, 212, 245, 277, 283, 296, 300, 305, 315, 316, 322
   hemorrhagic cystitis, 201–205, 209–212
   kidney, 6–10, 15, 177, 181–186, 189–191, 195–199, 243, 283, 321
   upper tract, 181, 315
   urethra, 233
   urinary tract, 181, 204, 205, 208, 211, 212, 245, 277, 283, 315, 322, 356
Blood-at-the-meatus, 64, 67, 96, 99
Blood culture, 118, 121, 136, 242, 322, 323
Blood supply, 17, 29, 33, 53, 62, 71, 72, 161, 167, 173, 192, 226, 303, 317, 318
Blood transfusion, 192, 201, 205
Blunt trauma, 57, 73–77, 80, 83, 95, 96, 102, 111, 233
   to bladder, 6, 37, 40, 42, 46, 52, 55, 56
   to kidney, 4, 6, 11, 12, 21, 37, 174
   to ureter, 6, 11, 22, 26, 37, 52, 55, 92, 174
Boari flap, 309, 310, 320
Bony pelvis, 330, 335

Bulbar urethral stricture, 61
Bypass, 4, 25, 37, 59, 173, 175, 183, 195–198, 306–309

C

Calculus, 92, 241, 243, 246, 247, 256, 284, 287, 326
   complications in, 248
   computed tomography, 242, 249, 250, 288
   during pregnancy, 258
   percutaneous stone removal, 248, 257, 258, 322
Catheterization, 12, 53, 56, 59, 85, 118, 121, 149, 173, 174, 298, 306, 359, 365, 372, 373
   in intraperitoneal bladder injury, 50
   in stricture, 54, 58, 64, 272, 285–288, 324
   in urinary retention, 65, 137, 281–290
   urinary tract infection, 136, 232, 272, 324, 368–371
Cavernosography, 97, 99, 110, 218
Ceftriaxone, 120
   in gonococcal urethritis, 140
Cephalosporin, 86, 121, 124, 149, 159
Chemotherapy, 209–211
Child, 6, 10, 12, 26, 27, 40, 42, 52, 55, 80–83, 116, 139, 178, 187, 225, 230, 232, 235, 237, 257, 258, 264, 265, 269, 281, 283, 285, 288, 290, 329, 333, 334, 335, 336, 342–347, 349, 353, 356, 359, 363–365, 368–371
   acute scrotum, 225, 230, 232, 235
   bladder trauma, 42, 52
   intersex states in, 343, 339
      ambiguous genitalia, 339
   newborn urologic evaluation, 67
   posterior urethral valves, 232, 283, 349, 359–361
   renal ultrasound, 6
   scrotal swelling, 146
   torsion of testicular appendages, 232, 237
Chills, 117, 323
Chlamydia infection, 140
Chronic bacterial prostatitis, 136
CIC; *see* Clean intermittent catheterization
Clean intermittent catheterization, 53, 56, 290, 321, 365, 368–373

Index

Closure, 15, 18, 32, 33, 82, 87, 89, 149, 162–165, 220, 267, 281, 282, 296–301, 311, 312, 317, 365, 372
   in exstrophy, 335–337
Clot retention, 201, 204, 205, 208, 283, 284, 287
Coagulation, 25, 28, 173, 176, 185, 204, 208, 223, 312, 323
   renal vein thrombosis, 177–179
Colic, 43, 47, 116, 131, 141, 173, 178, 190, 245, 264, 265, 269, 353
   renal, 15, 259
   ureteral, 15, 23, 241–263, 273, 274
Colles' fascia, 58, 77, 158
Complications, 3, 4, 10–12, 18–21, 25, 33, 35, 36, 53, 55, 58, 60, 67, 71, 85, 95, 102, 104, 105, 107, 110, 124, 132, 137, 151, 172, 175–177, 179, 190, 194, 195, 202, 203, 207, 219, 231, 236, 247, 253, 257, 272, 283, 287, 288, 290, 293, 295, 305, 310, 315, 316, 317, 319–324, 356, 360, 363, 368, 369, 371
   of bladder trauma, 53
   of BCG, 315–326
   of epididymitis, 78, 232
   of hemorrhagic cystitis, 203, 207
   of infection to the upper urinary tract, 124, 132
   of percutaneous nephrolithotomy, 198, 315, 320, 326
   of prostatitis, 137
   of renal embolism, 175–177
   of renal trauma, 10–12, 18–21
   of renal vein thrombosis, 175
   of trauma to external genitalia, 71, 85
   of trauma to the penis, 95, 102, 105, 107
   of ureteral trauma, 33, 35
   of urethritis, 137
Computed tomography, 28, 42, 47, 171, 182, 186, 188, 205, 242, 260, 288, 317, 365, 371
   of abscess, 158, 161
   perinephric, 122–126, 129, 132, 197, 259
   prostatic, 137, 138
   renal, 122–126, 132, 259
   in hydronephrosis, 249, 250, 265, 266
   in renal trauma, 3, 7, 11, 37, 199
Congenital adrenal hyperplasia, diagnosis of, 339, 340
Contaminated wound, 165
Contusion, 73, 74, 78–82, 91, 235
   bladder, 42, 46, 48, 58, 59
   renal, 3, 4, 8, 29, 42
   urethral, 42, 46, 58, 59, 96, 233
Corpora cavernosa, 110, 152, 155, 161, 218, 224
Corpus cavernosography, *see* cavernosography
Crush injury, 63, 64
Culture, 86, 136, 139, 143, 156, 159, 162, 283, 290, 345, 365
   in cystitis, 204
   in pyelonephritis, 118–122, 127, 128, 132, 242
   in renal abscess, 121, 122, 125
   in tuberculosis, 80, 324
   in urinary tract infection, 121, 125, 127, 132, 145, 204, 232, 322, 324
Cyclophosphamide, 276
   cystitis, 202–205, 209–211
Cycloserine, 323
Cystitis, 116, 117, 133, 204, 245, 286, 330
   cyclophosphamide-induced, 203, 209–211
   emphysematous, 115
   fungal, 244
   hemorrhagic, 201–205, 209–212
   radiation-induced, 202, 212
   viral, 203
Cystography, 33, 40–52, 65, 208, 297, 304, 305, 371, 374
   in bladder trauma, 45, 47, 51, 54–56
Cystoplasty, 310, 372
   augmentation, 39, 52, 53, 56, 299, 361, 363, 368–374
Cystoscopy, 51, 54, 96, 128, 161, 191, 205, 277, 289, 297, 308
Cystotomy, 33, 50, 59, 258, 290, 299, 314, 317
   in bladder injury, 48, 52, 64, 296

D

Deceleration injury, 6, 10, 11
Debridement, 15, 31, 59, 81, 82, 86, 87, 107, 110, 123, 162, 164, 317
   in Fournier's gangrene, 159–167
   in gunshot wound to the kidney, 10, 16, 32
   wound infection, 102
Diabetes mellitus, 54, 137, 148, 157, 167, 273, 279, 285, 286

Disligation of ureter, 31
Doxycycline,
    in Chlamydia infection, 140
    in gonococcal urethritis, 140
Drainage, 15, 16, 20, 25, 31–35, 42, 45–55, 58, 72, 82, 121–129, 132, 134, 137, 144, 145, 151, 158, 162, 165, 216, 220, 242, 254–258, 265, 271–275, 288–290, 298–300, 304–308, 312, 317–321, 324–326, 335, 336, 350, 353–360, 369, 371
Dressing, 12, 31, 82, 85, 92, 102, 110, 161, 162, 165, 167, 235, 333, 334
Dysraphism, 364, 372

E

Embolism, 176, 177, 180, 206, 215
    renal artery, 171–174, 179
Embolization, 191–196, 200, 208, 236, 268, 321
    of angiomyolipoma, 199
    of arterioureteral fistula, 198
    of renal trauma, 7, 12, 21, 199
Emphysematous cystitis, *see* cystitis, emphasematous
Emphysematous pyelonephritis, *see* pyelonephritis, emphysematous
Enterococcus, 118, 136
Enterocystoplasty, 52, 56, 372, 374
Epididymitis, 139, 232
    external genitalia trauma, 80, 81, 83
    exstrophy, 329, 333–336
    fever, 136, 139, 158, 232, 237
    in children, 139, 146, 232, 237, 238
    intersex conditions, 342–347
    posterior urethral valves, 349, 353, 356, 359, 360
    renal trauma, 6, 10, 12
    renal vein thrombosis, 178
    scrotal swelling, 146, 232, 236, 237
    scrotal ultrasound, 78
    testiscular torsion, 230
    urethritis, 135, 136, 139–145
    urinary retention, 281, 283, 285, 288, 290
Epididymo-orchitis, 135, 139–143, 146, 161, 225, 226, 232, 323
Epinephrine, 215, 219
Epispadias,
    exstrophy, 329–337
Epsilon aminocaproic, 208

Erection, 95–97, 101–110, 213–215, 218–224, 359, 369, 373
Erythromycin, 140
    in Chlamydia infection, 140
Escherichia coli, 150, 157
    in abscess, 132, 136
    in prostatitis, 136
    in pyelonephritis, 116, 132, 133
Excretory urography, 246, 248
Exstrophy, 329–337, 341
External genitalia, 71–78, 81, 84, 86, 89, 90, 93, 110, 157, 158, 167, 224, 339, 343
    penile, 73, 91, 110
    scrotal, 71–75, 78, 81–93, 158, 167
    testicular, 72–79, 87–93
    urethral, 110, 343
    anterior, 71, 85
    posterior, 85
Extravasation, 6, 7, 10, 28, 29, 33, 35, 40, 42, 43, 45, 47, 52, 58–60, 71, 96, 98–100, 158, 186, 267, 306, 310, 317, 318–321
    after bladder injury, 40, 42, 48, 52
    after renal trauma , 4, 5, 22
    after urethral injury, 58, 59, 96, 158
    contrast, 6, 28, 42–45, 47
    in renal trauma (*see* above)
    in urinary tract obstruction, 306, 310
    urinary, 7, 10, 29, 35, 50, 52, 71, 158, 320, 321

F

Failure to thrive, 4, 21, 35, 42, 62, 112, 118, 133, 175, 179, 180, 188–190, 201, 207–210, 216, 233, 235, 243, 251–254, 259, 262, 264, 270, 278, 281, 305, 321–325, 332, 337, 340
    in posterior urethral valves, 351, 359
Family history, 242, 331, 343
Female urethra, 288
    trauma to, 312
Fever, 80, 125, 131, 139, 151, 189, 194, 227, 232, 233, 237, 251, 256, 258, 265, 274, 306, 322, 371
    in prostatitis, 136, 137, 323
    in pyelonephritis, 117, 120, 121, 242–245, 369
Fistula, 53, 56, 105–107, 218, 220, 296
    arteriovenous, 21, 101, 196–200

Index

renal, 20, 21, 27, 33–37, 131, 189, 191, 195–200, 306–310, 320, 321, 326
ureteral, 27, 33–37, 51, 54, 187, 191, 195, 196, 200, 295–300, 305–310, 313, 314, 320, 321, 325, 326
ureterovaginal, 295, 299–314
urethral, 54, 58, 101, 110, 111, 162, 297–300, 311, 320, 321
Flank pain, 131, 176, 179, 194, 246, 248, 257, 260, 265, 272, 277, 319
  in pyelonephritis, 117, 173, 242–245, 259
  in ureteral injury, 27, 306
Flap, 17, 18, 30, 33–35, 61–64, 83, 85, 92, 165, 168, 299–302, 305, 309–313, 320
Fluoroquinolone, 118–121, 143, 149, 150, 155
  in bacterial prostatitis, 136
Foley catheter, 35, 42, 48, 50, 58, 162, 256, 288–290, 300, 354, 361
  in bladder trauma, 39, 45, 51–55
Foreign body, 116, 148, 150, 287, 297, 311
  in bladder trauma, 54, 55
Fournier's gangrene, 161
  coverage, 157, 163–167
  etiology and pathogenesis, 157
  management, 53, 56, 154, 157, 159, 167, 168
  presentation and diagnosis, 157, 158
Fracture, 5, 18, 40–42, 45, 46, 50, 54, 57, 58, 60, 63, 64, 65, 67, 68, 76, 95–99, 101, 102, 104, 105, 108, 233
  kidney, 5
  pelvic, 40–42, 45, 46, 50, 54, 55, 57, 64, 65, 67, 233
  penile, 58, 60, 67, 95–99, 101, 102, 104, 105
  renal trauma, 5

G

Gangrene, 53, 56, 107, 110–112, 147, 151, 154, 157–168, 195
Genital, 1, 4, 12, 40, 50, 57, 58, 64, 67, 71–89, 94, 95, 100, 101, 135–137, 139, 141, 143, 147, 151, 157–159, 164, 165, 167, 174, 184, 188, 195, 216, 263–265, 283, 286, 287, 305, 329, 332–334, 339–350, 353, 360
  ambiguous, 339, 340, 342, 344, 346, 347
  anomalies, 12, 50, 139, 237, 329, 332–336, 343, 360, 373
  external, 71, 74–79, 81, 86, 158, 343

female, 30, 58, 282, 288, 331, 340
gangrene, 147, 151
infections, 80, 135, 141, 145, 147, 151, 157, 167, 305
penis, 95–97, 100–107
priapism, 216
scrotum, 80, 81, 83
trauma, 78
Genitalia, 100, 136, 159, 238, 332
  ambiguous, 339, 340, 344–347
  external, 71–81, 84, 86, 89–93, 110, 157, 158, 167, 224, 339–344
  trauma, 58, 67, 71–81, 89–93, 101, 110, 157, 158, 333
Gentamicin, 120, 136, 149–156
Glycine, 361
Gonorrhea, 137, 232, 287
Gram-negative organisms, 122, 124, 150
Gunshot wound, 39, 57, 60, 68, 73, 75, 90–93, 101, 103, 106
  debridement, 10, 16, 32
  renal, 8, 10, 16, 27, 36
  ureteral, 10, 16, 26, 27, 32, 36

H

Hematoma, 29, 58, 78, 79, 86, 87, 97, 101, 110, 173, 235, 304
  in blunt trauma, 4, 6, 22, 46, 55, 73, 74, 92, 96, 102, 233
  pelvic, 41–50, 54, 55, 64, 82, 92, 189, 233
  perirenal, 7, 184, 186, 190, 197, 199
  retroperitoneal, 8, 10, 13, 22, 64, 181, 182, 186, 189–191, 197, 199
Hematuria, 136, 173, 176, 181, 206, 208, 236, 257–259, 265, 274, 277, 322, 360
  in cystitis, 116, 117, 201–205, 211, 244, 245
  in fistula, 21, 27, 51, 55, 58, 187–191, 195, 200
  in trauma, 4–8, 11, 12, 19, 21, 27, 41–43, 46, 51, 52, 55, 58, 178, 179, 188, 190, 195, 200, 207, 232, 237, 242–245, 264, 287, 290, 324, 369
Hemorrhage; see Bleeding, 3, 4, 8, 12, 15, 18, 21, 33, 42, 43, 50, 71, 74, 78, 161, 178–204, 208, 209, 243–250, 270, 290, 316
Hemorrhagic cystitis, 203, 205, 210, 212
  emergency options, 201
  etiology, 201

management, 201, 209, 211
pathology, 201
Herniated disk, 245
Hyperbaric oxygen therapy, 163, 206–208
in Fournier's gangrene, 163
Hydronephrosis, 127, 128, 187, 191, 248, 263, 269–273, 277, 281, 287, 297, 306, 352, 353, 357–361, 368, 372
after renal trauma, 21
computed tomography, 249, 250, 265, 266
of pregnancy, 257, 351
Hydroureter, 187, 351, 358
Hysterectomy, 51, 285, 296, 305, 306, 310–313

I

Imaging, 4–8, 12, 18, 21, 23, 29, 31, 45, 46, 52–55, 61, 67, 69, 72, 78, 89, 95–99, 102, 110, 115, 121, 127, 144, 174, 176, 190, 191, 195, 211, 230, 232, 237, 241–248, 258, 272, 283, 287, 319–322, 334, 343, 344, 368
computed tomography, 3, 28, 37, 42, 122, 126, 171, 197, 199, 205, 259
in hydronephrosis, 250, 265
scrotal, 91
Incision, 13, 31, 33, 50, 52, 64, 82, 87, 101, 102, 137, 144, 150, 159, 220, 231, 233, 266–268, 273, 289, 299, 300, 317, 355, 358
Infant; see Child, 177–180, 199, 226, 237, 238, 264, 269, 277, 332–334, 339, 342–346, 351–355, 359–361, 372
Infection, 26, 35, 48, 52–54, 57, 58, 71, 79, 80, 85, 86, 101, 102, 107, 113, 115–125, 127–132, 135–137, 139–141, 143–144, 147–154, 157–159, 161, 162, 164, 167, 203, 204, 209, 232, 235, 243, 245, 254–258, 264, 265, 269, 272–275, 281, 285, 288, 290, 296, 298, 299, 304, 305, 307–310, 315, 316, 318, 321–324, 329, 334, 336, 351, 358–360, 363, 368, 369, 371
epididymal, 232
genital, 135, 157
in trauma, 52, 232
in upper urinary tract obstruction, 264, 265, 269, 272–275
penile, 107, 148, 150–154
penile prosthesis, 147–155
prostatic, 136, 137, 285
renal, 35, 115–124, 127, 128, 131–134, 141, 154, 203, 209, 210, 232, 243, 245, 254–258, 262, 265, 269, 273–277, 281, 288, 290, 308, 310, 321, 351, 358–360, 363, 368, 369
upper urinary tract, 35, 115–117, 121–123, 127–134, 265, 269, 273–277, 315
Injury; see Trauma, 18, 27, 29, 63, 71–74, 78–86, 106, 158, 172, 179, 233, 259, 266, 291, 307, 319, 320
bladder, 6, 31, 33, 37–55, 58, 64–67, 116, 149, 283–287, 295–298, 305–310, 313–317, 322, 350, 362
external genital, 73, 75, 79, 87–91
kidney, 3–12, 19–25, 33, 37, 90, 174, 188, 283, 306, 308, 321, 350, 362
penile, 57, 58, 64, 67, 68, 73, 91, 95, 96, 99–102, 105, 109–112, 149, 153, 215, 218, 235
ureter, 6, 36
urethra, 37, 53, 64, 75, 99, 295
Intersex conditions,
diagnosis, 339, 343, 345
evaluation, 339, 345, 347
management, 339, 346, 347
Interstitial rupture of bladder, 48
Intraperitoneal rupture of bladder, 47, 48, 317

K

Kidney, 16, 34, 126, 130, 173, 177, 181–184, 187, 189, 251, 252, 263, 283, 306, 330, 332, 350, 353, 355, 362
angiography, 8, 21, 191, 196, 199, 243, 321
calculus of; see Renal calculus, 242, 243, 246, 247, 256, 288, 326
infection of, 35, 124, 125, 131, 135, 243, 254–258, 265, 277, 288, 308, 321, 329, 334, 359, 360
acute pyelonephritis, 118, 127, 128, 132
emphysematous pyelonephritis, 115, 128, 129
trauma; see Renal injury, 3–15, 19–25, 33–37, 90, 174, 175, 178, 180, 185–190, 195–200, 216, 221, 242, 244, 321, 334
Klebsiella, 118, 128, 130

L

Laceration, 4–12, 15, 18, 21, 22, 32, 33, 40–42, 47–55, 74, 76, 80, 82, 96, 102, 110, 174, 216, 224
Laparotomy, 4, 8, 10, 13, 31, 50, 53, 174, 209, 272, 273
Lower urinary tract, 117, 135, 139, 146, 201, 205, 282, 284, 335, 361, 365
  trauma to,
    anterior urethral, 57
    bladder, 48, 55, 313, 369
    posterior urethral, 57
    urethral, 57

M

Male urethra, 282, 288
  trauma to, 42, 289, 312
Membranous urethra, 53, 64, 68, 282, 284, 289
Metastasis, 198, 223
Metronidazole, 159
Microscopic examination, 242, 274
Microscopic hematuria, 41, 42, 173, 202
Multiple sclerosis, 52, 283, 286

N

Neobladder,
  rupture, 39, 53, 56
Neonate, 175, 178, 330, 331, 334, 345, 368
  ambiguous genitalia, 347
  exstrophy, 330, 331, 334
  intersex conditions, 345
  posterior urethral valves in, 361
  renal vein thrombosis, 175
  spina bifida, 368
Nephrectomy, 3, 8–15, 18, 21, 22, 123–129, 132, 134, 175, 188, 195, 196, 199, 245, 273, 306, 310, 320
Neurogenic bladder, 33, 52, 54, 123, 139, 149, 204, 232, 363, 371–374
Nitrofurantoin, 118
Nongonococcal urethritis, 140, 143
  Chlamydia trachomatis in, 145
  diagnostic of, 137, 139

O

Obstruction, 12, 27, 33, 35, 54, 55, 73, 121, 122, 126–128, 130, 196, 202, 204, 208, 215, 216, 232, 239, 241, 244–246, 248–253, 255–258, 261, 263, 265–267, 269–276, 282–286, 289, 290, 297, 305–307, 309, 310, 314, 315, 319, 349–351, 353, 354, 358–360
  bladder outlet, 54, 55, 204, 232, 283–285, 360
  fistula, 306
  in bladder trauma, 54
  in posterior urethral valves, 232, 283
  in renal trauma, 12,
  in upper urinary tract infection, 208, 263, 269, 273
  in ureteral trauma, 33, 122
  kidney, 258
  papillary necrosis, 263, 273–275, 279
  retroperitoneal fibrosis, 263, 269, 271, 279
  upper urinary tract, 35, 121, 122, 208, 265, 276, 283, 315, 349
  ureteral, 128
  ureteropelvic junction obstruction, 263, 277
  urethral, 349
Obstructive uropathy, 273, 351, 360–362
Ofloxacin, 119, 120, 133, 136, 140
Oligohydramnios, 350–352, 360
Orchitis, 54, 135, 139–146, 161, 225, 226, 232, 237, 238, 323

P

Pain, 27, 41, 51, 52, 54, 58, 72–74, 79, 85, 86, 101, 104, 117, 125, 131, 136, 137, 139, 141, 151, 158, 162, 173, 176, 179, 189, 190, 194, 202, 208, 213, 214, 218–220, 225–228, 230–233, 235–237, 241–246, 248, 251–258, 264, 265, 269, 272, 273, 275, 277, 281, 285–287, 290, 297, 306, 319, 336, 359, 369, 371
  abdominal, 41, 51, 117, 125, 189, 264, 265, 269, 273, 287, 371
  bladder, 281, 371
  flank, 27, 117, 131, 173, 176, 179, 194, 242, 243, 245, 246, 248, 257, 264, 265, 277, 306, 319
  genital, 158
  in bladder perforation, 371

in penile prosthesis infection, 151
in priapism, 213, 218, 219
in renal calculus disease, 241–243
in renal embolism, 171
in renal vein thrombosis, 176, 177
in retroperitoneal hemorrhage, 189, 190, 194
in upper tract hemorrhage, 189
in ureteropelvic junction obstruction, 264, 265
in urinary retention, 281, 285
kidney, 254
scrotal, 225, 227, 228, 232, 233, 236, 237
Palpation, 54, 141, 158, 230, 233
Papillary necrosis, 244, 246, 251, 263, 273–275, 279
Partial nephrectomy, 15, 195
Pelvic fracture, 45, 50, 55, 65, 69, 233
bladder injury, 40, 42, 54, 64
urethral injury, 41, 46, 57, 64, 67, 68
Pelvic hematoma, 41–46, 50, 54, 55, 64
Pelvis, 6, 10, 15, 28, 34, 40, 43, 45, 46, 50–52, 58, 67, 115, 122, 191, 253, 257, 266, 268, 270, 288, 305, 330, 332, 334, 335, 344, 358
fracture, 40–42, 45, 46, 50, 54, 57, 64, 65, 67
renal, 6, 10, 15, 34, 115, 122, 191, 253, 257, 268
Pendulous urethra, 57, 58, 61, 62
Penetrating injury, 6, 58, 74, 82, 102, 106, 172
Penicillin, 124, 159
Penile, 57–64, 67, 68, 73, 91, 95–112, 147–156, 161, 165, 168, 213–219, 222, 223, 235, 282, 284, 289
Penile prosthesis, 100, 147–156
Penile skin, 62, 64, 165, 168
Penis, 84, 100, 141, 151, 161, 162, 166–168, 219
fracture, 41, 96
injury, 41, 58, 67, 90, 95, 96, 101, 102, 105, 106, 110–112, 158
trauma, 41, 57, 58, 67, 75, 85, 92, 95–97, 101–112, 158, 289
Percutaneous drainage, 320
of abscess, 20, 126–129, 134, 145, 325, 326
of kidney, 326
Percutaneous nephrolithotomy, 198, 315, 320, 326

Percutaneous nephrostomy, 31, 121, 128, 134, 196, 208, 256, 258, 262, 265, 305–307, 310, 319, 320, 326
Perforation, 111
bladder, 40, 53, 56, 205, 289, 316, 317, 326, 369, 371, 374
during transurethral resection of the prostate, 315, 325
tumor resection, 324
ureteral, 25, 315–321, 325, 326
Perinephric abscess, 115, 124–128, 134, 245, 259
Periprosthetic, 148
scrotal, 144, 233
Perirenal abscess, 121, 134
Phimosis, 284, 287
Piperacillin, 120
Pneumothorax, 207, 321
Posterior urethral valves, 284, 350, 352, 355
anatomy, 349
clinical presentation, 232, 349, 351
evaluation, 232, 349, 354, 359–362
management, 283, 349, 359, 361
treatment, 232, 283, 349, 354, 357, 360, 361
Postobstructive diuresis, 283, 288, 290
Pregnancy, 116, 117, 123, 133, 182, 197, 244, 245, 258, 262, 324, 363, 369
hydronephrosis, 257, 351
Priapism,
etiology, 213, 214, 222
high flow, 224
incidence, 213–215, 222
ischemic, 213–221, 224
management of, 213, 214, 217–223
non-ischemic, 224
pathophysiology, 213, 215, 222, 224
Prolapse, 50, 284, 285, 288, 299
Prostate, 40, 41, 58, 64, 67, 92, 139, 146, 203, 218, 281, 287, 323
abscess, 135–138, 141, 244, 284
obstruction of, 204, 216, 244, 279, 282–284, 290
Prostatitis, 244, 323
acute, 135–137, 141, 145, 284, 285
chronic, 135, 136, 285
classification, 135, 145
diagnosis of, 136, 137, 145
management of, 145, 285
acute bacterial, 135
Prosthesis,
infection, 147–154

penile, 100, 147–156
Proteus, 118, 125, 128, 130, 150, 157, 370
Pseudomonas, 118, 130, 150, 157
Psoas hitch, 33, 34, 309, 310, 320
Pubic diastasis, 63, 335
Pubic ramus, 58
Pudendal artery, 71, 161
Pyelography, 173, 246, 272
    retrograde, 6, 128, 297, 306, 310
    in upper urinary tract obstruction, 265, 271
Pyelonephritis, 244
    acute, 116–123, 127, 128, 132, 133, 173, 242–245, 259, 288
    computed tomography, 122–124, 129, 132, 242, 259, 288
    diagnosis of, 117, 121–123, 127, 128, 133, 134, 173, 178, 242–245, 259, 288
    emphysematous, 115, 128, 129, 134
    imaging for, 115, 122
    signs and symptoms, 123, 128, 173, 369
    xanthogranulomatous, 115, 130, 134, 184
Pyonephrosis, 115, 127, 128, 262
    computed tomography, 122, 265, 288
Pyuria, 136, 173, 232, 237, 274

R

Radiography, 105
    bladder, 246
    renal, 126, 128, 246, 259, 260, 321
    in stone disease, 260
Reconstruction, 3, 8, 10, 12, 13, 15, 16, 18, 19, 30, 31, 35, 59–62, 64–67, 80, 83, 89, 162–165, 196, 218, 273, 320, 324, 334, 335, 365, 368
    bladder, 335
    genital, 165
    in renal injury, 3, 19, 22, 23
    penile, 62
    renal, 10, 15, 16, 19
    scrotal, 83, 162, 165
    spina bifida, 365
    ureteral, 30, 31, 320
    urethral, 60, 66, 67
    urinary tract, 365
Rectal examination, 41, 64
    in prostatitis, 136, 323
Reimplantation, 358
    in trauma, 33, 51, 88, 112
    ureteral, 32, 33, 51, 309, 310, 359
Renal abscess, 115, 121–125, 129, 134, 178, 189
Renal angiography, 8
Renal arteriovenous fistula, 198–200
Renal artery, 4, 6, 8, 11, 12, 18, 171–175, 179, 182, 183, 189, 191, 195, 243, 244, 247, 251, 263
    avulsion, 4, 8
    embolism, 71, 172, 174, 179
    thrombosis, 12, 171–174
Renal artery thrombosis, 12, 22, 171–174, 179, 180
Renal Calculus, 241, 326
Renal colic, 116, 141, 242, 244, 247, 249, 252–254, 257, 260–263, 273, 274, 353
    imaging, 241–250, 258, 259, 265
    interventions, 173, 241, 251, 255–258
Renal infarction, 171–175, 179, 184, 259
Renal parenchyma, 18, 115, 117, 122, 126–131, 189, 194, 203, 351
    laceration of, 6, 10
Renal pedicle,
    avulsion of, 8, 13
    trauma to, 8, 12, 13, 22, 23, 179
Renal pelvis, 6, 10, 15, 34, 115, 122, 191, 197, 253, 257, 261, 262, 268, 279
Renal trauma, 15, 17, 22, 23
    complications, 3, 4, 11, 12, 19, 21, 175, 180
    computed tomography, 3, 7, 11, 37, 199
    hematuria, 4–8, 11, 12, 19, 21, 27
    retroperitoneal hematoma, 8, 13
Renal ultrasound, 6
Renal vein, 171, 177–180, 184, 192, 236, 244, 247
    avulsion, 13
    injury, 6, 18, 175, 179
Renal vein thrombosis, 171, 175–180, 184, 244, 247
Retention; *see* Urinary retention, 65, 107, 137, 152, 201, 204–208, 233, 254, 281–291
Retrograde pyelography, 128
    in renal trauma, 6
Retrograde urethrography, 60, 62, 66, 99, 158
    in urethral trauma, 58–61, 65, 67
Retroperitoneal fibrosis, 190, 244, 263, 269–271, 278, 279
Retroperitoneal hematoma, 8, 10, 13, 22, 64, 181, 182

Rifampin, 151, 153, 323, 324
Rupture, 39–44, 46–48, 50, 52–55, 57, 58, 65, 73, 74, 76–79, 86–89, 95–100, 102, 104–106, 125, 181, 182, 185, 187, 189, 195, 233–235, 237, 243, 245, 248, 257, 316, 317
   bladder, 37–40, 43–58, 65, 100, 238, 245, 257, 316, 317, 325, 374
   forniceal, 248
   penis, 95, 97, 102
   renal pelvis, 257
   retroperitoneal hemorrhage, 182
   testis, 74, 76
   tunica albuginea, 76
   urethral, 43, 46, 50, 54, 57, 58, 65, 96–104, 110, 111, 233, 317

S

Scrotal, 57, 71–93, 102, 139–146, 149, 151, 156–168, 225–237, 343, 346
Scrotal swelling,
   in epididymitis, 146, 232, 236, 237
   in orchitis, 146, 232, 237
   in spermatic cord torsion, 87, 237
   in torsion of testicular appendages, 232, 236, 237
Scrotum, 144, 160, 161, 165–168, 236, 241, 332, 341
   acute, 73, 90, 139–143, 146, 158, 166, 225–238, 289
   injury, 41, 71–75, 78–84, 87–90, 101, 158, 233, 235
   laceration, 41, 74, 80, 82
   trauma, 41, 57, 60, 71–75, 78–89, 92, 97, 101, 107, 112, 158, 225–227, 232, 233, 237, 289
Segmental artery, 18, 195
Sepsis, 10, 27, 51, 117, 119, 121, 122, 127, 132, 133, 136, 147, 183, 186, 196, 242, 245, 257, 258, 272, 306, 308, 310, 315, 316, 323, 353
   after ureteral injury, 27
   BCG, 323
Serratia, 118, 150
Sexually transmitted disease, 137, 140, 145
Shock, 4, 6, 8, 26, 45, 52, 74, 79, 80, 121, 127, 190, 192, 196, 204, 206, 248, 258, 285, 286, 371
   hemorrhagic, 192, 206
   hypovolemic, 204
   in renal trauma, 4, 8
   septic, 121, 371
Shunt, 220, 368
Sickle cell disease, 116, 117, 273
   priapism, 215, 223
Skin, 50, 62, 64, 71, 76, 78, 80–83, 85–88, 102, 106, 107, 123, 124, 141, 142, 143, 148, 149, 150, 151, 153, 157–159, 161, 162, 164, 189, 205, 227, 228, 231, 235, 236, 255, 298, 299, 329, 345
   avulsion, 37, 92
   ecchymosis, 78
   gangrene, 107
   infection, 123
   in Fournier's gangrene, 157, 158, 161
   in penile prosthesis infection, 150
   loss, 86, 165
   penile, 62, 64, 165
   scrotal, 80, 82, 87, 141, 158, 159, 165, 167, 228, 235
Spermatic cord torsion, 72, 80, 82, 87, 89, 141, 144, 225, 231, 237
Spina bifida, 334, 370
   complications, 288, 363, 368–373
   diagnosis, 288, 363–365
   management, 288, 363–365, 368, 372–374
   pathogenesis, 363
Spiral computed tomography, 171, 265, 266
Spontaneous retroperitoneal hemorrhage, 197, 198
Spontaneous rupture, 182, 187, 195–200, 262
   of bladder, 56, 257
Stab wound, 8, 20, 21, 26, 27, 32, 39, 40, 300
Staphylococcus aureus, 80, 118
   in periprosthetic infection, 153
Stent, 6, 8, 12, 20, 40, 42, 52–55, 58, 64, 78, 98, 116, 123, 124, 127, 172–175, 179, 198, 199, 205, 209, 218, 228, 230, 233, 235, 265, 304, 316, 324, 330, 336, 340, 358, 361, 368–371
   ureteral, 16, 32, 34, 50, 118, 121, 122, 128, 155, 187, 191, 196, 241, 243, 248, 251, 256–258, 262, 267, 271–275, 278, 300, 306, 308, 320, 325, 359, 360
   in trauma, 10, 15, 23, 27, 28, 31–37, 48, 51, 54, 200, 242, 317–321
   in ureterovaginal fistula, 305, 307, 310
Straddle injury, 57

Index

Stricture, 33–35, 54, 57–64, 67, 68, 104, 158, 162, 263, 266, 272, 278, 279, 284–289, 308, 310, 314, 324–326, 356
Sulfamethoxazole, 119, 120, 133, 136, 151
Suprapubic tube, 33, 35, 56, 65, 102, 289, 300, 304, 317

T

Testicular torsion, 72–79, 86–93, 139–142, 146, 161, 203, 210, 225–238, 340, 341
Testicular appendage torsion, 231, 232
Testicular trauma, 73, 76, 89–93, 225, 233, 238
Thrombosis, 21, 104, 158, 176, 186, 215, 216
　renal artery, 6, 8, 11, 12, 22, 171–175, 179, 244, 247
　renal vein, 6, 171, 175–180, 184, 236, 244, 247
Torsion, 245
　spermatic cord, 141, 225, 231, 237
　testicular, 73, 74, 90, 139, 141, 225–237
　of testicular appendages, 231
Transureteroureterostomy, 34, 196, 310
Transurethral resection of prostate, 51
　complications of, 315, 316, 324, 325
Trauma, 1, 3–13, 15, 17, 19–21, 25–29, 31, 33, 35, 39–43, 45–49, 51–55, 57–65, 67, 71–81, 83, 85, 87–89, 95–97, 99, 101–103, 105, 107, 109, 157, 158, 171, 172, 174, 175, 178–179, 185, 186, 188, 190, 195, 207, 216, 218, 220, 221, 226, 227, 232, 233, 234, 235, 237, 242, 244, 245, 264, 269, 285–287, 289–290, 298, 316, 317, 319, 321, 324, 333, 334, 369
　bladder, 6, 33–37, 43–48, 52–59, 65–69, 216, 232, 238, 244, 245, 285, 286, 289, 290, 298, 312, 316, 317, 324, 333, 369
　external, 31, 39–42, 51, 55, 313
　genital, 64, 287, 334
　blunt, 4–8, 11, 12, 21–23, 26, 27, 36–42, 46, 48, 52, 55–59, 73–80, 83, 91, 92, 95–111, 172, 174, 199, 216, 233, 369
　pelvic, 289
　penile, 57–64, 67, 68, 73, 91, 95–112, 216, 218, 235, 285, 287, 289
　renal, 3–6, 5–7, 8, 9, 12, 13, 15, 17, 21, 22, 23, 27, 29, 37, 42, 72, 112, 171, 174, 175, 178, 185, 199, 216, 232, 242–245, 269, 333

　complications, 3, 4, 10–12, 19, 21, 25, 33–36, 172, 175, 179, 180, 190, 195, 200, 287, 290, 321, 369
　hematuria in, 188, 200
　retroperitoneal hematoma, 8, 10, 13
　scrotal, 71–75, 77, 78–93, 158, 225–227, 232–237
　testicular, 72–79, 87–93, 225–227, 232–238
　ureteral, 10, 22, 26–29, 33, 35, 48, 51, 79, 92, 244, 298, 313, 317, 321
　　diagnosis of, 15, 23–27, 31, 36, 37, 54, 195, 200, 242, 319
　　etiology of, 36, 195, 242
　urethral, 19, 41, 43, 46, 54, 59–62, 96–103, 110, 111, 216, 233, 286, 287, 290, 298, 317, 321
　　anterior, 57, 58, 61, 64, 67, 68, 71, 85
　　posterior, 42, 57, 58, 64–69, 85, 232, 285, 289, 291
Trimethoprim–sulfamethoxazole, 119, 120, 133, 136, 151
　classification, 25, 29
　diagnosis, 25, 27, 31, 37, 319
TUR; *see* Transurethral resection, 39, 52, 53, 95, 195, 201, 209, 255, 263, 272, 316, 329

U

Ultrasound, 6, 7, 52, 54, 61, 74, 78, 79, 131, 137, 158, 173, 175–179, 190, 192, 217–221, 229, 232, 233, 245, 246, 248, 249, 252, 257, 264, 265, 271, 277, 287, 317, 351, 352, 354, 360
　in children, 344
　in neonate, 330, 331, 345, 368
　in priapism, 217
　in renal colic, 353
　in renal vein thrombisos, 247
　renal, 6
　scrotal, 74, 78, 90, 91, 146, 158, 229, 232, 233, 237
Upper urinary tract, 115–119, 123–134, 181, 325, 330, 356, 357, 365
　trauma, 23, 35, 269, 334
　　obstruction, 35, 121, 122, 208, 263, 265, 269–279, 283, 315, 349

Ureter, 6, 10, 11, 15, 16, 25–36, 48, 50–52, 54, 55, 79, 115, 118, 121, 122, 128, 139, 174, 181, 187, 189, 191, 195, 196, 208, 209, 232, 241–244, 246–258, 267, 269–277, 288, 293, 295, 297–301, 303, 305–310, 315, 317–321, 324, 336, 350, 351, 353, 355, 357–359, 367, 368
  imaging, 6
  obstruction, 27, 33, 35
  trauma, 25–36
Ureteral calculus, 92, 247–250
Ureteral colic, 260, 261
Ureteral fistula, 37, 198, 200
Ureteral obstruction, 37, 122, 196, 241, 251, 252, 260–262, 276, 278, 309, 310, 315
  hydronephrosis, 128, 272, 273, 297, 306, 360
Ureteral perforation, 317–319, 325
Ureteral reimplantation, 33, 51, 309, 359
Ureteral stent, 16, 31–37, 121, 128, 155, 187, 191, 196–200, 242, 256, 257, 262, 33 267, 271, 300, 306–310, 319, 321, 325, 336
Ureteral Trauma, 26, 28, 33, 35
  classification, 25, 29
  diagnosis, 25, 27, 31, 37, 319
Ureteroenteric stricture, 263, 272, 279
Ureteropelvic junction, 11, 26, 34, 264
  injury, 6, 10, 37, 266, 318
  obstruction, 37, 241, 244, 263, 266, 277, 278, 353
Ureteroscopy, 257–259, 262, 266, 307, 315–320, 324, 325
Ureteroureterostomy, 33, 34, 196, 308, 310, 320
Ureterovaginal fistula, 55, 295, 299–314
Urethra, 19, 35, 41–43, 46, 50, 51, 53, 54, 57–67, 71, 75, 85, 96, 97, 99–104, 108, 110, 115, 132, 135–141, 143, 158, 161, 162, 167, 206, 216, 232, 233, 281–290, 295, 297, 298, 300, 304, 315–317, 320, 321, 324, 329, 343, 349–360, 365, 368
  female; see Female urethra, 35, 58, 96, 100, 101, 145, 282–284, 287, 311, 312, 316, 343
  male; see Male urethra, 35, 58, 96, 100, 101, 110, 111, 135, 137, 145, 167, 282, 283, 287–290, 311, 312, 316, 343, 349, 353, 361
  prolapse, 50, 284, 285, 288
  rupture, 65, 104
  trauma to, 19, 35, 37, 41, 43, 46, 51–54, 59–62, 75, 96–103, 110, 111, 216, 233, 286, 287, 290, 298, 312, 317, 321, 324
  anterior, 57, 58, 61, 64, 67, 68, 71, 85, 158
  posterior, 42, 57, 58, 64–69, 85, 232, 285, 289, 291, 316
Urethral stricture, 69, 104, 162, 284, 356
  after injury, 54, 61, 68, 158, 285, 287
Urethral valves, 353
  posterior, 232, 284, 351–357, 362
    etiology of, 283, 350, 360
    incidence of, 349
    management of, 283, 349, 359, 361
Urethritis, 135, 136, 141, 284
  gonococcal, 137–140, 145
  nongonococcal, 137–140, 143, 145
Urethroplasty, 62
  of urethral trauma, 61, 65–69
Urinalysis, 136, 141, 143, 258, 283
  in pyelonephritis, 118, 127, 242, 288
  in stone disease, 242, 288
  in trauma, 27, 232, 237, 242, 290
Urinary ascites, 28, 41, 52, 351
Urinary bladder; see Bladder, 39, 46, 50, 56, 211, 374
Urinary extravasation, 7, 10, 29, 35, 71, 158, 310, 321, 361
  after bladder injury, 50, 52
  after renal injury, 22
Urinary fistula, 20, 51, 320, 321
  ureterovaginal, 311, 313
  vesicovaginal, 54, 297, 311, 313
Urinary retention, 65, 281, 289, 291
  in benign prostatic hyperplasia, 287
  neurogenic, 285, 286
  spinal cord injury, 283–287
  treatment, 107, 137, 206, 233, 254, 283, 285, 288, 290
Urinary tract infection, 48, 53, 113, 115–117, 119, 121, 123, 125, 127, 129, 131, 135, 148, 204, 232, 264, 265, 269, 272–275, 318, 322, 324, 351, 368, 369, 371
  after trauma, 157, 158
  epididymitis, 139
  prostatitis, 136
  upper, 115, 116, 247
  urethritis, 135
Urinary tract obstruction, 239
  lower, 245, 251, 263
  upper, 251, 263, 265, 269–279

Urine culture, 118, 120, 283
  in stone disease, 242, 243
  in urinary tract infection, 125, 127, 136, 232
Urinoma, 10, 20, 35, 37, 296, 297, 316–321

V

Vagina, 30, 40–42, 51, 54, 56, 71–74, 77, 87, 95, 96, 116, 161, 225–228, 231–235, 284, 285, 288, 291, 296–313, 330, 344, 345, 363
Valve ablation, 355–362
Vancomycin, 124, 149–152
Vascular injury,
  renal, 3, 10–12, 18, 33, 320
Vomiting, 139, 189, 227, 251–254, 258, 265, 274, 275
  in pyelonephritis, 120, 243, 245, 369

W

White blood cell, 118, 227, 233

X

X-ray; *see* Radiography, 191, 204, 323
Xanthogranulomatous pyelonephritis, 115, 130, 134, 184